K. Reinhart K. Eyrich (Editors)

Clinical Aspects of O_2 Transport and Tissue Oxygenation

With 143 Figures and 24 Tables

Springer-Verlag Berlin Heidelberg New York
London Paris Tokyo Hong Kong

Prof. Dr. med. K. Reinhart
Prof. Dr. med. K. Eyrich

Freie Universität Berlin, Universitätsklinikum Steglitz
Klinik für Anästhesiologie und Operative Intensivmedizin
Hindenburgdamm 30, 1000 Berlin 45/FRG

Library of Congress Cataloging in Publication Data.
Clinical aspects of O_2-transport and tissue oxygenation / K. Reinhart, K. Eyrich (editors).
ISBN-13: 978-3-540-51470-1 e-ISBN-13: 978-3-642-83872-9
DOI: 10.1007/978-3-642-83872-9
1. Ischemia. 2. Tissue respiration. 3. Anesthesia. 4. CPR (First aid). 5. Respiratory therapy. I. Reinhart, K. II. Eyrich, K.
[DNLM: 1. Biological Transport. 2. Oxygen–physiology. 3. Oxygen Consumption. 4. Pulmonary Gas Exchange. 5. Respiratory Insufficiency–therapy. 6. Resuscitation. QV 312C641] RB144.C44 1989
616.2–dc20 DNLM/DLC for Library of Congress 89-21826 CIP

Typesetting: Brühlsche Universitätsdruckerei, Giessen
2119/3020-543210 – Printed on acid-free paper

List of Contributors

Ahnefeld, F. W., Prof. Dr.
Zentrum für Anaesthesiologie, Universität Ulm, Steinhövelstr. 9, 7900 Ulm, FRG

Baker, R. R., Dr.
Department of Anesthesiology, 619 South 19th Street, 941D THT Birmingham, Alabama 35233, USA

Bartlett, R. H., Prof.
The University of Michigan, General Surgery, 1500 E Medical Center Drive, Ann Arbor, Michigan 48109-0331, USA

Baumann, G., Prof. Dr.
I. Med. Klinik u. Poliklinik, Abt. für Kardiologie, Ismaninger Str. 22, 8000 München 80, FRG

Bersten, A., Dr.
Victoria Hospital Corporation, 375 South Street, Room 482 NW, London, Ontario N6A 4G5, Canada

Bredle, D., Prof. Dr.
Applied Physiology Research Lab, Kent State University, Kent, Ohio 44242, USA

Bryan-Brown, Ch. Dr.
Dep. of Anesthesiology, Montefiore Med. Center, 111 East 210th Street, Bronx, New York 10467, USA

Cabrol, C., Prof.
Département de Chirurgie Cardiovasculaire, Université de Paris VI, Hôpital de la Pitié-Salpétrière, Paris, France

Cain, S. M., Prof. Dr.
Dept. of Physiology and Biophysics, University of Alab., Birmingham, Alabama 35294, USA

Camporesi, E., Prof. Dr.
State University of N.Y., Health Science Center, 750 E. Street, Syracruse, NY 13210, USA

Cerretelli, P., Dr.
Département de Physiologie, Centre Médical Universitaire, Genève, Switzerland

Dantzker, D. R., Prof. Dr.
Div. of Pulmonary Medicine, The University of Texas, 6431 Fannin – Suite 1.274, Houston, Texas 77030, USA

Denison, D. M., Prof. Dr.
Lung Function Unit, Brompton Hospital, Fulham Road, London, SW3 6HP, England

Engstrom, P. C., Dr.
Department of Anesthesiology, 619 South 19th Street, 941D THT Birmingham, Alabama 35233, USA

Ernesti, U., Dr.
Istituto di Anestesia e Rianimazione, Università degli Studi di Milano, Ospedale Nuovo S. Gerardo, Monza (Mi), Italy

Falke, K. J., Prof. Dr.
Klinik für Anaesthesiologie und op. Intensivmedizin, Univ.-Klinikum R. Virchow, Spandauer Damm, 1000 Berlin 19, FRG

Felix, B., Prof. Dr.
1st Medical Department, Technical University of Munich, Division of Cardiology and Circulation, Ismaninger Strasse 22, 8000 München 80, FRG

Fumagalli, R., Dr.
Istituto di Anestesia e Rianimazione Università degli Studi di Milano, Ospedale Nuovo S. Gerardo, Monza (MI), Italy

Gaehtgens, P., Prof. Dr.
Institut für Physiologie, FU Berlin, Arnimalle 22, 1000 Berlin 33, FRG

Gattinoni, L., Prof. Dr.
Nuovo Ospedale S. Gerardo, I Serv. Di Anestesia e Rianim., Via G. Donizetti 106, I-20052 Monza (MI), Italy

Gazmuri, J., Dr.
Department of Medicine, University of Health Science / The Chicago Medical School, 3333 Green Bay Road, North Chicago, IL 60064, USA

Gelman, S., Prof.
Depart. of Anesthesia, Univ. of Alab., Birmingham, Alabama 35294, USA

Granger, D. N., Prof.
Dep. of Physiology, LSU Med. Center, P.O. Box 33932, Shreveport, LA 711303932, USA

Guitierrez, G., MD PhD
Associate Professor of Internal Medicine, Pulmonary Division, University of Texas Medical School at Houston, Texas, USA

Hannemann, L., Dr.
Klinik für Anaesthesiologie und op. Intensivmedizin, Univ.-Klinikum Steglitz, Hindenburgdamm 30, 1000 Berlin 45, FRG

Kretz, F. J., Dr.
Klinik für Anaesthesiologie und op. Intensivmedizim, Univ.-Klinikum Steglitz, Hindenburgdamm 30, 1000 Berlin 45, FRG

Kubes, P., Dr.
Dep. of Physiology, LSU Med. Center, P.O. Box 33932, Shreveport, LA 711303932, USA

Laverrière, M. C., Dr.
Dep. d'Anesth., Hopital Cantonal Univ., 24 - rue Micheli-du-Crest, CH-1211 Genève, Schweiz

Lennartz, H., Prof. Dr.
Department of Anesthesiology and Intensive Care, Clinical Center of Philipps-University, Baldingerstr. 1, 3550 Marburg, FRG

Lindner, K. H., Priv.-Doz., Dr.
Zentrum für Anaesthesiologie, Universität Ulm, Steinhövelstr. 9, 7900 Ulm, FRG

Marcolin, R., Dr.
Istituto di Anestesia e Rianimazione, Università degli Studi di Milano, Ospedale Nuovo S. Gerardo, Monza (MI), Italy

Marconi, C., Dr.
Istituto di Technologie Biomediche Avanzate, Consiglio Nazionale delle Ricerche, Milano, Italy

Matalon, S., Prof.
Department of Anesthesiology, University of Alab., Birmingham, Alabama 35294, USA

Mayr, O., Dr.
Klinik für Anaesthesiologie und op. Intensivmedizim, Univ.-Klinikum Steglitz, Hindenburgdamm 30, 1000 Berlin 45, FRG

Meyer, M., Prof. Dr.
Abteilung Physiologie, Max-Planck-Institut für Experimentelle Medizin, Göttingen, FRG

Nunn, J. F., Prof.
Clinical Research Centre, Division of Anaesthesia, Watford Road, Harrow, Middlesex HA1 3UJ, England

Perutz, M. F., Prof.
Medical Research Council, Hills Road, Cambridge, CB2 2QH, England

Pesenti, A., Dr.
Istituto di Anestesia e Rianimazione, Università degli Studi di Milano, Ospedale Nuovo S. Gerardo, Monza (MI), Italy

Priebe, H. J., Prof. Dr.
Klinik für Anaesth., Klinikum der Universität, 7800 Freiburg, FRG

Pugin, J., Dr.
Dep. d'Anesth., Hôpital Cantonal Univ., 24 - rue Micheli-du-Crest, CH-1211 Genève, Schweiz

Rackow, C., Dr.
Department of Medicine, University of Health Sciences, The Chicago Medical School, 3333 Green Bay Road, North Chicago, IL 60064, USA

Räsänen, J., Dr.
Dep. of Anesthesiology, Children's Hospital, University of Helsinki, SF-00290 Helsinki, Finland

Reinhart, K., Prof. Dr.
Klinik für Anaesthesiologie und op. Intensivmedizim, Univ.-Klinikum Steglitz, Hindenburgdamm 30, 1000 Berlin 45, FRG

Reiz, S., Prof.
Dept. of Anaesthesiology and Critical Care Medicine, Regionsjukhuset, S-901 85, Umeå, Sweden

Rieu, M., Dr.
Laboratoire de Physiologie des Adaptations, Université de Paris V, Faculté de Médecine Cochin Port-Royal, Paris, France

Rogers, M. C., Prof. Dr.
Dep. of Anesthesiology and Critical Care Medicine, The Johns Hopkins Hospital, Baltimore, Maryland 21205, USA

Romand, J.-A., Dr.
Dep. d'Anesth., Hôpital Cantonal Univ., 24 - rue Micheli-du-Crest, CH-1211 Genève, Schweiz

Rossaint, R., Dr.
Klinik für Anaesthesiologie und op. Intensivmedizin, Univ.-Klinikum R. Virchow, Spandauer Damm, 1000 Berlin 19, FRG

Rossi, G. P., Dr.
Ospedale Nuovo S. Gerardo, I Servizio Anestesia e Rianimazione, Via G. Donizetti, 106, 20052 Monza (MI), Italy

Scarani, F., Dr.
Istituto di Anestesia e Rianimazione, Università degli Studi di Milano, Ospedale Nuovo S. Gerardo - Monza (MI), Italy

Schachinger, H., Prof. Dr.
Ev. Krankenhaus, Virchowstr. 20, 4200 Oberhausen 1, FRG

Shaffner, H., Prof.
Dept. of Anesthesiology and Critical Care Medicine, The Johns Hopkins Medical Institutions, Baltimore, Maryland 21205, USA

Shah, D. M., Dr.
Dept. of Medicine, University of Health Sciences/The Chigaco Medical School, 333 Green Bay Road, North Chicago, IL 60064, USA

Sibbald, W. J., Prof. Dr.
Critical Care – Trauma Unit Victoria Hospital, 3375 South Street, London, Ontario – N6A 4G5, Canada

Siesjö, B. K., Prof.
Lab. f. Exp. Brain Res., Lund Hospital – Floor EA.5, S-22185 Lund, Sweden

Slama, K., Dr.
Freie Universität Berlin, Universitätsklinikum Rudolf Virchow, Institut für Anaesthesiologie, Spandauer Damm 130, 1000 Berlin 19, FRG

Striebel, H. W., Dr.
Klinik für Anaesthesiologie und op. Intensivmedizin, Univ.-Klinikum Steglitz, Hindenburgdamm 30, 1000 Berlin 45, FRG

Suter, P. M., Prof. Dr.
Dep. d'Anesth., Hôpital Cantonal Univ., 24 - rue Micheli-du-Crest,
CH-1211 Genève, Schweiz

Tarnow, J., Prof. Dr.
Zentrum für Anaesthesiologie, Universität, Moorenstr. 5, 4000 Düsseldorf,
FRG

Wan Lu, C. D., Dr.
State University of N.Y., Health Science Center, 750 E. Street, Syracuse,
NY 13210, USA

Weil, M. H., Prof.
Depart. of Medicine, The Chicago Medical School, 3333 Green Bay Road,
North Chicago, Illinois 60064, USA

West, J. B., Prof. Dr.
Section of Physiology, Dep. of Medicine, UCSD, La Jolla, California 92093,
USA

Contents

Physiology

Physiology

Mechanisms Regulating the Reactions of Human Hemoglobin with Oxygen and Carbon Monoxide

M. F. Perutz

Perspectives and Introduction

The reactions of hemoglobin with oxygen and carbon monoxide are subject to regulation by the heme and the residues surrounding it and by the effectors, also known as heterotopic ligands (H^+, Cl^-, CO_2, and 2,3-diphosphoglycerate), that regulate the equilibrium between its two forms, the oxy or R-structure with high and the deoxy or T-structure with low oxygen affinity. The stereochemical mechanisms of regulation have been studied for many years using a variety of methods. What is new since the subject was last surveyed [1] is determination of the crystal structures at resolutions sufficient to resolve individual atoms of the heme and its surroundings; such structures have now been determined for deoxy, oxy, and carbon monoxyhemoglobin, and for several analogues of transition states in the reaction with oxygen and carbon monoxide. In the past much useful information about the stereochemical mechanism of hemoglobin has come from the study of abnormal human hemoglobins. Now that the genes for the α and β chains of hemoglobin and for the single chain of myoglobin have been cloned in *E. coli,* directed mutagenesis has provided new tools for probing the reactions of these proteins with ligands. Finally, an (unsuccessful) search for possible antisickling drugs has led to the discovery of a family of compounds which are more powerful allosteric effectors than the natural one, 2,3-diphosphoglycerate, and combine with sites that are far removed from the diphosphoglycerate binding site.

In this review I shall describe the new insights into the allosteric mechanism provided by X-ray analysis at high resolution, or perhaps I should say, the refinement of the mechanism I proposed in 1970 [2]. At that time I suggested that combination of the heme iron with oxygen or carbon monoxide is accompanied by a shift of the iron atom and its attached histidine relative to the porphyrin. That shift causes changes in the tertiary structure of the subunits which lead to a rearrangement of the subunits from the quaternary deoxy or T-, to the oxy or R-structure. I proposed that the low oxygen affinity of the T-structure is due to additional bonds between the four subunits which take the form of hydrogen bonds between groups of opposite charge, also known as salt bridges, and that these bonds oppose the movement of the iron that is needed for the binding of oxygen. On oxygenation, these salt bridges are broken, with the release of the hydrogen ions that are linked to the Bohr effect. All these proposals have been confirmed, but certain aspects of my mechanism have remained unresolved. The structure of deoxyhemoglobin showed the ligand sites in the β-subunits to be obstructed by the distal valines, suggesting that no ligands can bind, but chemical studies showed the oxygen affinity of the β-hemes in the T-structure to be only slightly less than that of the α-hemes. X-ray analysis of a transition state analogue has now resolved this apparent contradiction. Another puzzle concerned the transmission of stereochemical effects from the hemes to the salt bridges. I proposed a system of levers which turned out to be wrong, but none of the studies of transition state analogues have suggested what the right mechanism could be. The partition coefficients of hemoglobin, and especially of myoglobin, between oxygen and carbon monoxide are much smaller than that of free heme. This is essential, because one mole of carbon monoxide is produced endogenously for each mole of porphyrin broken down. Directed mutagenesis has shown how myoglobin and the α-subunit discriminate between oxygen and carbon monoxide, but has left the mechanism of discrimination by the β-subunits obscure.

Common Features of Hemoglobins

All hemoglobins have similar structures. The globin chain has a characteristic fold that envelops the hemes in a deep pocket with its hydrophobic edges inside and its propionates facing the solvent. The chain is made up of seven or eight α-helical segments and an equal number of nonhelical ones placed at the corners between them and at the ends of the chain (Fig. 1). According to a notation introduced by Watson and Kendrew [3] the helices are named A to

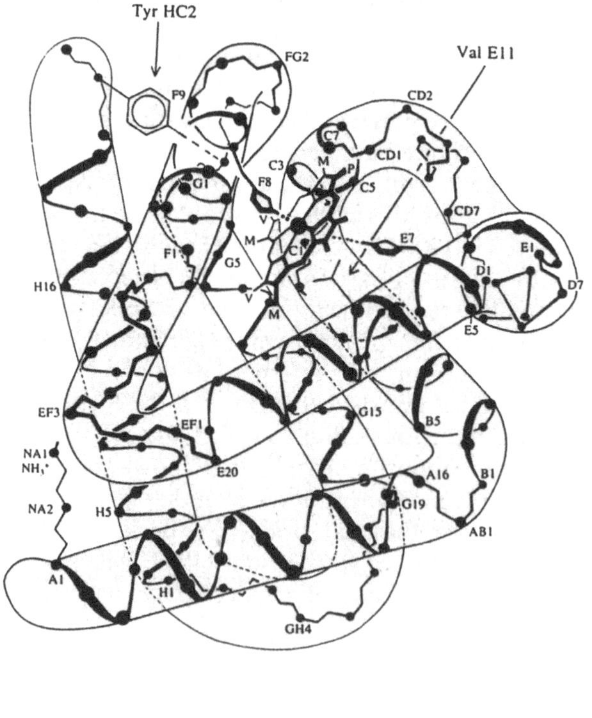

Fig. 1. Tertiary structure of β-chains of human hemoglobin, typical of hemoglobins and myoglobins of all other species. The figure also shows the proximal and distal histidines, marked F8 and E7, the distal valine E11, and the tyrosine HC2 which ties down the C-terminus by its hydrogen bond to the main chain carbonyl of valine FG5

H, starting from the amino end; the nonhelical segments that lie between helices are named AB, BC, CD, and so on. The nonhelical segments at the ends of the chain are called NA and HC. Residues within each segment are numbered from the amino end: A1, A2, CD1, CD2, and so on. Evolution has conserved this fold of the chain despite great divergence of the sequence: the only residues common to all hemoglobins are the proximal histidine F8 and the phenylalanine CD1, which wedges the hemes into its pocket. Most, but not all, globins also have a histidine on the distal (oxygen) side of the heme. Ionized residues are excluded from the interior of the globin chains, which is filled largely by hydrocarbon side chains, but some serines and threonines also occur there. The proximal and distal histidines (also called the heme-linked histidines) are potentially polar, but the proximal histidine does not ionize, and the pK_a of the distal one is so low ($\sim$5.5) that the fraction ionized in vivo is negligible.

Reaction with Oxygen and Change of Quaternary Structure

Hemoglobin combines with oxygen and carbon monoxide cooperatively. This cooperativity arises not primarily by any direct interaction between the active sites, but mainly by a change in equilibrium between the two alternative structures, T and R, at successive steps of ligand binding. The degree of cooperativity is expressed as the slope n at the midpoint of a plot of log $p(O_2)$ against log $y/1-y$, where y is the fractional saturation with oxygen or carbon monoxide. Cooperativity ensures that most of the molecules are either fully oxygenated or fully deoxygenated. This has first been demonstrated directly by Perella and his collaborators who devised a method of trapping the intermediates in the reaction of hemoglobin with carbon monoxide (Fig. 2).

The oxygen affinity of the R-structure is slightly larger than the average one of free α- and β-subunits; that of the T-structure is lower by the equivalent of the free energy of cooperativity. The oxygen equilibrium can be described by the oxygen association constants K_T and K_R, usually expressed in $(\mathrm{mmHg})^{-1}$, and by the equilibrium constant $L_o = [T]/[R]$ in the absence of oxygen. Imai has shown empirically that $\log K_T/K_R = A - 0.25 \log L_o$, where A is a constant, which leaves K_R and K_T as the only independent variables. K_T varies over a wide range as a function of $[H^+]$, $[Cl^-]$, $[CO_2]$ and [DPG]; K_R varies as a function of $[H^+]$ below pH 7, but is little affected by the other ligands [1, 7–13].

The T- and R-structures differ in the arrangement of the four subunits, referred to as the quaternary structure, and the conformation of the subunits, referred to as the tertiary structure. The quaternary R→T transition consists in a rotation of the dimer $\alpha_1\beta_1$ relative to the dimer $\alpha_2\beta_2$ by 12°–15° and a translation of one dimer relative to the other by 0.8 Å. The $\alpha\beta$ dimers move relative to each other at the symmetry-related contacts $\alpha_1\beta_2$ and $\alpha_2\beta_1$ and at the contacts $\alpha_1\alpha_2$ and $\beta_1\beta_2$; the contacts $\alpha_1\beta_1$ and $\alpha_2\beta_2$ remain rigid (Fig. 3).

The key questions for the understanding of hemoglobin function are these: How does the reaction with oxygen affect the stereochemistry at and around

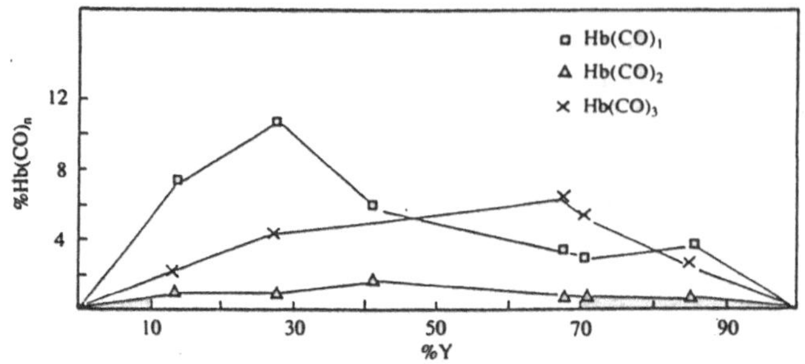

Fig. 2. Observed distribution of intermediates in the reaction of hemoglobin with CO as a function of percentage saturation with CO. The reaction showed a Hill's coefficient of 3.0. The concentration of intermediates was obtained after quenching the reaction of two solutions expelled into a mixing chamber from two separate syringes. Either one syringe was filled with deoxy and the other with carbonylhemoglobin, or one was filled with partially oxidized carbonylhemoglobin and the other with a solution of dithionite. After mixing, the solution was expelled into a cryochamber at −25 °C containing a tenfold molar excess of ferricyanide in an equal mixture of phosphate buffer and ethyleneglycol. Salt and ferricyanide were removed, and the different species separated by isoelectric focussing at −25 °C. Contrary to the claims of Gill et al. [4], the triligated species is significantly populated. The diligated species are nearly all of the type α(CO) β(CO)$\alpha\beta$. (From Perrella et al. [5, 6]

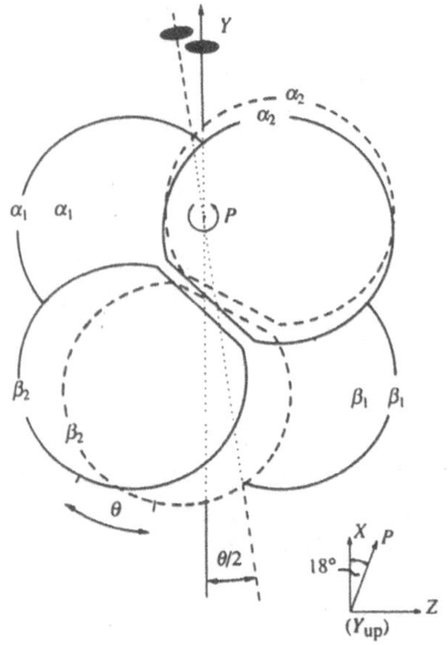

Fig. 3. Change of quaternary structure of mammalian hemoglobin on transition from deoxy or T *(full lines)* to oxy or R *(broken lines)*. The dimer $\alpha_2\beta_2$ turns by $\theta = 13°$ about the P axis; this entails a rotation of the dyad symmetry axis Y by $\theta/2 = 6.5°$. If the four subunits were identical, *P* would have to coincide with *X*. (From Baldwin and Chothia [14])

the heme so as to trigger the transition from the T- to the R-structure? What are the constraints of the T-structure and how do they lower the oxygen affinity? By what mechanisms do the heterotropic ligands influence the oxygen affinity? Single crystal X-ray analyses of deoxy and oxyhemoglobin, and of analogues of intermediates in the reactions with oxygen or carbon monoxide, together with chemical, spectroscopic, and magnetic studies, have furnished some of the answers.

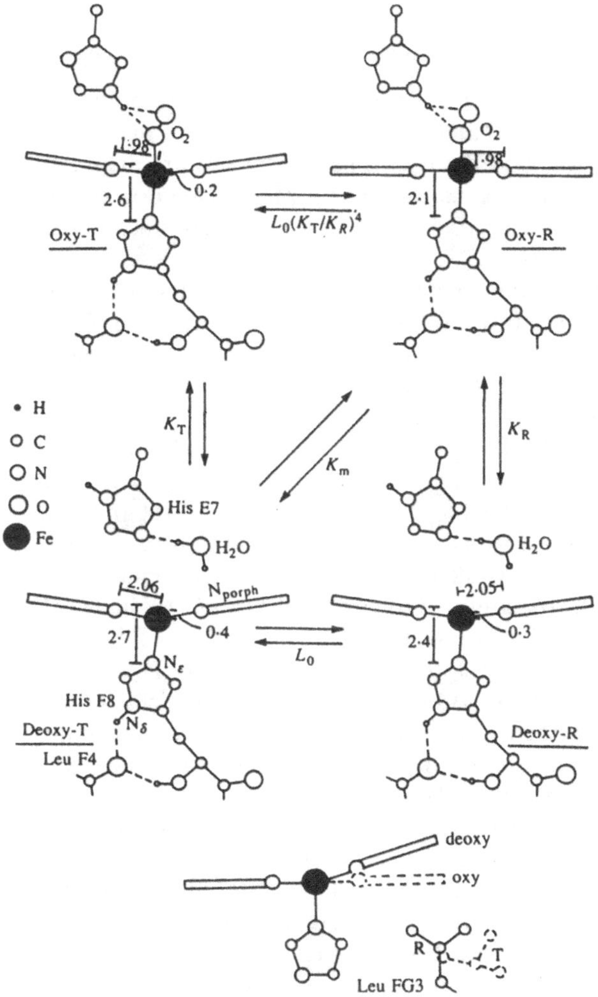

Fig. 4. Change of allosteric core on going from deoxy-T via oxy-T to oxy-R and from there via deoxy-R back to deoxy-T. The *vertical bars* indicate the distance of N_ε of the proximal histidine F8 from the mean plane of the porphyrin nitrogens and carbons (excluding β and γ carbons of the side chains). The *horizontal bar* gives the Fe-$N_{porphyrin}$ distance, and the figure to the right of the iron atoms in the lower two diagrams the displacement of the iron from the plane of the porphyrin nitrogens. L_0 is the allosteric constant in the absence of oxygen, K_T and K_R are the association constants with oxygen of the T- and R-structures, and K_m is the mean oxygen association constant. Note that the porphyrin is flat only in oxy-R and that the proximal histidine tilts relative to the haem normal in the T-structures. Note also the water molecule attached to the distal histidine in deoxy. The *bottom diagram* illustrates how the flattening of the porphyrin on going from deoxy to oxy exerts a leverage on leucine FG3 and valine FG5 which lie at the switching contact between the two structures; (from Perutz et al. 1987 [13]). The differences in heme geometry between deoxyhemoglobins in the T- and R-structures shown here are closely similar to those found between sterically hindered 2-methyl- and unhindered 1-methylimidazole iron porphyrin complexes. (Momenteau et al. [15])

Structural Mechanism

Changes in the Allosteric Core

Figure 4 summarizes the stereochemistry of the hemes in deoxyhemoglobin, oxyhemoglobin, and in two intermediates. In deoxy hemoglobin the iron is high spin ferrous ($S=2$) and five-coordinated. The iron atoms are displaced from the planes of the porphyrin nitrogens, and the porphyrins are domed. On oxygenation the iron becomes low-spin ferrous ($S=0$) and six-coordinated. The porphyrins flatten and the Fe-$N_{porphyrin}$ bond lengths contract from 2.06 to 1.98 Å, thus moving the iron atoms towards the porphyrin planes [1, 2]. As a result the proximal histidines come 0.5–0.6 Å closer to the porphyrin planes in oxy than in deoxyhemoglobin. Do these movements trigger the allosteric transitions between the R- and T-structures, and if so, how are the transitions initiated?

Semiliganded derivatives in the T-structure show that on combination of oxygen or carbon monoxide with the α-hemes, the irons move by 0.15 Å towards the plane of the porphyrin nitrogens while the doming of the pyrroles is preserved. The movements of the irons are transmitted to the proximal histidines and their adjoining residues, while the bulk of the protein remains unperturbed. Thus, perturbations are confined to what Gelin et al. [16] have called the "allosteric core." On loss of iron-linked H_2O and reduction of the irons of a ferric hemoglobin in the R-structure, the iron atoms move away from the plane of the porphyrin nitrogens by 0.2 Å and the porphyrins become domed; the movements are transmitted not just to the proximal histidines and their adjoining residues, but also to the $\alpha_1\beta_2$ and $\alpha_2\beta_1$ contacts which shift a short way towards their positions in the T-structure [13, 17].

There have been suggestions that the hydrogen bonds between N_σ of His F8 and the carbonyl of Leu F4 play a part in the allosteric mechanism. The lengths of these bonds may change in transition states, but they remain the same in deoxyhemoglobin and oxyhemoglobin. There has also been a suggestion that changes in charge transfer interaction between the porphyrin and Phe CD1 contribute to the free energy of cooperativity, but the distance between the phenylalanine side chain and the porphyrin is too large (3.8–4.1 Å) for such interactions to occur. *We are thus left with the distances of the Fe's and the proximal histidines from the porphyrin as the only determinants of the allosteric equilibrium visible in the α-subunits.* In the β-subunits, displacement of the distal valine relative to the heme is necessary in the T-structure before oxygen can bind. In the R-structure this steric hindrance is absent.

Changes in the Globin Chains

The α-Subunits

Since the $\alpha_1\beta_1$ contact undergoes no significant changes during the R→T transition, the atoms at this contact can serve as a reference frame for changes in tertiary structure elsewhere; except for residues G1–4 and H18–21, the B, G, and H helices were also found to be static. The largest movements relative to

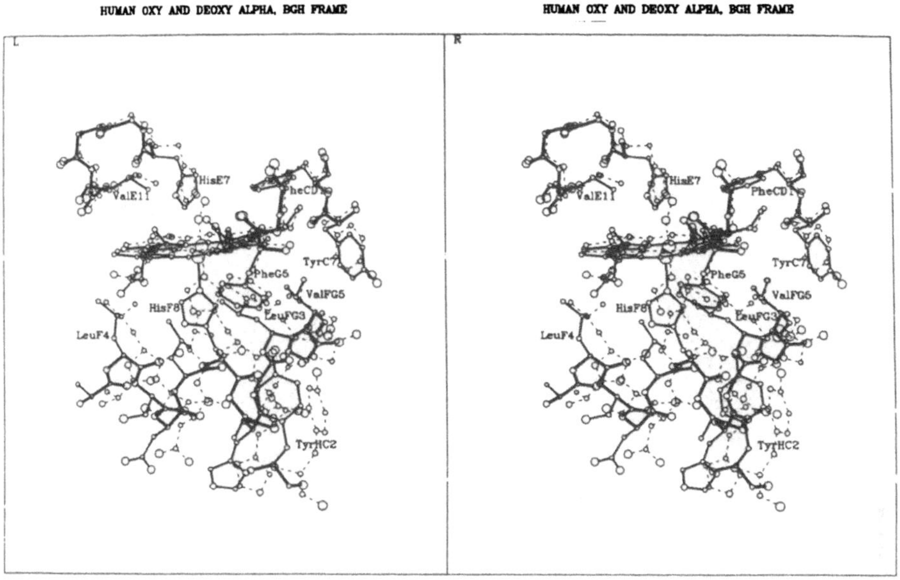

Fig. 5. Change of tertiary structure near the α-haem on going from deoxy-T *(full lines)* to oxy-R *(broken lines)*. Note how the proximal histidine straightens and moves closer to the porphyrin, carrying the residues in helix F with it. (From Perutz et al. [13])

either of these frames occur in helix F, in segment FG, and in residues G1–4, H18–21, and HC1–3. Figure 5 shows the heme environment of deoxyhemoglobin superimposed on that of oxyhemoglobin. It can be seen that on oxygenation helix Fα shifts towards the heme and to the right and carries the FG segment with it. In deoxyhemoglobin the imidazole of His F8 is tilted relative to the heme normal; in oxyhemoglobin the shift of helix F relative to deoxyhemoglobin aligns it with the heme normal. Taking as a reference frame residues F1–8, to which the heme is attached, the heme flattens and turns clockwise by 10°; the motion of its right-hand edge pushes down Leu FG3(91)α and Val FG5(93)α which form part of the $\alpha_1\beta_2$ contact where the quaternary switch occurs (Fig. 4). In the T-structure the N- and C-termini form the hydrogen bonds shown in Figs. 6–8. In the R-structure these hydrogen bonds are broken, and the terminal residues are seen only at a low level of electron density, implying that they are mobile.

The β-Subunits

Figure 9 shows that on oxygenation helix F moves towards the heme and in the direction of the FG segment, carrying that segment with it and aligning His F8 with the heme normal. The movement of F and FG is transmitted to residue G1 and dissipated beyond G5. The center of the heme moves further into its pocket along a line linking porphyrin N_1 to N_3, and the heme rotates about an axis close to the line linking N_2 to N_4. Referred to residues F1 to F6,

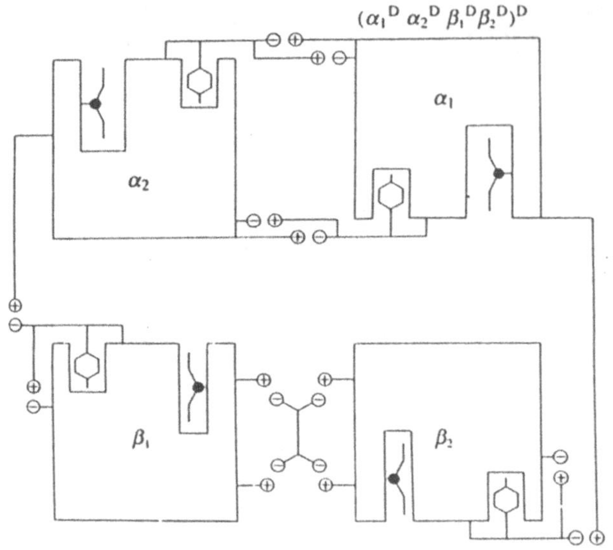

Fig. 6. Diagrammatic representation of salt bridges in the T-structure. Those at the *top* link the C-terminal Arg HC3(141)α_2 to Asp H9(126)α_1 and Lys H10(127)α_1. The others link the C-terminal His HC3 (146)β_1 to Asp FG1 (94)β_1 and Lys C5(40)α_2. The bridge between the β-subunits represents 2,3-diphosphoglycerate. (From Perutz [2])

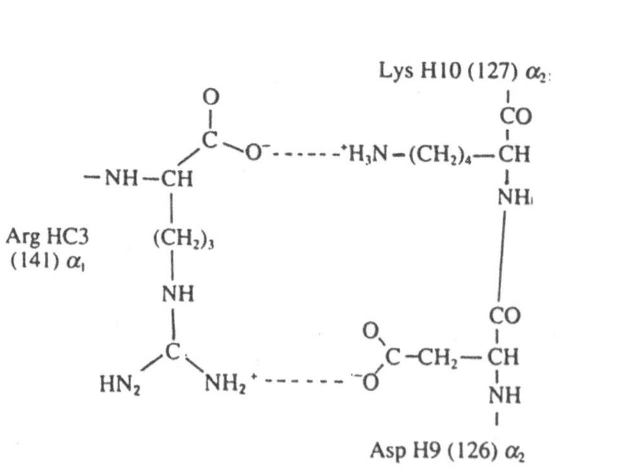

Fig. 7. Salt bridges between the α-chains in the T-structure

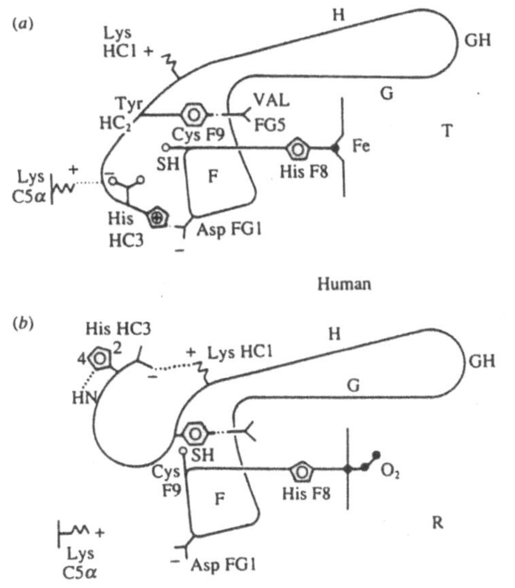

Fig. 8 a, b. Change in conformation of histidine HC3 (146)β and cysteine F9 (93)β on going from the T- to the R-structure. In the T-structure the imidazole of the histidine *donates* a hydrogen bond to Asp FG1 and is positively charged (pK_a = 8.0). Its carboxylate *accepts* a hydrogen bond from Lys C5α. The SH is cis to CO and points away from the heme. In the R-structure the imidazole *accepts* a hydrogen bond from the histidine's main chain NH and has a pK_a of 7.1 or below; and the C-terminal carboxylate accepts a weak hydrogen bond from Lys HC1. The SH group is cis to NH and in contact with Tyr HC2

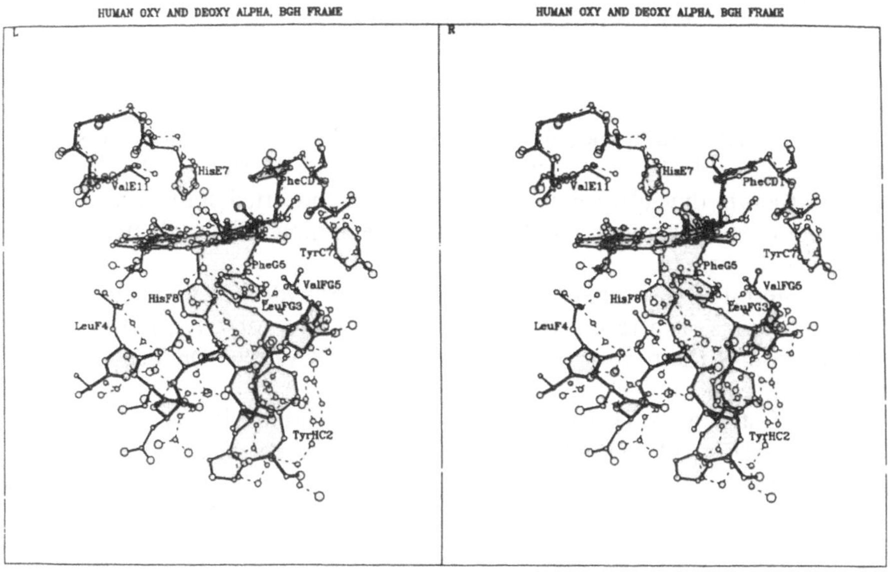

Fig. 9. Change of tertiary structure near the β-haem on going from deoxy-T *(full lines)* to oxy-R *(broken lines)*. Note how the heme moves to the right, into the heme pocket, and the distal valine and histidine make way for the bound oxygen. (From Perutz et al. [13])

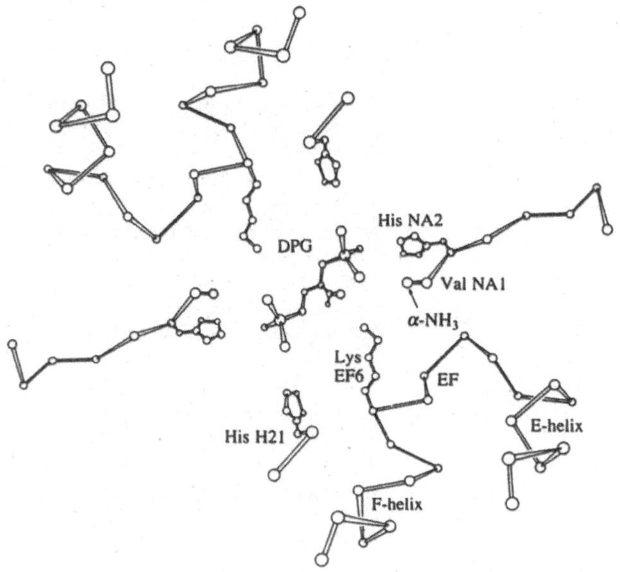

Fig. 10. Hydrogen bonds between 2,3-diphosphoglycerate and cationic groups of the β-chains in the T-structure. In the R-structure the gap between the EF corners closes and the N-termini move apart. (From Arnone [18])

the iron stays still and the porphyrin becomes coplanar with it. In the T-structure $C_\gamma H_3$ of Val E11(67) obstructs the ligand site at the iron; in the oxygenated R-structure that obstruction is cleared by a concerted shift of helices D and E and the CD segment together with the beginning of helix B, away from and across the heme.

The C-terminal histidines form different sets of hydrogen bonds in the T- and R-structures, as a result of which their pK_a's drop on oxygenation. The conformation of the reactive sulfhydryl groups of Cys F9(93)β also changes (Fig. 8) [13].

In the T-structure the two β-subunits form a binding site for 2,3-diphosphoglycerate (Fig. 10). In the R-structure the gap between the two β-chains becomes too narrow to accommodate it.

The Heterotropic Ligands

According to allosteric theory the low oxygen affinity of the T- as compared to that of the R-structures arises from increased energy and/or number of bonds between the subunits [19]. The contact areas and the number of bonds between segments $C\alpha_1$ and $FG\beta_2$ and between segments $C\beta_2$ and $FG\alpha_1$ are about equal in the R- and T-structures [14]; the C-terminal residues and DPG, on the other hand, form 14 salt bridges between the subunits which are absent in the R-structure (Fig. 7–10). The bond energies of the four pairs of salt bridges made by the C-terminal residues have been measured. Those formed by the C-terminal histidines and histidines H21(143) of the β-chains together contribute 7.6 kcal mol^{-1} [20], and those formed by arginine HC3(141)α contribute at least 4 kcal mol^{-1}, leaving only 300 cal mol^{-1} per salt bridge to be contributed by the remaining eight salt bridges, sufficient to account for the total free energy of cooperativity of 14.4 kcal/tetramer, because a salt bridge contributes usually at least 1 kcal mol^{-1} [21]. Absence of any of the bridges raises K_T and lowers L. The salt bridges keep the subunits rigidly in the tertiary deoxy structure and hinder the movement of the iron atoms into the planes of the porphyrin nitrogens and the flattening of the porphyrins themselves. This hindrance manifests itself in spectroscopic and magnetic differences between liganded hemoglobins in the two quaternary structures; these have recently been reviewed [13].

All the heterotropic ligands lower the oxygen affinity by forming additional hydrogen bonds that specifically stabilize and constrain the T-structure. The most important heterotropic ligands are protons. The linkage of proton uptake to oxygen release, and vice versa, is known as the Bohr effect. For each mole of oxygen released at pH 7.4 and 25 °C, human Hb takes up 0.2 moles H^+ in a deionized solution, 0.5 moles H^+ in 0.1 *M* Cl^-, and 0.7 moles H^+ in the presence of a molar excess of DPG [22, 23]. The identity of the residues that take up protons has been determined by X-ray crystallographic and chemical studies of normal and mutant hemoglobins. In deionized solutions all the protons are taken up by His HC3(146)β which donates a hydrogen bond to Asp FG1(94)β in the T-structure and accepts a hydrogen bond from its own main chain NH in the R-structure (Fig. 8). In consequence, its pK_a rises from 7.1 or less in oxyhemoglobin to 8.0 in deoxyhemoglobin [24, 25]. The binding of Cl^- by the T-structure raises the pK_a's of Val NA1(1)α (Fig. 7) and Lys EF6(82)β which contribute an additional 0.28 moles H^+ to the Bohr effect. DPG enters a cleft flanked by the N-termini and helices H of the β-chains and forms hydrogen bonds with Val NA1(1), His NA2(2), Lys EF6(82), and His H21(143) (Fig. 10). The rise in pK_a's of their cationic groups contributes 0.33 moles H^+ to the Bohr effect [22]. Carbon dioxide forms carbamino groups with Val NA1(1)α and β and these in turn make hydrogen bonds with cationic groups of the globin. All the groups that bind heterotropic ligands are at some distance from the hemes, consistent with the prediction by Monod et al. [26] that "no direct interaction need occur between the substrate of the protein and the regulatory metabolite which controls its activity."

In 0.1 *M* Tris HC1 + 0.1 *M* NaCl at pH 7.4 and 21.5 °C, the first mole of oxygen taken up releases 0.64 ($\pm$7) moles H^+, the second and third mole of oxygen combined release 1.62 ($\pm$27) moles H^+ and the fourth mole of oxygen releases only 0.05 ($\pm$6) moles H^+ [27]. How is their release related to the allosteric transition from T to R? Allosteric theory allows the equilibrium constant $L_i = [T]/[R]$ at the *i*th step of oxygenation to be calculated from $L_i = L_0\ (K_R/K_T)^i$. Under the above nonphysiological conditions $L_1 = 8.7 \times 10^4 \times 0.0073 = 633$ [8, 12]. Thus, more than one-quarter of the Bohr protons are discharged before $^1/_{600}$ of the Hb molecules have switched from T to

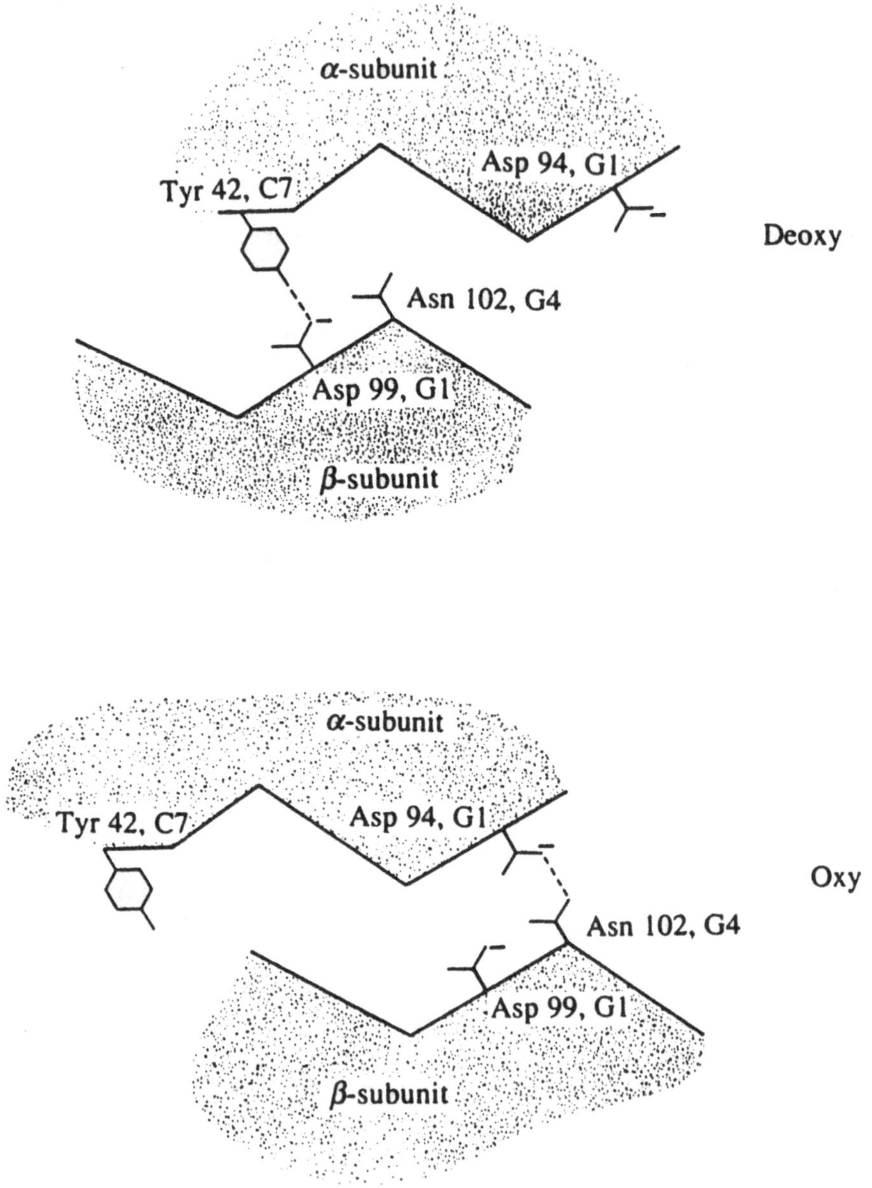

Fig. 11. The $\alpha_1\beta_2$ contact as a two-way switch, showing alternative hydrogen bonds stabilizing the deoxy-T and oxy-R structures

R, which implies that the hydrogen bonds responsible for H^+ discharge must break in the T-structure. The bulk of the protons are released in the T→R transition which takes place mostly at the second and third oxygenation steps. After the third oxygenation step $L_3 = 0.034$, leaving a little more than $^1/_{30}$ of the Hb molecules in the T-structure, which is roughly equivalent to the fraction of $^1/_{20}$ of the protons discharged at the fourth oxygenation step.

Effects of Abnormal Hemoglobins on Respiratory Function

Study of the abnormal human hemoglobins has taught us a great deal about the respiratory function. The $\alpha_1\beta_2$ contact acts as a two-way switch between the T- and R-structures. Each position of the switch is stabilized by a different set of hydrogen bonds. Disruption of any bond that stabilizes specifically the R-structure lowers the oxygen affinity and raises the allosteric constant L, and disruption of any bond that stabilizes the T-structure does the reverse. For example, hemoglobin Kansas [Asn G4(102)β→Thr] has a low oxygen affinity and low Hill's coefficient because the R-structure is destabilized (Fig. 11), while hemoglobin Kempsey [Asp G1(99)→Asn] has a high oxygen affinity and low Hill's coefficient because the T-structure is destabilized. Hill's coefficient is low in both hemoglobins on account of the bell-shaped curve that relates it to the allosteric constant L. Mutations that disrupt the C-terminal salt bridges in the T-structure also have high oxygen affinities and low Hill's coefficients. The surprise came when a mutation that disrupts hydrogen bonds common to *both* the R- and T-structures produced the same effect. This happens in hemoglobin Philly [Tyr C1(35)β→Phe] where the loss of the phenolic hydroxyl disrupts a network of hydrogen bonds at the $\alpha_1\beta_1$ contact which does not change in the T→R transition. It has since become clear that the loss of any bond, either between or within the subunits, even the creation of a cavity, relaxes the T-structure. This relaxation raises K_T and lowers L. K_R is unaffected, since it is almost the same as that of free α- and β-subunits or αβ dimers. In all instances changes in L are linked to changes in K_T; it is not possible to alter these parameters independently [28].

Directed Mutagenesis of Residues in the Heme Pockets

Despite the enormous amount of research done on the structure and function of hemoglobin, some of its most vital properties have remained ill understood. Free ferrous porphyrins are rapidly oxidized by oxygen, and their affinity for oxygen is several thousand times smaller than that for carbon monoxide. Globin keeps the iron ferrous, which is necessary because only ferrous iron combines reversibly with molecular oxygen; globin also discriminates in favor of oxygen and against carbon monoxide. A combination of directed mutagenesis and functional studies has recently clarified these problems.

In myoglobin and in the α-subunits of hemoglobin, N_ε of the distal histidine forms a hydrogen bond with the bound oxygen, but not with carbon monoxide; in the β-subunits that bond is either weak or absent (Fig. 12) [29,

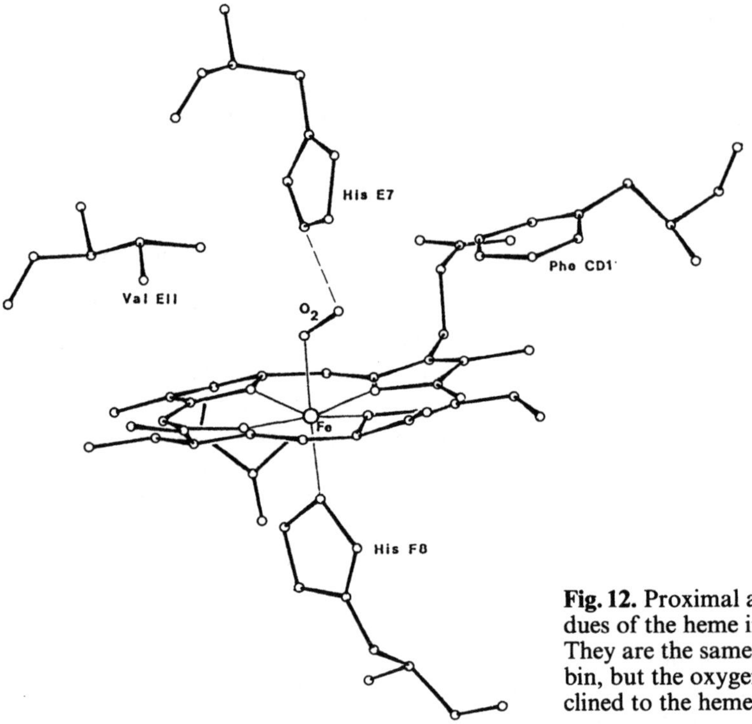

Fig. 12. Proximal and distal residues of the heme in myoglobin. They are the same in hemoglobin, but the oxygen is less inclined to the heme axis

30; X. Chang and B. Schoenborn, personal communication]. X-ray analysis shows that the distal histidine blocks access to the heme pocket [31]. Neither oxygen nor carbon monoxide can enter or leave unless the side chain of the distal histidine swings out of the way, which it can do only be elbowing the helix E to which it is attached, away from the heme. Thux, oxygen transport relies on the dynamics of the globin.

Olson et al. [32] have replaced the distal histidines in myoglobin and in the α- and β-subunits of hemoglobin by glycines, which opened access to the heme pockets, and have measured the resulting changes in the rates of association with and dissociation from oxygen, carbon monoxide, and a more bulky ligand, methylisocyanide. Their results are best analysed in terms of transition state theory [33]. If the transition state is product-like, any rise in affinity can be brought about mainly by a rise in the rate of association. If it is reactant-like, any rise in affinity can be achieved mainly by a drop in the rate of dissociation. These rules generally hold, even though neither rate gives directly the rate of formation or dissociation of the transition state.

The replacement of the distal histidine by glycine leaves the oxygen affinity and kinetic constants of the β-subunits unchanged within error; it *diminishes* the oxygen affinity of the α-subunits eightfold, equivalent to stabilization of the bound oxygen by hydrogen bonds with the histidines by the equivalent of

1.0 kcal mol^{-1}. The reduction in affinity is brought about by a 60-fold incrase in the dissociation (*off*) rate that more than compensates the 10-fold increase in association (*on*) rate due to the opening of the heme pocket. The acceleration brings the on-rate to a value of 15 ($\pm$5) $\times$ $10^7 s^{-1} M^{-1}$ which is close to Szabo's estimate [33] of 50 $\times$ $10^7 s^{-1} M^{-1}$ for a hypothetical globin in which that rate is limited only by diffusion into the heme pocket through a hole of 2.6 Å radius. The absence of any acceleration by the His→Gly replacement in the β-subunit implies that in native hemoglobin histidine E7β must be swinging in and out at least 10^9 times per second, while in myoglobin and in the α-subunits that rate appears to be about a hundred times slower. All the *off* rates are several orders of magnitude slower than the *on* rates, which indicates that the rate-limiting step for the *off* rates is rupture of the Fe-O bond rather than opening of the heme pocket.

Replacement of the distal histidine by glycine *increases* the affinity for carbon monoxide fourfold in the α-subunits, due largely to a rise in the *on* rates, and *decreases* it threefold in the β-subunits. In the native proteins, the *on* rates for carbon monoxide are slower by an order of magnitude than those for oxygen, whence the acceleration is likely to be due to the removal of static steric hindrance by the distal histidines within the heme pocket, rather than its function as a gate. If we multiply the decrease in oxygen affinity by the increase in affinity for carbon monoxide, we find that the distal histidine discriminates against carbon monoxide by the equivalent of about 2 kcal mol^{-1} in the α-subunits, but does not discriminate in the β-subunits.

The switch in quaternary structure from R to T reduces the oxygen affinity of hemoglobin by the equivalent of over 3 kcal per mole heme. Like the reduction in oxygen affinity due to the His→Gly replacement, it is brought about mainly by acceleration of the *off* rates. Hence all the evidence points to the transition state with oxygen being mainly reactant-like. By contrast, the decrease in carbon-monoxide affinity in the R→T transition is due to a drop in the *on* rates, consistent with the present evidence that transition state is mainly product-like.

What role does the distal valine play in the discrimination between oxygen and carbon monoxide? Its replacement by alanine increases both the *on* and *off* rates of oxygen with the α-subunits sevenfold and leaves those with the β-subunits unchanged. It increases the *on* rate of carbon monoxide with the α-subunits tenfold and leaves the *off* rates unchanged. Hence, the distal valine in the α-subunits discriminates against carbon monoxide by the equivalent of 1.3 kcal mol^{-1}, apparently by steric hindrance, but is ineffective in the β-subunits. However, this is only part of the story, because the results of Olson et al. [32] are confined to the R-structure. In the T-structure steric hindrance by the distal valine E11β plays a key role, which future experiments may quantify. Nevertheless, the mechanism of discrimination in the β-subunits remains a mystery.

Other evidence on the mechanism of discrimination between oxygen and carbon monoxide has come from recent crystal structure determinations. In synthetic model compounds that offer no steric hindrance to the ligands, oxygen binds with an Fe-O-O angle of 120°, while carbon monoxide lies on the heme axis. The heme pockets of myoglobin and hemoglobin seemed to be tailored to accommodate the bent oxygen and force the carbon monoxide off the heme axis, which might have accounted for their low carbon monoxide affinity. This is true in myoglobin, where carbon monoxide is seen in two orientations, with Fe-C-O inclined at either 120° or 140° to the heme axis [34]. On the other hand, recent X-ray analyses of human carbonmonoxyhemoglobins at 2.2–2.3 Å resolution have shown inclinations of less than 10°, too little to account for the observed energy of discrimination. There are no significant displacements of the distal residues, but the porphyrins are ruffled [50]. X-ray analysis of a synthetic "hindered pocket" iron porphyrin that has a carbon monoxide affinity lower than of the unhindered "picket fence" iron porphyrin by the equivalent of 1.2 kcal/mole shows similar geometry. Fe-C-O is inclined to the heme axis by only 7.5° and the porphyrin is markedly ruffled [35]. It looks as though in both the "hindered pocket" porphyrin and in hemoglobin a major part of the strain energy responsible for the low carbon monoxide affinity may be stored in the porphyrin.

According to the atomic models, replacement of valine E11β by isoleucine should block the oxygen site in both the T- and R-structures, but in fact isoleucine at E11 fails to inhibit oxygen binding: it merely shifts the entire equilibrium curve to the right, roughly halving the oxygen affinity, which implies a fourfold reduction of the affinity of the β-hemes if the α-hemes remain unaffected. It appears that both the T- and R-structures have enough flexibility to adjust the relative positions of the heme and the distal isoleucine sufficiently for ligands to bind, at a cost of only about 1.6 kcal/mole β-heme.

Computer simulations of the molecular dynamics of the exit of carbon monoxide from the interior of myoglobin suggest that there may be several alternative pathways in addition to that via the distal histidine [36], even though the latter is the most direct. Experimental evidence in support of the histidine as the door to the heme pocket comes from the structure of imidazole and phenylhydrazine myoglobin in which the side-chain of the distal histidine has been turned out of the heme pocket by the bulk of the ligand [37, 38] and from a recent crystal structure determination of ethylisocyanide-myoglobin that shows the side-chain of the distal histidine in two alternative positions, either in or out of the heme pocket, exactly as it would have to move to admit or release ligands [28]. The dynamic movements of the heme pocket are attested by NMR studies showing that phenylalanines CD1 and CD4, which wedge the heme into its pocket and are packed tightly between the heme and the distal helix E, flip over at rates faster than $10^4 s^{-1}$ [39]. They can do so only if the entire heme pocket breathes fast. The fast exchange of most main chain imino hydrogens with tritium also attests to the dynamic state of the hemoglobin molecule [40]. Oxygen has been found to quench the fluorescence of buried tryptophans in other close-packed proteins at velocities near the diffusion limit, which could not have happened unless the proteins' dynamic motion had opened gaps wide enough to let the oxygen pass [41, 42].

Springer et al. [43, 44] have studied the protection of the heme iron from oxidation by replacing the distal histidine in sperm whale myoglobin by ten different amino acid residues and shaking the deoxygenated myoglobin solutions in air in 75 mM potassium phosphate +25 mM EDTA pH 7.0 at 37 °C. All replacements reduced the oxygen affinity and accelerated autoxidation. Phenylalanine, methionine, and arginine produced the smallest accelerations (~50-fold); aspartate the largest (350-fold).

How can these results be interpreted? Paradoxically, combination with oxygen protects the heme iron from oxidation, as can be shown by performing the same experiments at several atmospheres of pure oxygen. Apparently oxidation occurs in that fraction of molecules which are deoxygenated at any one moment. The larger that fraction is at atmospheric oxygen pressure, the faster myoglobin autoxidizes. For example, replacement of the distal histidine by phenylalanine reduced the oxygen affinity 170-fold, so that a larger fraction of myoglobin molecules will have remained deoxygenated at atmospheric oxygen pressure and therefore have become autoxidized. However, this can be only part of the explanation, because the replacement of histidine by glycine reduces the oxygen affinity merely elevenfold, yet accelerates autoxidation over a hundredfold.

Autoxidation is catalysed by protons, hence the 350-fold acceleration by aspartate. I suggest that the distal histidine protects the ferrous heme iron by acting as a proton trap. The distal histidine has a pK_a of about 5.5; at neutral pH it is protonated only at N_σ which faces the solvent. Any proton entering the heme pocket of deoxymyoglobin would be bound by N_ε, and simultaneously N_σ would release its proton to the solvent. When the histidine side chain swings out of the heme pocket, the protons would interchange, restoring the previous state. No other amino acid side chain could function in this way. Evolution was a brilliant chemist.

Hemoglobin as a Drug Receptor

In a search for compounds that might prevent the aggregation of deoxyhemoglobin S in patients with sickle-cell anemia, two antilipidemic drugs, clofibric acid and its analogue bezafibrate, were found to lower the oxygen affinity of hemoglobin. X-ray analysis of crystals grown in the presence of these compounds showed that they combine with deoxy, but not with oxyhemoglobin. They stabilize the T-structure by combining with sites in the central cavity that are about 20 Å away from the DPG binding sites; their effects and that of DPG on the allosteric equilibrium are additive [45].

This discovery led I. Lalezari to synthesize a family of new compounds related to, but more active than bezafibrate [46]; one of these, L3, 4, 5 which has the formula shown below, has turned out to be the most powerful allosteric effector yet found (Fig. 13). At an effector concentration equimolar to heme and at pH 6, it lowers the oxygen affinity of solutions of human hemoglobin to a level found until now only in fish hemoglobins that exhibit a Root effect (Fig. 14). In such fish hemoglobins, the tension on the heme in the T-structure

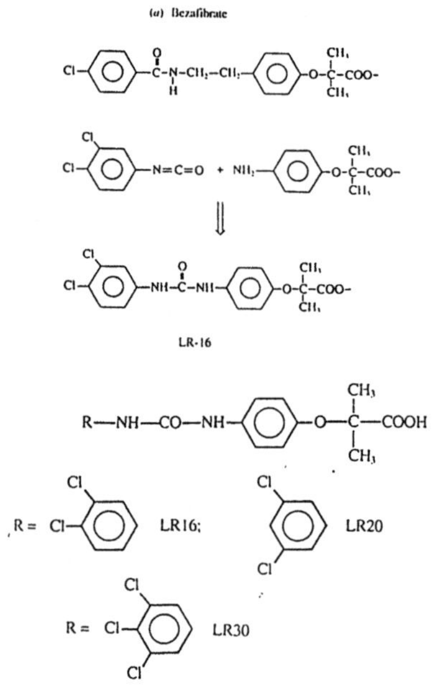

Fig. 13. Novel allosteric effectors of hemoglobin: bezafibrate, an antilipidemic drug, and compounds derived from it by Dr. I. Lalezari

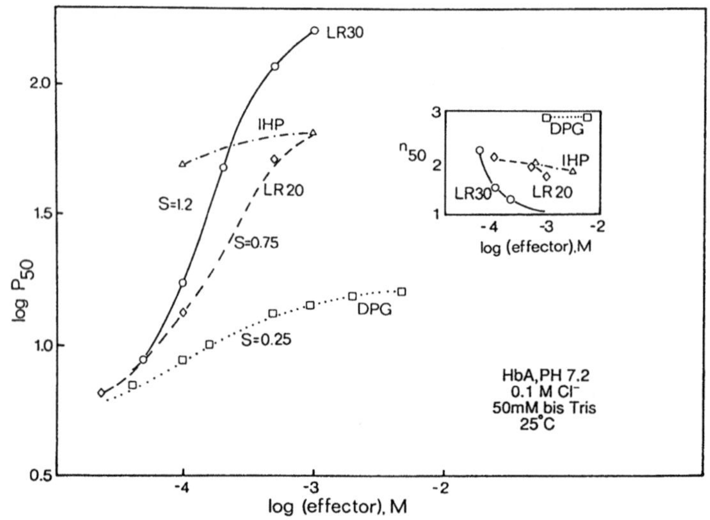

Fig. 14. Effect on partial pressure of oxygen at half saturation (P_{50}) of 2,3-diphosphoglycerate (DPG), inositol hexaphosphate (IHP), and two of Dr. Lalezari's synthetic effectors LR20 and LR30. The *inset* shows their effect on Hill's coefficient at half saturation. At 1 m*M* LR30 the hemoglobin is only half saturated at 2 × atmospheric oxygen pressure and its Hill's coefficient is near unity because the allosteric constant *L* is very large. (Courtesy of Dr. C. Poyart)

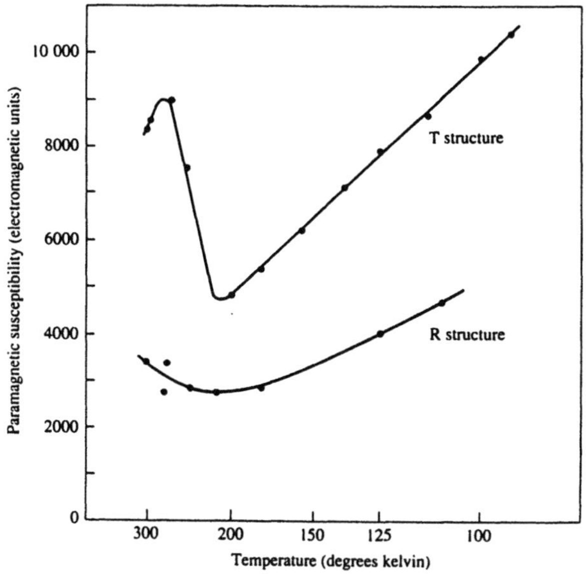

Fig. 15. Temperature dependence of paramagnetic susceptibility of carp azide methemoglobin in the R- and T-structures. Below about 200 K the susceptibility rises with falling temperature in accordance with Curie's law. Above that temperature a thermal equilibrium between a high and a low spin form masks that behavior, since the high spin form gains stability with rising temperature. It has longer Fe-N bond distances than the low spin form. Tension at the heme in the T-structure therefore shifts the equilibrium towards higher spin. (From Messana et al. [47])

that is associated with the low oxygen affinity has been demonstrated directly. In azidemethemoglobin the iron is in a thermal equilibrium between two different spin states that are characterized by different lengths of the iron nitrogen bonds; they are longer in the high spin than in the low spin state. In azidemethemoglobin of trout transition from the R- to the T-structure induces a transition to higher spin, equivalent to a stretching of the Fe-N bonds [47, 48]. This is manifested by an increase in paramagnetic susceptibility equivalent to a change in free energy of 1 kcal/mol (Fig. 15) and also by a change in optical spectra which show a rise in intensity of the high spin bands at 500 and 630 nm and a drop in intensity of the low spin bands at 540 and 570 nm. Until recently it was not possible to induce this transition in human azidemethemoglobin [49], but combination with the powerful new synthetic effector induced a difference spectrum identical to that of trout hemoglobin which demonstrates that the hemes are under tension also in human hemoglobin in the liganded T-state (Fig. 16). See also [51, 52].

X-ray analysis and oxygen equilibria show that four molecules of the effector combine with one molecule of human deoxyhemoglobin both in the crystal and in solution. One pair of symmetry-related binding sites is close to those of bezafibrate; the other pair is nearly at right angles to the first (Fig. 17). The four trichlorobenzene moieties form a parallel stack. Their close packing

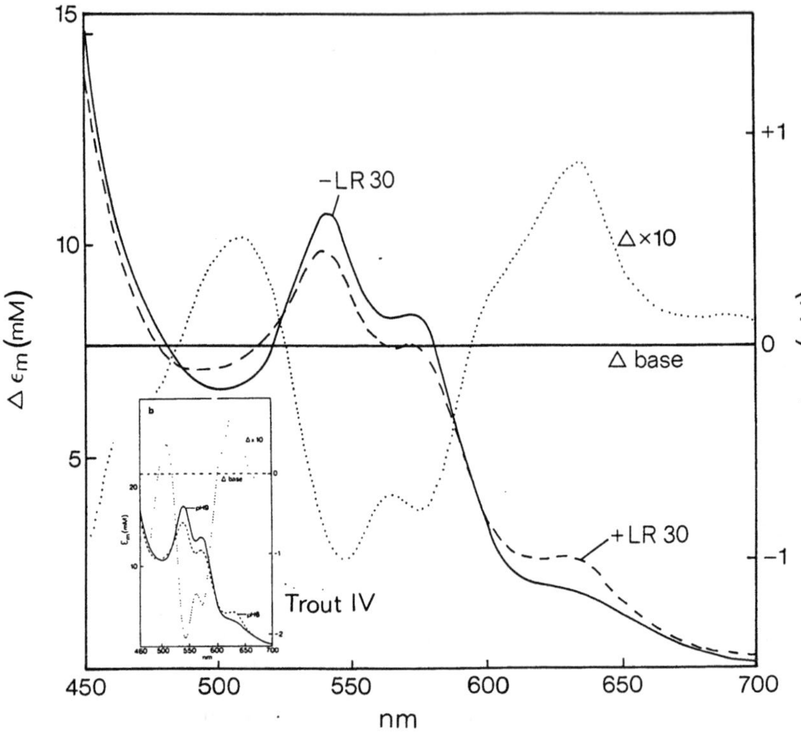

Fig. 16. Optical absorption spectra of human and trout IV azide methemoglobin in the R- and T-structures, showing the rise in intensity of the high spin bands at 500 and 630 nm and the fall of the low spin bands at 540 and 570 nm. *Full lines,* T-structure; *broken lines,* R-structure; *dotted lines,* difference spectra, 10 × enlarged

seems to dominate their mode of binding. The combination of human deoxyhemoglobin with the effectors induced no stereochemical changes at the allosteric core that were visible at 2.5 Å resolutiion and produced a decrease of the Fe-N_ε stretching frequency by only 1–2 cm^{-1} (Kitagawa, personal communication). Only in the liganded T-structure do the effectors make themselves felt at the hemes.

The work on drug binding by hemoglobin has led to generalizations that are relevant to the binding of effectors, transmitters, and drugs to other proteins. The stereochemistry of binding is determined by the available van der Waals space and, within that space, by interactions of a wide range of polarity, from strong hydrogen bonds between ionized groups of opposite charge to weak interactions between aromatic quadrupoles, and nonpolar interactions between aliphatic hydrocarbons. The detailed stereochemistry is governed by a tendency to maximize the sum of the energy of electrostatic interactions, for example, by aligning effectors relative to the protein so that the mutual polarizabilities are maximized. Drugs may influence the allosteric equilibrium of a protein receptor in the same direction as the natural effector even though they are chemically unrelated to it, because proteins may offer a variety of binding sites not used in nature [45].

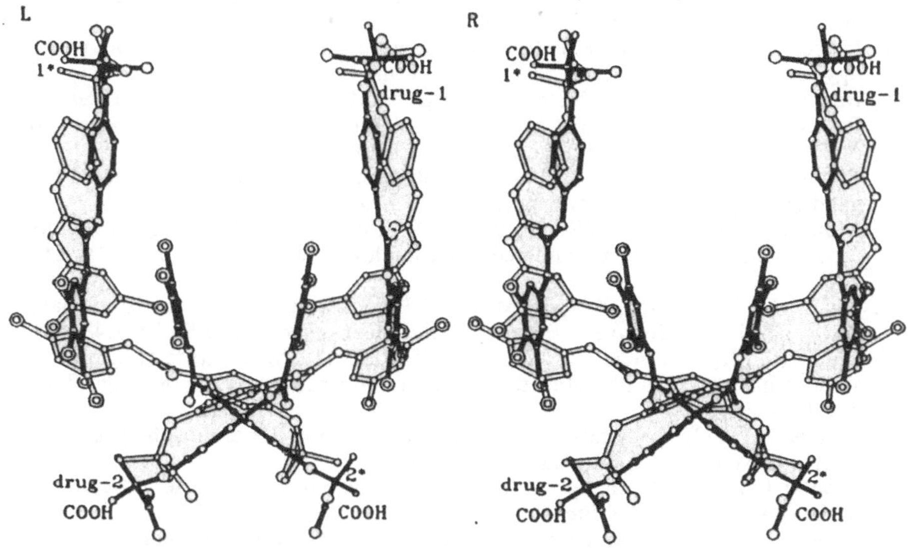

Fig. 17. Arrangement of the two effectors LR20 and LR30 in the central cavity of hemoglobin. The *vertical pairs* lie mainly between the two α-chains in sites that overlap those of bezafibrate. The other pairs occupy positions not taken up by bezafibrate, and the sites of the 3,5-dichloro derivative (LR20) differ from those occupied by the 3,4,5-trichloro derivative (LR30). The four trichlorobenzene moieties form a closely packed parallel stack right in the center of the hemoglobin molecule, while the dichlorobenzene moieties stack in separate pairs [53].

References

1. Perutz MF (1979) Regulation of oxygen affinity of hemoglobin: influence of structure of the globin on the heme. Ann Rev Biochem 48:327–386
2. Perutz MF (1970) Stereochemistry of cooperative effects in haemoglobin. Nature 228:726–739
3. Watson HC, Kendrew JC (1961) Comparison between the amino-acid sequences of sperm whale myoglobin and of human haemoglobin. Nature 190:670–672
4. Gill SJ, Di Cera E, Doyle ML, Robert CH (1988) New twists on an old story: hemoglobin. Trends Biochem Sci 13:465–467
5. Perrella M, Sabionedda L, Lamaja M, Rossi-Bernardi L (1986) The intermediate compounds between human hemoglobin and carbon monoxide at equilibrium and during approach to equilibrium. J Biol Chem 261:8391–8396
6. Perrella M, Colosimo A, Benazzi L, Samaja M, Rossi-Bernardi L (1988) Intermediate compounds between hemoglobin and carbon monoxide under equilibrium conditions. Symposium on Oxygen Binding and Heme Proteins, Asilomar Conference Grounds, Pacific Grove, California
7. Angel W-L, Karplus M, Poyart C, Burseaux E (1988) Analysis of proton release in oxygen binding by haemoglobin: implications for the cooperative mechanism. Biochemistry 27:1285–1301
8. Baldwin JM (1975) Structure and function of haemoglobin. Progr Biophys Mol Biol 29:225–320
9. Bunn HF, Forget GB (1985) Hemoglobin, molecular and clinical aspects. WB Saunders, Philadelphia, PA, USA

10. Fermi G, Perutz MF (1981) Atlas of molecular structures in biology: haemoglobin and myoglobin. Clarendon Press, Oxford
11. Dickerson RE, Geis I (1983) Hemoglobin: structure, function, evolution, pathology. Benjamin/Cummings Publishing Co, Kenlo Park
12. Imai K (1982) Allosteric effects in haemoglobin. Cambridge University Press
13. Perutz MF, Fermi G, Luisi B, Shaanan B, Liddington RC (1987) Stereochemistry of cooperative effects in hemoglobin. Accs Chem Res 20:309–321
14. Baldwin JM, Chothia C (1979) Haemoglobin: the structural changes related to ligand binding and its allosteric mechanism. J Mol Biol 129:183–191
15. Momenteau M, Scheidt WR, Eigenbrot CW, Reed CA (1988) A deoxymyoglobin model with a sterically unhindered axial imidazole. J Am Chem Soc 110:1207–1215
16. Gelin RG, Lee AW-M, Karplus M (1983) Hemoglobin tertiary structural change on ligand binding. Its role in the cooperative mechanism. J Mol Biol 171:489–559
17. Liddington R, Derewenda Z, Dodson G, Harris D (1988) Structure of liganded T-state of haemoglobin identifies the origin of cooperative oxygen binding. Nature 331:725–728
18. Arnone A (1972) X-ray diffraction study of binding of 2,3-diphosphoglycerate to human deoxyhaemoglobin. Nature 237:146–149
19. Monod J, Wyman J, Changeux JP (1965) On the nature of allosteric transitions: a plausible model. J Mol Biol 12:88–118
20. Louie C, Tran T, Englander JJ, Englander SW (1988) Allosteric energy at the hemoglobin β-chain C-terminus studied by hydrogen exchange. J Mol Biol 201:755–764
21. Fersht AR, Leatherbarrow RJ, Wells TNC (1986) Structure and activity of the tyrosyl-rRNA synthetase: the hydrogen bond in catalysis and specificity. Phil Trans Roy Soc A 317:305–320
22. Kilmartin JV (1974) Influence of DPG on the Bohr effect of human haemoglobin. FEBS Letts 38:147–148
23. Perutz MF, Kilmartin JV, Nishikura K, Fogg JH, Butler PJG, Rollema HS (1980) Identification of residues contributing to the Bohr effect of human haemoglobin. J Mol Biol 138:649–670
24. Kilmartin JV, Breen JJ, Roberts GCK, Ho C (1973) Direct measurement of the pK values of an alkaline Bohr group in human haemoglobin. Proc Nat Acad Sci USA 70:1246–1249
25. Matsukawa S, Itatani Y, Mawatari K, Shimokawa Y, Yoneyama Y (1978) Quantitative evaluation for the role β-146 His and β-143 His residues in the Bohr effect of human haemoglobin in the presence of 01 *M* chloride ion. J Biol Chem 259:11479–11486
26. Monod J, Changeux JP, Jacob F (1963) Allosteric proteins and molecular control systems. J Mol Biol 6:306–329
27. Chu AH, Turner BW, Ackers GK (1984) Effects of protons on the oxygen-linked subassembly in human haemoglobin. Biochemistry 23:604–617
28. Johnson KA, Olson JS, Phillips GN Jr (1989) The structure of myoglobinethyl isocyanide: histidine as a swinging door for ligand entry. J Mol Biol In the press
29. Phillips SEV, Schoenborn BP (1981) Neutron diffraction reveals oxygen-histidine hydrogen bond in myoglobin. Nature 292:81–82
30. Shaanan B (1983) Structure of human oxyhaemoglobin at 2.1 Å resolution. J Mol Biol 171:31–50
31. Perutz MF, Mathews FS (1966) An X-ray study of azide methaemoglobin. J Mol Biol 21:199–202
32. Olson JS, Mathews AJ, Rohlfs RJ, Springer BA, Edelberg KD, Sligar SG, Tame J, Renaud J-P, Nagai K (1988) The role of the distal histidine in myoglobin and haemoglobin. Nature 336:265–266
33. Szabo A (1978) The kinetic of haemoglobin and transition state theory. Proc Nat Acad Sci USA 75:2108–2111

34. Kuriyan J, Wilz S, Karplus M, Petsko GA (1986) X-ray structure and refinement of carbonmonoxy (FeII)-myoglobin at 1.5 Å resolution. J Mol Biol 192:133–154
35. Kim K, Fettinger J, Sessler JL, Cyr M, Hugdahl J, Collman JP, Ibers JA (1989) Structural characterisation of a sterically encumbered iron (II) porphyrin CO complex. J Amer Chem Soc 111:403–405
36. Elber R, Karplus M (1989) Molecular dynamics simulations of myoglobin. (To be published)
37. Bolognesi M, Cannillo E, Ascenzi P, Giacometti GM, Merli A, Brunori M (1982) Reactivity of ferric aplysia and sperm whale myoglobins towards imidazole: X-ray and binding study. J Mol Biol 158:301–315
38. Ringe D, Petsko GE, Kerr DE, de Montellano FRO (1984) Reaction of myoglobin with phenylhydrazine – a molecular doorstop. Biochemistry 23:2–4
39. Dalvit C, Wright PE (1987) Assignment of resonances in the ^{1}H nuclear magnetic resonance spectrum of the carbon monoxide complex of sperm whale myoglobin by phase-sensitive two-dimensional techniques. J Mol Biol 194:313–327
40. Englander SW, Kallenbach NR (1984) Hydrogen exchange and structural dynamics of proteins and nucleic acids. Q Rev Biophys 16:521–565
41. Calhoun DB, Vanderkooi JM, Woodrow GV III, Englander SW (1983) Penetration of dioxygen into proteins studied by quenching of phosphorescence and fluorescence. Biochemistry 22:1526–1532
42. Lakowicz JR, Weber G (1973) Quenching of protein fluorescence by oxygen: detection of structural fluctuations in proteins on the nanosecond time scale. Biochemistry 12:4171–4179
43. Springer BA, Egeberg KD, Sligar SG, Rohlfs RJ, Mathews AJ, Olson JS (1989a) Discrimination between oxygen and carbon monoxide and inhibition of autoxidation by myoglobin. J Biol Chem 264:3057–3060
44. Springer BA, Egeberg KD, Sligar SG, Rohlfs RJ, Mathews AJ, Olson JS (1989b) Site-directed mutagenesis of sperm whale myoglobin: role of His E7 and Val E11 in ligand binding. J Biol Chem (in the press)
45. Perutz MF, Fermi G, Abraham DJ, Poyart C, Bursaux E (1986) Hemoglobin as a receptor of drugs and peptides: X-ray studies of the stereochemistry of binding. J Amer Chem Soc 108:1064–1078
46. Lalezari I, Rahbar S, Lalezari P, Fermi G, Perutz MF (1988) LR16, a compound with potent effects on the oxygen affinity of hemoglobin, on blood cholesterol, and on low density lipoprotein. Proc Nat Acad Sci USA 85:6117–6121
47. Messana C, Cerdonio M, Shenkin P, Noble RW, Fermi G, Perutz RN, Perutz MF (1978) Influence of quaternary structure of the globin on thermal spin equilibria in different methaemoglobin derivatives. Biochemistry 17:3652–3662
48. Perutz MF, Sanders JKM, Chenery DH, Noble RW, Pennelly RR, Fung LW-M, Ho C, Giannini I, Pörschke D, Winckler H (1978) Interactions between the quaternary structure of the globin and the spin state of the heme in ferric mixed spin derivatives of hemoglobin. Biochemistry 17:3640–3652
49. Philo S, Dreyer U (1985) Quaternary structure has little influence on spin states in mixed-spin human methemoglobins. Biochemistry 24:2985–2991
50. Derewenda Z, Dodson G, Emsley P, Harris D, Nagai K, Perutz MF, Renaud J-P (1989) The stereochemistry of CO binding to normal adult and Cowtown haemoglobins. J Mol Biol (in the press)
51. Noble RW, DeYoung A, Vitale S, Cerdonio M, DiIorio EE (1989) Spin equilibria of human methemoglobin: effect of bezafibrate and inositol hexaphosphate as measured by susceptometry and visible spectroscopy. Biochemistra 28:5288–5292
52. Noble RW, DeYoung A, Rousseau DL (1989) Spin equilibrium in human methemoglobin: effects of inositol hexaphosphate and bezafibrate as measured by resonance Raman spectroscopy. Biochemistry 28:5293–5297
53. Lalezari I, Lalezari P, Poyart C, Marden M, Kister J, Bohn B, Fermi G, Perutz MF (1989) New effectors of human hemoglobin: structure and function. Submitted to Biochemistry

Physiology and Pathophysiology of Pulmonary Gas Exchange

J. B. West

The topic of the physiology and pathophysiology of pulmonary gas exchange which has been assigned to me is vast. In this presentation I propose to concentrate on recent advances in our understanding of ventilation-perfusion relationships in the lung, and to discuss how abnormalities in the matching of ventilation and blood flow affect gas exchange in several common types of lung disease.

It has been known for many years that mismatching of ventilation and blood flow is the commonest cause of hypoxemia in lung disease. However, this has always been a difficult topic to investigate because of its complexity. Part of the difficulty lies in the fact that the effects of uneven ventilation and blood flow on gas exchange are determined in part by the oxygen and carbon dioxide dissociation curves which are not only nonlinear but interdependent.

Krogh and Lindhard (1917) and Haldane (1922) recognized the importance of uneven ventilation and blood flow in the lung in determining gas exchange. However, it was not until the 1940s, when Fenn et al. (1946) and Riley and Cournand (1949) introduced the graphical analysis of pulmonary gas exchange, that the problem became tractable in quantitative terms. More recently, rapid advances in our knowledge have occurred as a result of the introduction of computer procedures to describe the oxygen and carbon dioxide dissociation curves (Kelman 1966, 1967). With these new techniques, it became possible to answer questions about pulmonary gas exchange which had been impossibly difficult before. The behavior of distributions of ventilation-perfusion ratios was analyzed (West 1969), and Wagner and his colleagues (1974a) introduced the multiple inert gas elimination technique which allowed, for the first time, information about the dispersion, number of modes, and shape of the distributions to be obtained.

Multiple Inert Gas Elimination Technique

When an inert gas dissolved in saline is steadily infused into the venous circulation, the proportion of the gas that is eliminated by the ventilation from the blood of the given lung unit depends only upon the solubility of the gas and the ventilation-perfusion ratio (VA/Q) (Kety 1951; Farhi 1967). The relationship is given by the following equation:

$$\frac{Pc'}{P\bar{v}} = \frac{\lambda}{\lambda + VA/Q},$$

where Pc′ is the partial pressure of the gas in end-capillary blood, and λ is the blood-gas partition coefficient. The end-capillary divided by the mixed venous partial pressure ($P\bar{v}$) is known as the "retention."

To use this technique in practice, a mixture of six gases (typically sulfur hexafluoride, ethane, cyclopropane, halothane, ether, and acetone) is dissolved in saline and infused into a peripheral vein at the rate of about 3 ml/min until a steady state of gas exchange has been established. This typically takes about 10 min. Samples of expired gas and arterial blood are then taken, and the gas concentrations are measured by gas chromatography. In addition, cardiac output and total ventilation are also measured. In patients who already have an indwelling pulmonary arterial catheter, such as those in the intensive care unit, a sample of mixed venous blood is also taken so that the arterial PO_2 and PCO_2 corresponding to the ventilation-perfusion distribution can be computed.

A graph is then constructed as shown in Fig. 1 (upper panel). This shows the data points for the inert gas retentions; these are joined by the *broken* line for clarity. Below this are the data points for excretion (partial pressure in mixed expired gas divided by partial pressure in venous blood) against solubility. The two *solid* lines show the values of retention and excretion for a lung with no ventilation-perfusion inequality but with the same overall ventilation and blood flow. In the normal lung from which these retention and excretion curves were derived, the broken and solid lines are very close together. However, the differences are more easily seen in Fig. 2 (upper panel) where the lung is diseased.

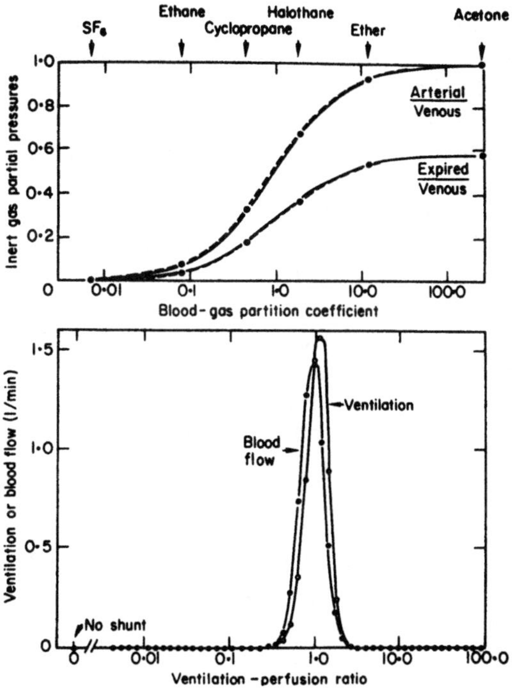

Fig. 1. Distribution of ventilation-perfusion ratios in a young normal subject determined with the multiple inert gas elimination technique. The *upper panel* shows data points for inert gas retention *(upper)* and excretion *(lower)*. *Broken lines* join the points for clarity. The two *solid lines* show the values of retention and excretion for a lung with no ventilation-perfusion inequality. The *lower panel* shows the recovered distribution of ventilation-perfusion ratios. (From Wagner et al. 1974b)

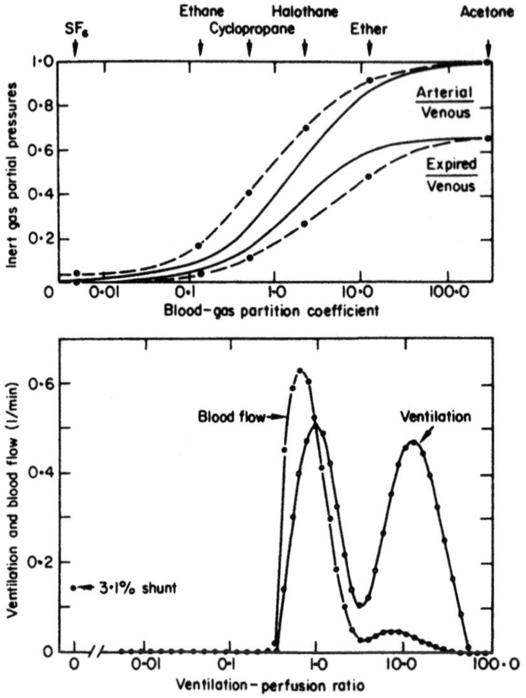

Fig. 2. Distribution of ventilation-perfusion ratios in a 60-year-old patient with chronic obstructive lung disease, predominantly emphysema. The *upper panel* shows the retention and excretion solubility curves; cf. Fig. 1. (From Wagner et al. 1977)

These graphs contain information about the distribution of ventilation-perfusion ratios in the lung. As an example, if a lung contains units that are perfused but not ventilated (shunt) these particularly increase the retention of the least soluble gas, sulfur hexafluoride. On the other hand, if the distribution contains large amounts of ventilation to lung units with extremely high ventilation-perfusion ratios, the retention of the very high solubility gases will be chiefly affected. When this technique is used in practice, the distribution of ventilation-perfusion ratios which is consistent with the measured pattern of inert gas retention and excretion is derived by an iterative process using a computer. It is not necessary to understand this sophisticated computer procedure to use the method.

The potential limitations of the transformation from retentions and excretions to distributions of ventilation-perfusion ratios have been explored in great detail (Evans and Wagner 1977). The recovered distributions are not unique, but in the clinical setting, the range of possible distributions compatible with the data is sufficiently small that confusion rarely arises. Other limitations include the fact that not more than three modes of a distribution can be recovered, and only smooth distributions can be obtained. However, in spite of these limitations, the technique gives much more information about the patterns of ventilation-perfusion distributions in patients with lung disease than has previously been available, and a good deal of additional insight has been afforded into conditions such as chronic obstructive lung disease, asthma, interstitial lung disease, pulmonary embolism, respiratory failure, and anesthesia.

Distributions in Normal Subjects

Figure 1 shows measured retention and excretion-solubility curves, and the resulting distribution of ventilation-perfusion ratios from a 22-year-old normal volunteer (Wagner et al. 1974b). It is clear from the upper panel that the retentions and excretions as indicated by the data points are almost superimposed on the solid lines for a homogeneous line. In other words, the lung of this young normal subject is behaving very like a lung with no ventilation-perfusion inequality. The lower panel shows the distribution of ventilation-perfusion ratios which is consistent with the measured retention and excretion data. Note that all the ventilation and blood flow are distributed to lung units with ventilation-perfusion ratios very near the normal value of about 1. For example, there was essentially no ventilation or blood flow to lung units outside the range of approximately 0.3 to 3.0 on the ventilation-perfusion scale.

An interesting finding in the normal subjects that we studied was that there was no shunt (blood flow to unventilated alveoli). It should be added that this technique is extremely sensitive to shunt in that a shunt of only about 0.5% of the cardiac output doubles the arterial concentration of sulfur hexafluoride. These results were a surprise to us and indicate that young normal subjects are ventilating essentially all of their alveoli.

When older subjects were investigated, we found that their recovered distributions of ventilation-perfusion ratios differed from those found in young people. Generally the distributions are broader, indicating that the lung is less successful in matching ventilation and blood flow. Occasionally a shoulder on the left of the blood flow distribution is seen indicating excessive amounts of blood flow to poorly ventilated lung units. The reason for this is not certain but may be the intermittent ventilation of lung units in dependent regions as a result of airway closure.

Chronic Obstructive Lung Disease

Figure 2 shows the distribution of ventilation-perfusion ratios from a patient with chronic obstructive lung disease who was believed to have predominately emphysema (Wagner et al. 1977). The patient was a 60-year-old man with a long history of increasing shortness of breath, little cough or sputum, large lung volumes, mild hypoxemia (arterial PO_2 63 torr), and a normal arterial PCO_2. The upper panel shows the measured retentions and excretions, and it can be seen that they deviated greatly from those predicted in a homogeneous lung with the same total ventilation and blood flow. Consistent with this, the lower panel shows a very abnormal distribution of ventilation-perfusion ratios compared with the normal pattern seen in Fig. 1. Note the broad bimodal distribution, the additional mode being a large amount of ventilation going to lung units with extremely high ventilation-perfusion ratios. In the classical

Riley analysis these would contribute alveolar dead space. It was interesting that there was relatively little blood flow to lung units having abnormally low ventilation-perfusion ratios, and the blood flow to unventilated lung (shunt) was only 3.1% of the cardiac output.

Presumably the additional mode of ventilation to lung units with very high ventilation-perfusion ratios can be explained by destruction of the capillary bed by the emphysematous process. This would be expected to result in regions which are ventilated but have very little blood flow. The fact that the arterial PO_2 was only slightly depressed is consistent with the fact that there was very little blood flow to lung units with low ventilation-perfusion ratios, and only a very small shunt. In fact the hypoxemia can be explained by the slight displacement of the main mode of blood flow to the left. This pattern is fairly consistently seen in patients with chronic obstructive lung disease with predominately emphysema, though exceptions do occur.

A different pattern is often seen in patients with severe chronic bronchitis. Figure 3 shows typical findings in a patient with chronic obstructive lung disease whose predominate lesion was severe bronchitis (Wagner et al. 1977). In this instance only the recovered distribution of ventilation-perfusion ratios is shown, but of course this was derived from the measured retention and excretion values as described for Figs. 1 and 2. It can be seen that the main abnormality in this patient was an abnormal mode of blood flow with a large amount of blood flow going to lung units with very low ventilation-perfusion ratios between 0.03 and 0.1. This explains the more severe hypoxemia in this type of patient, and in the Riley analysis, would be described as physiologic shunt. However, note that this patient had no blood flow to unventilated alveoli (shunt) in spite of the fact that there were clearly a large number of lung units which were very poorly ventilated.

Absence of shunt (or a very small amount) is a common finding in chronic obstructive lung disease where the lesion is predominately bronchitis, and we believe that it indicates that lung units distal to completely obstructed airways

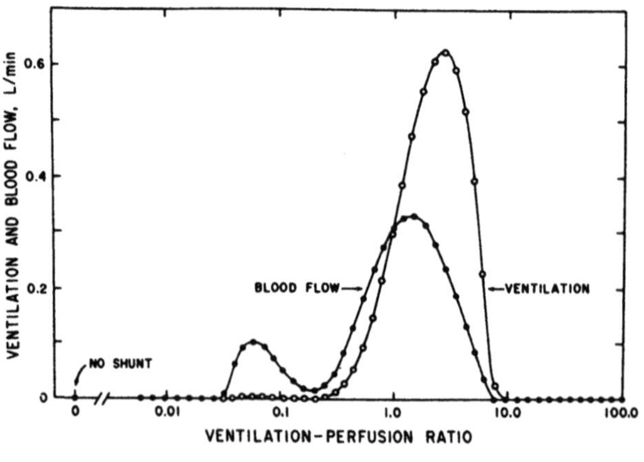

Fig. 3. Example of a distribution of ventilation-perfusion ratios in a patient with chronic obstructive disease, predominately chronic bronchitis; cf. Fig. 2. (From Wagner et al. 1977)

are being ventilated through collateral channels. The substantial amount of blood flow to units which low ventilation-perfusion ratios can presumably be explained by the diseased airways which are either partially or completely blocked by mucous gland hypertrophy, edema of the walls, retained secretions, or other mechanisms. It should be added that although patients with severe chronic bronchitis and chronic obstructive lung disease often show this pattern, there is a good deal of variability (Wagner et al. 1977). Of course most patients with chronic obstructive lung disease have a mixture of emphysema and chronic bronchitis with the result that mixed patterns are frequently obtained. Figures 2 and 3 were obtained from patients with relatively pure emphysema, on the one hand, and chronic bronchitis, on the other (as far as could be determined clinically), in order to clarify the pathophysiological basis of the gas exchange in these two common conditions.

Bronchial Asthma

A particularly interesting pattern of ventilation-perfusion ratios has been described in some patients with bronchial asthma (Wagner et al. 1978). An example is shown in Fig. 4, where it can be seen that there was a striking bimodal pattern with about one-quarter of the total blood flow going to lung units with ventilation-perfusion ratios in the region of 0.1. It is important to appreciate how rapidly the normal ratio becomes abnormal on this log scale. For example, these lung units had only one-tenth of their normal ventilation in relation to blood flow. However, note that there was no blood flow to unventilated units (shunt) in spite of the fact that many lung units were clearly extremely poorly ventilated. The mode of blood flow to lung units with low ventilation-perfusion ratios reduced the arterial PO_2 to 81 torr.

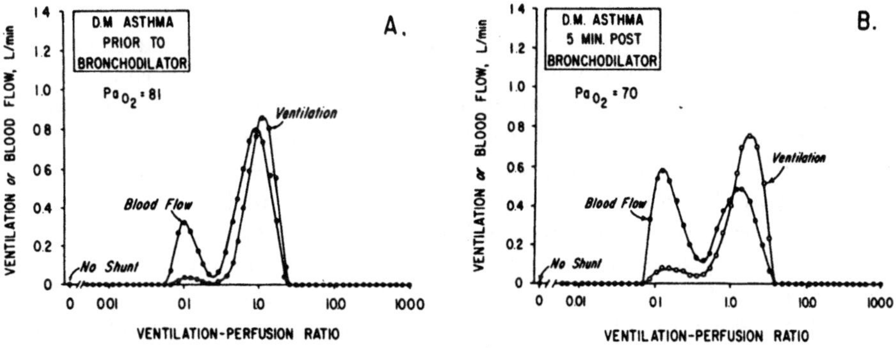

Fig. 4 A, B. Distribution of ventilation-perfusion ratios in a patient with asthma before (**A**) and after (**B**) the administration of isoproterenol by aerosol. Note the bimodal distribution, absence of shunt, and increase in blood flow to the lower mode after the bronchodilator. (From Wagner et al. 1978)

Figure 4 B shows how the distribution of ventilation-perfusion ratios was altered when the patient was given the bronchodilator isoproterenol by aerosol. It can be seen that there was a striking increase in the amount of blood flow to lung units with low ventilation-perfusion ratios, with the result that this mode of the distribution now received approximately one-half of the cardiac output. As a consequence, the arterial PO_2 fell from 81 to 70 torr. However, we found that the change shown in Fig. 4 B was short-lived. Five minutes later, that is 10 min after the administration of the drug, the distribution had returned to the pattern shown in Fig. 4 A. Naturally, the bronchodilator effects of the isoproterenol had a much longer duration.

These studies indicate that the decrease in arterial PO_2 which is often seen in asthmatics after bronchodilator therapy can be attributed to the increase in blood flow to lung units with low ventilation-perfusion ratios. The reason for this redistribution of blood flow is uncertain. It may be that the blood vessels supplying these poorly ventilated units dilate in response to the beta-adrenergic agonists. It is likely that the mediators released in the asthma attack affect the smooth muscle of the blood vessels as well as those of the airways, though surprisingly little attention has been given to the pulmonary circulation in asthma. If this is so, it may be that the bronchodilator drug also acts as a vasodilator, and this is the reason for the increase in blood flow to the poorly ventilated units.

Another possibility is that this increase in blood flow is caused by release of hypoxic pulmonary vasoconstriction in these areas of low alveolar PO_2. There is some evidence to support this. However, it is interesting that in this particular patient, the distribution of ventilation-perfusion ratios did not change when 100% oxygen was administered.

A particularly intriguing question is why these patients have such a marked bimodal distribution, and why they have so much blood flow to poorly ventilated units, but no shunt. Our initial expectation in this group of patients was that they would show a broad dispersion of ventilation-perfusion ratios. This is the pattern that one would expect if the asthmatic process narrowed some airways than others, and therefore decreased the venilation in some regions more than others. Although a broadened distribution *is* seen in some patients with asthma, especially those with very mild disease, a bimodal distribution is very frequent, even in some patients who appear to be in remission. The only way we can account for the existence of a clearly defined, second population of lung units is that these represent alveoli behind completely closed airways, and that they are being ventilated through collateral channels.

Note that the distribution shown in Fig. 4 B indicates that a very large proportion of the lung units are ventilated in this way. It was pointed out that about one-half of the cardiac outputs is going to these very poorly ventilated units, and unless we assume that these units are overperfused in relation to their volume (which seems very unlikely), the inevitable conclusion is that about one-half of the alveoli in the lung lie behind completely obstructed airways. This striking conclusion is at variance with many modern notions of the pathophysiology of asthma.

This pattern has now been seen repeatedly in patients with acute severe asthma. In a recent study by Roca et al. (1988) of ten patients with acute severe asthma requiring hospitalization, all the patients had bimodal distributions of ventilation-perfusion ratios consistent with extensive bronchial occlusion. This bimodal pattern gradually resolved over several days of hospitalization.

Pathological studies have always emphasized the importance of completely occluded airways in patients dying with acute severe asthma. For example, Dunnill (1960) reported on the appearances of the lungs of 20 patients dying in status asthmaticus. Mucus plugs in the airways and focus areas of collapse were described as "outstanding features." Indeed, Dunnill was so impressed by the degree of bronchial occlusion that he suggested that "bronchospasm plays little or no part ... in the pathogenesis of the asthmatic attack." He described one case in which both main bronchi were so tightly packed with viscid mucoid material that it could not be dislodged by a pressure of 5 feet of water. Other pathologists have described similar appearances in the lungs of patients who have died with acute asthma (Cardell 1956).

Some physicians have argued that these postmortem findings are misleading in that you might expect to see complete bronchial occlusion in terminally ill cases. Unfortunately, little is known about the histological appearances in patients with acute asthma who do not die of that disease because it is very seldom that lung tissue is available for examination. However, the autopsy findings fit so well with the physiological data from a variety of measurements that all the information taken together strongly supports the importance of completely occluded airways.

If many of the airways of a patient with asthma are completely blocked by mucus plugs, shed bronchial mucosal cells, and bronchial wall edema, this clearly affects our attitude towards management and prognosis. While the patient should be treated with bronchodilators such as beta-2 adrenergic agonists, theophylline, and steroids, recovery is bound to be very slow. The blocked airways will respond only gradually to treatment and the patient's ventilatory function will be severely compromised for a substantial time. Little is known about the mechanisms responsible for the abnormal mucus, edema, and shed bronchial mucosal cells which plug the airways. Presumably the chief therapeutic factors will be corticosteroids with attention to adequate hydration of the patient.

The fact that many of the airways in asthma are completely occluded may be a factor in the perceived increase in mortality of this disease, although there is considerable disagreement about the statistics. However, one possible reason for the increased mortality, if it exists, is the unwarranted expectation of physicians who predict that patients with asthma will respond rapidly to bronchodilators. Clearly, a patient with many or most of his airways completely occluded by mucus plugs will respond very slowly, and treatment will have to be maintained over a long period of time during which the patient may be very ill.

Another interesting feature of the distribution of ventilation-perfusion ratios shown in Fig. 4B is that despite one-half of the cardiac output going to lung units with very low ventilation-perfusion ratios, the arterial PO_2 was reasonably well maintained at 70 torr. One would certainly expect a much lower arterial PO_2 in the presence of so much mismatching of ventilation and blood flow. However, we were able to calculate the arterial PO_2 which was expected from the measured distribution of ventilation-perfusion ratios and it was very close to 70 torr. This agreement is not surprising. It simply means that the retention of oxygen was consistent with that of the six inert gases which we used to determine the distribution.

The apparent paradox of relatively mild hypoxemia and the presence of such striking ventilation-perfusion inequality can be explained by the increased cardiac output caused by the beta-1 effects of the isoproterenol on the heart. This caused an increase in the PO_2 of the mixed venous blood with the result that the effects of ventilation-perfusion inequality on oxygen transfer were substantially mitigated. Everybody is aware of the importance of overall ventilation in determining the arterial PO_2, but the role of cardiac output is frequently overlooked. It should be emphasized that, in the presence of ventilation-perfusion inequality, total cardiac output is an important determinant of the arterial PO_2.

Myocardial Infarction

Figure 5 shows a distribution of ventilation-perfusion ratios in a patient who developed a myocardial infarct and in whom there were signs of mild pulmonary edema including crackles at the lung bases. It can be seen that the main body of the distribution was broadened, there was a 6% shunt (blood flow to unventilated units), and also apparently some blood flow to units with extremely low ventilation-perfusion ratios. It should be pointed out that in a distribution of this type, the exact proportion of blood flow going to unventilated versus poorly ventilated units cannot be determined because of limitations in the discriminatory power of the technique. However, we can be confident of

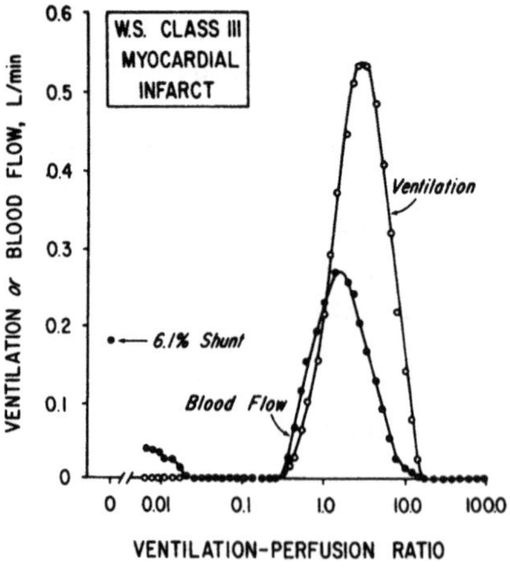

Fig. 5. Distribution of ventilation-perfusion ratios in a patient after a myocardial infarction. Class III refers to the American Heart Association classification, indicating that there were clinical signs of mild pulmonary edema. (From West 1977)

the total amount of blood flow going to very poorly ventilated and unventilated lung units.

An interesting feature of the distribution shown in Fig. 5 is that despite the relatively mild degree of ventilation-perfusion inequality, the arterial PO_2 was only 58 torr. This can be contrasted with the patient of Fig. 4 B where there was a much more abnormal distribution of ventilation-perfusion ratios, but the arterial PO_2 was decreased to only 70 torr. At first sight it is difficult to reconcile these two distributions with the arterial PO_2 values. The explanation again is in the cardiac output. The patient of Fig. 5 had a cardiac output of only 3 l/min as a result of the damaged myocardium. The PO_2 of mixed venous blood was measured via a Swan-Ganz catheter in the pulmonary artery, and this showed a PO_2 of only 29 torr, the normal value being about 40 torr. This is a substantial reduction of PO_2 on this steep part of the oxygen dissociation curve. As a result, this very low cardiac output, which depressed the PO_2 of mixed venous blood, resulted in a low arterial PO_2 in spite of the relatively mild degree of mismatching of ventilation and blood-flow. This is in obvious contrast to the situation in the asthmatic of Fig. 4 B, where a very large amount of ventilation-perfusion inequality only depressed the arterial PO_2 to 70 torr because the cardiac output was raised by the effects of the isoproterenol. Thus, a comparison of the distributions shown in Fig. 4 and 5 emphasized the important role of cardiac output in maintaining the arterial PO_2 in the presence of ventilation-perfusion inequality.

References

Cardell BS (1956) Pathological findings in death from asthma. Int Arch Allergy 9:189–199

Dunnill MS (1960) The pathology of asthma with special reference to changes in the bronchial mucosa. J Clin Pathol 13:27–33

Evans JW, Wagner PD (1977) Limits on V_A/Q distributions from analysis of experimental inert gas elimination. J Appl Physiol 42:889–898

Farhi L (1967) Elimination of inert gas by the lung. Respir Physiol 3:1–11

Fenn WO, Rahn H, Otis AB (1946) A theoretical study of the composition of alveolar air at altitude. Am J Physiol 146:637

Haldane JS (1922) Respiration. Yale University Press, New Haven

Kelman GR (1966) Digital computer subroutine for the conversion of oxygen tension into saturation. J Appl Physiol 21:1375–1376

Kelman GR (1967) Digital computer procedure for the conversion of PCO_2 into blood CO_2 content. Respir Physiol 3:335–343

Kety S (1951) The theory and applications of the exchange of inert gas at the lungs and tissues. Pharmacol Rev 3:1–41

Krogh A, Lindhard J (1917) The volume of the dead space in breathing and the mixing of gases in the lungs of man. J Physiol (Lond) 51:59

Riley R, Cournand A (1949) "Ideal" alveolar air and the analysis of ventilation-perfusion relationships in the lungs. J Appl Physiol 1:825–847

Roca J, Ramis LI, Rodriguez-Roisin R, Ballester E, Montserrat JM, Wagner PD (1988) Serial relationships between ventilation-perfusion inequality and spirometry in acute severe asthma requiring hospitalization. Am Rev Respir Dis 137:1055–1061

Wagner PD, Saltzman HA, West JB (1974 a) Measurement of continuous distributions of ventilation-perfusion ratios: theory. J Appl Physiol 36:588–599

Wagner PD, Laravuso RB, Uhl RR, West JB (1974b) Continuous distributions of ventilation-perfusion ratios in normal subjects breathing air and 100% O_2. J Clin Invest 54:54–68
Wagner PD, Dantzker DR, Dueck R, Clausen JL, West JB (1977) Ventilation-perfusion inequality in chronic obstructive pulmonary disease. J Clin Invest 59:203–216
Wagner PD, Dantzker DR, Iacovoni VE, Tomlin WC, West JB (1978) Ventilation-perfusion inequality in asymptomatic asthma. Am Rev Respir Dis 118:511–524
West JB (1969) Ventilation-perfusion inequality and overall gas exchange in computer models of the lung. Respir Physiol 7:88–110
West JB (1977) State of the art: ventilation-perfusion relationships. Am Rev Respir Dis 116:919–943

Oxygen Supply and Uses in Tissues

D. M. Denison

This paper introduces the following sequence of ideas, which are discussed in more detail below.

1. Molecular oxygen (O_2) is a mild, benign reducing agent which does little harm.
2. When it is activated it forms highly reactive oxygen radicals.
3. These are so destructive that almost all cells are equipped with protective enzymes which quench radicals as they form.
4. Those radicals that escape quenching cause random destructioin, i.e. "ageing."
5. More recently in evolution enzymes have developed which activate oxygen in close proximity to electrons or molecules that need to be consumed or modified.
6. The bulk use of oxygen in tissues is for the release of energy from foodstuffs, by oxidative phosphorylation in mitochondria.
7. This process has a Michaelis constant for oxygen that is as low as 1 mmHg and may be as low as 0.1 mmHg.
8. Therefore, it can be treated as if it were inexorable.
9. However, a significant fraction of the oxygen taken up by almost any cell is consumed by other enzymatic processes, in the making and breaking of a wide variety of critical neural transmitters, hormones, and structural proteins.
10. These processes have much higher Michaelis constants for oxygen and are therefore sensitive to local PO_2 variations that have no effect on oxidative phosphorylation.
11. These PO_2-sensitive processes are likely to explain many effects of hypoxia and oxygen toxicity in man.
12. Therefore, we would expect tissues to be provided with sufficient enzymes to quench oxygen radical formation at the highest PO_2 encountered naturally, sufficient mitochondrial oxidase to meet the highest normal demand for energy, sufficient other oxidases and oxygenases to meet the highest normal demands for manufacture and dismemberment, and sufficient blood flow to meet the bulk O_2-flow needs of the mitochondria, and the high-PO_2 needs of the other processes.
13. As the usable oxygen content and the time constant of equilibration of red cells are understood, a reasonable guess at the capillary density and blood flow can be made for any tissue whose mitochondrial and extra-mitochondrial oxygen requirements are known.

14. Significant volumes of tissue are oxygenated by direct diffusion through arterial and arteriolar walls.
15. The bulk of consumed oxygen diffuses through the arteriolar ends of capillaries, creating a small well-oxygenated cone in a territory otherwise held very close to local venous PO_2.
16. Some critical process with high KmO_2 may be preferentially located at the arteriolar ends of capillaries.
17. There are some advantages to perfusing damaged capillary beds with red-cell substitutes rather than blood.

In chemical reactions, partial or complete control of one or more electrons is transferred from one substance to another. The reactant losing control of the electron is "oxidized," and the material gaining control of the electron is reduced. A chemical's tendency to attract or repel electrons is measured by the voltage required to prevent a molar solution of the substance exchanging electrons with a molar solution of hydrogen. This scale, of oxidation-reduction or "redox" potentials ranges approximately from -3 to $+3$ volts, with hydrogen in the middle at 0 volts. On this scale molecular oxygen has a mild tendency to repel electrons, which is surprising.

Oxygen atoms have six electrons in their outer shell, and need two more two complete a stable octet. They attain stable states as diatomic oxygen molecules by sharing a pair of electrons with another oxygen atom. These molecules have the potential to accept four electrons from elsewhere. However, two of their own unpaired electrons are spinning the wrong way to make this coup likely. As a result molecular oxygen usually has to accept electrons singly. Since it has a mild tendency to repel them, only the more energetic electrons break through and thus molecular oxygen is not particularly reactive.

If an electron is successfully attached to an oxygen molecule the compound's chemical reactivity increases greatly. The superoxide ion (O_2^-) has an electron affinity at the oxidant extreme of the redox scale and rapidly draws in another electron, becoming a peroxide ion ($O_2^=$). In aqueous solutions this commonly exists as hydrogen peroxide (H_2O_2) that splits into highly reactive hydroxyl radicals (OH·), each of which immediately pulls an electron from the nearest available molecule to complete the reduction of the oxygen atoms.

In living cells, water is the most obvious source of electrons, but pulling an electron from a water molecule draws a proton with it, leaving another hydroxyl radical (OH·) as the residue. Thus, all four electrons involved in the complete reduction of diatomic oxygen must come ultimately from non-aqueous (i.e. solute) molecules that are oxidized in the process.

Life evolved in anaerobic environments where such events were very rare. That situation was transformed when the blue-green algae (the first organisms that photosynthesized) appeared. The oxygen liberated from CO_2, accumulated in the atmosphere and dissolved in cell sap, where it was activated by high-energy electrons generated randomly by cosmic rays, and by free radicals. The superoxide ions and their progeny created havoc by oxidizing solute molecules in their immediate vicinity. As a result, organisms evolved a series of protective enzymes, which had to be distributed ubiquitously. These enzymes (*superoxide dismutases, catalase,* and the other *peroxidases*), and the peroxysomes that contain some of them, appeared long before the evolution of mitochondria. Superoxide dismutases contain transition-metal prosthetic groups, much like the haem of haemoglobin, which attract superoxide ions and reduce them to hydrogen peroxide, in safe locations. Catalase and the other peroxidases, similarly ensure the safe conversion of hydrogen peroxide to water. Organs that have not evolved these enzymes are obligate anaerobes.

Although the protective enzymes may be placed strategically, at sites where free radicals are more likely to form, they cannot be ubiquitous at a molecular level, and some superoxide ions will form at unprotected sites, causing random oxidation with loss of cell information and control systems. This is thought to be one aspect of "ageing." Its likelihood is increased by raising local oxygen tensions, which also swamps the protective enzymes. That is the basis for hyperoxic enhancement of cytotoxic drugs and radiotherapy.

After the development of the quenching systems, other enzymes evolved that harnessed oxygen creatively. These enzymes fall into three groups: (a) the *oxidases* which use oxygen simply as an electron acceptor, ultimately turning it to water; (b) the *hydroxylases* (or *mixed function oxygenases*) which use one atom of the oxygen molecule as an electron acceptor, but take the other atom together with a proton, and insert them as a hydroxyl group (OH), directly into an organic molecule; and (c) the *oxygenases* which insert the entire oxygen molecule into an organic compound to make something new. Because of the ubiquity of the oxygen-using and quenching enzymes, non-enzymic reduction of oxygen in vivo is rare.

Something like 85%–90% of resting whole-body oxygen consumption is handled by a single enzyme, cytochrome c a3 oxidase, in mitochondria. It has a haem-like prosthetic group to attract oxygen, which it uses as the ultimate electron acceptor for many processes. It is also coupled to the phosphorylation of ADP to ATP which traps a good part of the energy released by electron transfer. This allows the Krebs cycle to proceed. For many years it was thought to be the only consumer of respired oxygen, perhaps because it employed much more than 90% of the oxygen consumption in easily studied exercising muscles.

Oxidative phosphorylation, like all the other enzyme-controlled operations on respired oxygen, roughly follows Michaelis-Menten kinetics. There is an approximately hyperbolic relation between the speed of the enzymatic action (VO_2) and the concentration of its substrate ($[O_2]$). As the reactions take place in simple aqueous solutions (mitochondrial fluid), there is an exact proportionality between $[O_2]$ and the more easily measured oxygen tension (PO_2). The hyperbolic curve relating VO_2 to PO_2 is generated by the appropriate Michaelis-Menten equation:

$$VO_2/VO_2\ \mathrm{max} = PO_2/\,(PO_2 + KmO_2)$$

and is described by the substrate concentration (PO_2) which the reaction proceeds at one-half its maximum velocity (VO_2 max). This concentration is called the Michaelis constant (for oxygen) or KmO_2 of the reaction.

The KmO_2 of oxidative phosphorylation is certainly as low as 1 mmHg and may be as low as 0.1 mmHg. That implies that, at all oxygen tensions above 3 mmHg, the major intracellular user of oxygen will proceed inexorably at full speed, other factors being equal. Thus, it will not be affected by variations in oxygen delivery unless intramitochondrial PO_2 falls below 3 mmHg. As the PO_2 gradients across mitochondrial walls are very small, the same statement applies to intracellular and interstitial PO_2. This suggests that any fall in VO_2 associated with a fall in oxygen delivery is more likely to be caused by some other effect of oxygen on electron transport or oxidative phosphorylation, rather than the immediate local fall of PO_2.

There are many other oxidases in mammalian cells, particularly in those organs (e.g. liver and kidney) concerned with elaborate biochemical transformations. They also have haem-like prosthetic groups and are often placed in the endoplasmic reticulum. They accept electrons from many processes, especially the breaking up of absorbed poisons and unwanted products of metabolism. As they are not coupled to any energy-trapping reactions, all of the energy released by electron transfer appears as heat. Most hydroxylases are used for similar purposes (i.e. detoxification) but some hydroxylases and the oxygenases are used in the manufacture and destruction of structural proteins, hormones, and neural transmitters. Almost all of the transmitters of the CNS are produced and deactivated by sequential insertions of respired oxygen. These particularly critical uses probably account for at most 2% of total oxygen consumption. However, the oxygenases, hydroxylases, and other oxidases, unlike cytochrome c a3, have Michaelis constants for oxygen that appear to range from about 5 to 250 mmHg. (Accurate information on these constants is still scanty.) This means they are much more sensitive to variations in oxygen delivery.

In addition, some cells, notably macrophages and leucocytes, can rapidly make and export short-lived and highly reactive partial-reduction products (oxygen radicals) from respired oxygen, in "respiratory bursts." These "Molotov cocktails" are made by enzyme complexes on the plasma membrane and oxidize their way through bacterial and other cell walls. Their manufacture raises the oxygen consumption of the white cell 10- to 20-fold, but their contribution to total oxygen consumption is slight except in fulminating infections. Their Michaelis constants are uncertain, but within the physiological range, and may limit host defences at hypoxic sites.

The information given so far helps to explain two of the most striking features of oxygen lack in man. The first of these is that the earliest effects of hypoxia (loss of night vision, impairment of sophisticated mental functions, and slight hyperventilation) appear when arterial PO_2 has fallen to 60–70 mmHg, arterial oxygen saturation has barely dropped at all, the mass despatch of oxygen from the aorta has hardly altered, and the mixed venous PO_2 has only fallen by 1–2 mmHg. In these circumstances, it is unlikely that oxidative phosphorylation has been affected at all. It is much more probable that these changes reflect reductions in processes with high KmO_2. Similarly, in brief profound hypoxia, when arterial PO_2 falls to 35–40 mmHg, consciousness is impaired and lost long before there is a detectable fall in whole-body oxygen uptake. This again suggests that oxidative phosphorylation is proceeding unabated, and loss of consciousness is due to the slowing of processes consuming low volumes of oxygen at high KmO_2. Conversely, the observation that healthy people at rest do not increase their CO_2 production measurably when they breathe pure oxygen implies their oxidative phosphorylation is not limited by oxygen delivery, but gives no clue about the state of the other oxygen-consuming processes which are not associated with the evolution of CO_2.

The facts given so far also allow some obvious predictions. We would expect tissues to be provided with sufficient enzymes to quench oxygen radical formation at the highest PO_2 encountered naturally. Since enzymes are expensive to make and maintain, there is no point in keeping them in excess quantities. Hyperoxia is not a natural hazard for terrestrial or aquatic animals. Conversely, accurate maps of the distribution of quenching enzymes might betray the normal PO_2 of tissues. They might also pin-point areas of excessive free-radical formation. We would expect a close correlation between mitochondrial density and maximum tissue oxidative phosphorylation. There ought also to be a close correlation between the concentrations and local reaction velocities of non-mitochondrial oxygen-consuming processes. However, as these are PO_2-sensitive there may be compensatory increases of enzyme density at areas of relatively low PO_2. This may be worth checking. Lastly, there ought to be sufficient blood flow to meet the bulk VO_2 demands of the mitochondria and the high PO_2 requirements of the high KmO_2 processes.

This brings us to the problems of oxygen transport and tissue capillarity. Red cells contain some 300 million haemoglobin molecules packed like marbles in a loose sack. Each molecule can carry four oxygen molecules (one for each monomer in the haemoglobin tetramer) of which, on average, three can be retrieved easily, and the fourth only at $PO_2 < 20$ mmHg. Making allowance for the haematocrit, each litre of arterial blood normally carries 200 ml of O_2 of which 150 ml are easily available. Working at an aerobic capacity of 3 l/min, a man requires a cardiac output of $3000/150 = 20$ l/min. Red cells have floppy cell walls and are loosely packed by design. They travel through capillaries narrower than themselves, rolling on their own membranes like tractors on their tracks. This mixes the haemoglobin molecules within, bringing fresh ones to the surface and accelerating gas exchange. In consequence, the equilibration time of the normal red cell in a normal capillary is about 1/3 s.

Parsimony demands that tissues do not have more capillaries than they need and do not waste red cells by allowing them to pass through the lungs unfilled, or through the tissues unemptied. Thus, in the lungs, for example, where the entire cardiac output during maximum exertion must be oxygenated at a single pass, the maximum blood flow of 20 l/min must be allowed a transit time of 1/3 s which requires a maximum pulmonary capillary blood volume of $20/180 = 111$ ml. On exercise the normal pulmonary capillary volume of an adult man (70 ml), as measured by other means, expands by 65% as pulmonary arterial pressure rises, so this figure (70·1.65–115 ml) accords well. Similarly, a capillary of 5 μm diameter has a cross-sectional area of roughly 20 m^2, so approximately 7 km of capillary are needed to contain the maximum volume of 115 ml. The surface area of this capillary would be close to 100 m^2 when fully deployed, which is in good agreement with independent estimates of alveolar membrane area. In the lung, of course, oxygen transfer bears no relation to local mitochondrial density.

In other tissues, Weibel and his collaborators, for example, have established clear-cut associations between maximum oxidative phosphorylation, mitochondrial density, and capillary density. *Variations* in these relationships need detailed study. Capillarity in excess of mitochondrial density implies some non-mitochondrial reason for increased blood flow, or an inefficiency in bulk oxygen delivery.

When Krogh and his mathematician colleague Erlanger first considered the problems of oxygen delivery to tissues, they were obliged by computational constraints to think of individual capillaries serving concentric cylinders of tissue. As blood passed along the capillary, they were forced to imagine oxygen leaving in equal quantities for each micron of capillary transit. This led to the concepts of the Krogh cyclinder and the so-called lethal corner, which was actually the rim of the Krogh cylinder, seen as the vulnerable zone likely to dictate blood flow to the cylinder.

Now, with improved computers and more information, different pictures of tissue oxygenation appear. First, various observations, notably those of Duling and Berne, indicate that considerable quantities of oxygen diffuse through pre-capillary vessel walls. This explains the lack of capillaries in the inner third of the aortic media, all of the media of smaller arteries and arterioles, and the immediate periarterial zones of many tissues. This is obvious in the retina, where the interior of the normal optic disc is white because it is served by diffusion from the central retinal artery, and so is avascular; and along the arteries that spread across the retina, which have pale capillary-free borders. Second, when blood finally arrives in a systemic capillary, the head of oxygen pressure is likely to drive the bulk of the oxygen out of the capillary and into the tissues very early indeed, where it is free to diffuse in all directions through the broad areas of cylinder, rather then wait in the narrow confines of the capillary. Third, directional patterns of blood flow in neighbouring capillaries may mean that the most vulnerable areas of tissue are not at the venous ends of individual capillaries. One consequence is that regions of high PO_2 will only exist very close to arteriolar walls and the arteriolar entrances to capillaries. These factors may not be important to the distribution and activity of very low KmO_2 mitochondria, but could be critical to the siting of high KmO_2 processes of hormone and transmitter production and deactivation. It may be worth looking for such evidence in careful detail.

Studies on blood flow through branching networks suggest that obstruction of one vessel diverts blood predominantly to neighbouring vessels where it may speed through too fast for oxygen equilibration. In general, it is likely that tissue oxygen levels are closely related to servant venous PO_2 but, as in the lung where alveolar-arterial O_2 gradients are generated by ventilation/perfusion inequality, so, in other organs, tissue-venous oxygen tension gradients are produced by metabolism/blood flow inequalities.

Various studies on blood flow suggest that red cells do not travel easily through all normal capillaries. Plasma skimmed from the blood stream passes down capillaries that red cells do not penetrate. Many factors, including hypoxia, make red cells stiffer, exaggerating such inequalities. Any destruction of a capillary bed forces blood to pass through the remaining bed more quickly. In addition, inflammatory responses in hypoxic blood and ischaemic tissues lead to reperfusion injury. Recent work suggests that infarct sizes in heart and brain can be reduced by perfusing the tissues with red cell substitutes rather than blood. They probably achieve this by four advantages: a much smaller particle size (0.1 cf 7 μm diameter), consequently briefer equilibration times, debateably better micro-rheological properties, and an absence of platelets and white cells that contribute to reperfusion injury. For many reasons, there is much renewed interest in red cell substitutes and grounds for believing more successful candidates will be produced in commercial quantities shortly. It may be that they will provide significant advances in our understanding and treatment of the distribution of oxygen to compromised tissues.

References

The supply and uses of oxygen in tissues is a vast topic. The following references may help entry into its literature:

Anderson HV, Nelson DL, Leimgruber PP, Roubin GS, Gruentzig AR (1986) Coronary artery perfusion during percutaneous transluminal coronary angioplasty. Prog Clin Biol Res 211:3–20

Autor A (ed) (1982) Pathology of oxygen. London, Academic Press

Denison DM (1981) The distribution and use of oxygen in tissues. In: Scadding JG, Cumming G, Thurlbeck WM (eds) Scientific foundations of respiratory medicine. Heinemann, London, pp 221–237

Denison DM (1981) High altitudes and hypoxia. In: Weiner JS, Edholm OG (eds) Principles and practice of human physiology. Academic Press, London, pp 241–307

Denison DM (1989) Artificial oxygen carriers. In: Kox W, Gamble J (eds) Fluid resuscitation. Ballière Tindall, London (in press)

Denison DM (1987) Time limits and the pulmonary capillary. Appl Cardiopulm Pathophysiol 1:93–99

Duling BR, Berne RM (1970) Longitudinal gradients in periarteriolar oxygen tension. A possible mechanism for the participation of oxygen in local regulation of blood flow. Circ Res 27:669–678

Duling BR, Klitzman B (1980) Local control of microvascular function: role in tissue oxygen supply. Ann Rev Physiol 42:373–382

Hakim TS, Macek AS (1988) Role of erythrocyte deformability in the acute pressor response in the pulmonary vasculature. Respir Physiol 72:95–108

Hakim TS, Malik AB (1988) Hypoxic vasoconstriction in blood- and plasma-perfused lungs. Respir Physiol 72:109–122

Halliwell B (1987) Oxidants and human disease: some new concepts. FASEB J 1:358–364

Halliwell B, Gutteridge JMC (1985) Free radicals in biology and medicine. Clarendon, Oxford

Stryer L (1988) Biochemistry. Freeman, New York, pp 397–426

Wayne RP (1985) Chemistry of the atmospheres. Clarendon, Oxford

Weibel ER (1984) The pathway for oxygen. Harvard University Press, London

Microcirculatory Control of Tissue Oxygenation

P. Gaehtgens

In contrast to other substrates of tissue metabolism, oxygen can be exchanged between the intra- and extravascular compartments without any significant restriction by the vascular walls. Due to lipid solubility and the diffusivity of oxygen in tissue fluids, diffusional barriers generally do not exist and oxygen exchange between the blood and the extravascular tissue is, therefore, largely a flow-limited phenomenon. As a consequence, tissue oxygenation depends strongly on the mechanisms which regulate the volume of the blood flow through the vessels of the microcirculation, determine the oxygen-carrying capacity of blood in the exchange vessels, and control the microvascular surface area available for exchange.

Recruitment

In the physiological adjustment matching oxygen supply to metabolic demand, the question of how regulation of blood flow and vascular exchange surface are interrelated has long been debated. In this discussion, the problem of recruitment has played a major role (Krogh 1919). According to the classical concept, in which oxygen exchange only took place in the true capillaries, the closing or opening of variable numbers of such exchange vessels would provide an efficient way to modulate the surface area available for oxygen exchange and thus the total amount of oxygen transported from the blood by a given gradient of partial pressure. A number of physiological experiments on isolated organs under well-controlled perfusion conditions have apparently confirmed the idea that the exchange surface area is not only variable but can be controlled independently of the hydraulic resistance to blood flow (Mellander and Johansson 1968).

Precapillary Sphincters

This has led to the postulation of two control mechanisms, which can be differentiated both in terms of the localization of the regulator within the vessel tree and the mode of physiological control. While blood flow is determined by the tone of the arteriolar resistance vessels, which display myogenic tone and are subject to both neurogenic and metabolic control, exchange surface area has been thought to be a function of the action of "precapillary sphincters" which are exposed to metabolic mechanisms (Folkow et al. 1971). This possibility of dual control has helped to explain the occurrence of situations in which changes of flow and exchange of principally flow-limited materials were dissociated, such as, e.g., under conditions of specific types of neurogenic stimulation or under pathophysiological conditions such as in, e.g., circulatory shock (Appelgren and Lewis 1972).

Direct microcirculatory observations in various living tissues have, during the past two decades, repeatedly shown that the concept of precapillary sphincters only applies to a few specific tissues, but cannot be regarded as a general morphological or functional entity. In particular, several investigations have clearly ruled out the existence or action of any sphincter-like structure in the skeletal muscle microcirculation (Eriksson and Lisander 1972), a tissue that had been in mind when the original concept of recruitment was developed and in which whole organ perfusion studies had revealed the occurrence of a dissociation between flow and exchange.

Capillary Contractility

Therefore, an even older concept was revitalized and the existence of independent capillary contractility was reinvestigated. Indeed, experiments mainly in cold-blooded animals showed that individual endothelial cells can be caused to contract by various stimuli, thereby causing transient arrest of blood flow because of protrusion of the cell nucleus into the capillary lumen (Weigelt 1982). On the other hand, physiological stimuli have so far not been shown to have such effects, and the phenomenon as such has not unequivocally been proven to occur in warm-blooded animal species. Although the details of this discussion have not been brought to a conclusive end, it appears that capillary contractility cannot be regarded as a general regulatory principle controlling the available surface area (Hammersen 1980). This is not to discount the possibility, however, that inspecific organs, particularly in cold-blooded animals, single capillary endothelial cells and/or pericytes may indeed show active changes of cell shape, thus affecting the effective size and configuration of the capillary lumen. Yet, definitive evidence in favor of this phenomenon to represent a consistent physiological mechanism determining capillary recruitment has not been presented so far.

With the possible exceptions mentioned, it is therefore justified to consider the arrangement of capillary vessels sensu strictiori as a largely passive system of tubes the perfusion of which is exclusively (at least over short periods of time) determined by the driving pressure available, the individual capillary geometry, and the rheological resistance offered by the flowing blood and its constituents. In this view, there is little or no room for active short-term adjustment of either capillary hydraulic resistance to flow or capillary surface area for exchange. How then can exchange of flow-limited materials such as oxygen vary independently of variations in blood flow rate? If capillary recruitment is uncertain and single capillary contractility does not occur to any relevant degree, other explanations for the occasional dissociation between flow and exchange are required.

The Network Concept

Recent microcirculatory research has increasingly focussed on the architectural organization of the terminal vascular bed and its relationship to both hemodynamic and exchange features. In the course of this approach the network concept of the microcirculation was developed by taking into account not only the substantial differences between the microvascular arrangement in different tissues, but also the mechanisms of communication between the vascular segments constituting such vessel networks. The concept also recognized the fact that neither blood flow nor transvascular exchange of materials occurs in a single identifiable section of the vascular system exclusively. The classical view, according to which the arterioles represent "the resistance vessels" and true capillaries represent "the exchange vessels," had been abandoned, since it became obvious that (a) practically all vessel sections contribute to a varying degree to the resistance to flow and, more importantly, to its regulation, and (b) exchange of oxygen across the vessel wall also occurs in precapillary arterioles (Duling and Berne 1970; Pittman et al. 1985), and exchange of other substances may even occur to a greater extent in the postcapillary venules. This also means that the correlation between the different microvessel categories, which had been proposed in a variety of classifying/ordering schemes, and specific physiological functions is, therefore, rather weak: even geometric or hemodynamic parameters (including diameter, length, flow velocity, and pressures) are found to exhibit a substantial dispersion within any identifiable subgroup of microvessels.

In those tissues where it has been performed, topological and morphometric analysis of the terminal vascular network showed a substantial asymmetry both of the arteriolar and venular subtrees in terms of number, length, and

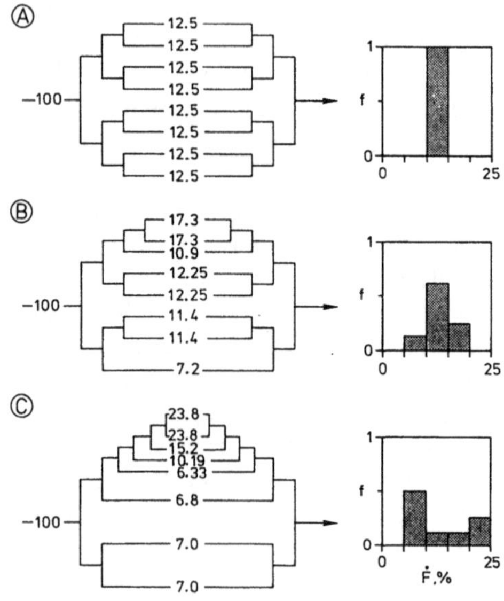

Fig. 1 A–C. Effect of increasing network asymmetry (from **A** to **C**) on the uniformity of red cell flux (Ḟ, in % of total influx) distribution. The calculations are based on the assumption of uniform volume flow in all eight capillaries of the networks, and on a uniformly applicable relationship between the distribution of volume flow and red cell flux at bifurcations. Flux heterogeneity is indicated in the histograms on the right (*f*, relative frequency). (From Gaehtgens 1989)

connectivity of the constituting vessel segments (Ley et al. 1986). As a consequence, perfusion of the complex network is characterized by a large degree of heterogeneity, the dispersion of arteriovenous path lengths being aggravated by that of vessel segment diameters, and thus vessel segment hindrance. Considerable dispersion of single pathway transit time can be predicted from these results, indicating that the complete network will act as an efficient mixer. This is obviated by evaluation of the distortion of a pulse of an intravascular indicator travelling from the feeding artery along the numerous pathways of the heterogeneous microvessel network.

In addition, the shape as well as the mean value of the transit time distribution is different for blood cells and plasma (Groom et al. 1957), indicating that different constituents of the blood travel along pathways exhibiting different velocities. Among other effects, this is caused by uneven distribution of red cells and plasma at each of the numerous consecutive branch points within a microvessel network, resulting in a rather heterogeneous dispersion of hematocrit between capillaries. Uneven red cell distribution at a bifurcation is caused by the difference in volume flow between the two daughter vessels; this difference is in turn a function of downstream resistance and thus of the number of dependent vessel segments. Therefore, the architectural asymmetry of a network has a large influence on the heterogeneity of red cell flux distribution in the network, as indicated schematically in Fig. 1.

Red cell concentration in each vascular segment, however, is a determinant of flow resistance (through the apparent viscosity) and of oxygen transport capacity (through the amount of oxygen bound to hemoglobin). In agreement with these considerations, measurements in single capillaries show substantial heterogeneity of all relevant oxygen transport parameters, notably capillary geometry, red cell flux, and entrance and exit oxygen saturation (Pittman and Okusa 1983). Furthermore, theoretical analysis shows that the importance of capillary hematocrit for oxygen delivery is not only related to the total oxygen-carrying capacity, but also to the spacing between the red cells following each other (Federspiel and Sarelius 1984). If a critical cell spacing is exceeded, oxygen flux at the capillary wall cannot be maintained constant and uniform. Therefore, substantial differences in single capillary O_2-supply efficiency may result from the observed effect of flow fractionation at bifurcations on capillary hematocrit.

Exchange Efficiency and Network Heterogeneity

It is evident from this discussion that the overall performance of a given network in terms of its ability to deliver oxygen to tissues is strongly influenced by its design as well as by the dispersion of hemodynamic parameters resulting from this design. Since substantial differences in design exist between tissues and these may be adapted to functional aspects through hitherto poorly understood growth processes, the relationship between flow distribution and the resulting tissue oxygenation must be considered separately for different organs. In the general case, however, the efficiency of a network to deliver materials,

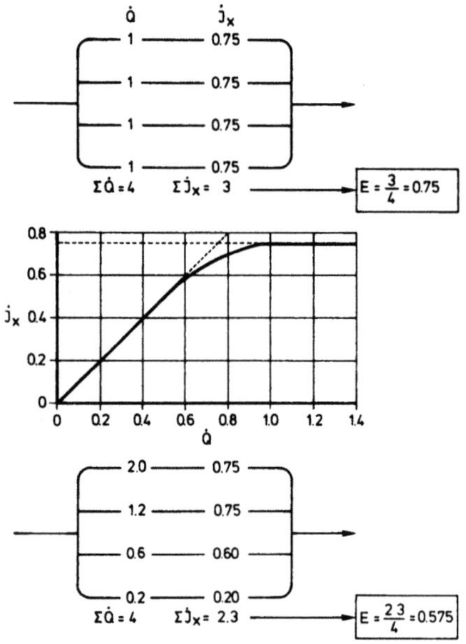

Fig. 2. Schematic illustration of the effect of network perfusion heterogeneity on the overall extraction (E) of a flow-limited substrate. The *middle panel* shows the theoretical relationship between flow ($\dot{Q}$) and the amount of substrate exchanged ($\dot{J}_x$). The *upper network* of four exchange vessels exhibits uniform flow distribution, the *lower network* shows substantial flow heterogeneity at the same total flow ($\Sigma\dot{Q}$)

whose intra/extravascular exchange mechanism is basically flow-limited, will strongly decrease with increasing degree of network heterogeneity, as schematically illustrated in Fig. 2. Since augmentation of delivery via individual vascular pathways cannot without limitation compensate for reduced delivery in alternative pathways, the extent of distributional heterogeneity represents an important determinant of overall supply efficiency of the vascular network.

Control of Heterogeneity?

On the other hand, alteration of the degree of heterogeneity represents a possible mechanism, whereby the relationship between blood flow and tissue oxygenation might be modified. The important but so far unresolved question is whether heterogeneity is purely an invariable consequence of network architecture, or whether it is subject to the control mechanisms which are turned on or off by tissue metabolism, neurogenic stimulation, or humoral/hormonal influences. If the latter possibility is true, microcirculatory control of tissue oxygenation may not only act through variation of total supply relative to total demand, but also through variation of supply dispersion.

The current state of knowledge provides no conclusive answer to this problem. In fact, existing evidence is not only limited, but also contradictory, and a considerable part of the problem arises from the necessity to define an appropriate quantitative parameter describing the extent of perfusional heterogeneity. If heterogeneity is expressed in terms of the coefficient of variation, some reports show remarkable constancy in the face of substantial variation of total flow (e.g., due to metabolic or pharmacological stimulation or due to alteration of ambient oxygen partial pressure). This is true both for measurements within the microvascular network (Damon and Duling 1985) and for measurements of local and regional blood flow (Piiper et al. 1985). Such data suggest that fractional flow dispersion, at the level of capillaries and precapillary arterioles, is independent of oxygen demand and not modified by the mechanisms controlling overall perfusion. On the other hand, other studies demonstrate indeed a decreased heterogeneity of flow dispersion among capillaries with increasing overall blood flow due to metabolic activation (Tyml 1989). If the latter observations can be confirmed to show a general mechanism of physiological relevance, then the control of oxygen supply to tissue must involve a rather complex and intricate pattern of local and regional communication between the single vascular elements of the microcirculatory network.

Intranetwork Communication

It is of great interest, therefore, that such mechanisms have indeed been identified by different approaches in different tissues and in experimental situations representing different stimuli (Fig. 3). On the one hand, it is known that local stimulation, e.g., by application of vasoactive substances, may lead to propagated responses of microvessels which may extend over considerable distances (several mm), thus involving several vessel segments (Duling and Berne 1970; Segal and Duling 1987). While the mechanism of signal transmission in such cases is not yet completely understood, its speed of propagation is sufficiently rapid to support conduction rather than diffusion of a chemical signal. The occurrence of such a phenomenon will, of course, prevent an increase of perfusional heterogeneity, which otherwise might result from a locally induced

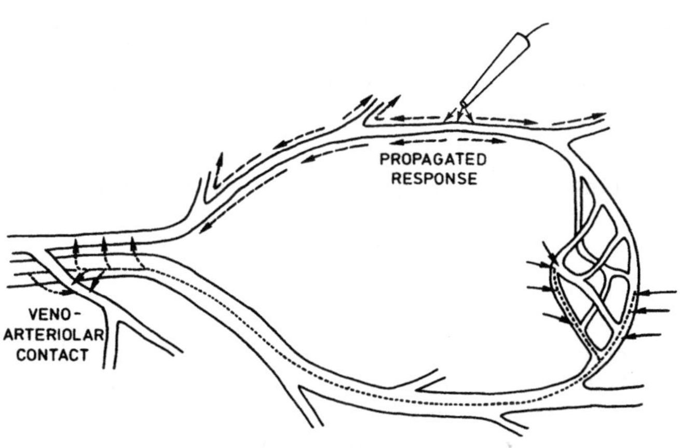

Fig. 3. Schematic drawing of a microvascular unit consisting of feeding arteriolar vessels, capillary network, and draining venules. Intraunit communication is indicated as due to propagated vasomotor response to a localized stimulus (micropipette), or due to diffusion of vasoactive material to the feed arteriole at venuloarteriolar contact site

vasocative stimulus reaching only a rather circumscript portion of the network. The smallest conceivable vascular unit within any network, consisting of a terminal arteriole and all dependent passive capillaries, must thereby be functionally coupled not only with neighboring units, but also with up- and even downstream control elements. As an example, a mechanism of propagation will also ensure the participation of vessel segments located beyond the direct reach of a vasoactive mediator generated in metabolically activated tissue. Such a mechanism would serve to homogenize a vasomotor response within a given network and thus help to limit the preexisting heterogeneity.

An additional mechanism of intranetwork communication limiting network heterogeneity results from the connectivity of the arterial and venous subtrees. Experiments have shown that not only oxygen, but also vasoactive substances can be exchanged by diffusion between microvessels crossing each other or running parallel at a small distance (Tigno et al. 1989). This provides the possibility of eliciting a vasoactive response of the feeding arteriole of a given unit of capillaries through a chemical signal generated in the tissue surrounding these capillaries. This type of "retrograde control" (Gaehtgens et al. 1989) would also serve to homogenize the response of a network to local stimuli, since in most tissues venous and arterial subtrees show considerable overlap; the capillaries supplied by a given arteriole are drained by several venules.

The combination of retrograde and conducted responses will almost certainly provide an efficient communication mechanism determining perfusional heterogeneity in the presence of changes in local microvascular conductivity. It could be added that even larger arteries feeding into the microcirculatory network may become involved by the phenomenon of ascending vasodilation which represents a response to endothelial stimulation by the increased blood flow through the vessel (Bassenge and Pohl 1986). Many of the communication phenomena described appear to involve the vascular endothelium which also participates in the adjustment of basal smooth muscle tone in the arteriolar microvessels (Pohl et al. 1987; Förstermann et al. 1987; Klotz et al. 1988). These abundant mechanisms of communication within and beyond the level of the microvascular network will clearly contribute to the control of perfusional heterogeneity during adjustments of blood supply to demand and will thus ensure the presence of controlled exchange efficiency for oxygen under physiological conditions.

Conclusion

The current state of understanding of tissue oxygenation via the microcirculation is far from complete. Many of the classical concepts explaining local, regional, and global regulation mechanisms have not survived the test of direct in vivo measurements without substantial modification, since quantitative discrepancies remain between data collected from whole organs and those obtained at the level of single capillaries. Supply heterogeneity of the microvascular network is now regarded as a significant feature of tissue oxygenation, the heterogeneity resulting from the dispersion of geometric, hemodynamic, and rheological properties of the microcirculation. It appears, furthermore, that oxygen can be exchanged through the walls of virtually all microvessels, and that network structure is therefore of substantial relevance. In addition, nonhomogeneity results from the uneven distribution of red cell fluxes, which by causing nonuniform red cell spacing may have an effect on oxygenation beyond that due to carrying capacity.

Since tissue oxygenation is extremely sensitive to network heterogeneity, its control through the complex regulatory mechanisms of blood flow would appear to be functionally important. It is indeed possible that the pronounced interaction between vasomotor control phenomena in the various categories of precapillary "resistance" vessels in the end allows for a coordinated response which also assures an effective control or at least limitation of the existing heterogeneity. If this were to prove true, signal transfer mechanisms between vessel sections within the microvascular network would represent the most important aspect of microcirculatory regulation of blood flow and tissue oxygenation.

References

Appelgren KL, Lewis DH (1972) Capillary flow and capillary transport in dog skeletal muscle in an experimental shock model. Europ Surg Res 4:46–54

Bassenge E, Pohl U (1986) Two principles of large artery dilation: indirect endothelium-mediated and direct smooth muscle relaxation. In: Magro A et al. (eds) Central and peripheral mechanisms of cardiovascular regulation. Plenum, New York, pp 163–196

Damon DH, Duling BR (1985) Evidence that capillary perfusion heterogeneity is not controlled in striated muscle. Am J Physiol 249:H386–H392

Duling BR, Berne RM (1970a) Longitudinal gradients in periarteriolar oxygen tension. Circ Res 27:669–678

Duling BR, Berne RM (1970b) Propagated vasodilation in the microcirculation of the hamster cheek pouch. Circ Res 26:163–170

Eriksson E, Lisander B (1972) Changes in precapillary resistance in skeletal muscle vessels studied by intravital microscopy. Acta Physiol Scand 84:295–305

Federspiel WJ, Sarelius IH (1984) An examination of the contribution of red cell spacing to the uniformity of oxygen flux at the capillary wall. Microvasc Res 27:273–285

Förstermann U, Dudel C, Frölich JC (1987) Endothelium-derived relaxing factor is likely to modulate the tone of resistance arteries in rabbit hindlimb in vivo. J Pharm Exp Therap 243:1055–1061

Folkow B, Sonnenschein RR, Wright DL (1971) Loci of neurogenic and metabolic effects on precapillary vessels of skeletal muscle. Acta Physiol Scand 81:459–471

Gaehtgens P (1989) Allgemeine Pathophysiologie der Mikrozirkulation. In: Rieger H, Schoop W (Hrsg) Handbuch der Inneren Medizin, vol 9. Springer, Berlin Heidelberg New York (in press)

Gaehtgens P, Tigno X, Thies K, Ley K (1989) Is there a retrograde control of arteriolar tone originating from capillaries? In: Grote J, Witzleb E (eds) Funktionsanalyse biologischer Systeme. F. Steiner, Stuttgart (in press)

Groom AC, Morris WB, Rowlands S (1957) The difference in circulation times of plasma and corpuscle in the cat. J Physiol 136:218–225

Hammersen F (1980) Endothelial contractility – does it exist? Adv Microcirc 9:95–134

Klotz KF, Pries AR, Schmucker P, Gaehtgens P (1988) The role of the endothelium in regulation of the local perfusion in skeletal muscle of the rat. Int J Micr Clin Exp Special Issue: S145 (Abstract)
Krogh A (1919) The supply of oxygen to the tissues and the regulation of the capillary circulation. J Physiol 52:457–474
Ley K, Pries AR, Gaehtgens P (1986) Topological structure of rat mesenteric microvessel networks. Microvasc Res 32:315–332
Mellander S, Johansson B (1968) Control of resistance, exchange, and capacitance functions in the peripheral circulation. Pharmacol Rev 20:117–196
Piiper J, Pendergast DR, Marconi C, Meyer M, Heisler N, Cerretelli P (1985) Blood flow distribution in dog gastrocnemius muscle at rest and during stimulation. J Appl Physiol 58:2068–2074
Pittman RN, Okusa MD (1983) Measurements of oxygen transport in single capillaries. In: Bicher HI, Bruley DF (eds) Oxygen transport to tissues, vol 4. Plenum, New York, pp 539–552
Pittman RN, Ellsworth ML, Swain DP (1985) Measurements of oxygen transport in skeletal muscle microcirculation. Proc Conf IEEE Eng Med Biol Soc: 536–540
Segal SS, Duling BR (1987) Propagation of vasodilation in resistance vessels of the hamster: development and review of a working hypothesis. Circ Res 61:II 20–25
Tigno XT, Ley K, Pries AR, Gaehtgens P (1989) Venulo-arteriolar communication and propagated response: a possible mechanism for local control of blood flow. Pflügers Arch Ges Physiol 414:450–456
Tyml K (1989) Redistribution of RBC flow in skeletal muscle in response to altered metabolism. Int J Micr Clin Exp 8 (Suppl I): 20-O (Abstract)
Weigelt H (1982) Die spezialisierte Endothelzelle – erregbare Zelle und mechanischer Effektor der Mikrozirkulation. Funkt Biol Med 1:53–60

Circulatory Compensation as a Response to Hypoxia *

D. L. Bredle

Introduction

The topic of circulatory responses to hypoxia can be very broad, depending on one's definition of terms, and quite complex regardless of how narrowly one tries to define terms. Not only are there are several categories of hypoxia, but the degree of severity can vary as well as the question of whether it is an acute or chronic situation. There are differences between species in their response to hypoxia which can become important when one tries to apply the results from animal research (where by necessity much of the experimental work has been done) to humans. Within the same species there can be differences in response between vascular regions and then differences between the arterial and venous sides of the same organ. There is the potential for a diseased or anesthetized patient to have a different response than a healthy, conscious subject. There are neural reflex and humoral responses, and there are local (often competing) vascular responses. The circulatory compensation to hypoxia, then, is not a simple, single response but the integration of all these variables. The use of laboratory animal models offers the chance to open the control loops involved and to analyze their components one piece at a time. In this brief review, I will focus primarily on what laboratory findings tell us about the circulatory responses to hypoxia. I hope to present a physiological framework for many of the presentations to follow which will delve more deeply into the recognition of and treatment for inadequate tissue oxygenation. I will first briefly mention the classifications of hypoxia, then discuss the local vascular effects of hypoxia, the chemoreceptor reflex effects, and finally the integrated response to hypoxia. For more detail on the circulatory adjustments to hypoxia there are excellent reviews by Heistad and Abboud (1980), Eyzaguirre et al. (1983), and Rowell and Blackmon (1987).

Classifications of Hypoxia

Hypoxia, which is defined as lower than normal amounts of oxygen in the lungs, blood, or tissue, can derive from a variety of causes. The four "classic" categories of hypoxia are (a) hypoxic hypoxia, in which arterial blood is poorly oxygenated due to low FiO_2 or pulmonary disease; (b) anemic hypoxia, in

* This work was supported by Grant #1F32 HL07790-01 from the National Heart, Lund, and Blood Institute of NIH, USA

which the blood cannot transport adequate oxygen due to hemoglobin abnormalities; (c) circulatory hypoxia, in which there is inadequate cardiac output or regional flow; and (d) histotoxic hypoxia, in which the tissues are incapable of using an otherwise adequate supply of O_2. It should be kept in mind that there can be mild hypoxemia (lower than normal arterial PO_2) without any real danger of tissue hypoxia, such as during travel to moderate altitude. On the other hand, there can be areas of tissue hypoxia without the usual clinical sign of hypoxemia. For this reason other variables, such as changes in cardiac output, O_2 extraction, or venous O_2 saturation, are being increasingly advocated for monitoring patient status. Most of the experimental studies which I will cite have produced a hypoxic state by lowering the FiO_2 and thereby lowering the arterial PO_2.

Local Vascular Effects of Hypoxemia

The uniquely local response of the vasculature to hypoxemia, though difficult to isolate from the net response of the body, has been studied in animal experiments in which an organ is perfused with hypoxic blood, while the rest of the body is maintained normoxic. As shown in Fig. 1, the typical response of arterioles to such perfusion is vasodilation (Daugherty et al. 1967; Heistad et al. 1975). The arterial PO_2 must drop severely (typically <40 torr) before any significant dilation occurs, and in this response all vascular beds are not created equal. Coronary and cerebral vessels dilate most strongly, those in skeletal muscle somewhat less, and renal vessels not at all, even when PO_2 is reduced to 20 torr. Cerebral blood flow in dogs increased when arterial PO_2 dropped below 50 torr and arterial PCO_2 was kept constant (Kogure et al. 1970). Similar vasodilation of cerebral arteries has been shown in humans, although it is more difficult to be sure of a purely local effect. Furthermore, if ventilation is stimulated by hypoxia it confuses the issue by changing an even stronger regulator, CO_2 (Shapiro et al. 1970). As can be seen in Fig. 2, a reduction of arterial PO_2 to below 50 torr caused an increase in cerebral flow as long as PCO_2 was kept constant. When hyperventilation reduced PCO_2, the vasoconstrictive effects of hypocapnia counterbalanced the vasodilator effects of hypoxia and cerebral flow returned to the level measured at normoxic conditions.

Coronary vessels likewise dilate under hypoxic conditions (Berne and Rubio 1979). Unlike the brain, however, the heart is always extracting a high percentage of the delivered O_2, so it must rely on increased flow to meet increased metabolic demands. The sensitivity of the arterioles of the heart and brain to hypoxia helps provide a continuously adequate O_2 supply to these vital organs which cannot incur a significant O_2 debt. The local effect of oxygen on the vasculature appears to follow a wide spectrum, so that when arterial PO_2 is raised above normal, there is arteriolar vasoconstriction. Therefore, the possibility exists for a paradoxical type of circulatory hypoxia, "hyperoxic hypoxia," if reduced flow or maldistribution of the flow overwhelms the increased O_2 driving pressure (Bourdeau-Martini et al. 1974; Bredle et al. 1988 a).

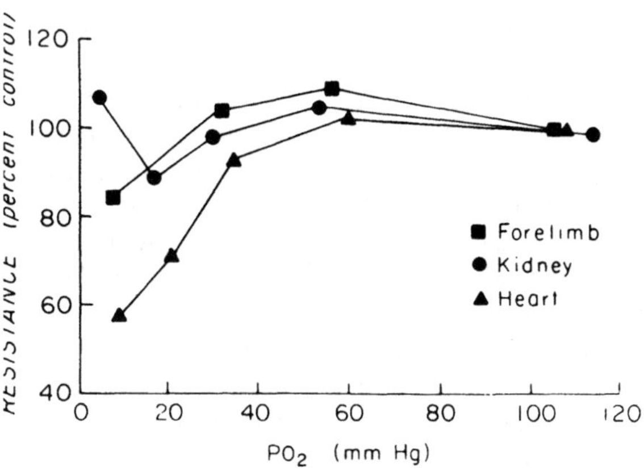

Fig. 1. Local vascular response in three organs to perfusion with blood of varying PO_2 while rest of the body was normoxic. [From Daugherty et al. (1967) with permission]

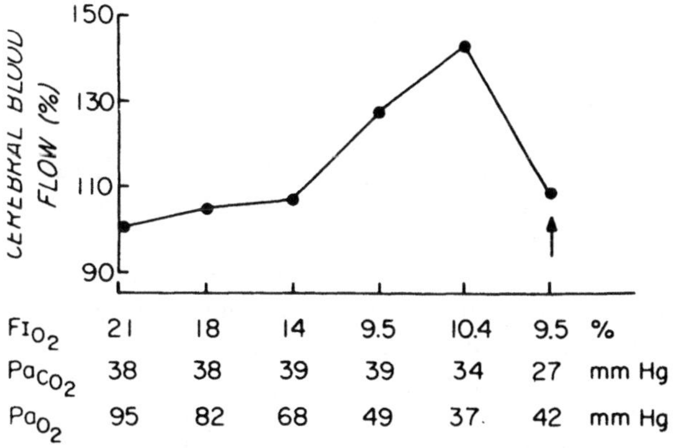

Fig. 2. Increases in cerebral blood flow in humans as FiO_2 is reduced and $PaCO_2$ kept constant by adding CO_2 to inspired air (first 4 points). No CO_2 was added for last two points. Hyperventilation and hypocapnia reduced cerebral flow (the last point). [From Shapiro et al. (1970) with permission]

Canine skeletal muscle regions dilated when perfused with hypoxic blood (Daugherty et al. 1967; Bachofen et al. 1971). Similarly in human forearm (mostly muscle), vasodilation occurred when the arterial PO_2 dropped below 30 torr (Richardson et al. 1967). This was considered to be a strictly local effect because it was unaffected by alpha- or beta-adrenergic blockade or local sympathetic neural blockade (Black and Roddie 1958). Heistad et al. (1975) have shown that the metabolic requirement of muscle is important in determining its local response to hypoxia. Resting canine gracilis muscle vasoconstricted in response to angiotensin when it was hypoxic, but the myocardium did not. When the gracilis was contracting and its arterial PO_2 was reduced, the vasoconstrictor effect of norepinephrine was abolished. Such selective inhibition of the local effects of vasoconstrictor agents in hypoxia would appear to favor redistribution of the cardiac output to organs that are active and dependent upon oxygen for their metabolism.

The vasodilation associated with low PO_2 is generally believed to be mediated by the local production of metabolites rather than a direct effect of oxygen on vascular smooth muscle (Berne et al. 1981). No specific oxygen receptor has been identified in vascular smooth muscle. O_2 levels may alter sarcolemmal membrane permeability to sodium and potassium ions (Bohr 1978; Detar 1980). Alternatively, hypoxia may cause the release of vasoactive substances such as adenosine, prostaglandins, or ATP (Forrester 1981). The local vascular effect of hypoxia, in summary, is differential in that it tends to dilate the vessels in vital and active organs. One can teleologically argue that there is an attempt to maintain O_2 delivery to these regions in a time of dwindling supply. Such dilation, however, would tend to reduce arterial pressure unless offset by reflexes which will be discussed below.

The pulmonary circulation, contrary to the systemic circulation, responds to decreased PO_2 with vasoconstriction. This response depends more on the alveolar PO_2 than on the PO_2 within the pulmonary vessels (Marshall and Marshall 1983). One result of the vasoconstriction is to redistribute blood within the lungs to regions where better ventilation/perfusion matching will accomplish better oxygenation. Such vasoconstriction would of course be of little benefit in situations where all lung regions are equally hypoxic.

Reflex Effects of Hypoxemia

The afferent limb of the hypoxic neural reflex begins with the peripheral chemoreceptors, sensory bodies that monitor changes in the chemical composition of their immediate environment (Eyzaguirre et al. 1983). The primary peripheral chemoreceptors are located in highly perfused regions of the carotid artery bifurcations near the carotid sinus baroreceptors. Of somewhat lesser importance are a second group of chemoreceptors located on the aortic arch. Low arterial PO_2 stimulates the firing rate of the chemoreceptors, particularly when PCO_2 is increased and pH reduced. Therefore, chemoreceptor stimulation is greater during hypoxemia due to hypoventilation than it is during hypoxemia combined with hyperventilation when CO_2 is being eliminated and PCO_2 reduced (Rowell 1986).

The results of chemoreceptor stimulation are: (a) constriction in skeletal muscle, mesenteric, and renal vessels (but vasodilation in heart and skin) from increased sympathetic drive (Heistad et al. 1975; Hackett et al. 1972); (b) bradycardia from increased vagal activity (Daly and Scott 1962); (c) positive inotropic response in the myocardium (Vatner and Rutherford 1978); and (d) increased respiratory drive. Most of the information on the reflex effects of hypoxia, as for the local effects, has come from animal studies in which the feedback control loop is opened, either by independently perfusing or stimulating the chemoreceptors or by normoxic perfusion of an isolated region during hypoxic ventilation.

Recent work of the latter sort from our laboratory has shown canine hindlimb resistance to almost double when PaO_2 was ~ 25 torr but the muscle was perfused with normoxic blood (Fig. 3; Bredle et al. 1988 b). This increase in resistance was well sustained throughout 40 min hypoxia; there was little evidence for local autoregulatory escape from the reflex vasoconstriction as long as the leg remained normoxic. In addition, vasoconstriction was even stronger

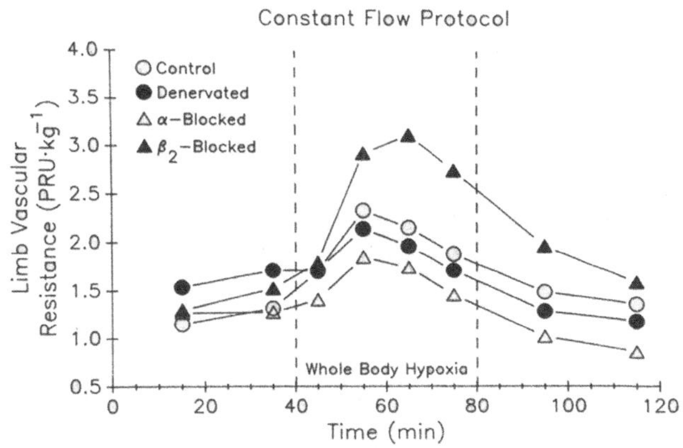

ʼig. 3. Canine hindlimb vascular resistance for normoxic muscle in whole-body hypɔxia. *Significant difference ($P<0.05$) from preceding value in same group; ▼$P<0.05$ between groups. [From Bredle et al. (1988b) with permission]

ollowing beta$_2$-adrenergic blockade, indicating the existence of some beta$_2$-nediated vasodilation during the hypoxic vasoconstriction. Perhaps even nore interesting, the hypoxic vasoconstriction persisted even in the presence ɪf alpha-adrenergic blockade (Bredle et al. 1988c) or denervation (Bredle et l. 1989), which suggests the role of nonsympathetic humoral constrictor gents such as vasopressin or angiotensin. Of interest, too, in these experinents was our finding that O_2 demand was increased in resting skeletal muscle n hypoxia as evidenced by an increase in oxygen uptake IN the normoxic limb vhen both alpha- and beta$_2$-adrenergic receptors were intact. This would inlicate that muscle does not subserve more "vital" organs as far as reducing O_2 lemand during limited supply.

In contracting canine gracilis muscle, local vasodilator mechanisms were ble to overcome the neural reflex vasoconstriction of moderate hypoxia but ıot that of brief severe hypoxia (Costin and Skinner 1971). Evidently, even the ıigh state of metabolic activity in the contracting muscle was not enough to ɪvercome the reflex vasoconstriction when the viability of the organism was hreatened.

The teleological supposition for the reflex bradycardia during hypoxia is ɔ spare the heart by reducing oxygen demand. Whether or not this actually ccurs is questionable, but at least one can assume that a given cardiac output ; more efficiently achieved by a lower rate and higher stroke volume. The seɛctive vasoconstriction would help redistribute blood to organs of high metbolic requirement, though vasodilation of the skin does not quite fit the sceario of preFerential distribution to vital organs. The increased peripheral reistance and positive inotropic effect work towards maintaining arterial presure in the face of the hypotensive local effects mentioned above. The pressor ɛsponse of the chemoreceptors in man has been clearly demonstrated by comaring the hypoxic response in normal subjects with a group of patients who

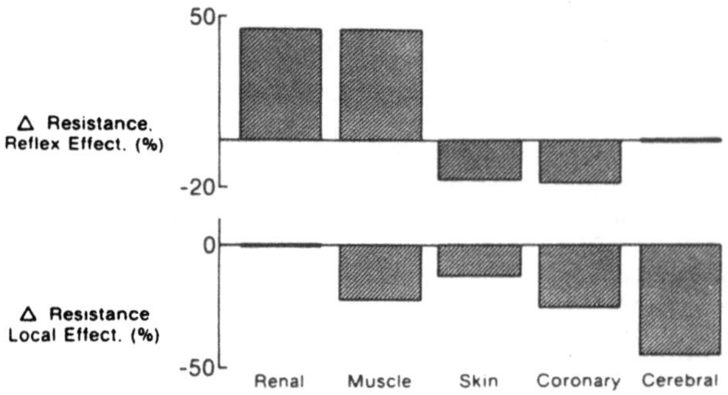

ig. 4. Vascular response to hypoxemia for chemoreceptor reflex *(top)* and local dilator effect *(bottom)*. Reflex effects are responses to maximal chemoreceptor stimulation in anesthetized, ventilated, normotensive dogs. Local effects are from perfusion with arterial PO_2 of 30 torr. [From Heistad and Abboud (1980) with permission]

had undergone carotid body resection (Lugliani et al. 1973). The normals maintained arterial pressure when breathing 10% O_2, whereas in the absence of functioning chemoreceptors arterial pressure decreased significantly.

The increase in respiratory drive from chemoreceptor stimulation, interestingly, leads to attenuation or even reversal of some of these reflex responses. If an animal is allowed to breathe spontaneously during hypoxia, hyperventilation lowers PCO_2 and reduces the carotid body afferent activity, as mentioned above. Furthermore, pulmonary stretch receptors are stimulated which reduces the sympathetic vasomotor outflow and the cardiac vagal activity. The selective vasoconstriction is reduced (Rutherford and Vatner 1978) and the bradycardia can become tachycardia (Daly and Scott 1962).

The predominant effect of hypoxemia by way of the neural reflex from chemoreceptors is selective vasoconstriction of certain regions, primarily skeletal muscle and abdominal visceral areas. Additionally, cardiac output tends to increase, particularly when ventilation increases. These effects combine to oppose the drop in pressure that would be caused by local hypoxic vasodilation. Taken together, the neural reflex and the local effect ostensibly tend to redistribute blood toward the vital organs. A composite histogram of the separate local and reflex effects in several regions is shown in Fig. 4 (Heistad and Abboud 1980). The local cerebral vasodilation is unopposed by any reflex chemoreceptor response. The coronary and skin vessels dilate from both the local and reflex effects. Renal vessels constrict due to the chemoreceptor reflex, and constriction in resting skeletal muscle due to the reflex effect is relatively stronger than dilation due to the local effects.

Integrated Responses to Hypoxia

It is of course the net effect of the simultaneous local and reflex responses to hypoxia that is of most interest to the clinician in dealing with patients. When the various responses to hypoxia are integrated, the most consistent effect is increased cardiac output which helps to maintain O_2 delivery throughout the body, followed by some degree of redistribution of blood flow to active tissue. A marked increase in cardiac output that is not dependent on hyperventilation has been shown in man (Richardson et al. 1967) and several anesthetized or conscious animal models (see Eyzaguirre et al. 1983). Both heart rate and stroke volume are increased, and these responses can occur even after carotid body resection (Sylvester et al. 1979). This type of result has prompted the hypothesis that there is a central pressor effect of hypoxia, that is, perfusion of the brain with hypoxic blood, particularly at lower than normal perfusion pressures, causes an increase in systemic arterial pressure independent of peripheral chemoreceptor activity (Heistad and Abboud 1980). While the balance of reflex and local effects of hypoxia typically keeps systemic arterial pressure from being significantly altered, pulmonary arterial pressure is usually increased (Grover et al. 1983).

Increased sympathetic nervous and hormonal activity from hypoxemia have been convincingly demonstrated in laboratory studies (Korner et al. 1967; Rose et al. 1983; Sylvester et al. 1979). In spontaneously breathing rabbits, increased splanchnic nerve activity (Iriki and Simon 1973) and decreased portal and renal blood flow (Chalmers et al. 1967) have been shown. In unanesthetized sheep, hypocapnic hypoxia increased arterial catecholamines by 2.5 times (and cardiac output by 26%), while hypercapnic hypoxia caused a 37-fold increase in catecholamines (and a 61% increase in cardiac output; Davidson et al. 1986). In the latter study, absolute blood flow was increased to the brain, heart, diaphragm, and nonrespiratory skeletal muscle, but not to the spleen, kidneys, and gastrointestinal tract.

In anesthetized, ventilated dogs, cardiac output increased 15% with mild hypoxia ($PaO_2 \sim 40$ torr) and it increased 65% during severe hypoxia ($PaO_2 \sim 24$ torr; Adachi et al. 1976). With mild hypoxia absolute flow was increased to the heart, liver, and diaphragm (Fig. 5). When calculated as fractional distribution of cardiac output, only the liver and diaphragm increased while skin and ileum decreased (Fig. 6). During the more severe hypoxia, absolute flow increased to all regions except skeletal muscle and skin, and the fraction of cardiac output increased to heart, liver, and brain. Other investigators, however, have shown that skeletal muscle will vasodilate and increase blood flow if the hypoxia is prolonged (Cain and Chapler 1979). Even at that point, the presence of some constrictor tone remaining in the muscle was illustrated by hyperemia upon reoxygenation. The importance of alpha-adrenergic receptors was shown by the lack of reflex vasoconstriction in muscle following alpha-adrenergic blockade (Cain and Chapler 1980). Furthermore, most of the alpha-blocked dogs could not tolerate 40 min of severe hypoxia ($PaO_2 \sim 26$ torr) due to marked hypotension. The lack of changes in various regional blood flows during moderate hypoxia is consistent with the metabolic theory of microvascular regulation which holds that adequate tissue oxygenation is achieved with changes at the exchange vessel level before changes at the resistance level occur (Granger et al. 1976). Thus, of the regional circula-

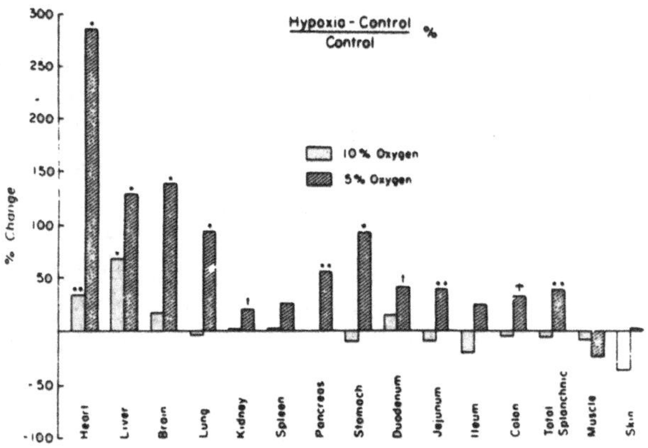

Fig. 5. Percentage change during hypoxia of absolute blood flow to organs and tissues (per 100 g) compared with control (normoxic) distribution. $*P<0.01$; $**P<0.05$; $^{+}P<0.10$. [From Adachi et al. (1976) with permission]

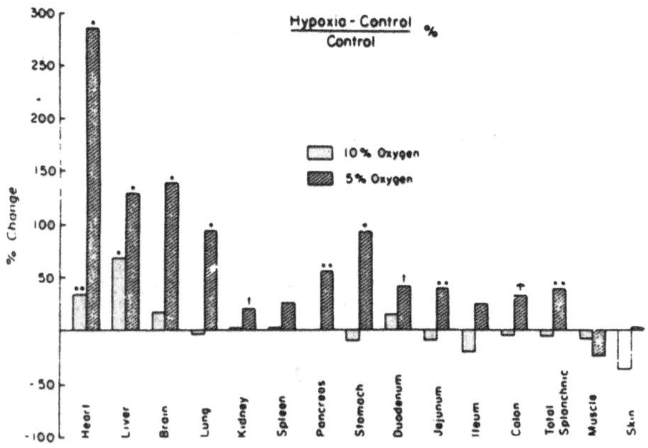

Fig. 6. Percentage change during hypoxia of fractional distribution of cardiac output compared with control (normoxic) distribution. $*P<0.01$; $**P<0.05$; $^{+}P<0.10$. [From Adachi et al. (1976) with permission]

tions which have been observed, the coronary flow exhibits the most dramatic changes during hypoxia.

The precise involvement of sympathetic discharge in hypoxia in humans has been more obscure. In healthy, resting, spontaneously breathing humans, Rowell and Blackmon (1986) found very little evidence for hypoxemic stimulation of sympathetic outflow to splanchnic organs, skin, or skeletal muscle. Rowell (1986) concluded that the activation of arterial chemoreceptors in moderate hypoxemia ($PaO_2 \sim 27$–34 torr) had a varied response on ventilation, ranging from weak to powerful among individuals, yet little increase in sympathetic vasoconstrictor traffic to major organs. He further reasoned that vasoconstriction would serve no useful purpose as long as increased cardiac output maintained flow to the heart and brain. This may be true until a level of hypoxia is reached in which O_2 delivery to the vital organs no longer meets their O_2 demand. These same investigators found that, in contrast to the situation at rest, during exercise plasma norepinephrine and presumably sympathetic nervous activity did increase to a greater extent in hypoxemia than in normoxia (Rowell et al. 1984). Nevertheless, splanchnic blood flow during the combination exercise/hypoxia was not reduced as it typically is during exercise alone. As for modeling the hypoxic response of the critically ill patient, I would submit that the healthy, exercising human may not be as representative of the anesthetized, ventilated patient as is an animal in a similar state.

Summary

This brief survey has presented the complexities of the circulatory responses to hypoxia as determined primarily from studies of laboratory animals. Generalizations are indeed risky, as mentioned in the opening paragraph. Nevertheless, a few conclusions can be drawn:

1. The local vascular effect of hypoxic vasodilation is probably common to all but the pulmonary vessels, yet it appears to be strongest in active tissues (heart, brain, working skeletal muscle) that are dependent on oxygen for their metabolism.
2. A chemoreceptor reflex produces an increase in cardiac contractility as well as selective vasoconstriction (in resting muscle, splanchnic regions) that supports arterial pressure and some degree of redistribution of cardiac output.
3. The integrated response to hypoxia involves a balance of the above effects along with some modification by central pressor effects and lung mechanoreceptors. The overall cardiovascular response includes an increase in cardiac output and selective vasodilation and vasoconstriction in an attempt to maintain O_2 delivery and perfusion pressure to all organs, but with some degree of preference to the heart and brain.

References

Adachi H, Strauss HW, Ochi H, Wagner HN (1976) The effect of hypoxia on the regional distribution of cardiac output in the dog. Circ Res 39:314–319

Bachofen M, Gage A, Bachofen H (1971) Vascular response to changes in blood oxygen tension under various blood flow rates. Am J Physiol 220(6):1786–1792

Berne RM, Rubio R (1979) Coronary circulation. In: Berne RM, Sperelakis N, Geiger SR (eds) Handbook of physiology, sect 2: the heart, vol I. Am Physiol Soc, Bethesda MD, pp 873–952

Berne RM, Winn HR, Rubio R (1981) Metabolic regulation of cerebral blood flow. In: Vanhoutte PM, Leusen I (eds) Vasodilatation. Raven, New York, pp 231–241

Black JE, Roddie IC (1958) The mechanism of the changes in forearm vascular resistance during hypoxia. J Physiol (Lond) 143:226–235

Bohr DF (1978) Vascular smooth muscle. In: Johnson PC (ed) Peripheral circulation. Wiley, New York, pp 13–43

Bourdeau-Martini J, Odoroff CL, Honig CR (1974) Dual effect of oxygen on magnitude and uniformity of coronary intercapillary distance. Am J Physiol 226:800–810
Bredle DL, Bradley WE, Chapler CK, Cain SM (1988 a) Muscle perfusion and oxygenation during local hyperoxia. J Appl Physiol 65:2057–2062
Bredle DL, Chapler CK, Cain SM (1988 b) Metabolic and circulatory responses of normoxic skeletal muscle to whole-body hypoxia. J Appl Physiol 65:2063–2068
Bredle DL, Chapler CK, Cain SM (1988 c) Metabolic and circulatory responses of normoxic skeletal muscle to whole body hypoxia and alpha blockade. Physiologist 31(4):A147 (abstract)
Bredle DL, Chapler CK, Cain SM (1989) Central reflex effects of hypoxia on muscle oxygenation. Adv Exp Med Biol (in press)
Cain SM, Chapler CK (1979) Oxygen extraction by canine hindlimb during hypoxic hypoxia. J Appl Physiol 46:1023–1028
Cain SM, Chapler CK (1980) O_2 extraction by canine hindlimb during alpha-adrenergic blockade and hypoxic hypoxia. J Appl Physiol 48:630–635
Chalmers JP, Korner PI, White SW (1967) Local and reflex factors affecting the distribution of the peripheral blood flow during arterial hypoxia in the rabbit. J Physiol (London) 192:537–548
Costin JC, Skinner NS (1971) Competition between vasoconstrictor and vasodilator mechanism in skeletal muscle. Am J Physiol 220(2):462–466
Daly M de B, Scott MJ (1962) An analysis of the primary cardiovascular reflex effects of stimulation of the carotid body chemoreceptors in the dog. J Physiol (London) 162:555–573
Daugherty RM, Scott JB, Dabney JM, Haddy FJ (1967) Local effects of O_2 and CO_2 on limb, renal, and coronary vascular resistances. Am J Physiol 213:1102–1110
Davidson D, Stalcup SA, Mellins RB (1986) Systemic hemodynamics affecting cardiac output during hypocapnic and hypercapnic hypoxia. J Appl Physiol 60:1230–1236
Detar R (1980) Mechanism of physiological hypoxia-induced depression of vascular smooth muscle contraction. Am J Physiol (Heart Circ) 238:H761–H769
Eyzaguirre C, Fitzgerald RS, Lahiri S, Zapata P (1983) Arterial chemoreceptors. In: Shepherd JT, Abboud FM, Geiger SR (eds) Handbook of Physiology, sect 2. The Cardiovascular System, vol III. Peripheral Circulation and Organ Blood Flow, part 2. Amer Physiol Soc, Bethesda MD, pp 557–621
Forrester T (1981) Adenosine or adenosine triphosphate? In: Vanhoutte PM, Leusen I (eds) Vasodilatation. Raven Press, New York, pp 205–229
Granger HJ, Goodman AH, Granger DN (1976) Role of resistance and exchange vessels in local control of skeletal muscle oxygenation in the dog. Circ Res 38:379–385
Grover RF, Wagner WW, McMurtry IF, Reeves JT (1983) Pulmonary circulation. In: Shepherd JT, Abboud FM, Geiger SR (eds) Handbook of Physiology, sect 2. The Cardiovascular System, vol III. Peripheral Circulation and Organ Blood Flow, part 2. Amer Physiol Soc. Bethesda MD, pp 103–136
Hackett JB, Abboud FM, Mark AL, Schmid PG, Heistad DD (1972) Coronary vascular responses to stimulation of chemoreceptors and baroreceptors: evidence for activation of vagal cholinergic innervation. Circ Res 31:8
Heistad DD, Abboud FM, Mark AL, Schmid PG (1975) Response of muscular and cutaneous vessels to physiologic stimulation of chemoreceptors Proc Soc Exp Biol Med 148:198
Heistad DD, Abboud FM (1980) Circulatory adjustments to hypoxia. Circulation 61:463–470
Iriki M, Simon E (1973) Differential autonomic control of regional circulatory reflexes evoked by thermal stimulation and by hypoxia. Aust J Exp Biol Med Sci 51:283–293
Kogure FJ, Scheinberg P, Reinmuth OM, Fujishima M, Busto R (1970) Mechanisms of cerebral vasodilatation in hypoxia. J Appl Physiol 29:223–229

Korner PI, Chalmers JF, White SW (1967) Some mechanisms of reflex control of the circulation by the sympatho-adrenal system. Circ Res 20, 21 [Suppl III]:157–172
Lugliani F, Whipp BJ, Wasserman K (1973) A role for the carotid body in cardiovascular control in man. Chest 63:744
Marshall C, Marshall B (1983) Site and sensitivity for stimulation of hypoxic pulmonary vasoconstriction. J Appl Physiol 55:711–716
Richardson DW, Kontos HA, Raper AJ, Patterson JL (1967) Modification by beta-adrenergic blockade of the circulatory responses to acute hypoxia in man. J Clin Invest 46:77–85
Rose CE, Kimmel DP, Godine RL, Kaiser DL, Carey RM (1983) Synergistic effects of acute hypoxemia and hypercapnic acidosis in conscious dogs. Circ Res 53:202–213
Rowell LB (1986) Human circulation, regulation during physical stress. Oxford University Press, New York
Rowell LB, Blackmon JR (1986) Lack of sympathetic vasoconstriction in hypoxemic humans at rest. Am J Physiol (Heart Circ) 251:H562–570
Rowell LB, Blackmon JR (1987) Human Calovascular adjustments to acute hypoxaemia. Clin Physiol 7:349–376
Rowell LB, Blackmon JR (1988) Venomotor responses during central and local hypoxia. Am J Physiol (Heart Circ) 255:H760–H764
Rowell LB, Blackmon JR, Kenny MA, Escourrou P (1984) Splanchnic vasomotor and metabolic adjustments to hypoxia and exercise in humans. Am J Physiol (Heart Circ) 247:H251–H258
Rutherford JD, Vatner SF (1978) Integrated carotid chemoreceptor and pulmonary inflation reflex control of peripheral vasoactivity in conscious dogs. Circ Res 43:200
Shapiro W, Wasserman AJ, Baker JP, Patterson JL (1970) Cerebrovascular response to acute hypocapnic and eucapnic hypoxia in normal men. J Clin Invest 49:2362–2368
Sylvester JF, Scharf SM, Gilbert RD, Fitzgerald RS Traystman RJ (1979) Hypoxic and CO hypoxia in dogs: hemodynamics, carotid reflexes, and catecholamines. Am J Physiol (Heart Circ) 236:H22–H28
Vatner SF, Rutherford JD (1978) Control of myocardial contractile state By carotid chemo- and baroreceptor and pulmonary inflation reflexes in conscious dogs. J Clin Invest 61:1593

Oxygen Transport and Oxygen Uptake on the Summit of Mount Everest

J. B. West

Why go to the trouble, time, and expense of organizing a medical research expedition to the summit of Mount Everest? The reason is an interest in how the human body tolerates extreme oxygen deprivation. Every physician who works in the intensive care environment, or sees patients with severe lung disease, knows that a common problem is severe hypoxemia. Our hope was that by looking at normal man under conditions of extremely severe oxygen lack, we could better understand how a patient can tolerate the hypoxemia of severe lung disease.

There is good reason to believe that a climber near the summit of Mt. Everest is very close to the limits of oxygen tolerance. Data to support this contention are shown in Fig. 1. These were the measurements available to us prior to our expedition in 1981, and they show that as the altitude increases (and barometric pressure decreases) maximal oxygen uptake declines rapidly (Pugh et al. 1964). If one is bold enough to extrapolate the line to the barometric pressure of the summit of Mt. Everest, a very interesting prediction emerges. It appears that all the oxygen available will be required for basal oxygen uptake. It therefore becomes very difficult to understand how climbers can reach the summit of Mt. Everest without supplementary oxygen, a feat first accomplished by the two European climbers Reinhold Messner and Peter Habeler in 1978.

We therefore designed the American Medical Research Expedition to Everest to obtain physiological measurements at extreme altitudes including, if possible, on the summit itself (West 1985). Naturally this was a very ambi-

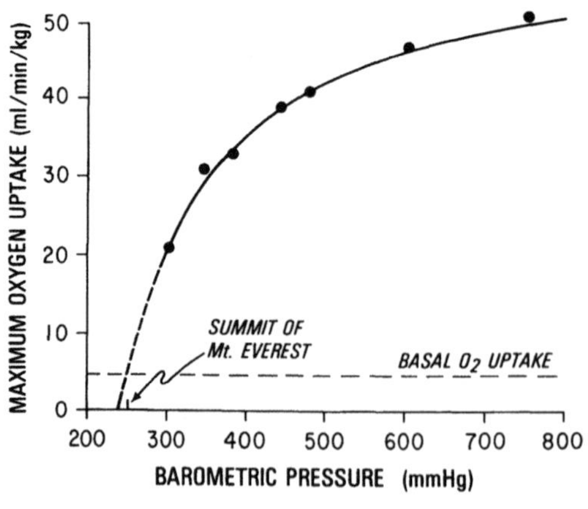

Fig. 1. Data available prior to our expedition showing maximal oxygen uptake against barometric pressure. The plot suggests that all the oxygen available at the Everest summit would be required for basal oxygen uptake. (From West and Wagner 1980)

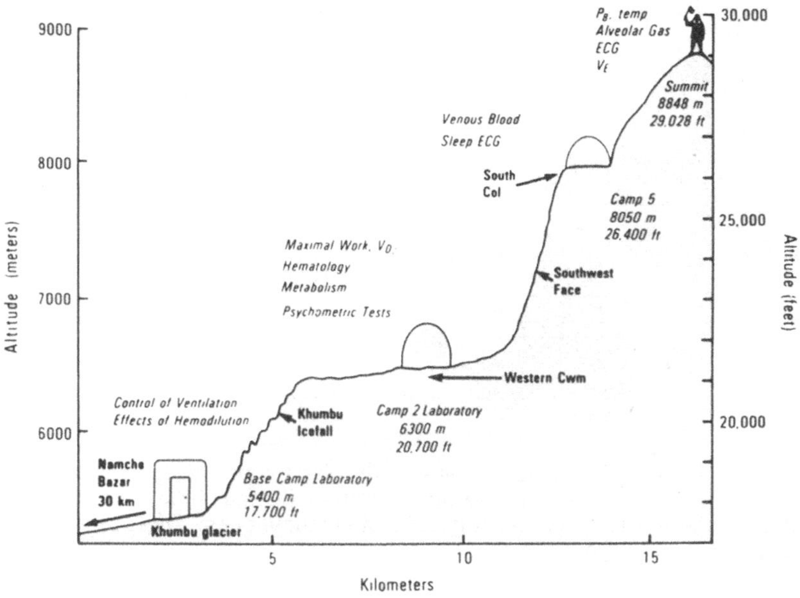

Fig. 2. Researchprojects carried out during the 1981 American Medical Research Expedition to Everest. Note that measurements were carried out at the Base Camp (5400 m), Camp 2 (6300 m), Camp 5 (8050 m), and the summit (8848 m)

tious plan. It is still very difficult to climb Mt. Everest, and when we looked back on the six expeditions immediately prior to our own, we found that none of them had been successful in reaching the summit. However, our expedition was extremely fortunate, and we obtained the first physiological measurements above 8000 m.

The design of the expedition is shown in Fig. 2. Our plan was to make measurements at the Base Camp where we had a prefabricated laboratory hut (5400 m), in the Western Cwm where we had a "Weatherport" laboratory at Camp 2 at an altitude of 6300 m, at Camp 5 (8050 m) just above the South Col, and finally on the summit itself (8848 m). Almost all the planned experimental program was completed, and measurements obtained on the Everest summit included alveolar gas samples, direct measurement of barometric pressure and temperature, and electrocardiogram. In addition, maximal oxygen uptake for the summit inspired PO_2 was obtained by giving well-acclimatized subjects low oxygen mixtures to breathe in the main laboratory at Camp 2. Figure 3 shows Dr. Christopher Pizzo sitting on the summit of Mt. Everest taking alveolar gas samples from himself.

There is space here to describe only some of the major findings and I shall concentrate on the measurements on the summit because they are of particular interest. When human beings go to high altitude, there is an increase in ventilation as a result of stimulation of the peripheral chemoreceptors by the hypoxemia. We recognized that this was one of the most important features of acclimatization at extreme altitude, and so we were careful to obtain good mea-

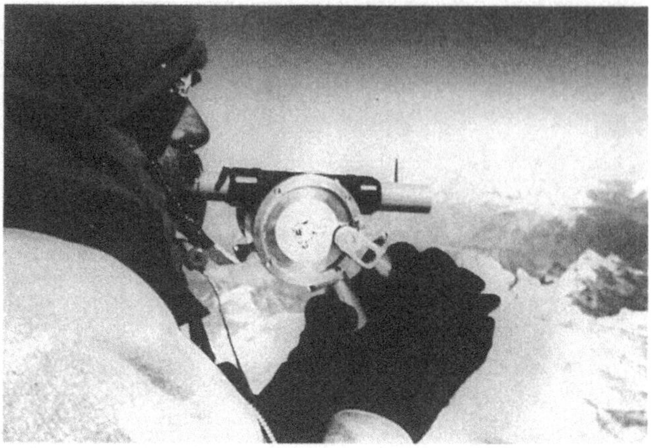

Fig. 3. Christopher Pizzo, MD taking samples of alveolar gas on the summit of Mt. Everest, 24 October, 1981. At the end of a full expiration, he pulled the lever that allowed the end-expired gas to be collected in a small aluminum can. These cans were brought back to UC San Diego for analysis

surements of alveolar PCO_2 as a measure of the degree of hyperventilation. Figure 4 shows the alveolar PCO_2 plotted against barometric pressure at increasing altitudes (West et al. 1983 b). The triangles show the means of the results obtained on our expedition, while the circles are data from previous measurements. It can be seen that as the barometric pressure decreases, the PCO_2 falls in a roughly linear fashion reaching the astonishingly low value of about 7.5 torr on the Everest summit. The normal value at sea level is 40 torr, and these remarkable findings emphasize the extraordinary degree of hyperventilation that a successful well-acclimatized climber develops.

When the alveolar PO_2 and PCO_2 were plotted on an oxygen carbon dioxide diagram as shown in Fig. 5, an interesting result emerged. Sea level is at the top right and the summit of Mt. Everest at the bottom left. It can be seen that both the alveolar PO_2 and PCO_2 fall as subjects go to higher and higher altitudes. The PO_2 falls because of the reduction of PO_2 in inspired air as altitude increases, and the PCO_2 falls because of the increasing hyperventilation. The interesting point is that once a climber exceeds an altitude of about 7000 m, the alveolar PO_2 remains approximately constant at about 35 torr. In other words, the successful climber defends the alveolar PO_2 against the falling value in the environment around him. He does this by the process of extreme hyperventilation, and this appears to be one of the most important features of the acclimatization process to extreme altitude.

Although Fig. 5 indicates that the alveolar PO_2 is kept up reasonably well at a value of 35 torr, a more important question is what happens to the arterial PO_2. With present-day technology it is difficult to see how one could take a sample of arterial blood on the summit of Mt. Everest. We therefore calculated the arterial PO_2 from the Bohr integration along the pulmonary capillary us-

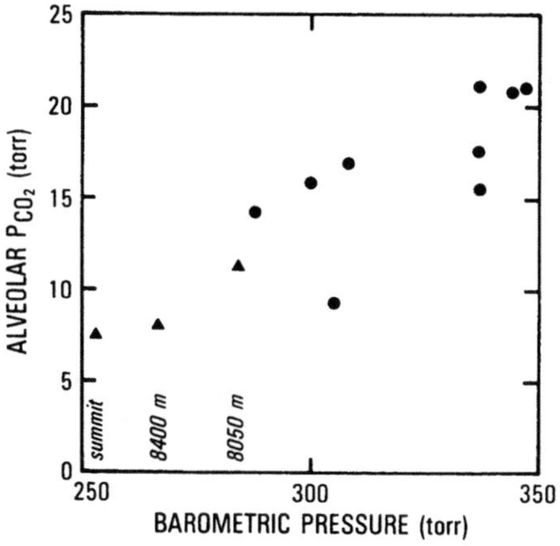

Fig. 4. Relation between alveolar PCO_2 and barometric pressure at extreme altitudes. Note that the value on the Everest summit was about 7.5 torr. (From West et al. 1983b)

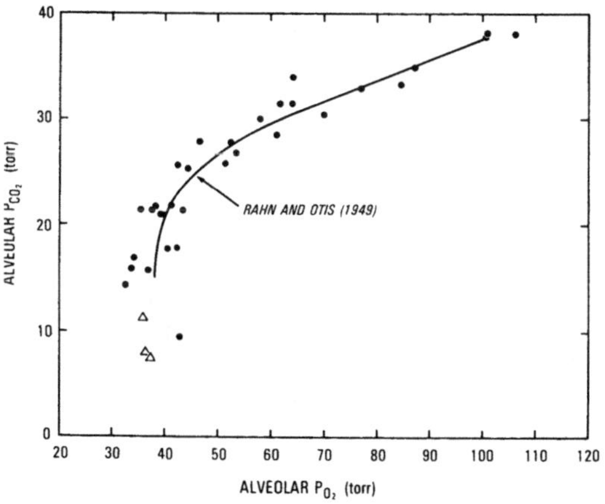

Fig. 5. O_2–CO_2 diagram showing alveolar gas composition in acclimatized subjects as altitude increases (*top right* to *bottom left*). Note that at extreme altitudes, hyperventilation defends the alveolar PO_2 at a value of about 35 torr. (From West et al. 1983b)

ing the alveolar gas and venous data that we had available. Figure 6 shows the time course of PO_2 along the pulmonary capillary at sea level. Note that the blood comes into the lung with a PO_2 of about 40 torr, and the capillary PO_2 rises very rapidly, approaching very close to the alveolar value after about one-third of the time available for oxygenation. There is essentially no PO_2 difference between alveolar gas and end-capillary blood.

Figure 7 shows the same calculations made for Pizzo on the summit of Mt. Everest (West et al. 1983b). It can be seen that the blood comes into the lung with a PO_2 of only about 21 torr, and the PO_2 rises very slowly, reaching a value of only 28 torr at the end of the capillary. Note the large PO_2 difference between alveolar gas and end-capillary blood, indicating diffusion limitation of oxygen uptake, something which never (or hardly ever) occurs in the normal lung at sea level. In other words, the lung is ill-prepared for oxygen uptake under the extraordinary conditions of the summit of Mt. Everest.

Although we were unable to take arterial blood on the summit, this was done in a simulated ascent of Mt. Everest known as Operation Everest II in

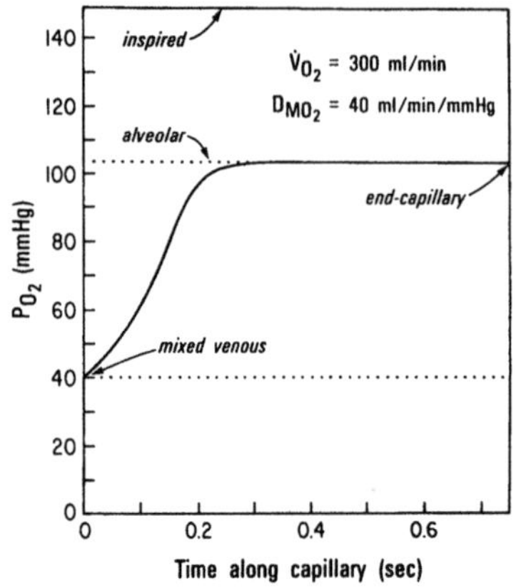

Fig. 6. Bohr integration showing changes in PO_2 along the pulmonary capillary at sea level. (From West and Wagner 1980)

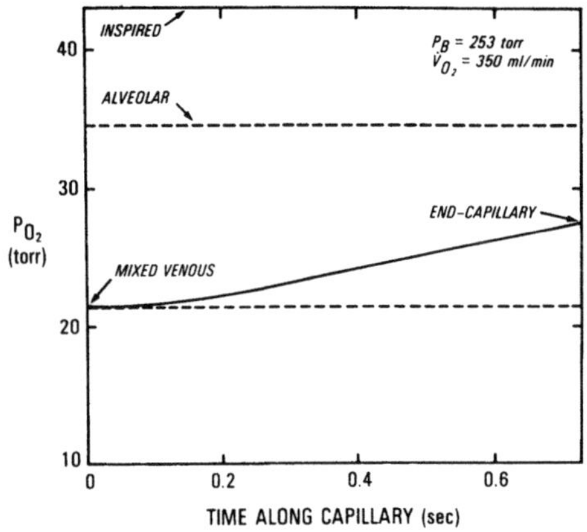

Fig. 7. Bohr integration for a climber resting on the summit of Mt. Everest using data obtained on the expedition. (From West et al. 1983b)

1985 (Sutton et al. 1988). Eight subjects were confined to a low pressure chamber for 40 days and nights, and at the end of that period samples of arterial blood were taken under conditions simulating the Everest summit. The arterial PO_2 during mild exercise was 28 torr, the same as that calculated using our expedition data.

We were particularly interested to know what happened to the acid-base status of the climbers at extreme altitude because of the extremely low levels of alveolar PCO_2. Fortunately two physicians who reached the summit were able to take venous blood samples from each other during the morning after their successful climb. This allowed us to measure their base excess (-7.2 m*M*), and, knowing the alveolar and therefore arterial PCO_2 on the summit, the arterial pH could be derived. Figure 8 shows the Siggaard-Andersen diagram, indicating that the arterial pH on the summit was between 7.7 and 7.8, an extraordinary degree of respiratory alkalosis.

Table 1 summarizes the alveolar gas and arterial blood values for a resting climber on the summit of Mt. Everest, as best we can determine them. We ob-

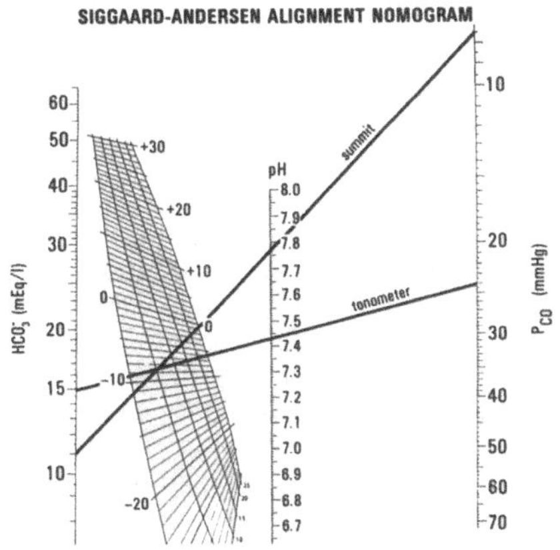

Fig. 8. Siggaard-Andersen monogram showing that the calculated arterial pH on the summit exceeded 7.7. (From West et al. 1983b)

Table 1. Alveolar gas and estimated arterial blood values on the summit of Mt. Everest

Altitude	Barometric pressure (mm Hg)	Inspired PO_2 (mm Hg)	Alveolar PO_2 (mm Hg)	Arterial PO_2 (mm Hg)	Arterial PCO_2 (mm Hg)	Arterial pH
8848 m (summit)	253	43	35	28	7.5	>7.7
Sea level	760	149	100	95	40	7.40

tained the first direct measurement of barometric pressure which was 253 torr (West et al. 1983c). Incidentally this was a surprise to some physiologists who had predicted a much lower value based on the Standard Atmosphere tables. These are the tables that are used to calibrate altimeters and low pressure chambers, but it has been recognized for many years that the barometric pressures on Mt. Everest are higher. Indeed Paul Bert calculated a barometric pressure on the Everest summit of 248 torr in 1878 (see Bert 1943)! Interestingly it can be shown that if the barometric pressure on the summit of Mt. Everest were as low as the Standard Atmosphere predicts (246 torr), it would not be possible for man to reach the summit without supplementary oxygen (West 1983).

Knowing the barometric pressure on the summit, the inspired PO_2 can be calculated as 43 torr. Table 1 and Fig. 5 show that the alveolar PO_2 ist kept up fairly well at 35 torr. However, the arterial PO_2 is very much lower at 28 torr because of diffusion-limitation of oxygen transfer across the blood-gas barrier as shown in Fig. 7. The alveolar (and therefore arterial) PCO_2 is extraordinarily low at 7.5 torr (Fig. 4), and the calculated arterial pH exceeds 7.7 (Fig. 8). I often ask physicians who frequently see patients in the intensive care unit whether they have ever encountered such deranged blood gases as are seen in a normal subject on the summit of Mt. Everest. Probably not. It is re-

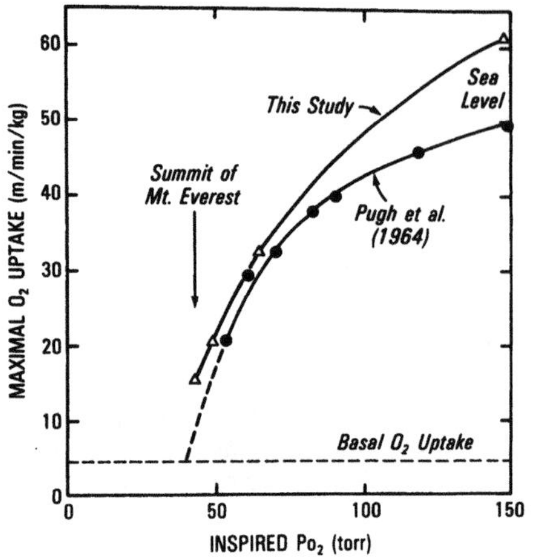

Fig. 9. Maximal oxygen uptake against inspired PO_2. The *lower line* shows the same data as in Fig. 1. The *upper line* shows results obtained during the American Medical Research Expedition to Everest and indicate that the maximal oxygen uptake for the summit is just over 1 l/min. (From West et al. 1983 a)

markable that a climber can not only survive these extraordinary values but actually walk slowly to the summit under these conditions.

As indicated at the beginning of this article, we were perplexed by the ability of Messner and Habeler to reach the summit without supplementary oxygen, given the data shown in Fig. 1. We therefore made careful measurements of maximal oxygen uptake at different altitudes, and the results are shown in Fig. 9. This shows the data of Fig. 1 with the addition of new data from the 1981 expedition (West et al. 1983 a). It can be seen that the maximal oxygen uptake measured for the inspired PO_2 of the summit was 15.3 ml/min/kg or 1.07 l/min. This is a very limited maximal oxygen uptake being equivalent to that obtained during slow walking on sea level. However, it is apparently just sufficient to account for the ability of a climber to reach the summit of Mt. Everest without supplementary oxygen. Messner reported that during the first "oxygenless" ascent in 1978, the last 100 m took more than 1 h to climb, and this very slow climbing rate is consistent with this maximal oxygen uptake.

Incidentally the logistics of measuring the maximal oxygen uptake for the summit conditions were interesting. It was clearly impossible to take a bicycle ergometer and place it on the summit. Instead, we made measurements on the well-acclimatized climbers in the Camp 2 laboratory at an altitude of 6300 m (barometric pressure 350 torr). To obtain the same inspired PO_2 as the summit, the subjects breathed 14% oxygen, giving an inspired PO_2 of 42.5 torr. Since very large volumes of inspired gas were required because of the enormous ventilations at these great altitudes, the supply of 14% oxygen posed a problem. This was solved by having subjects pedal on the ergometer at a moderate rate, and collecting their expired gas in large meteorological balloons. The carbon dioxide was scrubbed out with soda lime, the PO_2 was adjusted to the correct value by adding air, and the gas was given back to the subjects for the measurement of maximal oxygen uptake. It is worth noting that the maximal oxygen uptake measured on the "summit" during the simulated ascent of Operation Everest II was almost identical.

Recently we have given a great deal of thought to some of the consequences of the severe respiratory alkalosis measured at extreme altitude. This was unexpected; indeed in a theoretical study carried out prior to the expedition in an attempt to identify the most important variables to measure, we assumed that there would be full compensation of the respiratory alkalosis (that is an arterial pH of 7.4 for the prevailing PCO_2) at an altitude of 7620 m (25 000 ft.). In the event, the climbers showed some uncompensated respiratory alkalosis even while residing at the Advanced Base Camp 2 at an altitude of 6300 m where the mean arterial pH was 7.45. As indicated above, the arterial pH on the summit exceeded 7.7.

Initially, we thought that the extreme respiratory alkalosis was simply an inevitable consequence of the enormous hyperventilation required to maintain the alveolar PO_2. However, it is now clear that the alkalosis has other important implications. One is to greatly increase the oxygen affinity of the hemoglobin and thus the loading of oxygen by the pulmonary capillaries. While it is true that the increased affinity also interferes with the unloading of oxygen by peripheral capillaries, modelling studies show that when the oxygen uptake is diffusion-limited in the lungs at high altitude, the benefits of enhanced loading outweigh the disadvantages of unloading (Bencowitz et al. 1982). It is interesting that many animals who live in an oxygen-deprived environment have an increased oxygen affinity of their hemoglobin.

Although it is clear that the initiating factor for the respiratory alkalosis is the extreme hyperventilation which depresses the arterial PCO_2, the question arises of why the kidney does not excrete sufficient bicarbonate to restore the pH to near normal, or in other words why is there not full metabolic compensation? The answer is not clear, although there is evidence that bicarbonate excretion is very slow at these great altitudes. For example, the base excess values measured on the two summiters when they were at an altitude of 8050 m (Camp 5) were almost the same as the mean values for the expedition members living at an altitude of 6300 m in Camp 2.

One possible clue to the cause of the slow bicarbonate excretion comes from measurements of serum osmolality of the expedition members at sea level, 5400 m and 6300 m as shown in Fig. 10. Note that the people living at an altitude of 6300 m had a significantly higher serum osmolality than the control values at sea level (Blume et al. 1984). This chronic volume depletion occurred in spite of adequate fluids to drink and a reasonably normal life style. In fact most of the day was spent working in the Camp 2 laboratory. An interesting feature of these data was that the plasma arginine-vasopressin concentrations remained unchanged from sea level to 6300 m in spite of the hyperosmolality. A likely factor in the chronic dehydration was the large insensible loss of fluid at these great altitudes as a result of the hyperventilation. However, the failure of the vasopressin levels to change suggests that there was some abnormality of body fluid regulation.

It is known that the kidney is slow to correct an alkalosis in the presence of volume depletion. Given the options of restoring fluid balance or correcting acid-base balance, the kidney normally gives a higher priority to fluid balance.

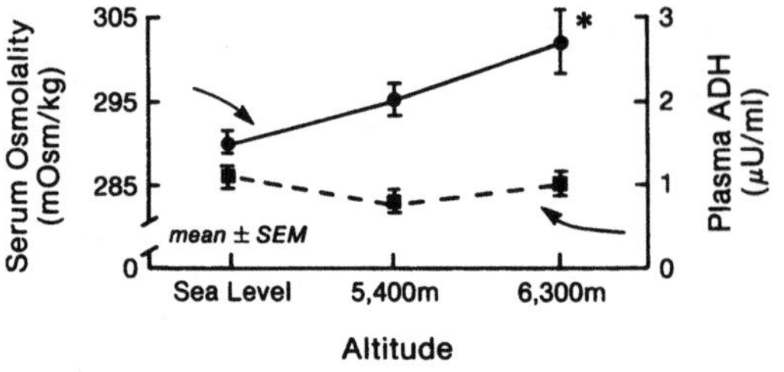

Fig. 10. Serum osmolality and plasma argenine-vasopressin in climbers at sea level, 5400 m, and 6300 m. Note that there was volume depletion at 6300 m but no rise in plasma vasopressin. (From Blume et al. 1984)

The reason for this is that in order to correct the respiratory alkalosis, bicarbonate ion excretion must be increased (or absorption decreased) and this entails the loss of a cation which inevitably aggravates the hyperosmolality. This may be part of the explanation for the slow metabolic compensation of the respiratory alkalosis at very great altitudes in the presence of volume depletion. Incidentally, we know that the kidney *can* greatly increase the excretion of bicarbonate in the subjects living at an altitude of 6300 m because this is what occurred when they were given acetazolamide (Hackett et al. 1985). It is also worth noting that Gonzales et al. (1988) have recently shown, in a chronically hypoxic rat model, that metabolic compensation of respiratory alkalosis is slow in the presence of severe hypoxia. Thus, it may be that hypoxia per se also plays a role in the slow metabolic compensation of respiratory alkalosis at high altitude.

In conclusion measurements from the 1981 American Medical Research Expedition to Everest have clarified how man can tolerate the extreme oxygen deprivation at very great altitudes. One of the most important features of the acclimatization process is hyperventilation which reduces the alveolar PCO_2 to less than 8 torr in well-acclimatized subjects. Even so the arterial PO_2 is less than 30 torr. The hyperventilation causes a marked respiratory alkalosis, which increases the oxygen affinity of the hemoglobin and assists in the loading of the oxygen by the pulmonary capillaries. The respiratory alkalosis is partly the result of slow excretion of bicarbonate by the kidneys, possibly related to chronic volume depletion. The maximal oxygen uptake on the summit is just over 1 l/min which is apparently just sufficient to allow a climber to reach the summit without supplementary oxygen.

References

Bencowitz HZ, Wagner PD, West JB (1982) Effect of change in P50 on exercise tolerance at high altitude: a theoretical study. J Appl Physiol: Respir Environ Exerc Physiol 53:1487–1495

Bert P (1943) Barometric pressure. Researches in experimental physiology. College Book, Columbus/Oh. Translation of: La pression barométrique. Masson, Paris, 1878

Blume FD, Boyer SH, Braverman LE, Cohen A (1984) Impaired osmoregulation at high altitude. J AMA 252:1580–1585

Gonzales NC, Clancy RL, Albrecht T (1988) Compensation of hypocapnic alkalosis induced after acclimatization to simulated altitude in rats. Physiologist 31:A146 (abstr)

Hackett PH, Schoene RB, Winslow RM, Peters RM Jr, West JB (1985) Acetazolamide and exercise in sojourners to 6300 meters – a preliminary study. Med Sci Sports Exerc 17:593–597

Pugh LCGE, Gill MG, Lahiri S, Milledge JS, Ward MP, West JB (1964) Muscular exercise at great altitude. J Appl Physiol 19:431–440

Sutton JR, Reeves JT, Wagner PD, Groves BM, Cymerman A, Malconian MK, Rock PB, Young PM, Watter SD, Houston CS (1988) Operation Everest II: oxygen transport during exercise at extreme simulated altitude. J Appl Physiol 64:1309–1321

West JB (1983) Climbing Mt Everest without supplementary oxygen: an analysis of maximal exercise during extreme hypoxia. Respir Physiol 52:265–279

West JB (1985) Everest – the testing place. McGraw-Hill, New York

West JB, Wagner PD (1980) Predicted gas exchange on the summit of Mt Everest. Respir Physiol 42:1–16

West JB, Boyer SJ, Graber DJ, Hackett PH, Maret KH, Milledge JS, Peters RM Jr, Pizzo CJ, Samaja M, Sarnquist FH, Schoene RB, Winslow RM (1983 a) Maximal exercise at extreme altitudes on Mount Everest. J Appl Physiol: Respir Environ Exerc Physiol 55:688–698

West JB, Hackett PH, Maret KH, Milledge JS, Peters RM Jr, Pizzo CJ, Winslow RM (1983 b) Pulmonary gas exchange on the summit of Mt Everest. J Appl Physiol: Respir Environ Exerc Physiol 55:678–687

West JB, Lahiri S, Maret KH, Peters RM Jr, Pizzo CJ (1983 c) Barometric pressures at extreme altitudes on Mt. Everest: physiological significance. J Appl Physiol: Respir Environ Exerc Physiol 54:1188–1194

Lung Structure and Function in ARDS *

L. Gattinoni, A. Pesenti, R. Fumagalli, G. P. Rossi, F. Scarani, R. Marcolin, and U. Ernesti

Introduction

The acute respiratory failure (ARF) due to diffused inflammation of the pulmonary parenchyma, otherwise known as adult respiratory distress syndrome (ARDS), leads to increased extravascular lung water with a consequent increase in the density of the lungs. Computerized tomography (CT) may detect the density change of pulmonary parenchyma without interference due to overlying or underlying structures. In the past few years we have made a consecutive study of several ARDS patients using a CT scan. In this chapter we will describe:

1. The diagnostic value of the CT scan in ARDS
2. The morphological pattern of the syndrome
3. The CT scan variations in response to changes of positive end expiratory pressure (PEEP) and to body positioning

Moreover, we have developed a technique for quantitative analysis of CT images. We also describe the relationship we have found between the lung anatomy, as revealed by CT, and the physiological variables routinely measured in these ARDS patients.

Diagnostic Value

In a large series of ARDS patients (more than 80) CT allowed detection of alterations that were not visible with conventional X-rays, i.e., bullae, abscesses and, more importantly, localized tension pneumothoraces (strictly anterior or posterior), not detected by the anteroposterior chest X-rays. However, the chest X-rays and the CT images give the same information relative to the total amount of edema, if the chest X-ray is read using standardized procedure, as done by Pistolesi and Halperin [1]. The X-ray score and the average CT scan density show, in fact, a high degree of correlation. In our opinion, CT in ARDS is mainly indicated in cases where there is clinical suspicion of pneumothorax not evident on the chest X-ray.

* Supported in part by C.N.R., 87.00750.57, Rome, Italy

Morphological Pattern in ARF

Typically in the ARDS lung, the lesions (densities) are distributed nonhomogeneously, being mainly seen in the dependent lung regions, while the nondependent (ventral) regions maintain normal density (i.e., an air/tissue ratio with in normal limits [2–4]). However, it is important to recall that, in ARDS patients, the CT scan is usually done with the lung inflated to a pressure of at least 5 cm H_2O. The concept of "normal density," referring to normal lung scanned at an inflation pressure of 0 cm H_2O, is therefore called into question.

Morphological Response to PEEP

When ARDS patients undergo an increase in PEEP, lung density decreases, to various degrees. It is obviously important to define the regions of the lung where this decrease in density occurs. If the region was inflated before the PEEP increase, the decrease in density is merely due to overinflation; if the region was gasless before application of PEEP, the decrease in density is due to recruitment of pulmonary units. In a large number of ARDS patients, we found that approximately 15% of the original lung mass is recruited when PEEP is increased by 10 cm H_2O. The PEEP response is more evident at the base and hilum of the lung and less evident at the apex [4].

Morphological Response to Positioning

When the patient's position was changed from supine to prone, we found almost without exception a dramatic change in the distributioin of the densities. The dorsal regions tend to clear, while the ventral regions become dense. These variations occur in the time required to turn the patient and perform a new scan, i.e., 5 to 10 min. The average density does not change and the variations in density distribution are somehow independent of gas exchange modifications [5, 6].

Quantitative Analysis of the CT Scan

Over the past few years we have developed a method for quantitative analysis of CT images [7–9], based on the frequency distribution of the CT numbers. Coupled with determination of the pulmonary gas volumes by helium dilution, this allows estimation of the following variables:

1. Lung weight: the weight of the whole lungs, including the blood and the edema, if any. In normal subjects we found a lung weight ranging from 800 to 1200 g, varying according to sex and height. In a given patient, it is possible to estimate the "expected normal lung weight," and to compute the excess weight as a percentage of the expected.

2. Mass of tissue normally inflated: the mass of tissue where the gas/tissue ratio is within normal limits (90% gas: 10% tissue to 50% gas: 50% tissue). In the normal lung more than 80% of the total mass is within the above limits.
3. Mass of poorly inflated tissue: the mass of the lung where the air/tissue ratio is between 50% gas: 50% tissue and 10% gas: 90% tissue. In the normal lung 15% of the total mass is within these limits.
4. Mass of noninflated tissue: the mass of the lung where the air/tissue ratio is between 10% gas: 90% tissue and 0% gas: 100% tissue. In the normal lung 5% of the mass is within these limits.
5. Recruitment. This is computed as the mass of tissue which shifts, with PEEP, from the non- or poorly inflated category to the normally inflated category. Computation of recruitment is independent of hyperinflation.

Relationship Between the Physiological Variables and the Anatomic Variables Derived from the CT Scan

Lung Weight in ARF

In ARDS patients we found an average lung weight of 2600 ± 1200 g [8], which is well in agreement with the lung weight found in an earlier study at autopsy (2500 g) [10]. The excess lung weight was about 200% of the normal. These values markedly exceed the values of extravascular lung water found in ARDS [11]. However, it is important to recall that extravascular lung water is measured only in well-perfused lung regions, whereas in cases of hypoperfusion the amount of extravascular lung water is underestimated. The excess lung weight is strictly related to the mean pulmonary artery pressure. It is tempting to speculate that in ARDS lung the increased vascular pressures cause an increase of edema; however, it is possible that the edema itself may cause an increase of vascular pressures via vascular compression.

Relationship Between Lung Compliance and Anatomy

Reportedly, decreased lung compliance is considered a marker of ARDS. In a series of 22 ARDS patients, we correlated the compliances derived from the pressure–volume (PV) curve of the lung with the anatomic variables obtained at different pressures on the PV curve, as computed by the CT scan.

We found that the compliances are strictly related to the mass of lung tissue normally inflated, independently of the mass of non- or poorly inflated tissue. The compliances are then an estimate of the residual "healthy" lung, which maintains a normal air/tissue ratio. The specific compliance, in these patients, was normal or higher than normal. We concluded that the decreased compliance in ARDS is not due to a "stiff" lung but simply to a "small" residual healthy lung, which is the only thing "seen" by the PV curve.

Relationship Between Gas Exchange and Anatomy

We found a strictly significant correlation between the hypoxemia and shunt fraction and the mass of noninflated tissue. We can not discriminate between edema, atelectasis, or consolidation on the basis of the CT scan. However, whatever the nature of the densities, they appear to be the main cause of the shunt-related hypoxemia.

Effects of PEEP

The mechanism of PEEP is still being debated. The CT scan has revealed the morphological equivalent of the recruitment [4]; moreover, a quantitative analysis of CT scan images has shown that the anatomical recruitment is significantly associated with a decreased hypoxemia and shunt. These findings suggest that the immediate effect of PEEP is the recruitment of pulmonary units from the noninflated compartment to the inflated compartment. It is reasonable to think that such units are atelectatic, as it is unlikely that edema or consolidation will clear in a few minutes.

Effects of Positioning

In all the patients studied for the effects of positioning, we observed an apparent migration of the densities from the dorsal to the ventral lung regions when the patients were shifted from the supine to the prone position. This phenomenon also occurs in normal subjects, the only difference being quantitative. The clearing of the dorsal regions could theoretically be attributed to reabsorption of edema, while the simultaneous increase in density in the ventral regions could be due to the development of a new edema. However, this hypothesis is unlikely, due to the shortness of the period in which these phenomena occur. In experimental animals, in fact, the reabsorption of edema requires days [12]. It is also unlikely, for physical reasons, that the interstitial edema freely crosses the interstitial spaces. The available body of data [13] suggests that the density redistribution is due to the opening of pulmonary units which are decompressed (dorsal regions) and to the simultaneous closure of the units which are compressed (ventral regions). The lung weight, which is three times the normal, probably plays a key role in this compression and decompression.

Lung Model in Acute Respiratory Failure

From the CT scan data and the physiological variables measured, we may hypothesize the following sequence of phenomena during ARF. The first alteration is interstitial edema due to capillary lesions. The dense edema accumulates in the lung independently of the force of gravity. However, when the excess mass reaches a critical value (100%–150%), the dependent regions of the lung collapse due to the weight of the overlying structures. Consequently shunt-related hypoxemia develops. This induces an increase of cardiac output associated with pulmonary hypertension. The increased vascular pressure may further increase the edema. While the gas volume decreases the compliance decreases, since it is the mass of normally inflated tissue being reduced. The effects of PEEP on this system are immediate and probably consist in the reopening of pulmonary units which have been collapsed by the weight of the overlying structures. The same regions reopen when the effects of gravity are modified by changing position. It is then possible that the PEEP response and the positioning response share a common mechanism, i.e., reopening of compression atelectasis. Further studies are needed to clarify this. However, in a series of ten patients in whom we compared PEEP and positioning effects, we found a high degree of correlation between these two phenomena.

In additioin to its diagnostic value in ARF, CT is in our opinion a powerful tool for physiopathological investigation.

References

1. Gattinoni L, Pistolesi M, Rossi F, Bombino M, Bellato V, Miniati M (1987) Portable X-rays versus CT scan in ARDS. Am Rev Respir Dis 135:A214 (Suppl)
2. Maunder RJ, Shuman WP, McHugh JW, Marglin SI, Butler J (1986) Preservation of normal lung regions in the adult respiratory distress syndrome. Analysis by computed tomography. JAMA 55:2463–2465
3. Gattinoni L, Pesenti A (1987) ARDS: the nonhomogeneous lung; facts and hypothesis. Intensive & Critical Care Digest 6:1–4
4. Gattinoni L, Mascheroni D, Torresin R, Marcolin R, Fumagalli R, Vesconi S, Rossi GP, Rossi F, Baglioni S, Bassi F, Nastri G, Pesenti A (1986) Morphological response to positive end-expiratory pressure in acute respiratory failure. Computerized tomography study. Intensive Care Med 12:137–142
5. Mascheroni D, Marcolin R, Giuffrida A, Pesenti A, Torresin A, Gattinoni L (1987) Prone position affects lung densities distribution in ARDS. Am Rev Respir Dis A10:135S
6. Langer M, Mascheroni D, Marcolin R, Gattinoni L (1988) The prone position in ARDS patients. A clinical study. Chest 94:103–107
7. Gattinoni L, Pesenti A, Avalli L, Rossi F, Bombino M (1987) Pressure volume curve of total respiratory system in acute respiratory failure. Computed tomographic scan study. Am Rev Respir Dis 136:730–736
8. Gattinoni L, Pesenti A, Bombino M et al. (1988) Relationships between lung computed tomographic density, gas exchange and PEEP in acute respiratory failure. Anesthesiology 69:824–832
9. Gattinoni L, Pesenti A, Baglioni S, Vitale G, Rivolta M, Pelosi P (1988) Inflammatory pulmonary edema and positive end-respiratory pressure: correlations between imaging and physiological studies. J Thorac Imag 3(3):59–64
10. Zapol WM, Trelstad RL, Coffey JW, Tsai I, Salvador RA (1979) Pulmonary fibrosis in severe acute respiratory failure. Am Rev Respir Dis 119:547–554
11. Sibbald WJ, Short AK, Warshawski FJ, Cunningham DG, Chung H (1985) Thermal dye measurements of extravascular lung water in critically ill patients. Chest 87:585–592
12. Stoub NC (1988) New concepts about the pathophysiology of pulmonary edema. Journal Thorac Imag 3:8–14
13. Gattinoni L, Pelosi P, Vitale G, Pesenti A, D'Andrea L, Mascheroni D (1989) Lung computed tomographic densities: redistribution from supine to prone position in acute respiratory failure. Submitted for publication

Supply Dependency of Oxygen Uptake *

S. M. Cain

A puzzling and disturbing finding in certain patients with adult respiratory distress syndrome (ARDS) or sepsis is that their oxygen (O_2) uptake appears to vary directly with total O_2 delivery (total O_2 delivery is defined as the product of cardiac output and arterial O_2 content). The more usual situation is that O_2 extraction in the periphery varies inversely with O_2 delivery so that O_2 uptake remains approximately constant. In these certain patients, if delivery to the periphery is increased, O_2 uptake will increase or, if delivery decreases, O_2 uptake falls. This is puzzling because it is not the normal response of O_2 uptake when cardiac output and arterial O_2 content are both in acceptable ranges, as they often are in such patients. This is disturbing because when abnormal supply dependency of O_2 uptake is found, it appears to be a dire prognostic sign. In this paper, I will expand on the essential differences between normal or physiological O_2 supply dependency and its abnormal or pathological manifestation. Following that, I will present some evidence that the pathological form is a very bad prognostic sign. Finally, I will report the results from some animal experiments in which we tried to reproduce the defect in peripheral O_2 extraction that is the hallmark of pathological O_2 supply dependency and speculate on why it may occur.

Figure 1 illustrates the two kinds of O_2 supply dependency. In its physiological form, as O_2 delivery is lowered, O_2 uptake does not change until a critical value of delivery is reached. Below that point, O_2 uptake becomes a linear function of delivery. If time is allowed for circulatory adjustments to occur [4], O_2 extraction increases with each lowering of delivery until the critical value is reached. This presumably marks the physiological limit for using the O_2 reserve in blood. Given the necessity for a PO_2 gradient to move O_2 from the capillary to the tissue interior and the likelihood that all perfusion heterogeneity cannot be eliminated, all of the O_2 cannot be extracted from the perfusing blood even in a highly vascular organ such as skeletal muscle. The empiric O_2 extraction limit in canine hindlimb muscles is 0.93 with supply dependency evident as extraction approaches 0.80 [7]. Although the relationship depicted in Fig. 1 is almost certainly a curvilinear one, experimental data can be closely approximated by fitting two straight lines, one to the plateau where O_2 uptake is independent of delivery and another to the data in the zone of supply depen-

* Support for this work was obtained from Grants HL 26927 and HL 07790 from the National Heart, Lung, and Blood Institute of NIH and by a grant from Fisons plc, Loughborough, England, UK

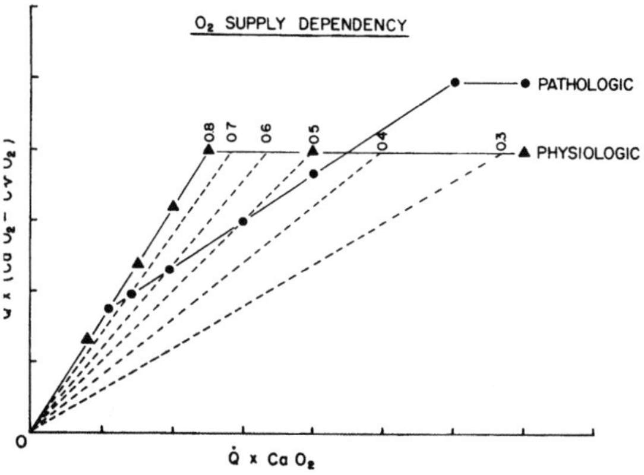

Fig. 1. Schematic representation of the relationships between O_2 uptake (Q × [CaO_2-CvO_2]) and total O_2 delivery (Q × CaO_2) in physiologic and pathologic O_2 supply dependency (from [8])

dency. This provides an index of the efficacy with which the peripheral tissues can utilize a limited supply of O_2 by the point of intersection of the two lines, the critical O_2 extraction ratio. In the physiological example, O_2 extraction increases as delivery is decreased until O_2 uptake begins to fall below the critical O_2 extraction ratio. Extrapolation of the dependent line shows its origin to be very close to zero. With no O_2 delivery, there obviously should be no O_2 uptake.

Contrast that situation with the one for the pathological form of O_2 supply dependency shown in Fig. 1. First, O_2 demands are generally higher in patients who display abnormal O_2 supply dependency. With ARDS and sepsis, for example, patients are often agitated and may be febrile as well. Aside from these more obvious reasons for elevated O_2 needs, there may be other more occult ones such as increased extramitochondrial O_2 use in formation of reactive O_2 metabolites [1, 17]. Whereas increased O_2 demand in the normal situation speeds the mobilization of capillary reserve to promote O_2 extraction [11], there is evidence that this compensatory mechanism is not as effective in patients who show abnormal O_2 supply dependency. Although straight lines have again been used to illustrate the pathological case of O_2 supply dependency, the truth might be better served by a more pronounced curvilinear relationship. Furthermore, there is also some doubt that a plateau can be found. These reservations will be discussed in light of some recent findings in animal experiments that will be described later.

The description that was just given is much clearer than the real situation. Many factors bear on the lack of clarity presented by real patients in a real clinical setting. First, both kinds of O_2 supply dependency can coexist. If a septic patient, for example, has not been aggressively treated to convert a hypodynamic state to a hyperdynamic one, then the shock and reduced peripheral perfusion could lower O_2 delivery well into the zone of supply dependency that would limit O_2 uptake in even the normal situation. The group led by Carlson at Wayne State University used fluid loading to increase cardiac output and O_2 delivery. In those patients who had elevated blood lactate levels, O_2 uptake increased and lactate levels decreased [10, 13]. Elevated blood lac-

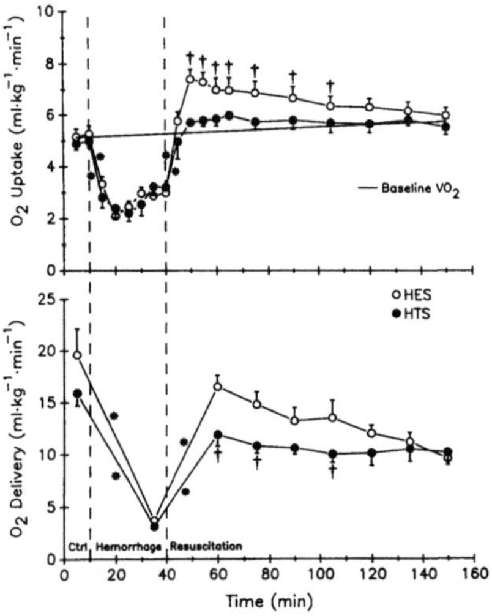

Fig. 2. Whole body O_2 uptake *(top panel)* and O_2 delivery *(bottom panel)* in two groups of six dogs during hemorrhage and after resuscitation with either hypertonic saline solution (HTS) or hydroxyethyl starch solution (HES). (From [16])

tate levels would indicate stimulation of anaerobic metabolism imposed by a limitation in O_2 delivery so that these findings implied that there was a straightforward reversal of a supply limitation. To support this idea, in these same studies patients without elevated lactate levels did not increase O_2 uptake with fluid loading. The question of whether all was right with these patients other than this straightforward correction of an insufficient supply of O_2 lies in the fact that O_2 extraction never exceeded 0.30 on the average in any group in either of the two studies. If more O_2 was available in the blood, then why did the distribution of flow at the microcirculatory level in the peripheral tissues not readjust to shorten diffusion distances and promote better extraction rather than require increased blood flow before O_2 uptake could be raised?

When we made anesthetized dogs hypovolemic by hemorrhage to a mean arterial pressure of 40 mmHg, O_2 delivery was lowered past the critical point and O_2 uptake fell until the dogs were resuscitated, as shown in Fig. 2. In these experiments we compared a small volume (5 ml/kg) of hypertonic saline (HTS) to a more conventional replacement of shed volume with hydroxyethyl starch solution (HES). In Fig. 3, while O_2 delivery was below critical, O_2 extraction increased to almost 0.80 and remained over 0.50 during the entire recovery period. In these same experiments we progressively lowered blood flow to the isolated hindlimb muscles and those results are shown in Fig. 4. In this case there was actually a slightly negative slope above the critical delivery level but it is plain that O_2 extraction increased as delivery was lowered until a critical extraction of nearly 0.80 was reached. In yet other studies in anesthetized dogs, O_2 demand was stimulated by uncoupling of oxidative phosphorylation with 2,4-dinitrophenol and O_2 delivery was decreased by ventilation with hypoxic gas mixtures [9]. Figure 5 shows that resistance in the hindlimb muscles did not start to fall until O_2 extraction exceeded 0.50. This illustrated very well that in the normal animal, the first line of defense against a decrease in the ratio of O_2 supply to demand is to increase utilization of the O_2 reserve held in blood

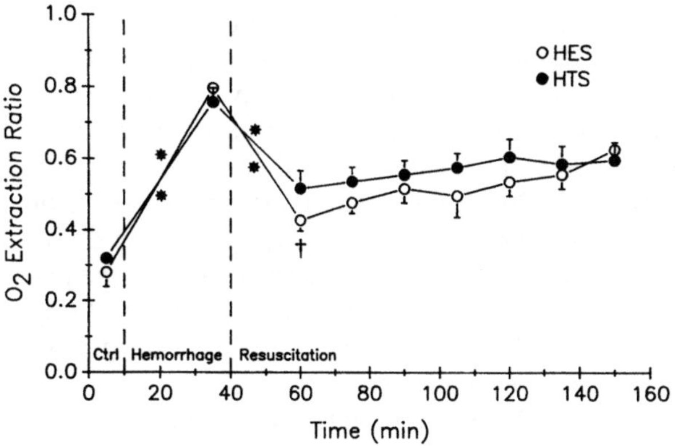

Fig. 3. Whole body O_2 extraction ratio in the same experiments as in Fig. 2. (From [16])

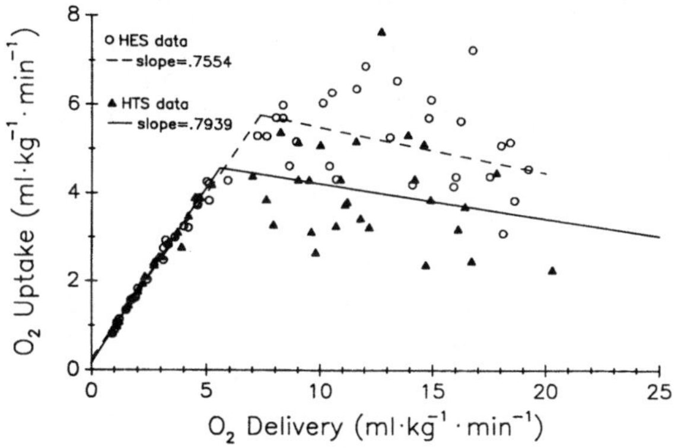

Fig. 4. Limb O_2 uptake shown as a function of limb O_2 delivery with progressive lowering of blood flow to pump-perfused, vascularly isolated, hindlimb after resuscitation of dogs from hemorrhage with either HES or HTS. (From [16])

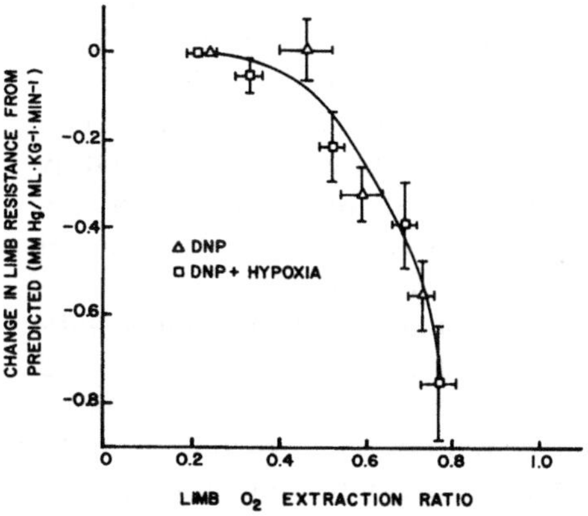

Fig. 5. Change in limb vascular resistance as a function of the O_2 extraction ratio when O_2 demand has been increased with 2,4-dinitrophenol (DNP) and O_2 supply has been decreased by hypoxic hypoxia (from [9])

rather than increasing regional blood flow. The difference between the results of these animal studies and those in septic patients is due to the presence of the septic condition and not to the difference between a patient and an animal model.

This apparent inability to increase O_2 extraction to meet an apparently unsatisfied O_2 demand, or "pathological O_2 supply dependency," as I have called it, is somehow related to the multiorgan failure that contributes to the very high mortality in patients with ARDS and sepsis. Not very many patient studies have tried to assess this relationship. In a retrospective study, Gutierrez and Pohil [12] examined consecutive admissions to an intensive care unit and selected 30 in whom serial measurements of O_2 uptake and delivery were made. Most had ARDS or sepsis or both. In 20 of their cases there was evidence of O_2 supply dependency in that O_2 uptake decreased with any decrease in delivery and there was no increase in O_2 extraction. In the other ten cases, the patients were able to keep O_2 uptake constant by increasing extraction. Only 30% of the first group survived their illness but 70% of the second group, those without O_2 supply dependency, eventually recovered.

A prospective study by Bihari et al. [2] also showed that an impaired ability of peripheral tissues to extract O_2 was associated with a dire prognosis for recovery. They infused the vasodilator prostacyclin into 27 critically ill patients who had acute respiratory failure. This treatment increased O_2 delivery similarly in all the patients but of the 27, 13 increased their O_2 uptake and 14 did not. All of those exhibiting O_2 supply dependency died whereas those who did not show supply dependency survived. In a small group of healthy volunteers, treatment with prostacyclin also increased O_2 delivery but this group showed no tendency to increase O_2 uptake with delivery. The authors suggested that supply dependency indicated inadequate tissue oxygenation and a substantial oxygen debt in those patients who subsequently died. They went on to suggest that this may have been an important contributing mechanism to the irreversible multiple organ failure which was ultimately responsible for their death. Another interpretation of their data might indicate with equal justification that improving O_2 delivery did not improve recoverability. If the increase in O_2 uptake that these patients experienced was attributable to improved tissue oxygenation, then it would be reasonable to suppose that it should have led to less multiple organ failure. In this particular study, a negative base excess value of 6 mmol/l in the nonsurviving patients became more negative with prostacyclin treatment, whereas it converted from slightly negative to slightly positive in the patients who survived. The authors did not measure blood lactate but these findings were consistent with severe tissue hypoxia that was not reversed by improved oxygenation in the nonsurviving patients.

Recognition of abnormal O_2 supply dependency and its possible significance originated from studies, both prospective and retrospective, conducted at the bedside of patients with ARDS or sepsis. As valuable as this has been, further advances require that the condition be reproduced in an animal model so that studies under more carefully controlled conditions and with more invasive interventions can be done. In this manner, we can increase the probability of finding the mechanisms of pathological O_2 supply dependency and either preventing or correcting it.

A clear demonstration of a lessened ability of the peripheral tissues to extract O_2 has been made in anesthetized dogs that have been made septic, either by injection of live bacteria or endotoxin. In one such study, Nelson et al. [14] used a strain of *Pseudomonas aeruginosa* that was isolated from a septicemic patient. They then progressively lowered O_2 delivery by controlled hemorrhage. With the multiple points along a relationship describing O_2 uptake as a function of O_2 delivery, they were able to identify the critical delivery point below which O_2 uptake began to decrease with any further lowering of delivery. This was taken as the point of intersection of two straight lines fitted to the plateau and to the supply-dependent zones of the relationship. They also found the critical O_2 delivery at which blood lactate levels began to increase. Both of these values were compared with those obtained in another group of dogs that were treated similarly but were not injected with live bacteria. The critical values were similar for either the decrease in O_2 uptake or for the increase in blood lactate. In the case of the bacteremic group, the critical delivery level was 11.4 ml/kg/min as compared with 7.4 ml/kg/min in the control group. By taking the ratio of O_2 uptake to delivery at the critical point, the critical O_2 extraction ratio can be calculated. This was 0.51 vs 0.71 for the bacteremic and control groups respectively. Impaired O_2 extraction as a result of bacteremia was clearly shown.

The same group went on to investigate both whole body and regional critical O_2 extraction in anesthetized dogs given a bolus injection of *Escherichia coli* endotoxin in two other studies [15, 18]. They obtained similar results to the bacteremia study in the whole body, again using progressive controlled hemorrhage as the means to lower total O_2 delivery. In one study, they also examined critical O_2 extraction in an isolated, autoperfused section of gut [15]. They found that O_2 extraction was impaired in the gut section to a similar extent as in the whole body, 0.47 and 0.54 respectively for the endotoxic group vs 0.69 and 0.78 for gut and whole body respectively in a control group. In the context of whole body O_2 delivery, however, gut became supply dependent at a higher value than did the whole body. This implied that the gut was receiving a proportionately smaller share of cardiac output. In the other study [18], they examined resting skeletal muscle of the hindlimb in a similarly designed experiment. Contrary to the results of the gut, muscle showed no impairment as total O_2 delivery was progressively lowered by hemorrhaging the whole animal. They also found that muscle did not increase its share of cardiac output in endotoxic shock as some had suggested. However, they did find that whole body and muscle O_2 uptake increased after endotoxin treatment. We presently have no knowledge about regional distribution of blood flow or regional capabilities for O_2 extraction in patients with sepsis or ARDS, thus this illustrates the potential utility of animal models.

In a joint study with this group, we have examined the effect of endotoxin on resting skeletal muscle of anesthetized dogs with a different question in mind [3]. With hemorrhage of the whole animal, other regulatory factors that might affect hemodynamics and metabolism of resting muscle may be brought into play as baroreceptor activity, among other things, is increased. To circumvent such additional factors, we pump-perfused the hindlimb musculature so that flow could be controlled. In addition, we wished to ascertain whether an elevated PO_2 might overcome any impairment of O_2 extraction on the hypothesis that abnormal diffusion limitation as a result of endotoxin treatment

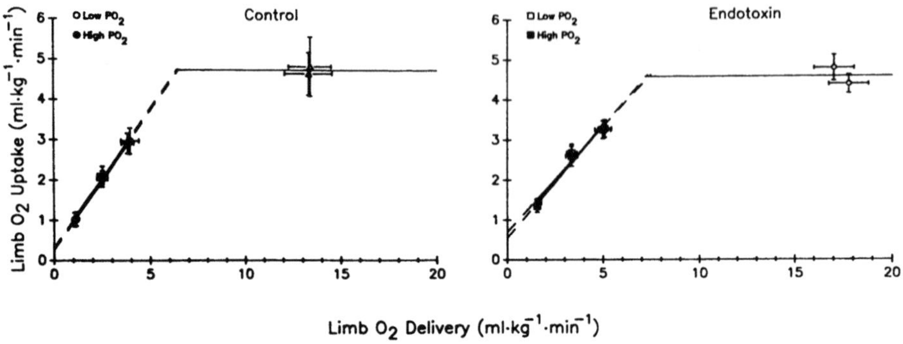

Fig. 6. Limb O_2 uptake as a function of O_2 delivery at normoxic and at flow-limited conditions in a group of control animals (*left panel, n* = 6) and in a group given endotoxin (*right panel, n* = 6). Low arterial PO_2 was ~60 torr and high PO_2 was ~200 torr (from [3])

might be the cause. From the earlier results, we knew that the limb muscle would show a plateau value so that one measurement at adequate O_2 delivery levels would suffice to establish it. We then lowered blood flow to the vascularly isolated but innervated limb below the critical level in three stages. A membrane oxygenator in the line allowed us to set the arterial inflow PO_2 at either 60 or 200 torr. For each animal, a normoxic control level was established with blood flow to the limb set at approximately 90 ml/kg/min. Following that, flow was lowered to about 30, 20, and 10 ml/kg/min at 15-min intervals. The sequence was repeated with the other PO_2 setting and the order was reversed with each experiment. One group of six served as controls and another group of six was given a bolus injection of *E. coli* endotoxin. After the initial hypotensive reaction, the endotoxin group was given sufficient donor red cells, suspended in dextran solution, to restore cardiac output and mean arterial blood pressure to normal values and these were maintained at those levels throughout the experiment.

O_2 uptake by the limb is shown as a function of O_2 delivery in Fig. 6. A straight line was fitted to the supply-dependent values for each animal and the intersection with the normoxic level of O_2 uptake was noted. From the line fitted to the mean data points for the control group at the left of the figure, the critical O_2 delivery was about 6 ml/kg/min and there was no difference between high and low PO_2. In the endotoxic group, the slope of the line was less so that there was a positive intercept on the ordinate and the critical delivery value was a little greater than 7 ml/kg/min. The difference proved to be significant ($P < 0.05$). As in the control group, no difference was seen between high and low arterial PO_2 values.

The ratio of the plateau O_2 uptake to the critical O_2 delivery value gave the critical O_2 extraction ratios, which are shown in Fig. 7. The value of 0.72 agreed quite well with the value found in the earlier study. Although it was unchanged by the high PO_2, the variability in the data was increased. We surmise that this may be the result of some direct effects of higher PO_2 on vascular

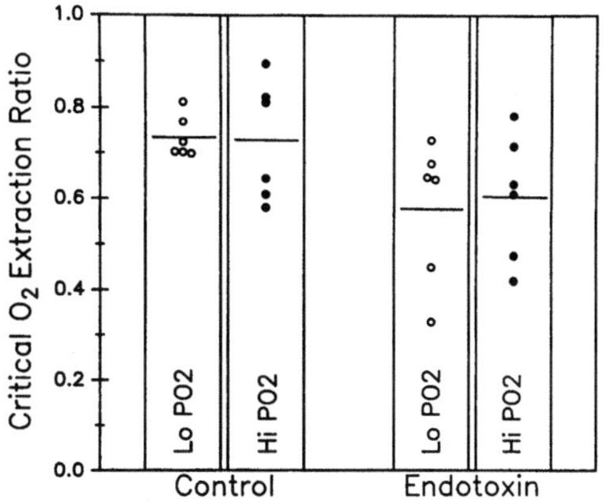

Fig. 7. Critical O_2 extraction in the limbs of control and endotoxic groups at the two levels of arterial PO_2 (from [3])

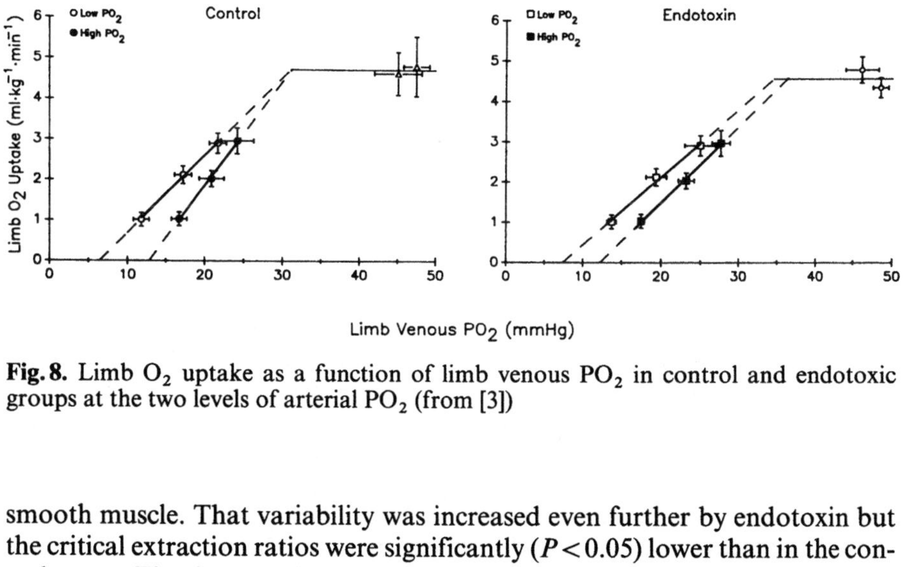

Fig. 8. Limb O_2 uptake as a function of limb venous PO_2 in control and endotoxic groups at the two levels of arterial PO_2 (from [3])

smooth muscle. That variability was increased even further by endotoxin but the critical extraction ratios were significantly ($P<0.05$) lower than in the control group. That increase in variability is one of the difficulties of the endotoxin model. Each dog had an individual reaction to the bolus of endotoxin that covered a range from mild to severe, as well as we could judge by the degree of hypotension that ensued. Nevertheless, a similar or worse variability must certainly occur in even a carefully selected patient population.

The reason that increased arterial PO_2 did not aid O_2 extraction may be partially explained by the results in Fig. 8. Limb O_2 uptake is shown in this figure as a function of limb venous PO_2. First, consistent with the higher critical O_2 delivery values with endotoxin, the critical venous PO_2 was also significantly higher ($P<0.05$) by about 5 torr. The extrapolation to the abscissa indicates that some form of functional shunting was also taking place. Anatomic shunts are not thought to occur in canine skeletal muscle. To explain how O_2 uptake could fall to zero while there was still a PO_2 of about 10 torr left in venous blood, there are several possibilities. For example, transit time was too

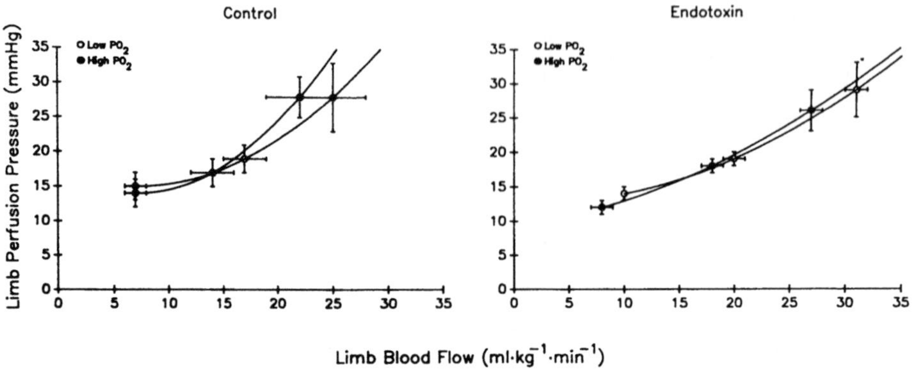

Fig. 9. Mean values ($\pm$SE) of limb perfusion pressure and blood flow in the control *(left panel)* and endotoxin treated *(right panel)* groups (from [3])

short to allow diffusion of O_2 out of the capillary. This may have been due to a large diffusion barrier at the capillary wall, which some investigators feel is normally present. Given the facts that the venous PO_2 became higher with higher arterial PO_2 and lower flow, we think that the best explanation is pre-capillary diffusion across adjacent arterioles and venules, a process that is known to occur. This is a diffusional shunt, therefore, which would prevent an elevated arterial PO_2 from aiding any impaired diffusion at the capillary level because it would largely be dissipated before reaching that level.

In earlier discussions [5, 6, 8] of the possible origins of pathological O_2 supply dependency, the loss of vascular reactivity and autoregulatory capacity were suggested to be important functional correlates. In their study of gut segments in endotoxic dogs, Nelson et al. [14] saw reactive hyperemia practically disappear. In muscle, on the other hand, Samsel et al. [18] said that vigorous reactive hyperemia was present at all times in their endotoxic dogs. Another and more classical way to look at autoregulatory function is shown in Fig. 9. Average pressure-flow points are shown for the two groups of dogs. Autoregulation is the process by which muscle attempts to maintain flow constant with changes in perfusion pressure. The steeper curve and lesser range of flows seen in the control group indicates that autoregulatory function was better than in the endotoxic group. This different conclusion from the one reached by Nelson et al. [15] may be attributed to a more sensitive index of autoregulatory function.

It seems clear from the results we obtained and from the earlier studies that were just cited, that muscle probably does not contribute strongly to the pathological disturbance in the ability of peripheral tissues to extract O_2 in the septic condition, whereas gut probably does. Nevertheless, our studies showed that signs of functional disturbance in O_2 delivery to skeletal muscle can be detected in the endotoxic animal. This information may take on critical importance in the case of respiratory muscles. Any functional disturbance in them may contribute to the mandatory use of mechanical ventilation in ARDS and septic patients.

The question must be asked, however, "Are our determinations of a critical O_2 delivery or extraction ratio in animal models the same kind of information that has been forthcoming from studies of patients?" The reason for asking is that most of the information obtained from patients does not include an entire range of O_2 delivery values, for obvious reasons, and most often they do not approach the low values at which O_2 extraction ratios are increased to 0.5 or greater as they were at the critical levels in the animal studies. More typically, abnormal O_2 supply dependency has been identified with O_2 extractions of 0.3. Some reason for that can be found in the last group of animal experiments that I will describe next.

The experiments were similar to those just described except that, instead of only three points in the supply-dependent zone, we obtained nine points from very low O_2 delivery rates to above the normal found in the anesthetized dog. We wished to describe the O_2 uptake-O_2 delivery relationship for the limb muscles much more completely. Once again a control group of six dogs was compared with another group of six given endotoxin together with sufficient red cells and dextran to restore mean arterial pressure and cardiac output to acceptable levels. Figure 10 shows O_2 uptake as a function of delivery. The experimental points obtained for individual dogs are connected by straight lines, but all of the data were fitted with a third-order regression equation. This acknowledged the fact that this is really a curvilinear relationship that can only be approximated by two straight lines. If we had used the latter analysis, the control group would have shown a line in the so-called plateau region with a slightly negative slope, whereas the endotoxin group showed a flat or even a slightly positive slope above the critical threshold of delivery. A more marked curvilinearity and greater variability in the data are also evident in the endotoxic group.

When O_2 extraction is shown as a function of O_2 delivery, as in Fig. 11, another difference between the two group becomes evident. Extraction changes in an almost linear fashion with delivery in the control group but not in the endotoxic group. There is much more flattenning as the higher ranges of de-

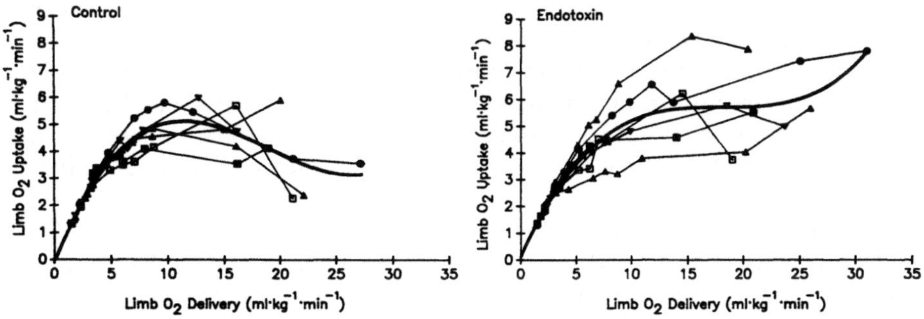

Fig. 10. O_2 uptake as O_2 delivery was progressively lowered in pump-perfused, vascularly isolated limbs of two groups of dogs, control *(left panel)* and endotoxin treated *(right panel)*. The *thicker line* is the curve fitted by a third-order regression equation to all of the data

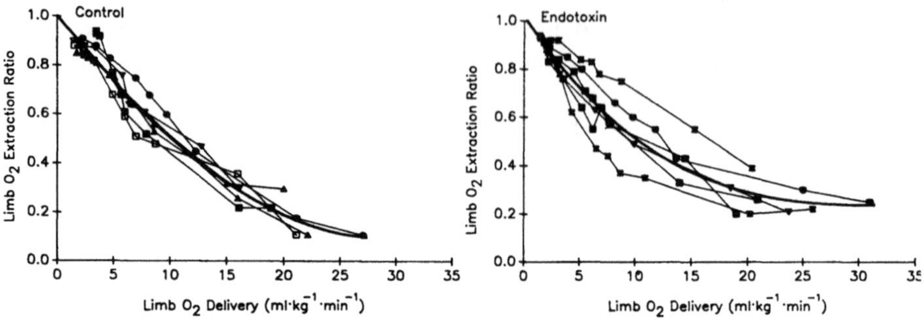

Fig. 11. Limb O_2 extraction ratio as a function of O_2 delivery in the same experiments shown in Fig. 10

livery are approached and the relationship becomes quite flat above a delivery of about 15 ml/kg/min and at an extraction of about 0.25. The slight increase in O_2 uptake with any increase in delivery at levels above the usual critical value and with an extraction that stays fixed near 0.3 is a very close approximation of the type of data obtained from patients with abnormal O_2 supply dependency. If the dogs in our endotoxic group were able to increase extraction almost as much as the normal dogs at low O_2 delivery rates, why would they not extract more if they were supply dependent at a higher delivery rate? That is the question that now challenges us. One answer may lie in the injury rendered to the endothelium and vascular control mechanisms by the various immune and defense reactions elicited by a septic challenge. That might explain a failure to recruit more capillary surface area but it would not explain an increase in O_2 uptake with an increase in supply at relatively high rates of O_2 delivery. This was seen in one-half of the endotoxic dogs and in only one of the control groups. An uncoupling of oxidative phosphorylation because of mitochondrial injury is certainly a possible explanation for this aspect of supply dependency. Supportive evidence for this can be found. Yet another explanation is that continuing formation of reactive O_2 metabolites through extramitochondrial pathways may account for the increase. Because the oxidases responsible for the formation of reactive O_2 metabolites generally have a lesser affinity for O_2 than does cytochrome oxidase, they would desaturate at higher values of PO_2 and could contribute to the shallow slope of supply dependence typically seen in the higher ranges of O_2 delivery. Whether their O_2 use is quantitatively sufficient to account for the amount of change that is seen is unknown at this time but their possible role deserves a closer examination.

In summary, disturbances in the ability of peripheral tissues to extract O_2 can be produced in dogs treated with endotoxin. Other animal models such as sheep or even rats with cecal ligation offer other advantages, depending on the experimental goals. All of them provide us with opportunities to make experimental interventions designed not only to discover the mechanisms of unusual O_2 supply dependency, but to discover why so many of the patients who exhibit it die. The very high mortality associated with this condition in ARDS and sepsis imparts a definite urgency to continuing research with animal models to provide a rational basis for the treatment of such patients.

References

1. Babior BM (1984) The respiratory burst of phagocytes. J Clin Invest 73:599–601
2. Bihari D, Smithies M, Gimson A, Tinker J (1987) The effects of vasodilation with prostacyclin on oxygen delivery and uptake in critically ill patients. N Engl J Med 317:397–403
3. Bredle DL, Samsel RW, Schumacker PT, Cain SM (1989) Critical O_2 delivery to skeletal muscle at high and low PO_2 in endotoxemic dogs. J Appl Physiol (in press)
4. Cain SM (1978) Effects of time and vasoconstrictor tone on O_2 extraction during hypoxic hypoxia. J Appl Physiol 45:219–224
5. Cain SM (1984) Supply dependency of oxygen uptake in ARDS: myth or reality? Am J Med Sci 288:119–124
6. Cain SM (1986) Assessment of tissue oxygenation. Crit Care Clin 2:537–550
7. Cain SM (1988) Tolerable limits of hypoxia in muscle. In: Sutton JR, Coates C, Houston CS (eds) Hypoxia: the tolerable limits. Benchmark, Indianapolis, Ind., chap 7
8. Cain SM (1989) Mechanisms of limited oxygen delivery in sepsis and adult respiratory distress syndrome. In: Reinhart K, Eyrich K (eds) Sepsis – an interdisciplinary challenge. Springer, Berlin Heidelberg New York, pp 281–294
9. Cain SM, Chapler CK (1985) Circulatory responses to 2,4-dinitrophenol in dog limb during normoxia and hypoxia. J Appl Physiol 59:698–705
10. Gilbert EM, Haupt MT, Mandanas RY, Huaringa AJ, Carlson RW (1986) The effect of fluid loading, blood transfusion, and catecholamine infusion on oxygen delivery and consumption in patients with sepsis. Am Rev Respir Dis 134:873–878
11. Granger HJ, Shepherd AP (1979) Dynamics and control of the microcirculation. Adv Biomed Eng 7:1–63
12. Gutierrez G, Pohil RJ (1986) Oxygen consumption is linearly related to O_2 supply in critically ill patients. J Crit Care 1:45–53
13. Haupt MT, Gilbert EM, Carlson RW (1985) Fluid loading increases oxygen consumption in septic patients. Am Rev Respir Dis 131:912–916
14. Nelson DP, Beyer C, Samsel RW, Wood LDH, Schumacker PT (1987) Pathological supply dependence of O_2 uptake during bacteremia in dogs. J Appl Physiol 63:1487–1492
15. Nelson DP, Samsel RW, Wood LDH, Schumacker PT (1988) Pathologic supply dependence of systemic and intestinal O_2 uptake during endotoxemia in dogs. J Appl Physiol 64:2410–2419
16. Reinhart K, Rudolph T, Bredle DL, Cain SM (1989) O_2 uptake in bled dogs after resuscitation with hypertonic saline or hydroxyethylstarch. Am J Physiol 257(Heart Circ Physiol 26):H238–H243
17. Reiss M, Roos D (1978) Differences in oxygen metabolism of phagocytosing monocytes and neutrophils. J Clin Invest 61:480–488
18. Samsel RW, Nelson DP, Sander WP, Wood LDH, Schumacker PT (1988) Effect of endotoxin on systemic and skeletal muscle O_2 extraction. J Appl Physiol 65:1377–1382

O_2 Transport and Tissue Oxygenation in the Critically Ill

C. W. Bryan-Brown and G. Gutierrez

Introduction

The normal physiology of oxygen transport and tissue oxygenation were basically understood after the work of Krogh (1919 a, b) and Barcroft (1920). The requirements of the transport system were listed as:

1. Hemoglobin (deficit = anemia)
2. Oxygenation (deficit = hypoxia)
3. Flow (deficit = low cardiac output)

It was also understood that distribution of blood flow could affect oxygenation. Probably under the influence of Haldane, a Lancet (Anonymous 1920) editorial even gave the suggestion that hemoglobin might not release oxygen as easily as usual. This showed that "affinity" hypoxia was a consideration even 70 years ago.

As far as tissue oxygenation was concerned, there were basically three methods of increasing the supply to tissues in need:

1. Recruitment of nonconducting capillaries
2. Increased diameter of conducting capillaries
3. Decreased transit time through conducting capillaries

The more the clear and rational premises of our forebears are examined, the less easy it becomes to find rational hypotheses on which to develop therapeutic approaches to the management of the critically ill (Bryan-Brown 1987). This confusion is further compounded by acute illness, so that it becomes difficult to define the optimum or even minimal parameters of arterial oxygen tension (PaO_2) hemoglobin concentration ([Hb]), cardiac output, and the position of the oxyhemoglobin dissociation curve needed to give a patient the best chances of survival. In addition, it may well turn out that a decreased transit time of the erythrocyte through a tissue may not give it time to deliver its oxygen load efficiently (Gutierrez 1986).

What is different about oxygenation in the critically ill? One of the earliest recognized phenomenon was that oxygen utilization ($\dot{V}O_2$) is increased. Over the past 20 years, clinical research has shown that the delivery system becomes less competent, and a greater oxygen transport ($\dot{T}O_2$) is needed to maintain the same $\dot{V}O_2$.

In the early 1970s, we would watch septic patients with ever-increasing $\dot{T}O_2$ and diminishing extraction ratios ($\dot{V}O_2/\dot{T}O_2$) with forebodings that were usually correct. The patients did not recover (Bryan-Brown 1988 a), and died with multisystem organ failure. The thinking quickly turned to oxygen conformity. The critically ill, particularly septic, patients needed not only a much greater $\dot{T}O_2$ but also had a supply dependency over and above normal. We seemed to demonstrate that $\dot{V}O_2$ was determined by $\dot{T}O_2$. This idea was intriguingly developed by Peirce (1977), who suggested that, man, normally an *oxygen regulator*, became an *oxygen conformer* in shock states – a reversion to a more primitive vertebrate physiology, as found in fishes.

The phenomenon of oxygen conformity may well have looked convincing because $\dot{V}O_2$ and $\dot{T}O_2$ were calculated with very short time cardiac output measurements. In patients on high levels of ventilatory support, cardiac output measurements were shown by Snyder and Powner (1982) to vary by as much as 70%. During these "snapshot views" mixed venous oxygen content ($C\bar{v}O_2$) is unlikely to change, and $\dot{V}O_2$ and $\dot{T}O_2$ would go up and down together, following changes in cardiac output, not changes in metabolism.

It now appears that a major part of the problem is a combination of greater cellular energy requirements and inefficient oxygenation in the tissues (Cain 1984; Taylor et al. 1987).

Cellular Changes

Increased Metabolism

The majority of "resting" cellular energy is spent on pumping substances across membranes, either against gradients or faster than passive diffusion would normally allow (Hochachka 1986; Hochachka and Guppy 1987). If the cell membranes are rendered more permeable to unwanted substances, the energy and oxygen requirements are increased to keep the ion and other pumps working at a greater rate to maintain a normal consistency of the cytosol. If oxygen delivery is not increased to meet this demand, hypoxia will further vitiate the cell, increasing the damage. Thus, the mediators of shock, e.g., the monokines, amines, complement factors, and arachidonic acid metabolites, increase the need for oxygen by the cell. It has been noted that the toxicity of polyene antibiotics on the medullary thick ascending loop of Henle (a poisoning by increasing membrane permeability) can be reduced when the reabsorptive function of the cell is countered by ouabain (Brezis et al. 1984 a, b). This oxygen-sensitive part of the kidney is thus able to maintain vital function if no energy is used for its special functions.

Other vital energy-requiring reactions for repair and maintenance (generally protein synthesis) are also needed to maintain cellular viability, although their contribution to the increased metabolism is probably less than the acute processes that prevent cell death from acute changes in membrane permeability.

Adenosine Triphosphate (ATP) Turnover

When cells are undergoing metabolically active processes, ATP levels are not found to fall until the balance between oxygen requirements and oxygen supply has fallen extremely low (Clark et al. 1987). At this point a major portion of the creatine phosphate (PCr) stored in the cell will have been used up in the creatine kinase (CK) reaction.

$$PCr + ADP + H^+ \leftrightarrow ATP + Cr$$

PCr would seem to be an unnecessary product to have available for the spatial buffering of cytosolic ATP concentration, given that aerobically derived ATP levels change little during moderate muscular activity. In a laboratory model, Connett (1988) were able to show that the absence of PCr would cause but a 3% variation in ATP concentrations.

A "phosphocreatine shuttle," where energy is transported within the cell by the diffusion of PCr, may be a mechanism for coupling mitochondrial energy production with the sites of utilization when these are at a distance, such as in the neuron or muscle cell. During muscle contraction (an event that does not in and of itself use oxygen) adenosine diphosphate (ADP) is produced, and is immediately converted by the CK reaction to ATP. Creatine is then phosphorylated again from mitochondrial sources (Bessman and Geiger 1981). Further development of the "shuttle" model by Meyer et al. (1984) indicates that "spatial" buffering by PCr is probably unnecessary for supplying a constant amount of ATP for cell function.

An exciting new idea has emerged recently that PCr provides the mechanism for buffering the concentrations of ADP and adenine monophosphate (AMP) (Funk et al. 1988). The effect of sudden energy use in the absence of PCr might produce a 3% variation in concentration of ATP, but this would become a fourfold variation in ADP and 16-fold for AMP. ADP and AMP both increase glycolytic activity by stimulating both the phosphofructokinase and pyruvate kinase reactions. The need for "temporal" buffering of these products of ATP hydrolysis becomes apparent. Without PCr, the mean cytosolic concentrations over time would increase. This will give rise to overactive glycolysis. Another problem may arise from increased activity of the adenylate kinase reaction:

$$2\,ADP \leftrightarrow ATP + AMP$$

This further amplifies the production of AMP, and initiates the depletion of the adenylate pool. The accumulation of AMP leads to accelerated glycolysis and lactate production.

Perhaps as a defense against excessive glycolysis, skeletal muscle and other tissues contain the enzyme AMP deaminase, that converts AMP to inosine monophosphate. This deamination occurs more readily in the presence of acidosis. AMP can also be metabolized by 5′-nucleotidase to adenosine, which may diffuse out the cell, further depleting the nucleotide pool. When adenosine diffuses out of the cell it acts as a potent vasodilator, and therefore may provide the already well-perfused tissue with further blood.

The Hyperdynamic State

Thus, the ingredients of the hyperdynamic state can be brought together:

1. Increased metabolic work to maintain ionic gradients
2. Increased glycolysis and lactate production
3. Increased blood flow to tissues with loss of autoregulation and development of a "steal" phenomenon in damaged tissues

Circulatory Support

In their clinical studies on shock patients, Shoemaker et al. (1987) have shown that adequacy of the circulation and oxygen transport to the tissue defined the parameters that predict survival. In addition, hypovolemia is not reliably assessed by even advanced clinical monitoring (Shippy et al. 1984). Both supranormal blood volume and oxygen transport may be needed to maximize survival in shock (Bland et al. 1985). In high-risk patients undergoing surgery, Shoemaker et al. (1988 b) demonstrated that periods of low oxygen uptake, leading to an oxygen debt, were followed by both lethal and nonlethal organ failure. When the trial of prospectively increasing oxygen delivery to supranormal values was performed, surgical morbidity and mortality were markedly improved (Shoemaker et al. 1988 a).

Thus, supplying the circulatory needs of the critically ill patient with increased $\dot{T}O_2$, cardiac output, and blood volume has a salutary effect on survival. Just volume loading of the circulation may be sufficient to increase $\dot{V}O_2$ (Haupt et al. 1985). The vasodilatation, loss of autoregulation, and increased oxygen requirement are satisfied with more delivery.

Pharmacologic Support and Hypovolemia

When the circulation begins to fail or the oxygen transport system becomes insufficient, it has long been recognized (Wiggers and Werle 1942) that the circulation is preferentially diverted to organs that are most supply dependent – e.g., the heart and brain. A simple monitor of this phenomenon has been the measurement of big toe temperature (Joly and Weil 1969). Peripheral and cutaneous circulation is reduced. Another monitor of decreasing skin perfusion is the transcutaneous oxygen electrode. The oxygen tension falls as cutaneous blood flow decreases (Tremper and Shoemaker 1981; Barker and Tremper 1985).

Splanchnic (Kessler et al. 1984; Rowell and Johnson 1984), renal (Brenner et al. 1986), and cutaneous vasoconstriction are the natural defense mechanisms against inadequate oxygen delivery, and this is mediated in large part by the sympathetic nervous system. Considerable hypovolemia can be present before there is an elevation of splanchnic vascular resistance (Price et al. 1966). When using adrenergic drugs, there is therefore the problem of enhancing vascular tone. The result could be to reduce renal meduallary and hepatic blood flow, possibly converting organ insufficiency to failure. Some drugs (e.g., ergotamine) mobilize the circulation by peripheral vasoconstriction, while others (e.g., etilofrine) constrict the splanchnic veins (Stanton-Hicks et al. 1987).

Balancing cardiovascular function with catecholamine support may require very delicate manipulation to keep as many organ systems as possible adequately perfused (Mueller 1986). Afterload reduction to increase cardiac output should also result in increased oxygen uptake. A greater $\dot{T}O_2$ to resting muscle or peripheral vasular beds, as occurs in hepatic cirrhosis, is not necessarily accompanied by increased $\dot{V}O_2$ (Ito et al. 1988). The patient in liver failure appears to have lost control over distribution of the circulation and thus compensates with a hyperdynamic circulation.

Oxygen Transport

Oxygen Tension

The philosophy of "if some is good, more is better" has constantly been an issue in oxygenation. Soon after oxygen was discovered, John Hunter (1776) was suggesting that "the dephlogisticated air recently discovered by Dr. Priestley be more efficacious than common air" for resuscitation. He also proclaimed its ready availability in "bottles and bladders." It seems strange that nearly a century later (Birch 1869) oxygenated bread was being touted as a suitable method of administration. William Osler (1912) was very dubious of the merits of treating pneumonia with oxygen, probably because of recent work on oxygen toxicity to the lungs.

Boerema et al. (1960) demonstrated that at 3 ATA there would be sufficient tension to dissolve enough oxygen in the blood stream to make hemoglobin unnecessary. The man breathing normal air, on the other hand, would theoretically require a cardiac output of over 100 l/min to deliver enough oxygen if hemoglobin were not present (Comroe 1974). Where, between these extremes, should the oxygen tension be to provide the 2 mmHg (0.26 kPa) needed at the mitochondrial end of the transport system (Chance 1965)?

For the critically ill an argument can be made for a great variety of arterial oxygen tensions (PaO_2), mostly depending on circumstance. Inspired oxygen fractions (FiO_2) as low as 0.27 (at sea level) have been shown to interfere witz the ciliary clearance of mucus from the trachea (Laurenzi et al. 1968). On the other hand, oxygen-related clinical pathophysiological disorders of lung function have not been shown to have a significant effect on outcome if the inspired fraction is kept below 0.50. An operational view would probably recommend keeping the PaO_2 above 70 mmHg (9.3 kPa), and using whatever airway maneuvers, including a high FiO_2, to do this. If a PaO_2 can be maintained above 70 mmHg (9.3 kPa) the FiO_2 should be reduced to the 0.35–0.40 range.

The arguments for keeping the PaO_2 at least at 70 mmHg (9.3 kPa) during acute illness are mostly theoretical (Bryan-Brown 1988 b) and based on normal physiology. At this PaO_2 the only organ that should need to recruit blood flow in the microcirculation is the heart, as myocardial oxygen extraction is always near the critical level. As the hemoglobin is well over 90% saturated at this oxygen tension, all other organs should be able to function normally without more cardiac output by extracting more oxygen. Operationally a higher PaO_2 could be beneficial when some organ system is malfunctioning, (e.g., cardiac arrhythmias, depression of the S-T segment, or confusion) and should be tried. If the patient has severe anemia or an otherwise compromised oxygen transport system, a higher PaO_2 is justifiable. On the other hand, unnecessarily high PaO_2 levels may so upset the microcirculation, that small areas of hypoxia arise in tissues due to maldistribution (Carlsson et al. 1985; Lund et al. 1979).

Hemoglobin

Two factors should be considered, oxyhemoglobin dissociation and concentration. The former can probably be dismissed for lack of evidence that patient outcome can be significantly altered by manipulating the affinity of hemoglobin oxygen. For the majority of patients a normal oxyhemoglobin dissociation curve (P_{50} = 27 mmHg, 3.6 kPa) would appear to be optimal and a left shift probably best avoided (Klocke 1987; Gutierrez and Andry 1989).

The minimal acceptable hemoglobin concentration for presurgical and acutely ill patients has long been a source of Delphic opinion, with very little hard data (Rawstron 1976). For a general principle, Carson et al. (1988) were able to demonstrate that anemia was associated with an increased operative mortality, but as many of the patients were bleeding, hypovolemia was not taken into account. In a more discriminating review of data, Shoemaker et al. (1982) were able to show that a [Hb] above 12 $g \cdot dl^{-1}$ favored survival, but a red cell mass at least at the predicted normal was more important.

From the experimental observations of Richardson and Guyton (1959) and Guyton and Richardson (1961), it appears that the optimum hematocrit for delivering oxygen for the least work is 40%–44%. At this level viscosity and content are in balance. Lower hematocrits, produced by isovolemic hemodilution, may be beneficial if there are restrictions in the cardiovascular system. Messmer et al. (1972) introduced this as a deliberate technique, but its value in peripheral vascular disease has been questioned (Wolfe et al. 1985). Cain (1977) was able to show in an isovolemic anemic canine model that VO_2 increased as the hematocrit fell below 27%. This appeared to be due to increased myocardial utilization. When the hematocrit had fallen below 19% in man, Chang et al. (1983) found that they were unable to elevate subnormal wound oxygen tensions by fluid loading. At this level wound healing could be impaired. The restoration of the blood volume would restore wound oxygen tensions normal at higher Hcts.

Extreme Anemia

Miculicz (1890, cited in DaCosta and Kalteyer 1901) noted that when surgical patients had [Hb] less than 20% of normal (2.9 $g \cdot dl^{-1}$ or Hct = 9%), they developed pulmonary edema and died. He therefore would not operate on patients with an [Hb] less than 30% of normal (4.4 $g \cdot dl^{-1}$ or Hct = 14%). This was the lowest [Hb] ever found acceptable in a preoperative patient! As the patients concerned would probably have been breathing anesthetic mixtures with air as a carrier gas, the figures are truly remarkable.

Cain (1977) found that when dogs were isovolemically rendered progressively more anemic, at the critical point (when $\dot{T}O_2$ becomes insufficient to maintain $\dot{V}O_2$, the mixed venous oxygen tension was surprisingly high). It is also shown in similarly treated rats by Borgström et al. (1975), that when the hemoglobin concentration fell below 50% of normal, cerebral blood flow increased more than would have been expected to supply oxygen, i.e., the extraction ratio fell. As the transit time of the red cell in the microcirculation is markedly reduced, Gutierrez (1986) postulated that the oxygen delivery was rendered inefficient because the red cell did not have time to equilibrate with the tissue oxygen tension. An interesting phenomenon pointed out by Cain (1977) was that at the critical point, $\dot{T}O_2$ was the same, whether produced by anemia or hypoxic hypoxia. Gutierrez et al. (1989) found that venous oxygen tension is an unreliable guide to tissue oxygenation under conditions of extreme hypoxia. Therefore, it is possible that muscle oxygen tensions were similar at equivalently low $\dot{T}O_2$ values in hypoxemia and anemia.

The data in man are mainly derived from patients who refuse blood transfusion as a matter of conscience or belief. One of the findings, often to the author's surprise, was that once the circulation was adequately loaded the mixed venous oxygen tension was at a normal or supranormal level (Nearman and Eckhauser 1983; Lichtenstein et al. 1988). Cooling the patient also allowed for the oxygen requirements to be met by the stressed $\dot{T}O_2$.

Summary

Oxygen transport and utilization in the critically ill is stresed by an increased metabolic load, in part produced by the need to maintain ionic equilibrium in the face of increased cell membrane permeability. Cellular metabolic disorder, possibly produced by impairment of the phosphocreatine "shuttle," gives rise to greater transient concentrations of ADP and AMP. Glycolysis, lactic acid production, and depletion of the adenylate pool may result. There is also a loss of autoregulation of the microcirculation, which leads to a need for a greater $\dot{T}O_2$ to supply oxygen needs.

The most successful therapy has been to increase $\dot{T}O_2$ to above normal levels and increase or maintain the circulating blood volume. Pharmacological support of the circulation may make further damage if the extra cardiac output does not get distributed where it is needed. Optimal [Hb] is probably around normal for most patients, and the PaO_2 should be at least 70 mmHg (9.3 kPa).

References

Anonymous (1920) The therapeutic use of oxygen (editorial). Lancet II:365

Barcroft J (1920) On anoxaemia. Lancet II:485–489

Barker SH, Tremper KK (1985) Transcutaneous oxygen tension: a physiological variable for monitoring oxygenation. J Clin Monit 2:130–134

Bessman SP, Geiger PH (1981) Transport of energy in muscle: the phosphorylcreatine shuttle. Science 211:448–452

Birch SB (1869) Some remarks on the exhibition of oxygen as a therapeutic, in connection with a new agreeable and easy form of administration by the stomach. Lancet I:492–493

Bland RD, Shoemaker WC, Abraham E, Cobo JC (1985) Hemodynamic and oxygen transport patterns in surviving and non-surviving postoperative patients. Crit Care Med 13:85–91

Boerema I, Meyne NG, Brummelkamp WK, Bouma S, Mensch MH, Kamermans F, Stern Hanf M, Van Aalderen W (1960) Life without blood. J Cardiovasc Surg 1:133–146

Borgström L, Jóhannsson H, Siesjö BK (1975) The influence of acute normovolemic anemia on cerebral blood flow and oxygen consumption of anesthetized rats. Acta Physiol Scand 93:505

Brenner BM, Zatz R, Ichikawa I (1986) The renal circulation. In: Brenner BM, Rector RF Jr (eds) The kidney. Saunders, Philadelphia, pp 93–123

Brezis MS, Rosen K, Spokes K, Silva P, Epstein FH (1984a) Transport dependent anoxic cell injury in the isolated perfused rat kidney. Am J Pathol 116:327–341

Brezis M, Rosen S, Silva P, Spokes K, Epstein FH (1984b) Polyene toxicity in renal medulla: injury mediated by transport activity. Science 224:60–68

Bryan-Brown CW (1987) Oxygen transport variables and the management of the critically ill: rationalization in pursuit of uncertainty? In: Bryan-Brown CW, Ayres SM (eds) New horizons II. Oxygen transport and utilization. Soc Crit Care Med, Fullerton, Ca, pp 1–12

Bryan-Brown CW (1988a) Current status of multisystem organ failure and possible directions for the future. In: Kvetan V, Askanazi J (eds) Management of patients with multisystem organ failure. Saunders, Philadelphia, pp 237–245 (Anesthesiology clinics of North America, vol 6[1]

Bryan-Brown CW (1988b) Blood flow to organs: parameters for function and survival in critical illness. Crit Care Med 16:170–178

Cain SM (1977) Oxygen delivery and uptake in dogs during anemic and hypoxic hypoxia. J Appl Physiol 42:228

Cain SM (1984) Supply dependency of oxygen uptake in ARDS: myth or reality? Am J Med Sci 288:119–121

Carlsson C, Eintrei C, Ödman S, Lund N (1985) Effects of increases in the inspired oxygen fraction on brain surface oxygen pressure fields and regional cerebral blood flow. Acta Anaesthesiol Scand 29 [Suppl 80]:86

Carson JL, Poses RM, Spence RK, Bonavita G (1988) Severity of anaemia and operative mortality and morbidity. Lancet I:727–729

Chance B (1965) Reaction of oxygen with the respiratory chain in cells and tissues. J Gen Physiol 49:163–188

Chang N, Goodson WH III, Gotrup F, Hunt TK (1983) Direct measurement of wound and tissue oxygen tension in postoperative patients. Ann Surg 197:470–478

Clark BJ, Smith D, Chance B (1987) Metabolic consequences of oxygen transport studied with phosphorus nuclear magnetic spectroscopy. In: Bryan-Brown CW, Ayres SM (eds) New horizons. II Oxygen transport and utilization. Soc Crit Care Med, Fullerton Ca, pp 145–170

Comroe JH (ed) (1974) Physiology of respiration, 2nd edn. Year Book Medical, Chicago, pp 183–196

Connett RJ (1988) Analysis of metabolic control: new insights using scaled creatine kinase mode. Am J Physiol 254:R949

DaCosta JC, Kalteyer FS (1901) The changes induced by ether as an anaesthetic. Ann Surg 34:329–360

Funk C, Clark A Jr, Connett RJ (1988) How phosphocreatine buffers cyclic changes in ATP demand in working muscle. Addendum to ISOTT Proceedings, Ottawa

Gutierrez G (1986) The rate of oxygen release and its effects on capillary O_2 tension: a mathematical analysis. Respir Physiol 63:79–96

Gutierrez G, Andry JM (1989) Increased hemoglobin O_2 affinity does not improve O_2 consumption in hypoxemia. J Appl Physiol 66:837–843

Gutierrez G, Lund N, Acero AL, Marini C (1989) The relationship of venous PO_2 to muscle PO_2 during hypoxemia. J Appl Physiol 67:1093–1099

Guyton AC, Richardson TQ (1961) Effect of hematocrit on venous return. Circ Res 9:157–163

Haupt MT, Gilbert EM, Carlson RW (1985) Fluid loading increases oxygen consumption in septic patients with lactic acidosis. Am Rev Respir Dis 131:912–916

Hochachka PW (1986) Defense strategies against hypoxia and hypothermia. Science 231:234–241

Hochachka PW, Guppy M (1987) Metabolic arrest and the control of biological time. Harvard university Press, pp 10–35

Ito K, Ramirez-Schon G, Shah PM, Del Guercio LRM (1988) Functioning hepatic cell mass and the hyperdynamic state of cirrhosis. Surg Gynecol Obstet 167:180–186

Joly H, Weil MH (1969) Temperature of the great toe as an indication of the severity of shock. Circulation 39:131–138

Kessler M, Hoper J, Harrison KD, Skilasinska K, Klovekorn WP, Sebening F, Volkholz HJ, Beier I, Kernbach C, Rettig V, Richter H (1984) Tissue O_2 supply under normal and pathological conditions. Adv Exp Med Biol 169:68–80

Klocke RA (1987) Oxygen transport for the red cell to the mitochondrion. In: Bryan-Brown CW, Ayres SM (eds) New horizons. II. Oxygen transport and utilization. Soc Crit Care Med, Fullerton Ca, pp 239–270

Krogh A (1919 a) The number and distribution of capillaries in muscle with calculations of the oxygen pressure head necessary for supplying the tissue. J Appl Physiol 52:409–415

Krogh A (1919 b) The supply of oxygen to the tissues and the regulation of capillary circulation. J Physiol 52:457–474

Laurenzi GA, Vin S, Guaraneri JJ (1968) Adverse effect of oxygen on tracheal mucus flow. N Engl J Med 279:333

Lichtenstein A, Eckhart WF, Swanson KH, Vacanti CA, Zapol WM (1988) Unplanned intraoperative and postoperative hemodilution: oxygen transport and consumption during severe anemia. Anesthesiology 69:119–122

Lund N, Lewis DH, Löfström JB, Odman S (1979) Skeletal muscle oxygen tension: a comparison of normal humans and critically ill patients. Microvasc Res 17(3):S22

Messmer K, Sunder-Plassman L, Klovekorn WP, Holper K (1972) Circulatory significance of hemodilution: rheologic changes and limitations. Adv Microcirc 4:1–77

Meyer RA, Sweeney HL, Kushmerick M (1984) A simple analysis of the "phosphocreatine shuttle." Am J Physiol 246:C365–377

Mueller HS (1986) Catecholamine support of the critically ill cardiac patient. Inotropic agents versus vasopressor: alpha- or beta-adrenergic agonists or both? Intensive Crit Care Digest 5:36–39

Nearman HS, Eckhauser ML (1983) Postoperative management of a severely anemic Jehovah's Witness. Crit Care Med 11:142–143

Osler W (ed) (1912) The principles and practice of medicine. Appleton, New York, p 101

Peirce EC II (1977) Extracorporeal membrane oxygenation for acute respiratory insufficiency: current status. In: Bregman E (ed) Mechanical support of the failing heart and lungs. Appleton, New York, pp 143–163

Price HL, Deutsch S, Marshall BE, Stephen GW, Behar MG, Neufeld H (1966) Hemodynamic and metabolic effects of hemorrhage in man, with particular reference to the splanchnic circulation. Circ Res 18:469–474

Rawstron RE (1976) Preoperative hemoglobin levels. Anaesth Intensive Care 4:175–185

Richardson TQ, Guyton AC (1959) Effects of polycythemia and anemia on cardiac output and other circulatory factors. Am J Physiol 197:1167–1170

Rowell LB, Johnson JM (1984) Role of the splanchnic circulation in reflex control of the cardiovascular system. In: Shepherd AP, Granger DN (eds) Physiology of the intestinal circulation. Raven, New York, pp 153–163

Shippy CR, Appel PL, Shoemaker WC (1984) Reliability of clinical monitoring to assess blood volume in critically ill patients. Crit Care Med 12:107–112

Shoemaker WC, Appel PL, Bland R, Hopkins JA, Chang P (1982) Clinical trial of an algorithm for prediction in acute circulatory failure. Crit Care Med 10:390–397

Shoemaker WC, Appel PL, Kram HB (1987) The role of oxygen transport patterns in the pathophysiology, prediction of outcome and therapy of shock and critical illness. In: Bryan-Brown CW, Ayres SM (eds) New horizons. II. Oxygen transport and utilization. Soc Crit Care Med, Fullerton Ca, pp 65–92

Shoemaker WC, Appel PL, Kram HB (1988 a) Tissue oxygen debt as a determinant of lethal and non-lethal postoperative organ failure. Crit Care Med 16:1117–1120

Shoemaker WC, Appel PL, Kram HB, Waxman K, Lee TS (1988 b) Prospective trial of supranormal values of survivors as therapeutic goals in high risk surgical patients. Chest 94:1176–1186

Snyder JV, Powner DJ (1982) Effects of mechanical ventilation on the measurement of cardiac output by thermodilution. Crit Care Med 10:677–682

Stanton-Hicks M, Hock A, Stumeier KD, Arndt JO (1987) Venoconstrictor agents mobilize blood from different sources and increase intrathoracic filling during epidural anesthesia in supine humans. Anesthesiology 66:317–322

Taylor AE, Hernandez L, Perry M, Smith M, Womack BS (1987) Overview of tissue oxygen utilization. In: Bryan-Brown CW, Ayres SM (eds) New horizons. II. Oxygen transport and utilization. Soc Crit Care Med, Fullerton Ca, pp 13–23

Tremper KK, Shoemaker WC (1981) Transcutaneous oxygen monitoring of critically ill adults with and without low flow shock. Crit Care Med 9:706–709

Wiggers CJ, Werle JM (1942) Cardiac and peripheral resistance factors as determinants of circulatory failure in hemorrhagic shock. Am J Physiol 136:421–432

Wolfe JHN, Waller DG, Chapman MG, Blackford HN, Prout WG (1985) The effect of hemodilution upon patients with intermittent claudication. Surg Gynecol Obstet 160:347–351

The Role of Tissue Hypoxia in Multiple Organ Failure*

W. J. Sibbald, A. Bersten, and F. S. Rutledge

Introduction

The metabolic theory of circulatory control proposes that the regulated variable is tissue oxygen (O_2) flux [1, 2] and that the primary function of the circulation is to, thereby, continuously couple blood flow to cellular O_2 need. In order to establish a framework for the subsequent discussion of the role of tissue hypoxia in multiple systems organ failure (MSOF), we will briefly review the normal processes responsible for appropriately matching tissue O_2 delivery (DO_2) with O_2 need, i.e., the intrinsic control of the cardiovascular system [1].

Conceptually, intact metabolic autoregulation requires that tissue DO_2 increase during periods of increased tissue O_2 need to prevent tissue hypoxia [1, 2]. This compensation is normally achieved by: (a) a decrease in precapillary sphincter tone which facilitates augmented O_2 extraction (O_2E) by increasing perfused capillary surface area; (b) a decrease in arteriolar tone which augments regional blood flows (Q), provided that arterial perfusion pressures are not concurrently depressed; and (c) an increase in systemic Q, i.e., cardiac output (CO). A further role may be attributed to the control of arteriolar tone, as changes in this autoregulatory process also affect the number of perfused capillaries during periods of high resting tone [3]. In individual organs, there is variability in the compensatory circulatory mechanisms used to maintain tissue O_2 availability. Thus, an increase in microregional O_2E is the most important response of the intestinal microcirculation to increased O_2 needs [1], while the heart primarily responds to an increased O_2 need with an increase in Q at all of the systemic, regional, and microregional levels [4]. At the whole-body level, the integration of these varied circulatory changes which subserve tissue DO_2 is associated with an increase in venous return which thereby supports the increase in systemic Q [2].

Following adequate "ebb" phase resuscitation, the "flow" phase of early MSOF secondary to sepsis is typically a hypermetabolic state [5]. The measurable increase of systemic VO_2 in MSOF has been correlated with augmented metabolic activity created by the normal inflammatory response to tissue injury, and, therefore, has origin in an increase in neutrophil chemotaxis and phagocytosis. Remote from the primary focus of inflammatory injury,

* Work reported herein was supported by grants from the Medical Research Council of Canada and the Ontario Heart and Stroke Foundation

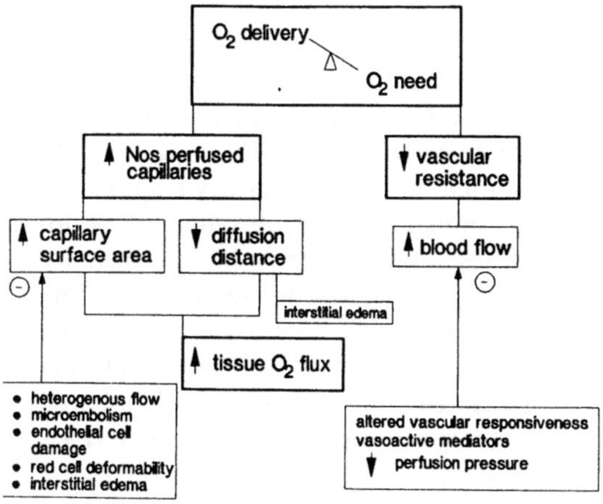

Fig. 1

pyrexia, an increase in heart work, acute phase protein synthesis, muscle catabolism, and the maintenance of cellular osmotic integrity further increase tissue O_2 needs in septic-MSOF [5–8]. These heightened tissue needs for O_2 and other nutrients in septic-MSOF will augment the adverse sequelae of any abnormality in the circulatory control of tissue DO_2 on organ function and cellular integrity.

The goal of this review is to analyze evidence supporting the hypothesis that the progression of MSOF is related to the effects of cellular hypoxia. This will be done by reviewing both whole body and isolated organ studies which have examined the relationship between tissue O_2 need and O_2 availability in MSOF secondary to sepsis. Although many different processes may be operative, it is our belief that the final common pathway of the diverse clinical insults that underly the development of MSOF is a failure of metabolic autoregulation, and, therefore, the development of tissue injury due to hypoxia.

Hypoxia may result in tissue injury through a number of mechanisms. Of sufficient duration, cellular hypoxia on any of a circulatory (stagnant), hypoxic anemic or histiotoxic basis will result in irreversible damage to the cellular metabolic machinery, and necrosis will thereby ensue. Hypoxia followed by reperfusion is also an important mechanism of human disease through the generation of toxic reactive oxygen species (ROS) in excess of normal tissue antioxidant defence mechanisms. The histology of hypoxic-ischemic versus hypoxic-reperfusion injury is remarkably similar. Thus, pathological studies describing tissue injury on an ischemic basis cannot often distinguish between hypoxic and hypoxic-reperfusion mechanisms. In addition to pathological studies, organ injury secondary to hypoxia may also be inferred from studies in isolated organs which demonstrate biochemical evidence of anaerobic metabolism and/or depressed whole organ function.

Whole Body Studies

A number of clinical studies in patients with septic MSOF have demonstrated a strong linkage between the level of systemic DO_2, biochemical evidence of anaerobic metabolism, and the subsequent development of MSOF. Thus, Abraham and coworkers correlated an augmented central circulatory response to increased tissue O_2 needs, i.e., increased systemic DO_2, and outcome following trauma or during sepsis; nonsurvivors of these illnesses were characterized by a lower systemic DO_2 than were survivors [9]. The concept that a "supranormal" systemic DO_2 was positively correlated with survival and negatively correlated with an increase in arterial (lactate) was confirmed by Rashkin in normotensive ARDS patients [10]. Despite an increase in systemic Q and systemic DO_2, Fowler further demonstrated a direct correlation between death and arterial acidemia in ARDS patients [11]; the decreased pH in Fowler's study may have reflected the presence of excessive anaerobic metabolism consequent upon a failure at any of the central, regional, or microcirculatory levels of the circulation to ensure an adequate tissue DO_2 to maintain the aerobic state. Subsequently, Bihari and coworkers demonstrated that an infusion of prostacyclin uncovered a "covert O_2 debt" in nonsurvivors of MSOF [12]. Further evidence that tissue hypoxia may be a fundamental characteristic of diseases which could progress to MSOF was provided by Grum with the demonstration of elevated levels of ATP degradation products in critically-ill patients [13]. In a similar group of critically ill patients, Liaw found that tissue high-energy phosphate stores were depressed and proposed that mitochondrial dysfunction due to tissue O_2 lack was the cause of this observation [14]. From these clinical studies at the "whole-body" level, it seems reasonable to conclude that a failure of metabolic autoregulation to maintain adequate tissue O_2 flux is characteristic of the sequence of events which result in MSOF, and ultimately death, in critically ill patients.

Single Organ Studies

The remainder of this review will focus on individual organ studies which would support the hypothesis that MSOF is related to the cumulative effects of multiorgan injury on a hypoxic basis. In isolated organ studies, injury secondary to hypoxia may be inferred by a demonstration of depressed function or the identification of pathological characteristics felt typical of hypoxic-ischemic injury. Potential mechanisms for such injury will be explored and the possibility of therapeutic intervention will be briefly discussed.

The Myocardium

It has been proposed that depressed biventricular contractility in sepsis [15] and septic shock [16] is caused by a circulating MDF [17]. However, it is also possible that hypoxic-induced cellular injury also contributes to a depression of ventricular contractile reserve in septic-MSOF.

Despite an increase in Q heart, we found widespread but patchy necrosis of myofibrils in a nonhypotensive septic model characterized by depressed ventricular contractile reserve [18]. In clinical studies of septic shock, similar pathological characteristics have also been described in the heart, albeit to a greater extent [19]. However, biochemical evaluation of myocardial metabolism has not universally demonstrated supportive evidence of significant myocardial hypoxia in sepsis. Dhainaut found that net myocardial lactate production by the myocardium characterized only the minority of patients studied with septic shock in whom myocardial metabolism was evaluated following catheterization of the coronary sinus [20]. Such "whole-organ" studies may, however, not reflect the presence of subtle, yet significant alterations in aerobic/anaerobic conditions at the microregional or cellular level [21]. Thus, in our studies, we have consistently found patchy myocardial necrosis in hyperdynamic sepsis [18] and further noted that the presence of hypoxic conditions in the myocardium, as evidenced by net transmyocardial lactate production, was accompanied by a failure to augment systemic Q to the heightened levels typical of sepsis (unpublished).

If hypoxic injury to the myocardium occurs in sepsis, what could be the mechanism? It is unlikely that hypoxic injury occurs due to a direct "toxic" effect of sepsis or due to an increase in any of the phlogistic mediators associated with this disease on mitochondrial function. Dawson reported that sepsis augmented rather than damaged mitochondrial function up to 4 h after death in a murine model of endotoxemia [22]. Further, at both the central and regional levels of myocardial O_2 flux, few studies have documented any significant depression in DO_2. Both Cunnion [23] and Dhainaut [20] demonstrated an increase in coronary sinus blood flows in clinical studies of septic shock, although evidence that inefficient myocardial O_2 utilization characterized patients with septic shock was described [23]. Our description of a patchy distribution to myofibrillar injury in an hyperdynamic septic model in the presence of both an elevated systemic Q and Q heart, inferred a primary microcirculatory basis for metabolic "dysregulation" within the myocardium during normotensive sepsis. In support of this concept, both the Cunnion [23] and Dhainaut [20] studies demonstrated a depression of myocardial O_2E. This data suggested the probability of a significant defect in O_2 exchange within the coronary microcirculation, as has been demonstrated in whole body O_2E studies of patients with septic-MSOF [24]. We feel that regional heterogeneity in myocardial blood flows, and hence in myocardial O_2E during septic-MSOF, may well result in significant hypoxic-induced injury to the myocardium and, therefore, in depressed biventricular contractility [25]. A similar mechanism contributing to myocardial dysfunction in acute ischemic heart disease has been proposed by Conway and Weiss [26].

Although inefficient myocardial O_2E has been proposed in human [23] and animal [25] models of sepsis and septic shock, thereby implicating a microregional defect in O_2 flux within the myocardium, the demonstration that ATP levels were elevated in the heart of a murine peritonitis model was used to argue for the adequacy of net myocardial DO_2 to subserve O_2 needs [27]. However, recent NMR studies of skeletal muscle in a small animal model of sepsis have demonstrated that the effects of significant intracellular hypoxia could be found despite normal ATP levels, the latter which were maintained at the expense of the high-energy storage compound PC_r [28].

Although our data [18, 25] may require that alternate modes of injury other than hypoxia be considered to explain the patchy tissue injury in the septic myocardium, a plausible explanation would be that significant heterogeneity in LV blood flows at the microregional level during sepsis result in focal cell hypoxia that may well be undetected in the earliest stages of septic-MSOF by the more global evaluations of myocardial metabolism [21, 26]. Whether such injury occurs on the basis of reperfusion, or for other reasons, cannot yet be concluded.

The Kidney

A number of hyperdynamic septic animal models have evaluated the (sepsis × renal function) interaction on organ function. Following cecal ligation and puncture in rats, Townsend's laboratory described a fall in renal energy charge in association with a decrease in both the effective renal plasma flow and glomerular filtration rate [29]. This data may indicate that renal dysfunction on an hypoxic basis followed a hypoperfusion-induced fall in DO_2 kidney during these septic studies. Notwithstanding the likelihood of significant variation in para-amino hippuric acid clearance during sepsis, these data [30] also did not support previous conclusions that Q kidney was equivocally altered during sepsis [31, 32]. Thus, other studies have described an unchanged Q kidney in similar hyperdynamic septic models using radioactive microspheres to measure changes in the distribution of organ Q [32, 33]. It may be concluded that Q kidney is not usually in hyperdynamic sepsis, although autoregulation of Q kidney through the normal ranges of arterial perfusing pressure may well be abnormal in sepsis.

Richmond et al. examined the effectiveness of fluid loading in maintaining renal function following cecal ligation and perforation in sheep [34]. Animals on maintenance fluids failed to increase CO and developed an increase in plasma renin with a concurrent fall in creatinine clearance. These changes were prevented in a cohort group of animals who were fluid-loaded, while microsphere-determined Q kidney was unchanged in similarly treated animals [35]. However, when the septic insult was more severe, a fluid loaded, hyperdynamic, and normotensive state failed to prevent the onset of renal failure in this septic sheep model [36]. In the latter study, the findings of an increase in plasma renin, a high urinary osmolality and a fall in free-water clearance suggested that the kidney perceived a hypoperfused state despite normal arterial perfusion pressures and an increase in systemic Q. Therefore, although Q kidney may be increased in hyperdynamic sepsis, functional studies support the concept that DO_2 kidney may, generally, be insufficient to meet the increased renal metabolic needs noted in this disease. This would, therefore, establish a process by which hypoxic-induced cell injury in the kidney could contribute to renal dysfunction in sepsis, however, whether alterations in DO_2 kidney at the microregional level could account for the hypoxic-induced fall in renal energy charge noted in Townsend's study [29] has not been further examined in the septic kidney.

The Liver

Similar to the kidney, a fall in effective hepatic blood flow in septic rats has been correlated with a fall in energy charge and an elevation in the lactate to pyruvate ratio [31, 37, 38]. This data supported the concept that a hypoxic insult may underly the hepatic dysfunction in sepsis and MSOF, despite a systemic normotensive and hyperdynamic state, since the depression in Q liver preceded the change in energy charge [31]. In contrast, other studies have reported a sustained increase in Q liver when radiolabelled microspheres were used to measure organ Q [32, 39]. However, depending on the calculated portal flows in these latter microsphere experiments, total Q liver may have been either decreased or unchanged [32].

We consider it probable that DO_2 liver is, therefore, frequently depressed in hyperdynamic sepsis. A depression in hepatic DO_2 may occur secondary to a decrease in any or all of the hepatic arterial flow, portal vein flow, or in portal vein O_2 saturation in hyperdynamic sepsis. The liver is also vulnerable to a further depression in DO_2 as a consequence of therapy employed in the treatment of sepsis. For example, we found that PEEP therapy in septic sheep reduced hepatic arterial flows out of proportion to any concurrent decrease in systemic Q [39], while Beyer found that hepatic tissue O_2 tensions also fell with the application of PEEP [40].

In combination with an increase in hepatic O_2 need consequent upon the augmented synthesis of acute-phase proteins in sepsis, and a likely fall in portal vein O_2 saturation due to an increase in gut O_2 extraction, it is probable that hepatic DO_2 is frequently depressed below hepatic O_2 need in hyperdynamic sepsis. This conclusion is further supported by pathologic studies of the liver in a model of hyperdynamic sepsis which demonstrated evidence of tissue injury, apparently on an ischemic basis [18]. Thus, hepatic dysfunction in sepsis could well be initiated, or aggravated, by the development of hypoxia at the cellular level.

The Bowel

The splanchnic circulation normally participates in the defence of tissue DO_2 to heart and brain during states of globally reduced O_2 availability through a diversion in its flow to the vital organs. Within the circulatory system, this organ is well-suited for such compensation, since it normally demonstrates considerable O_2E reserve. Although abnormalities in Q bowel in septic-MSOF have not been as extensively studies as in other organs, some inferences can be made from available data.

In clinical studies, Dahn found that splanchnic O_2 consumption was increased in septic patients and that the prerequisite increase in O_2 availability was principally supported by an increase in O_2E rather than an increase in local DO_2 [7].

In a number of animal models of hyperdynamic sepsis, Q bowel has been either unchanged [32] or increased from the nonseptic state [33, 35, 39]. While the adequacy of changes in Q bowel to match bowel O_2 need with DO_2, thereby to prevent hypoxic-ischemic injury, has not been documented in these septic models, cyclooxygenase inhibition has been reported to further augment Q bowel in sepsis [41]. The latter study suggested that circulating vasoconstrictor prostanoids in sepsis may prevent appropriate arterial vasodilation within the gut circulation. A potential explanation of the beneficial effects of prostacyclin on systemic VO_2 described by Bihari [12] is afforded by a study of endotoxic shock which demonstrated an increase in Q bowel, together with a reduction in the release of MDF and lysosomal hydrolase, with prostacyclin infusion [42]. Thus, an increase in splanchnic blood flow at a low enough dose of prostacyclin to avoid further arterial hypotension attenuated the release of these mediators in the latter study [42].

At the microregional level, Nelson postulated that the supply/dependency of O_2 consumption found in the small bowel in sepsis was due to increased heterogeneity of intraorgan flows, consequent upon altered microvascular flow control [43]. Kuchta suggested that a circulatory factor, rather than tissue or endothelial factors, was the principal mechanism underlying this altered vascular responsiveness in sepsis [44]. These latter studies reinforced the potential for the participation by one or more humoral mediators in the development of a significant DO_2 debt in the gut. Not only do these studies suggest a mediator-based depression in splanchnic tissue DO_2 relative to O_2 need, but when combined with Nelson's observations that the septic gut is characterized by a deficit in O_2E at the microregional level [43], it also suggests that therapy directed toward improving gut flows could improve survival in sepsis [45].

The Pancreas

In both endotoxic [30] and hyperdynamic [33, 35] septic models, an absolute depression in Q pancreas has been a consistent finding. In a large clinical autopsy series of patients with MSOF, Coalson described a 16% incidence of pancreatitis which was unsuspected prior to death [46]. Subsequently, Nicod et al. described an increase in lipase and immunoreactive trypsin an average of 6 days after the onset of ARDS, and suggested that hypoxic injury to the pancreas was the cause of this clinical evidence for organ injury [47]. We found the histology of the pancreas in hyperdynamic sepsis was characterized by more severe tissue injury than noted in other organs, possibly because of the additive effect of a depression in DO_2 pancreas at both the regional and microregional levels [18].

The exocrine pancreas is at particular risk from ischemia because of its small vascular surface area [48]. Pancreatic O_2 consumption normally becomes supply-dependent when flow falls 30% below resting values [49], a decrease typical of hyperdynamic sepsis is reported animal studies [34, 35]. Since

Few studies have evaluated the mechanisms potentially contributing to a decrease in Q pancreas, hence DO_2, in hyperdynamic, nonhypotensive sepsis, we can only speculate as to the probable cause. Pancreatic blood flow could be depressed by vasoconstrictive putative mediators released in sepsis. Alternatively, an increase in resistance to venous return from the splanchnic bed may increase pancreatic venous pressure which could depress pancreatic blood flow secondary to an increase in vascular resistance.

Reactive Hyperemia in Sepsis

Reactive hyperemia is a phenomenon which defines the ability of a specific organ's circulation to increase Q consequent upon a metabolic stimulus, i.e., hypoxia [3], and hence should allow assessment of the extent to which local DO_2 could increase to meet tissue O_2 needs. Depressed reactive hyperemia indicates depressed metabolic autoregulation and usually also implies the presence of a significant O_2 debt. Proposed mechanisms of the ascending vasodilation, which is characteristic of reactive hyperemia, capillary to arteriole to artery, include a flow-dependent vasodilation, endothelial cell-mediated vasodilation, and retrograde electrical conduction along the arteriole [3].

A recent report describing the loss of reactive hyperemia in septic patients prior to the development of MSOF [50] has reinforced the concept that MSOF may develop consequent upon a failure at any of the three levels of the circulation, thereby resulting in inadequate tissue O_2 flux and the subsequent development of significant O_2 debt. Depressed reactive hyperemia has also been described in animal studies of sepsis. Thus, coincident with the development of a defect in O_2E in bowel, Nelson described a concurrent loss of reactive hyperemia in gut [43] as defined by an inability to further augment flow to bowel following an ischemic stimulus [3]. This latter finding was particularly important since the gut normally has a large vasodilator reserve [4]. The loss of normal vasodilator reserve has been associated with hypoxic cell injury in patients with cardiac disease, and could certainly further support other studies previously reviewed which demonstrated not only an imbalance between tissue O_2 supply and demand in septic-MSOF, but also little available compensation to increase tissue DO_2 in times of increased O_2 need.

The etiology of a depressed tissue DO_2 reserve at the level of the regional circulations in sepsis remains speculative. Excessive tissue edema due to an increase in systemic microvascular permeability in sepsis [51] may blunt reactive hyperemia [52], while the altered peripheral vascular responsiveness found in sepsis could also depress this important response to a cellular O_2 debt.

Linkage to Other Clinical Observations in MSOF

A unifying theme concerning the genesis of MSOF is that sepsis results in numerous inflammatory processes that may both increase local metabolic rate and alter local metabolic autoregulatory function. At best, it is probable that the resulting hyperdynamic state marginally delivers adequate O_2 to meet augmented local demand owing to total impairment of regional redistribution of blood flows, primary dysfunction of the central control of DO_2, and finally impaired microregional O_2E.

Although many conditions have been correlated with the development of MSOF, infection remains the most common, if not a ubiquitous, cause [53–56]. Among other factors, Pine found that associated variables including shock, alcoholism, bowel infarction, and age greater than 65 years, predicted mortality in patients with intraabdominal sepsis [56]. Hence, MSOF and death may follow when delayed resuscitation results in tissue hypoxic-ischemic injury, or when the elderly are unable to appropriately augment central DO_2 because of associated coronary artery disease [57]. The description of bowel infarction as a risk factor for mortality in sepsis may also emphasize the importance of regional DO_2 to the gut in this disease. Other factors have also been causally related to the development of MSOF by establishing a process of "secondary" tissue injury [58]. Thus, translocation of bacteria and/or endotoxin from the gut of critically ill patients has been implicated in the development of MSOF in patients without a well-defined septic focus [59] and may result if increased gut permeability were to occur on an hypoxic basis. The finding of unrecognized pancreatitis in ARDS patients [47], perhaps on an ischemic basis, suggests that this disease may also complicate and perpetuate MSOF, by virtue of the relationship between pancreatitis and acute lung injury.

Conclusion

It is clear that MSOF complicating sepsis may develop in the presence of, and progress despite of, maintenance of a systemic DO_2 which is physiologically considered "supranormal," and apparently sufficient to maintain arterial lactates within normal ranges. As suggested by some, this may therapeutically dictate support of an increase in CO, hence systemic DO_2, until no further increase in whole body VO_2 is demonstrable [24]. However, it is more likely that the progression of septic-MSOF despite a "supranormal" systemic DO_2 is evidence for the presence of a fundamental abnormality at other levels of the circulation which participate in maintaining adequacy of metabolic autoregulation, such as the regional vascular beds determining flow distribution to various organs and/or the specific microcirculations which determine intraorgan DO_2.

MSOF may be characterized by significant abnormalities in circulatory function at all levels of the schema describing the circulatory control of tissue O_2 flux, and evidence of disordered metabolic autoregulation has been clinically recognized as pathological supply/dependency of whole-body O_2 consumption (VO_2) [12, 22, 23]. While it seems to us unclear which specific regional microcirculations primarily account for this latter finding, Nelson and coworkers suggested that the small bowel is an important site [43]. Other levels of the circulation may also contribute to impaired tissue DO_2 in MSOF. Thus, abnormalities in regional vascular tone during sepsis-associated MSOF [60] may prevent appropriate interorgan redistribution of flows at baseline or during therapy normally designed to increase DO_2, i.e., PEEP, while myocardial dysfunction may also result in failure to adequately increase the CO and thereby systemic DO_2.

An increase in skeletal muscle blood flow is a common finding in human sepsis [61], and is commonly accompanied by an increase in CO. The latter is, in part, secondary to an increase in venous return following the redistribution of flow towards a tissue with a fast time constant of venous return [62, 63]. Clearly, this increase in muscle DO_2 does not ensure an appropriate increase in systemic Q and, therefore, an adequate O_2 availability to all organs. Thus, maldistribution of flow at the microcirculatory and regional levels complicates septic-MSOF and may be the result of alterations in vascular tone secondary to circulatory mediators which override the normal ability of tissue ischemia to effect appropriate metabolic vasodilation [64].

MSOF complicating sepsis is, therefore, likely due to the summed effects of a depression in tissue DO_2 and other toxic mediators on local organ function. Clinically, this is collectively represented by impaired homeostasis. Since current evidence supports the concept that widespread tissue ischemia characterizes multiple systems organ failure (MSOF) [10, 22, 30], it is reasonable to assume that circulatory dysfunction secondary to metabolic "dysregulation," and resulting in tissue hypoxia, is important in the genesis of this syndrome. Tissue hypoxia must complicate the inability to sustain tissue O_2 flux at the levels dictated by cellular metabolic activity and ischemic necrosis undoubtedly follows. What is unknown is the role of sustained hypoxic versus reperfusion injury in the final genesis of tissue damage. Further, the various cytokines released in sepsis, such as TNF, not only perturb metabolic autoregulation but may have also direct cellular effects, and their participation in the process leading to MSOF remains to be clarified. Although an integrated picture of the participation of the many factors governing tissue O_2 flux in septic-MSOF remains ill-defined, hypoxic cell injury seems to be a consistent and important end-point in the pathogenesis of the septic-MSOF syndrome.

References

1. Shepherd AP, Granger DN (1984) Metabolic regulation of the intestinal circulation. In: Physiology of the intestinal circulation. Raven, New York, pp 33–47
2. Shepherd AP, Granger HJ, Smith EE et al. (1973) Local control of tissue oxygen delivery and its contribution to the regulation of cardiac output. Am J Physiol 225:747–755
3. Duling BR, Hogan RD, Langille BL et al. (1987) Vasomotor control: functional hyperemia and beyond. Fed Proc 46:251–263
4. Mellander S, Johansson B (1968) Control of resistance and comparitance functions in the peripheral circulation. Pharmacol Rev 20:117–196
5. Cerra FB (1987) Hypermetabolism, organ failure and metabolic support. Surgery 101:1–14
6. Cuthbertson D, Tilstone WJ (1969) Metabolism during the post-injury period. Adv Clin Chem 12:1–55
7. Dahn MS, Lange P, Lobdell K et al. (1987) Splanchnic and total body oxygen consumption differences in septic and injured patients. Surgery 101:69–80

8. Stoner HB (1986) Metabolism after trauma and in sepsis. Circ Shock 19:75–87
9. Abraham E, Bland RD, Cobo JC et al. (1984) Sequential cardiorespiratory patterns associated with outcome in septic shock. Chest 85:75–80
10. Rashkin MC, Bosken C, Baughman RP (1985) Oxygen delivery in critically ill patients: relationship to blood lactate and survival. Chest 87:580–584
11. Fowler AA, Hamman RF, Zerbe GO et al. (1985) Adult respiratory distress syndrome – prognosis after onset. Am Rev Respir Dis 132:472–478
12. Bihari D, Smithies M, Gimson A et al. (1987) The effects of vasodilation with prostacyclin on oxygen delivery and uptake in critically ill patients. N Engl J Med 317:397–403
13. Grum CM, Simon RH, Dantzker DR et al. (1985) Evidence for adenosine triphosphate degradation in critically ill patients. Chest 88:763–767
14. Liaw K-Y (1985) Effect of injury, sepsis, and parenteral nutrition on high-energy phosphate in human liver and muscle. Journal of Parentual and Entual Nutrition 9:28–33
15. Raper RF, Sibbald WJ, Driedger AA et al. (1988) Relative myocardial depression in normotensive sepsis. J Crit Care 4(1):9–18
16. Parker MM, Shelhamer JH, Bacarach SL et al. (1984) Profound but reversible myocardial depression in patients with septic shock. Ann Intern Med 100:483–490
17. Parillo JE, Burch C, Shelhamer JH et al. (1985) A circulating myocardial depressant substance in humans with septic shock. J Clin Invest 76:1539–1553
18. Hersch H, Gnidec AA, Bersten AD et al. Widespread tissue injury antedates significant biochemical organ failure in normotensive, hyperdynamic sepsis. Surgery (In Press) (submitted)
19. McGovern VJ, Tiler DJ (1980) Shock: a clinicopathological correlation. Masson, New York, pp 1–176
20. Dhainaut J-F, Huyghebaert M-F, Monsallier J-F et al. (1987) Coronary hemodynamics and myocardial metabolism of lactate, free fatty acids, glucose and ketones in patients with septic shock. Circulation 75:533–541
21. Barlow CH, Chance B (1976) Ischemic areas in perfused rat hearts: measurement by NADH fluorescent photography. Science 193:909–910
22. Dawson KL, Geller ER, Kirkpatrick JR (1988) Enhancement of mitochondrial function in sepsis. Arch Surg 123:241–244
23. Cunnion RE, Schaer GL, Parker MM et al. (1986) The coronary circulation in human septic shock. Circulation 73:637–644
24. Schumacker PT, Cain SM (1987) The concept of a critical oxygen delivery. Int Care Med 13:223–229
25. Bersten A, Hersch M, Neal A et al. (1988) Adequate myocardial O_2 transport fails to prevent LV failure in a non-hypotensive model of sepsis. Chest 94:473
26. Conway RS, Weiss HR (1982) Role of propranolol in improvement of the relationship between O_2 supply and consumption in an ischemic region of the dog heart. J Clin Invest 70:320
27. Pasque MK, Murphy CE, Vantrigt P et al. (1983) Myocardial adenosine triphosphate levels during early sepsis. Arch Surg 118:1437–1440
28. Jacobs DO, Maris J, Fried R et al. (1988) In vivo phosphorus 31 magnetic resonance spectroscopy of rat hind limb skeletal muscle during sepsis. Arch Surg 123:1425–1428
29. Haybron DM, Townsend MC, Hampton WW et al. (1987) Alterations in renal perfusion and renal energy charge in murine peritonitis. Arch Surg 122:328–331
30. Brenner M, Schaer GL, Mallory DL et al. (1987) Determination of renal blood flow in septic and critically ill patients using a newly designed renal vein catheter. Crit Care Med 15:435
31. Townsend MC, Hampton WW, Haybron DM et al. (1986) Effective organ blood flow and bioenergy status in murine peritonitis. Surgery 100:205–212
32. Fish RE, Lang CH, Spitzer JA (1986) Regional blood flow during continuous low-dose endotoxin infusion. Circ Shock 18:267–275

33. Lang CH, Bagby GJ, Ferguson JL et al. (1984) Cardiac output and redistribution of organ blood flow in hypermetabolic species. Am J Physiol 246:R331–R337
34. Richmond JM, Walker JF, Avila A et al. (1985) Renal and cardiovascular response to non-hypotensive sepsis in a large animal model with peritonitis. Surgery 97:205–213
35. Raper RF, Rutledge FS, Hobson S et al. (1986) Organ blood flow in high output normotensive sepsis. Crit Care Med 14:440
36. Walker FJ, Cumming AD, Lindsay RM et al. (1986) The renal response produced by non-hypotenisve sepsis in a large animal model. Am J Kidney Dis 8:88–97
37. Asher EF, Garrison RN, Ratcliffe EJ et al. (1983) Endotoxin, cellular function, and nutrient blood flow. Arch Surg 118:441–445
38. Garrison RN, Ratcliffe DJ, Fry DE (1982) Hepatocellular function and nutrient blood flow in experimental peritonitis. Surgery 92:713–719
39. Bersten AD, Gnidec A, Neal A et al. (1988) Hyperdynamic sepsis modifies the regional vascular responses to PEEP. Crit Care Med 16:394
40. Beyer J, Beckenlechner P, Messmer K (1982) The influence of PEEP ventilation on organ blood flow and peripheral oxygen delivery. Int Care Med 8:75–80
41. Schuette AH, Huttemeier PC, Hill RD et al. (1984) Regional blood flow and pulmonary thromboxane release after sublethal endotoxin infusion in sheep. Surgery 95:444–453
42. Lefer AM, Tabas J, Smith EF (1980) Salutary effects of prostacyclin in endotoxic shock. Pharmacology 21:206–212
43. Nelson DP, Samsel RW, Wood LDH et al. (1988) Pathological supply dependence of systemic and interstitial O_2 uptake during endotoxemia. J Appl Physiol 64:2410–2419
44. Kuchta KF, Fink MP, Morrissey PE et al. (1988) Vascular reactivity in the rat isolated perfused mesentery is not affected by prior in vitro administration of endotoxin. Crit Care Med 16:421
45. Krausz MM, Utzunomiya T, Feuerstein G et al. (1981) Prostacyclin reversal of lethal endotoxin in dogs. J Clin Invest 67:1118–1125
46. Coalson JJ (1985) Pathology of sepsis, septic shock and multiple organ failure. In: Sibbald WJ, Sprung CL (eds) Perspectives on sepsis and septic shock. New Horizon SCCM, Fullerton Calif., USA, pp 27–59
47. Nicod L, Leuenberger PH, Seydoux C et al. (1985) Evidence for pancreas injury in adult respiratory distress syndrome. Am Rev Respir Dis 131:696–699
48. Vetterlein F, Petho A, Schmidt G (1987) Morphometric investigation of the microvascular system of pancreatic exocrine and endocrine tissue in the rat. Microvasc Res 34:231–238
49. Kvietys PR, McLendon JM, Buckley GB et al. (1982) Pancreatic circulation: intrinsic regulation. Am J Physiol 242:G596-602
50. Hartl WH, Cunther B, Inthorn D et al. (1988) Reactive hyperemia in patients with septic conditions. Surgery 103:440–444
51. Avila A, Warshawski F, Sibbald WJ et al. (1985) Peripheral lymph flow in sheep with bacterial peritonitis: evidence for increased peripheral microvascular permeability accompanying sepsis. Surgery 97:685–695
53. Bell RC, Coalson JJ, Smith JD et al. (1983) Multiple organ system failure and infection in adult respiratory distress syndrome. Ann Intern Med 99:29308
54. Fry DE, Pearlstein L, Fulton RL et al. (1980) Multiple system organ failure – the role of uncontrolled infection. Arch Surg 115:136–140
55. McMenamy RH, Birkhahn R, Oswald G et al. (1981) Multiple systemic organ failure: 1. The basal state. J Trauma 21:99–114
52. Zelis R, Lee G, Mason DT (1974) Influence of experimental edema on metabolically determined blood flow. Circ Res 34:482–490
56. Pine RW, Wertz MJ, Lennard S et al. (1983) Determinants of organ malfunction or death in patients with intra-abdominal sepsis. Arch Surg 118:242–249

57. Raper RF, Cunningham DG, Driedger AA et al. (1988) The effect of coronary artery disease on the biventricular hemodynamic response to human hyperdynamic sepsis. Chest 94:507–511
58. Bersten AD, Sibbald WJ (1989) Acute lung injury in septic shock. In Crit Care Clinics B. Cohen (ed) W.B. Saunders, Philadelphia, pp 49–79
59. Carrico CJ, Meakins JL, Marshall JC et al. (1986) Multiple-organ-failure syndrome. Arch Surg 14:196–208
60. Chernow B, Roth BL (1986) Pharmacologic manipulation of the peripheral vasculature in shock: clinical and experimental approaches. Circ Shock 18:141–155
61. Finley RJ, Holliday RL, Lefcoe M et al. (1975) Capillary muscle blood flow in human sepsis. Surgery 78:87
62. Caldini P, Permutt S, Waddell JA et al. (1974) Effect of epinephrine on pressure, flow, and volume relationships in the systemic circulation of dogs. Circ Res 34:606–623
63. Rothe CF (1983) Venous system: physiology of the capacitance vessels. In: Shepherd JT, Abboud FM (eds) The cardiovascular system, Sect 2, pt 1. American Physiological Society, Bethesda, M.D., pp 397–452 (Handbook of physiology, vol 3)
64. Aversano T, Becker LC (1985) Persistence of coronary vasodilator reserve despite functionally significant flow reduction. Am J Physiol 248:H403–H411

Mechanisms and Modifications of Hyperoxic Injury to the Mammalian Pulmonary Surfactant System

S. Matalon, R. R. Baker, and P. C. Engstrom

Introduction and Purpose

Oxygen is an indispensable therapeutic agent used extensively in clinical medicine for the mitigation of arterial hypoxemia in patients with a variety of pulmonary and cardiac diseases. Unfortunately, the usefulness of oxygen therapy is limited by its well-documented toxicity to the central nervous and pulmonary systems. When oxygen is inspired at pressures less than 3 atmospheres absolute (3 ATA), the pulmonary system is the most important target organ [1]. Numerous studies on different species have demonstrated that prolonged, continuous exposure to high concentrations of oxygen (>95%) at atmospheric pressure results in progressive injury to the alveolar epithelium [2], capillary endothelium [3, 4], and pulmonary interstitial space [5]. The increased permeability of the blood-gas barrier to solute and solvent leads to the formation of noncardiogenic interstitial and alveolar edema, atelectasis, hypoxemia, and hypercapnia, and causes the death of the animals from hypoxemia or respiratory acidosis [2, 6].

Many of the physiological and pathological manifestations present in animals suffering from pulmonary oxygen toxicity are also seen in patients with either neonatal or adult respiratory distress syndrome. In the former (NRDS), there is a primary deficiency of pulmonary surfactant due to immaturity [7]. In the latter (ARDS), surfactant deficiency may be either primary or secondary [8].

These observations have led many investigators to question whether exposure of animals to hyperoxia damages the pulmonary surfactant system and, if so, whether the development of a surfactant-deficient state is an important contributor to the pathogenesis of pulmonary oxygen toxicity. Early studies on the effects of hyperoxia on the pulmonary surfactant system yielded contradictory results (for review see [1]). More recent findings, however, using sensitive and specific physiological, biochemical, and biophysical indices of surfactant function, indicate that exposure to hyperoxia compromises all components of the surfactant system.

The purpose of this article is to review the current knowledge on hyperoxic injury to the pulmonary surfactant system. Our discussion will include physiological, biochemical, and biophysical studies in whole animals, perfused lungs, and isolated type II pneumocytes. In addition, we will present results of our most recent studies on mitigation of hyperoxic injury by increasing alveolar surfactant levels in rabbits. These data offer considerable insight into the biochemical and biophysical mechanisms by which increased concentrations of oxygen in the inspired gas damage the pulmonary surfactant system and lead to respiratory failure.

The Pulmonary Surfactant System: Structure and Function

Biochemical Composition

The biochemical composition and physiological function of pulmonary surfactant have been the subject of many excellent reviews [9–11]. The brief description in this section will only touch on key points relevant to the subject matter of this review.

The biochemical composition of pulmonary surfactant is shown in Table 1. Surfactant is a complex mixture of phospholipids and proteins. It contains a large amount of phosphatidylcholine (~80% by weight); more than 60% of PC contains fully saturated acyl groups (dipalmitoylphosphatidylcholine, DPPC). In addition pulmonary surfactant contains a relatively high fraction of phosphatidylglycerol (~7%) and small amounts of phosphatidylethanolamine, sphingomyelin, and phosphatidylserine. Thus, its composition differs markedly from that of lung tissue and cell membranes.

Two classes of specific apoproteins, not found in serum, have been identified in lung surfactant. The first one appears to consist of a single hydrophilic

Table 1. Biochemical composition of surfactant. (Modified from [33])

Component	% Composition by weight in bronchoalveolar lavage
Phospholipids	90
Neutral lipids	6
Proteins	
SP-A (26 to 36 kDa)	2
SP-B, SP-C (4 to 18 kDa)	2

Phospholipid content of bronchoalveolar lavage and lung tissue in rabbits (% by weight)

Phospholipid class	Lavage	Lung tissue
Saturated (DPPC)	80.9	50.5
Unsaturated	30.9	18.6
Phosphatidylglycerol (PG)	7.1	1.7
Phosphatidylthanolamine (PE)	3.2	21.2
Sphingomyelin (SPH)	1.4	10.8
Phosphatidylserine (PS)	0.5	7.3
Phosphatidylinositol (PI)	3.2	4.6
Others	3.8	4.2
Saturated as % of total phosphatidylcholine (DPPC/PC)	61.6	36.6

native protein, referred to as surfactant apoprotein A (SP-A); SP-A plays a role in surfactant recycling and secretion and enhances the adsorption properties of surfactant [13, 14]. However, it is worth noting that a lipid extract of pulmonary surfactant which lacks SP-A still exhibits all major biophysical properties of natural surfactant [15]. The second class consists of a number of hydrophobic proteins (referred to as SP-B and SP-C) which are necessary for optimum surfactant biophysical activity [16]. It is the unique combination of lipids and the specific apoproteins that confers surfactant its unique surface-tension reducing properties.

Surfactant Metabolism and Physiological Function

Current evidence indicates that surfactant phospholipids are synthesized in the endoplasmic reticulum of alveolar type II pneumocytes and packaged and stored in the lamellar bodies [17]. Surfactant apoproteins follow the same general pathway. Pulmonary surfactant is then secreted from the type II pneumocytes into the alveolar lumen where it assumes a variety of physical forms, including the monomolecular surface film, which is responsible for biophysical activity. Surfactant is being continuously recycled by the alveolar type II cells and macrophages with a half-life of approximately 20 h [18, 19]. Hyperoxic injury to the alveolar type II cells considerably prolongs clearance time [20].

The most important property of pulmonary surfactant is its ability to lower the surface-tension of the gas-blood interface, thus increasing lung compliance and minimizing the work of breathing. In the presence of surfactant, the surface tension of an air-liquid interface changes proportionally with its surface area. This property promotes alveolar stability by equalizing the pressure among alveoli of different sizes (see Fig. 1). A low surface tension also decreases the driving force for solvent flux and thus helps to maintain alveoli free from fluid [21]. Abnormal surfactant function results in atelectasis, right to left shunt, hypoxemia refractory to oxygen, and pulmonary edema, and may lead to death from respiratory failure. We will now review the physiological, biochemical, and biophysical evidence indicating that hyperoxia damages the pulmonary surfactant system.

Effects of Hyperoxia on the Pulmonary Surfactant System: In Vivo Studies

One of the first in vivo studies investigating the effects of hyperoxia on the pulmonary surfactant system was performed by Caldwell et al. [22]. These investigators exposed conscious dogs to 100% O_2 at 1 ATA for periods ranging from 30 h till death. They then measured the surface tension of endobronchial washings and minced lungs in a Wilhelmy balance. Their findings indicate that the endobronchial washings of animals who died from oxygen toxicity had increased minimum surface tension and exhibited decreased hysteresis. However, endobronchial washings of dogs killed after breathing 100% O_2 for up to 54 h had normal surfactant function.

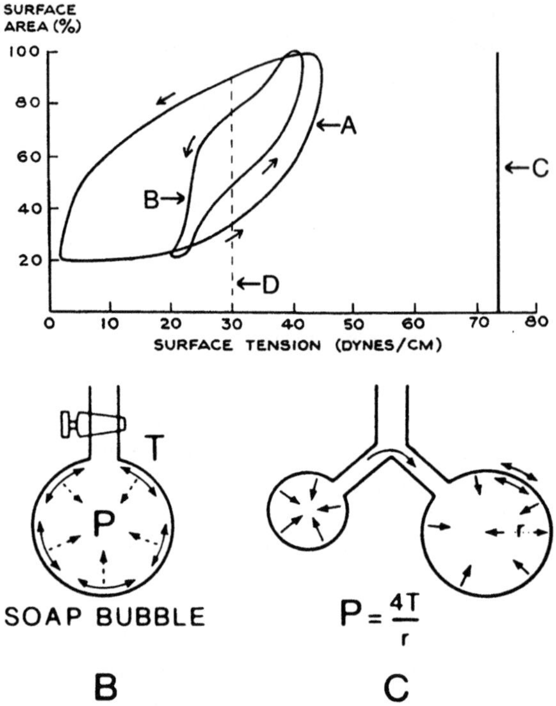

Fig. 1 a. Surface tension-area relationships of water (*C*), water with detergent (*D*), alveolar washings from a normal lung (*A*), and from an infant that died from RDS (*B*). Measurements were obtained in a Langmuir-Wilhelmy balance. Washings from the normal lung show a change in surface tension with area (hysteresis), with different values of surface tension obtained during expansion or contraction of the surface film. The minimum surface tension is less than 3 dynes/cm. Washings from the surfactant-deficient lung (*B*) show decreased amount of hysteresis and a minimum surface tension of 20 dynes/cm; (modified from [49]). **b** Effects of surface tension on bubble stability. Because of the existing air-liquid interface, the generated surface tension acts on the surface of the bubble, trying to reduce the surface area. The resulting pressure inside the bubble is calculated from Laplace's Law $P = 4T/r$ where P is the pressure, T is the surface tension, and r is the bubble radius. Because of the pressure difference, smaller bubbles would tend to collapse into bigger ones. Similar relationships can be obtained across alveoli. Surfactant helps alveoli of different sizes to coexist by reducing the surface tension as a function of the surface area (see **a**)

In a similar study, Morgan et al. [23] exposed dogs to 100% O_2 at 1 ATA for periods ranging from 44 to 52 h, and measured the surface activity and lipid composition of endobronchial lung washings. Lung washings from dogs without pulmonary edema and respiratory distress showed decreased DPPC/PC ratios, but normal minimum surface tensions. At later stages of exposure, when the hyperoxic injury to the blood-gas barrier was severe enough to cause the accumulation of protein-rich pulmonary edema in the alveolar space, endobronchial washings had higher than control levels of lipid and protein, markedly decreased DPPC/PC ratios, and abnormally high surface tensions.

The results of these two studies suggest that hyperoxic injury to the pulmonary surfactant system occurs at the terminal stages of exposure, after the development of severe injury to the blood-gas barrier and the flooding of the alveolar space.

A different conclusion can be drawn from the studies of Gross and Smith [24]. Gross and Smith exposed mice to 100% O_2 and measured the amounts of phospholipids in bronchoalveolar lavage and lung tissue between 42 and 72 h in O_2. Their results indicate a gradual decline in both PC and DPPC in alveolar lavage starting after 48 h in O_2, a time at which all mice were alive and alert and did not have pulmonary edema. The ratio of DPPC/PC remained unchanged throughout the exposure. PC and DPPC turnover rates, as calculated by measurements of specific activities of these substances in the bronchoalveolar lavage, following an intraperitoneal injection of [^{3}H] glycerol were also decreased between 48 and 72 h in 100 O_2. In contrast, PC values in lung tissue remained unchanged throughout the exposure; DPPC levels in lung tissue decreased by 15% after 96 h in O_2 but the decrease was much smaller than the one seen in the bronchoalveolar lavage (36%). The authors concluded that hyperoxia decreased both the synthesis and secretion of surfactant before the onset of lethal injury to the blood-gas barrier.

The data of Morgan et al. [22] and Gross and Smith [24] clearly point out that information on the status of lung surfactant should be derived from biochemical and biophysical studies of lung lavage and not lung tissue. This fact may explain the findings of Fujiwara et al. [25], who reported that hyperoxia altered neither the composition nor the minimum surface tension of pulmonary surfactant. As shown in Table 1 the PC and DPPC content of lung tissue is more indicative of cell membrane lipid composition than of surfactant.

The main shortcoming of the studies reviewed so far is that they did not attempt to correlate physiological changes in lung function with the appearance of decreased levels of phospholipids in the bronchoalveolar lavage. The experiments of Holm et al. [26] addressed this issue and are discussed in detail below.

In previous studies, Matalon et al. [2] have shown that rabbits exposed to 100% O_2 for 64 h have normal gas exchange, no evidence of alveolar and interstitial edema, but increased alveolar permeability to solute. Using this model Holm et al. [26] studied the development of lung injury to the pulmonary surfactant system, its progression, and eventual recovery when rabbits were returned to room air after 64 h in 100% O_2. Their results are shown in Table 2 and Figs. 2–5. After 64 h in 100% O_2, there was a 30% decrease in alveolar phospholipid levels and a threefold increase in alveolar protein levels. In spite of these changes, lung volumes, lung compliance, minimum surface tension of the bronchoalveolar lavage, arterial blood gases, and lung wet/dry weight ratios remained normal. However, 24 h after return to room air breathing, the rabbits developed arterial hypoxemia pulmonary edema, decreased lung volumes, and compliance. At that time alveolar phospholipid and protein levels were one-half and eight times their control values respectively. Measurements of specific lipid classes showed no changes in the fractions of PC and

Table 2. Physiological, biochemical, and biophysical changes in rabbits exposed to 100% O_2 for 64 h and returned to room air for the indicated intervals. (Modified from [26])

	Control	64 h 100% O_2	64 h 100% O_2 + 24 h air	64 h 100% O_2 + 200 h air
(DPPC/PC)	71	75	77	75
(Pr; mg/kg)	7.4±3.5	27.7±4.7*	56.0±3.5*	10.5±2.6
Pr/PL (mg/μmoles)	0.85	4.5	12.4	0.80
W_L/W_D	4.1±0.3	4.5±0.2	6.3±0.2*	4.6±0.2
TLC (ml/kg)	37±2	35±1	23±3*	35±2
T_{min} (dyn/cm)	1±0.2	5±2	30±2*	1±0.2

$\bar{x} \pm 1$ SEM; $n > 5$; * = significantly different from control ($P < 0.05$); PL, total phospholipid in bronchoalveolar lavage; PC, phosphatidylcholine; DPPC, desaturated phosphatidylcholine; Pr, protein; W_L/W_D, lung wet and dry weight; TLC, total lung capacity; T_{min}, minimum surface tension

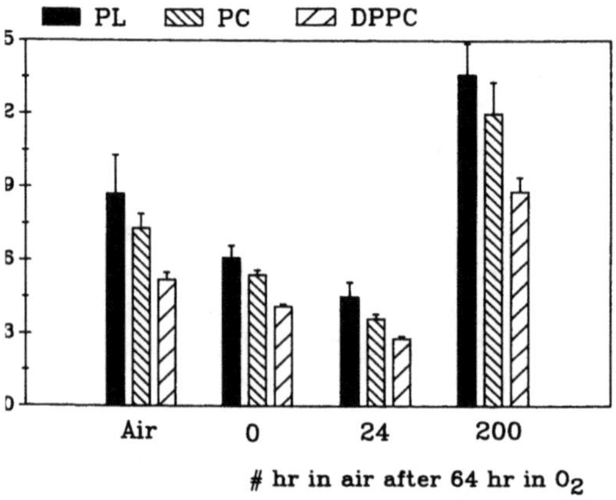

Fig. 2. Amounts of different lipids in the bronchoalveolar lavage of rabbits exposed to 64 h of 100% O_2 and then returned to room air for the indicated time periods. *PL*, total phospholipids; *PC*, phosphatidylcholine; *DPPC*, disaturated phosphatidylcholine. Values are means ± SE, $n \geq 5$. All values are significantly different from their corresponding air levels ($P < 0.05$)

DPPC. Measurements of minimum surface tension of the bronchoalveolar lavage using an oscillating balance showed high minimum surface tensions not consistent with normal physiological function (Fig. 4). These findings indicate that during hyperoxic exposure biochemical alterations in the pulmonary surfactant system occur before the compromise in gas exchange and the manifestations of a surfactant deficient state.

In summary, the majority of studies suggest that exposure to hyperoxia injures the pulmonary surfactant system. Because of the large amounts of alveolar stores and the slow turnover of alveolar surfactant, the physiological sequaelae of this injury may not appear till sometime later. Also, in comparing the results of different studies, one should always keep in mind the well-documented differences in the response of various species to hyperoxia [1]. We will

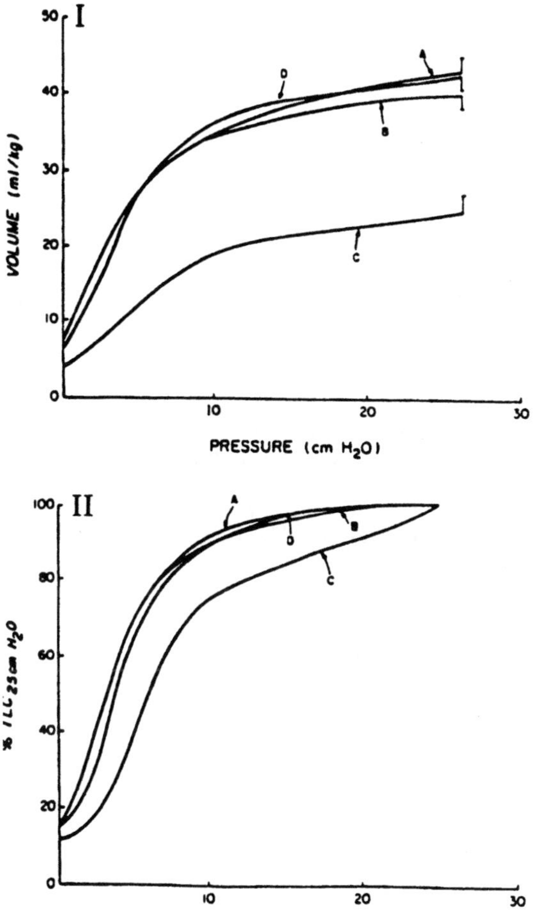

Fig. 3 I, II. Descending limbs of quasistatic, open-chested, lung pressure volume relationships of air filled lungs. **I** Volumes expressed as ml/kg of body weight at the onset of exposure. *A*, control, no exposure; *B*, 64 h in 100% O_2; *C*, 64 h in O_2 and 24 h in air; *D*, 64 h in O_2 and 200 h in air. **II** Volumes are expressed as percent of total lung capacities (TLC). TLC was defined as the volume at 25 cm H_2O distending pressure. Values are means for $n \geq 5$; *vertical bars* in the upper panel are SE for TLC values. Rabbits exposed to 64 h in O_2 and 24 h in air (*C*) have a lower lung compliance than the rest of the groups. (From [26] with permission)

now discuss the possible mechanisms by which hyperoxia may impair surfactant function.

Mechanisms of Hyperoxic Injury to the Pulmonary Surfactant System

Gershman et al. [27] first proposed that oxygen-induced damage was the result of increased production of free radicals. The incomplete reduction of oxygen

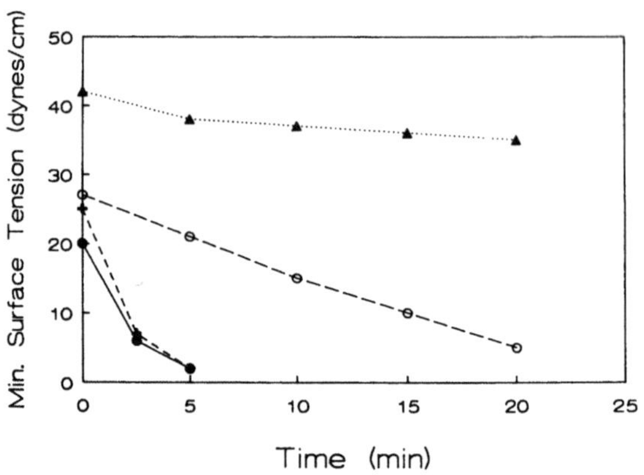

Fig. 4. Surface tension vs time plots for bronchoalveolar lavages as measured on an oscillating bubble apparatus. All samples were concentrated to a standard lipid concentration of 1.0 μmol/ml. ●---●, control, no exposure; ○---○, 64 h in O_2; △····△, 64 h in O_2 + 24 h in air; +---+, 64 h in O_2 + 200 h in air. Each *point* represents the mean value for at least three determinations from different rabbits. The *x*-axis represents the bubble pulsation time. (From [26] with permission)

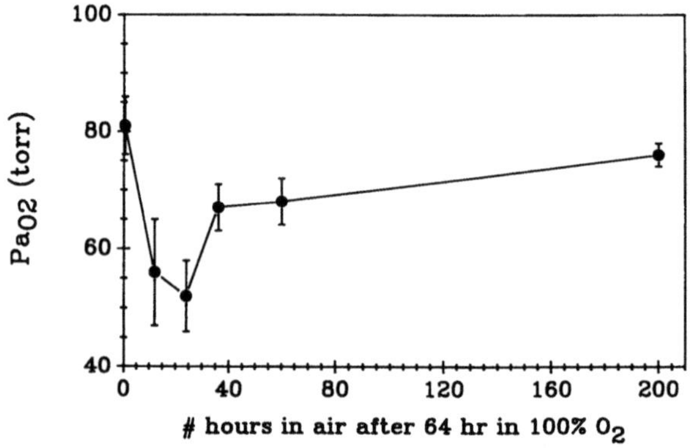

Fig. 5. Partial pressure of oxygen in the arterial blood (PaO_2) of rabbits exposed to 64 h in O_2 and then returned to room air. PaO_2 was normal immediately upon return to room air but declined to around 50 torr by 24 h. Surviving rabbits had normal PaO_2 values after 200 h in air. Mean values ±1 SEM; $n \geq 4$

leads to the production of superoxide anions, hydrogen peroxide, and hydroxyl radicals [28]. These very reactive species are known to cause lipid peroxidation, protein inactivation, destruction of DNA, and ultimately cell and animal death [29]. Several investigators have shown that hyperoxia increases production of these toxic species in lung homogenates and lung cells [29, 30]. Thus, exposure to hyperoxia may damage the alveolar type II pneumocytes and impair their ability to synthesize and secrete surfactant in the alveolar hypophase. In addition, the increased amounts of protein that enter the alveolar space due to the oxygen-induced damage to the alveolar epithelium

[2] may interfere with normal surfactant function by limiting its ability to adsorb to the surface and lower the surface tension in the alveolar hypophase. These two potential mechanisms are discussed in detail below.

Effects of Hyperoxia on Surfactant Metabolism

In their previously cited study, Gross and Smith [24] also assessed the effects of hyperoxia on surfactant metabolism. These investigators exposed mice to 60 h of 100% O_2, an exposure period that resulted in significant alterations of phospholipid levels in the bronchoalveolar lavage, removed their lungs, and measured the rates of incorporation of ^{3}H-glycerol and ^{14}C-palmitate into DPPC by 0.5 mm slices in vitro. The rates of incorporation of both agents decreased by about 50% after 60 h in 100% O_2. Using similar methodology, Välimäki et al. [31] reported decreased incorporation of [^{14}C] methionine into PC by rat lung slices through the N-methyltransferase pathway after a 60 h exposure. By contrast, increased incorporation was seen by liver slices of these rats. More detailed studies on this topic were conducted by Gilder and McSherry [32], who measured the effects of hyperoxia (3 h in 100% O_2 at 3 ATA) on the two pathways of PC synthesis, both in lung slices and in vivo. They reported that the incorporation of both ^{14}C-choline and ^{14}C-palmitate into PC by lung slices were reduced, the latter to a much greater extent. Measurements of specific activities of the PC content of lung and alveolar fluid after the instillation of ^{14}C-choline and ^{3}H-palmitic acid into rats showed that hyperbaric hyperoxia markedly inhibited PC synthesis from palmitic acid, but had a much smaller effect on the choline pathway. The authors concluded that hyperbaric hyperoxia damages the surfactant system by inhibiting the acylation pathway.

The above cited in vitro studies were performed using lung tissue slices where the surfactant-producing type II pneumocytes make up only 10% of the total cell population. Holm et al. [33] were the first to investigate the effects of hyperoxia on surfactant metabolism by freshly isolated type II pneumocytes. Rabbits were exposed to 100% O_2 for 64 h and then returned to room air. These rabbits were then killed immediately upon return to room air and at 24, 72, and 200 h later. Their lungs were removed and type II pneumocytes were isolated using elastase and trypsin digestion of the lung tissue and purification of the crude lung homogenate by density centrifugation. These investigators measured the rate of incorporation of ^{14}C-choline into PC, as an index of surfactant synthesis, cellular lipid content, and the specific activity of glycerol 3-phosphate (G-3-P) acyltransferase, an enzyme that catalyzes one of the early reactions of phosphoglyceride biosynthesis. Their results showed that alterations in alveolar phospholipid levels in vivo correlated consistently with cellular lipid metabolic changes measured in isolated type II pneumocytes (Table 3). In particular, alveolar pneumocytes isolated from lungs of rabbits exposed to 100% O_2 for 64 h exhibited a 60% decrease in PC synthesis, cell lipid content, and G-3-P acyltransferase activity. All variables then followed a pattern of recovery to normal, and ultimately above normal levels beginning

Table 3. Cellular lipid metabolic changes. (Modified from [33])

Surfactant index	Control	64 h in 100% O_2	64 h in 100% O_2 plus		
			24 h in air	72 h in air	200 h in air
Rate in choline incorporation into phosphatidylcholine (nmol · 10^6 cells^{-1} · h^{-1})	0.49±0.029	0.197±0.065*	0.260±0.095*	0.638±0.095	0.881±0.147*
G-3-P acyltransferase activity (nmol · min^{-1} · mg^{-1})	2.5±0.60	1.23±0.26*	1.36±0.26*	–	2.96±0.40
PL in lavage (μ*M*)	17.5±3	12±0.1*	9±1.2*	–	28±5*
PL in type II cells (nmol/10^6 cells)	50±3	28±4*	29±*	–	83±3*

PL, total phospholipid levels; values are means±SE; $n=5$ in all cases; * significantly different from control ($P<0.05$ or less)

at approximately 3 days after return to room air. These findings suggest that oxygen-induced changes in type II cell surfactant biosynthesis may account, at least, in part, for observed changes in lung phospholipid levels in vivo [26]. More recent results from our laboratories indicate that partially reduced oxygen species, produced by the action of xanthine oxidase on xanthine, also decrease choline and palmitate incorporation into freshly isolated type II cells and their G-3-P content in a dose-dependent fashion [34, 35].

In summary, the data presented indicate that exposure to hyperoxia affects surfactant biosynthesis by the type II cells, and that these changes may be responsible, at least in part, for the observed changes in lung phospholipid levels in vivo. It seems that several steps in the surfactant biosynthetic chain are involved, although knowledge of the precise mechanisms is still deficient.

Inactivation of Lung Surfactant by Plasma Proteins

Results from several studies suggest that plasma proteins, hemoglobin, and cell membranes are capable of inhibiting the ability of surfactants to reach a minimum surface tension upon compression by either forming complexes with surfactant molecules or by competing with surfactant molecules for space at the air-liquid interface [36–38]. Seeger et al. [36] reported that rabbits with permeability-type (high protein content) pulmonary edema had lower lung compliance and higher minimum surface tension in the bronchoalveolar lavage than rabbits with an equivalent amount of cardiogenic (low protein content) edema. Holm and Notter [37] quantified the effects of increasing alveolar protein levels on surfactant function in isolated lungs. The results of their studies

Table 4. Effects of exogenous proteins on surfactant (LS) dynamic surface tension lowering in vitro. (From [38])

LS concentration (mg/ml)	Albumin concentration (mg/ml)	T_{min} (dyne/cm)
0.5	–	< 1
–	100	45
0.5	20	21
2.0	200	< 1

A bubble was formed in an oscillating bubble apparatus at the indicated air-liquid interface. The bubble was then pulsated at 20 cycles/min for 20 min at which point the minimum surface tension was recorded

indicated that intratracheal instillation of plasma proteins caused lung mechanical dysfunction which was made even more severe when the lungs were first made partially surfactant deficient. Moreover, the mechanical abnormalities present in these lungs were almost abolished following the administration of exogenous surfactant. Holm et al. [38] also demonstrated that the protein-induced inhibition of the natural surfactant function observed at lower phospholipid concentrations was completely abolished when the surfactant concentration was increased (Table 4). In addition, this resistance to inhibitors was maintained even when the protein to lipid ratio was increased fivefold.

This last finding indicates that the protein-induced inhibition of surfactant activity depends upon the lipid/protein ratios. As previously pointed out, hyperoxia decreases surfactant synthesis and increases the amount of protein in the alveolar space. The combination of these two factors leads to the development of a surfactant-deficient state. The practical relevance of this finding is that the functional surfactant deficiency present in hyperoxia may be alleviated by the instillation of exogenous surfactant.

Mitigation of Hyperoxic Injury by Surfactant Replacement

Observations suggesting that exposure to hyperoxia damages the pulmonary surfactant system have generated considerable interest in assessing to what extent the development of pulmonary pathophysiology in oxygen toxicity results from the existence of a surfactant-deficient state. To address this question Matalon and coworkers [39–41] studied the efficacy of exogenous surfactant in mitigating hyperoxic injury to the mammalian lung in vivo.

In the first study [39], surfactant was administered after the development of sublethal injury to the blood-gas barrier. Rabbits were exposed to 100% O_2 for 64 h and then returned to room air for 24 h. At that time, rabbits exhibit an adult respiratory distress syndrome (ARDS)-type injury characterized by hypoxemia refractory to oxygen, increased alveolar permeability, and abnormal lung mechanics. At the end of a 64 h exposure to 100% O_2, the rabbits were anesthetized and 125 mg of calf lung surfactant extract (CLSE), dissolved in 6–8 ml of 0.15 *M* sterile NaCl ($\sim$170 μmol of lipid) were instilled in the lungs through the trachea. CLSE was obtained by chloroform-methanol extraction of cell-free bronchoalveolar lavage of lungs of freshly killed calves [38]. It consists of 99% lipid and 1% protein including the low molecular weight hydrophobic apoproteins (SP-B, SP-C). This extract has been shown to significantly improve lung mechanics both in premature lambs and infants with RDS [42, 43]. The rabbits were rotated slowly during the instillation procedure through a 360° arc to enhance the distribution of instillate among the different lung fields. A second instillation was given 12 h after return to room air to maintain high lipid levels in the alveolar space. Control rabbits received an equal volume of saline under similar conditions.

The distribution of lung surfactant among the different lung fields was assessed by adding a small amount of Evans Blue in the instillate, killing the rabbits immediately after instillation, and inspecting the different lung lobes for the presence of dye. There was intense staining of the dorsal and medial sections of the upper, middle, and lower lobes in both lungs. Transverse sections of the lower lobes showed staining around the main bronchi, with its intensity diminishing toward the periphery. These findings are consistent with nonuniform distribution of surfactant among the different fields. In a more recent study, Engstrom et al. [41] assessed the interlobar and intralobar distribution of CLSE in rabbits exposed to hyperoxia by adding ^{14}C-DPPC liposomes into the CLSE to be instilled. Rabbits were killed 24 h after instillation and the tissue-associated radioactivity was measured using standard techniques. Their results indicate that the right lower lobe received most of the CLSE (30% of the instillate, corrected for the weight of the tissue), while the left upper lobe received the least (10%). In spite of these differences, all areas of the lung received surfactant and there were no differences in the distribution between air and hyperoxia.

The beneficial effects of surfactant replacement on gas exchange and lung mechanics are shown in Table 5 and Figs. 6 and 7. Surfactant instillation prevented the development of abnormal lung mechanics and alveolar collapse and significantly decreased the amount of protein in the bronchoalveolar lavage. Moreover, the mortality from respiratory failure decreased from 45% to 10%.

It is interesting to note that both surfactant- and saline-instilled rabbits were hypoxemic 24 h after the end of the exposure ($PaO_2 \sim 55$ torr; see Table 5). However, at that time, after breathing 100% O_2 for 30 min, the mean PaO_2 of the surfactant group was higher than 400 torr while the corresponding value in the saline group was only 200 torr. These data suggest that the hypoxemia in the surfactant group was caused by areas of low ventilation/perfusion ratio while in the saline group by a right-to-left shunt. As expected, surfactant instillation alleviated the surfactant-deficient state and prevented alveoli from collapsing.

Table 5. Effects of surfactant treatment on hyperoxic lung injury

	Control (unexposed)	64 h in 100% O_2+24 h in air		
		Un-treated	Saline treated	Surfactant treated
Aveloar phospholipid (mg/kg)	6.5±1.2	3.4±0.5*	4.5±0.8*	26±3.0$^+$
Alveolar protein (mg/kg)	7.4±3.5	56±3.5*	60±2.0*	35±3.0$^+$
Minimum surface tension (m*N*/m)	1.0±0.2	30±2.0*	26±2.0*	1.0±0.2$^+$
Lung wet/dry weight	4.1±0.3	6.2±0.2*	6.6±0.3*	5.6±0.1*$^{,+}$
Total lung capacity (ml)	80±4.0	48±6.0*	57±2.0*	88±4.0*$^{,+}$
PaO_2 (torr):				
$FiO_2=0.21$	80±3.0	56±9.0*	52±6.0*	54±3.0*
$FiO_2=1.0$	474±16	200±40*	197±55*	446±31$^+$

Values are means±SE; $n \geqq 4$. Rabbits were exposed to 100% O_2 for 64 h and then returned to room air. Two boluses of CLSE (125 mg each) suspended in saline were instilled intratracheally immediately upon return to room air and 12 h later. Untreated rabbits received no instillations. * Significantly different from control, $P<0.05$; $^+$ significantly different from saline-treated animals, $P<0.05$

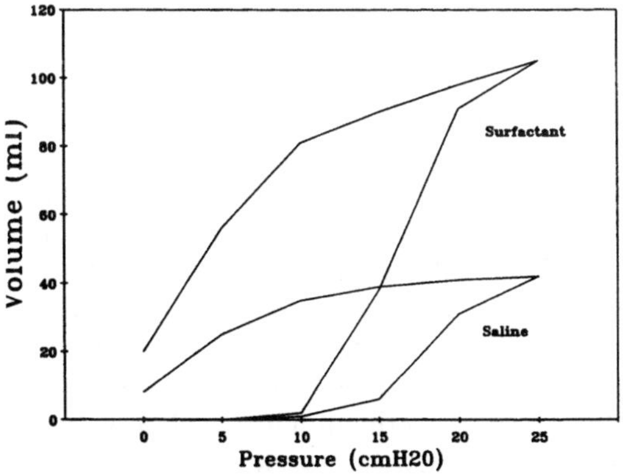

Fig. 6. Quasistatic, open-chested lung pressure-volume relationships for representative rabbits that received either two boluses of calf lung surfactant extract (CLSE) or saline. Both rabbits were exposed to 100% O_2 for 64 h followed by 24 h in room air. After being completely collapsed, the lungs were inflated slowly to 25 cmH_2O of distending pressure, maintained at that pressure for 3–5 min to allow stress-relaxation to occur, and then deflated to zero distending pressure. The rabbit that received saline had low lung volumes and decreased hysteresis, consistent with the existence of functional surfactant deficiency. (From [39] with permission)

In the study of Matalon et al. [39], surfactant was instilled after a significant degree of lung injury had developed. Loewen et al. [40] investigated whether prophylactic administration of exogenous lung surfactant could prevent or at least minimize the onset of hyperoxic lung injury. These authors exposed rabbits to 100% O_2 and instilled intratracheally multiple doses of 125 mg of CLSE, dissolved in 10 ml of sterile saline, as described by Matalon

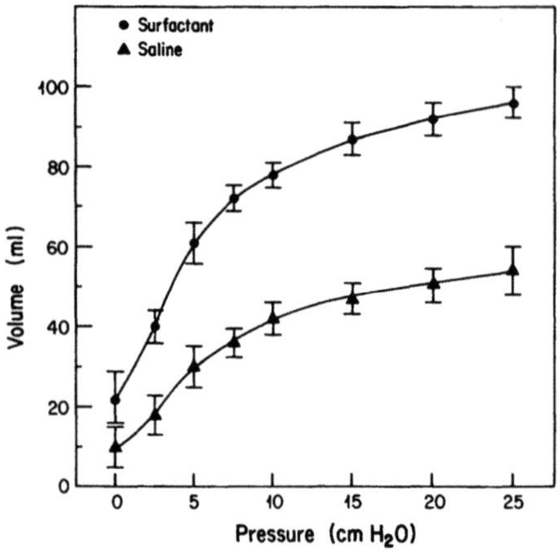

Fig. 7. Deflation limbs of quasistatic pressure-volume relationships for surfactant ($n=7$) and saline ($n=5$) instilled rabbits. Rabbits were exposed to 100% O_2 for 64 h followed by 24 h in air. Immediately after exposure and 12 h later the rabbits were instilled with either 125 mg of CLSE or an equal volume of saline. CLSE-treated rabbits had significantly higher lung volumes throughout the pressure range. Each curve was calculated by averaging the value of each animal at the indicated pressures. Values are means ± 1 SE. (From [39] with permission)

et al. [39]. The first instillation was performed after 24 h in O_2, a time at which no physiological or biochemical injury could be detected; subsequent instillations were performed every 24 h thereafter. CLSE-instilled rabbits survived considerably longer in 100% O_2 when compared with saline controls (120 ± 4 h vs 102 ± 4 h; $\bar{x} \pm 1$ SE; $n \geqq 10$; $P < 0.005$). In addition, after 72 h in O_2, CLSE-instilled rabbits had lower levels of alveolar protein and lung wet/dry weight ratios and higher total lung capacities compared with either saline or uninstilled rabbits (see Table 6). Since CLSE has no measurable antioxidant activity [44], its protective effects on the alveolar epithelium are probably due to the maintenance of normal lung mechanics. However, it should be kept in mind that the pathophysiology of hyperoxic lung injury is multifaceted and involves damage to all components of the blood-gas barrier. Instillation of exogenous surfactant in animals breathing 100% O_2 can only delay the onset of respiratory failure.

Development of Oxygen Tolerance by Increasing Endogenous Surfactant Levels

Heretofore the development of oxygen tolerance has been thought to be associated with increased levels of antioxidant enzymes (superoxide dismutase and catalase) in lung cells [29, 45]. In a recent study, Baker et al. [46] investigated whether rabbits with increased levels of endogenous surfactant are more resistant to the toxic effects of hyperoxia. Like Holm et al. [33], Baker et al. [46] exposed rabbits to 100% O_2 for 64 h and then returned them to room air for

Table 6. Physiological and biochemical variables after 72 h in 100% O_2 or 66 h in air. (From [48])

	72 h in 100% O_2		66 h in air
	Surfactant	Saline	Unexposed and uninstilled[a]
Pa_{O_2} (torr)	333±28*,* (19)	281±29** (18)	79±3 (5)
P_L (µm/kg)	12.5±1.5*,** (7)	5±1** (8)	8.7±1.6 (5)
Pr (mg/kg)	24±3*,** (7)	52±8** (8)	7.4±3 (5)
T_{min} (dyn/cm)	2±1* (7)	26±1** (8)	2±1 (5)
TLC (ml/kg)	41±2* (5)	25±3.5** (4)	42±1 (5)
C_L (ml/cm H_2O)	4.4±0.2 (5)	4.3±0.2 (4)	4.8±0.1 (5)
W_L/W_D	5.9±0.2*,** (7)	6.5±0.3** (6)	4.1±0.3 (5)

Values are means ± SE with the number of animals in parentheses. Pa_{O_2}, partial pressure of oxygen in the arterial blood; P_L, Pr, total phospholipid and protein amounts in the bronchoalveolar lavage; T_{min}, minimum surface tension of the bronchoalveolar lavage; TLC, total lung capacity; C_L, lung compliance (measured as the slope of the linear portion of the pressure-volume curve); W_L/W_D, lung wet/dry weights; * $P<0.05$ compared with the corresponding saline value; ** $P<0.05$ compared with the corresponding uninstilled air value
[a] From [26]

8 days (preexposed). At this time, they had normal gas exchange and alveolar permeability to solute and increased levels of lavageable alveolar phospholipids compared with control rabbits breathing air (26±2 vs 12±µmol/kg). Preexposed rabbits survived significantly longer than control rabbits when reexposed to 100% O_2 (166±24 vs 80±6 h; $n=7$; $P<0.05$) and had signifi-

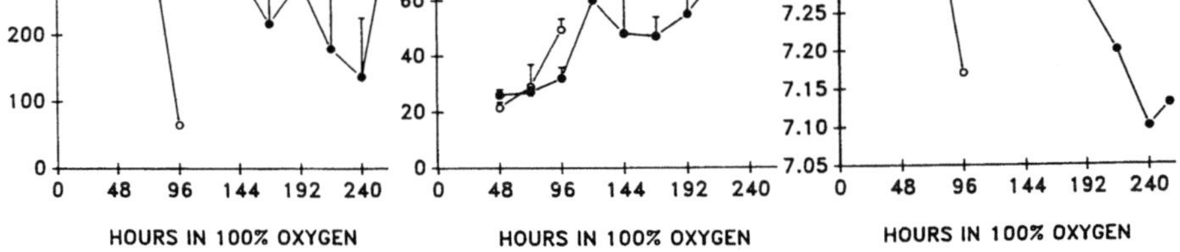

Fig. 8. Serial arterial blood gas determinations in control ($n=7$) and preexposed ($n=2$) rabbits during reexposure to 100% O_2. Values are means ±SE; $n \geq 3$ for up to 192 h in 100% O_2. Pa_{O_2}, arterial O_2 partial pressure; Pa_{CO_2}, arterial CO_2 partial pressure; pH, arterial pH value. (From [46] with permission)

cantly higher values of total lavageable phospholipids after 72 h in 100% O_2 (15±2 vs 5±2 µmol/kg). Control rabbits developed arterial hypoxemia after 72 h in 100% O_2 (Fig. 8). On the other hand, preexposed rabbits maintained arterial PO_2 values >200 torr throughout the hyperoxic exposure and developed progressive respiratory acidosis (Fig. 8). Specific activities of CuZn and Mn superoxide dismutase, catalase, and glutathione peroxidase in lung homogenates and isolated alveolar type II pneumocytes of preexposed rabbits were unchanged from those of controls before O_2 reexposure, and after 72 h in 100% O_2. This is the first report indicating that animals may develop tolerance to hyperoxia without a previous increase in their antioxidant enzyme levels. Furthermore, these results are consistent with the notion that pulmonary surfactant may play an important role in the development of oxygen tolerance.

Conclusions

The purpose of this article has been to review the current knowledge on hyperoxic injury to the pulmonary surfactant system. The existing evidence suggests that continuous prolonged exposure to 100% O_2 damages the type II pneumocytes, resulting in decreased synthesis and secretion of surfactant in the alveolar hypophase. This injury appears before the onset of pulmonary edema and respiratory failure. Plasma proteins entering the alveolar space, because of the increased alveolar permeability to solute, contribute to the development of a surfactant-deficient state by competing with surfactant for the air-water interface. At the terminal stages of exposure, bronchoalveolar lavages exhibit very high minimum surface tensions which are incompatible with normal physiological function.

Instillation of exogenous surfactant during hyperoxic exposure increases lung phospholipid levels, decreases minimum surface tension, and restores lung mechanics to their normal values. In addition, it considerably prolongs survival time and delays the onset of hypoxemia. Rabbits with increased levels of endogenous surfactant, but normal levels of lung antioxidant enzyme levels, are resistant to the toxic effects of hyperoxia. These findings indicate that injury to the pulmonary surfactant system plays an important role in the pathogenesis of hyperoxic lung injury.

Acknowledgements. This project was supported by NIH grant HL31197 and a Career Investigator Award cosponsored by the American Lung and Alabama Lung Associations. Mr. Baker and Dr. Engstrom were partially supported by NIH Training Grant HT32HL07553. The authors would like to thank Mrs. Charlotte Shaw for the excellent editorial assistance in the preparation of this manuscript and Melinda Johansson for her graphics.

References

1. Clark JM, Lambertsen CJ (1971) Pulmonary oxygen toxicity: a review. Pharmacol Rev 23:37–133
2. Matalon S, Egan EA (1981) Effects of 100% O_2 breathing on permeability of alveolar epithelium to solute. J Appl Physiol 50:859–863

3. Matalon S, Cesar MC (1985) Effects of oxygen breathing on the capillary filtration coefficient in rabbit lungs. Microvasc Res 29:70–80
4. Kistler GS, Caldwell PRB, Weibel ER (1967) Development of fine structural damage to alveolar and capillary lining cells in oxygen poisoned rat lungs. J Cell Biol 32:605–622
5. Matalon S, Egan EA (1984) Interstitial fluid volumes and albumin spaces in pulmonary oxygen toxicity. J Appl Physiol 57:1767–1772
6. Matalon S, Nesarajah HS, Farhi LE (1982) Pulmonary and circulating changes in conscious sheep exposed to 100% O_2 at 1 ATA. J Appl Physiol 53:110–116
7. Avery ME, Mead J (1959) Surface properties in relation to atelectasis and hyaline membrane disease. Am J Dis Child 97:517–523
8. Rinaldo JE, Rogers RM (1982) Adult respiratory distress syndrome, changing concepts of lung injury and repair. N Engl J Med 15:900–909
9. Wright JR, Clements JA (1987) Metabolism and turnover of lung surfactant. Am Rev Respir Dis 135:426–444
10. Roony SA (1985) The surfactant and lung phospholipid biochemistry. Am Rev Respir Dis 131:439–460
11. Notter RH, Finkelstein JN (1984) Pulmonary surfactant: an interdisciplinary approach. J Appl Physiol 57:1613–1624
12. Holm BA (1987) The role of pulmonary surfactant in hyperoxic lung injury. Thesis, University of Rochester, Rochester New York
13. Dobbs LG, Wright JR, Hagwood S, Gonzalez R, Venstrom K, Nellenbogen J (1987) Pulmonary surfactant and its components inhibit secretion of phosphatidylcholine from cultured rat alveolar type II cells. Proc Natl Acad Sci USA 84:1010–1014
14. Wright JR, Wagner RE, Hagwood S, Dobbs L, Clements JA (1987) Surfactant apoprotein $M_r = 26\,000$–$36\,000$ enhances uptake of liposomes by type II cells. J Biol Chem 262:2888–2894
15. Egan EA, Notter RH, Kwong MS, Shapiro DL (1983) Natural and artificial lung surfactant replacement therapy in premature lambs. J Appl Physiol 55:875–883
16. Whitsett JA, Ohning BL, Ross G, Mouth J, Weaver T, Holm BA, Shapiro DL, Notter RH (1986) Hydrophobic surfactant-associated protein in whole lung surfactant and its importance for biophysical activity in lung surfactant extracts used for replacement therapy. Pediatr Res 20:460–467
17. Massaro GD, Massaro D (1972) Granular pneumocytes. Electron microscopic radioautographic evidence of intracellular protein transport. Am Rev Respir Dis 105:927–931
18. Baritussio AG, Magoon MW, Goerke J, Clements JA (1981) Precursor-product relationship between rabbit type II cell lamellar bodies and alveolar surface active material. Surfactant turnover time. Biochim Biophys Acta 666:382–393
19. Jobe A, Kirkpatrick E, Gluck L (1978) Labeling of phospholipids in the surfactant and subcellular fractions of rabbit lung. J Biol Chem 253:3810–3816
20. Holm BA, Tonucci D, Matalon S (1989) Clearance of exogenous surfactant in hyperoxic lung injury. FASEB J 3:A546 (Abstract)
21. Raj JU (1985) Alveolar liquid pressure in excised air-inflated lungs of mature and immature fetal rabbits. Physiologist 28:349 (Abstract)
22. Caldwell PRB, Giammona ST, Lee WL, Bondurant S (1965) Effect of oxygen breathing at one atmosphere on the surface activity of lung extracts in dogs. Ann NY Acad Sci 121:823–828
23. Morgan TE, Finley TN, Huber GL, Fialkow H (1965) Alterations in pulmonary surface active lipids during exposure to increased oxygen tension. J Clin Invest 44:1737–1744
24. Gross NJ, Smith DM (1981) Impaired surfactant phospholipid metabolism in hyperoxic mouse lungs. J Appl Physiol 51:1198–1203
25. Fujiwara T, Adams FH, Seto K (1964) Lipids and surface tension of extracts of normal and oxygen-treated guinea pig lungs. J Pediatr 65:45

26. Holm BA, Notter RH, Siegle J, Matalon S (1985) Pulmonary physiological and surfactant changes during injury and recovery from hyperoxia. J Appl Physiol 59:1402–1409
27. Gerschman R, Gilbert DL, Nye SW, Dwyer P, Fenn WO (1954) Oxygen poisoning and X-irradiation: a mechanism in common. Science 119:623–626
28. Fridovich I (1978) The biology of oxygen radicals. The superoxide radical is an agent of oxygen toxicity; superoxide dismutases provide an important defense. Science 201:875–880
29. Freeman BA, Crapo JD (1982) Biology of disease: free radicals and tissue injury. Lab Invest 47(5):412–426
30. Turrens JF, Freeman BA, Carpo JD (1982) Hyperoxia increases H_2O_2 release by lung mitochondria and microsomes. Arch Biochem Biophys 327:411–421
31. Välimäki M, Pelliniemi J, Nirnikoski J (1975) Oxygen-induced changes in pulmonary phospholipids in the rat. J Appl Physiol 39:780–787
32. Gilder H, McSherry CK (1974) Mechanisms of oxygen inhibition on pulmonary surfactant synthesis. Surgery 76:72–79
33. Holm BA, Matalon S, Finkelstein JN, Notter RH (1988) Type II pneumocyte changes during hyperoxic lung injury and recovery. J Appl Physiol 65:2672–2678
34. Baker RR, Holm BA, Engstrom PC, Matalon S (1989) Extracellular and intracellular oxygen radicals decrease surfactant production in vitro. FASEB J 3:A536
35. Holm BA, Cavanaugh C, Baker RR, Matalon S (1984) Effects of reactive O_2 metabolites on type II surfactant synthesis. Am Rev Respir Dis 139:A504
36. Seeger W, Stohr G, Wolf HRD, Neuhof H (1985) Alteration of surfactant function due to protein leakage: special interaction with fibrin monomes. J Appl Physiol 58:326–338
37. Holm BA, Notter RH (1987) Effects of hemoglobin and cell membrane lipids on pulmonary surfactant activity. J Appl Physiol 63:1434–1442
38. Holm BA, Notter RH, Finkelstein JN (1985) Surface property changes from interactions of albumin with natural lung surfactant and extracted lung lipids. Chem Phys Lipids 38:287–298
39. Matalon S, Holm BA, Notter RH (1987) Mitigation of pulmonary hyperoxic injury by administration of exogenous surfactant. J Appl Physiol 62(2):756–761
40. Loewen GM, Holm BA, Milanowski L, Wild LM, Notter RH, Matalon S (1989) Alveolar hyperoxic injury in rabbits receiving exogenous surfactant. J Appl Physiol 66:1087–1092
41. Engstrom PC, Holm BA, Matalon S (1989) Surfactant replacement attenuates the increase in alveolar permeability in hyperoxia. J Appl Physiol 67(2):688–693
42. Egan EA, Notter RH, Kwong MC, Shapiro DL (1983) Natural and artificial lung surfactant replacement therapy in premature lambs. J Appl Physiol 55:875–883
43. Kwong MC, Egan EA, Notter RH, Shapiro DL (1985) Double-blind clinical trial of calf lung surfactant extract for the prevention of hyaline membrane disease in extremely premature infants. Pediatrics 76:585–592
44. Matalon S, Holm BA, Baker RR, Freeman BA (1988) Antioxidant properties of surfactant replacement mixtures. Am Rev Respir Dis 137:80
45. Crapo JD, Barry BE, Foscue HA, Shelburne J (1980) Structural and biochemical changes in rat lungs occurring during exposures to lethal and adaptive doses of oxygen. Am Rev Respir Dis 122:123–143
46. Baker RR, Holm BA, Panus PC, Matalon S (1989) Development of O_2 tolerance in rabbits without an increase in antioxidant enzymes. J Appl Physiol 66:1679–1684

Interaction Between Circulating Granulocytes and Xanthine Oxidase-Derived Oxidants in the Postischemic Intestine *

P. Kubes and D. N. Granger

In 1981, it was first postulated that xanthine oxidase derived oxidants play an integral role in the microvascular injury associated with the reperfusion of ischemic tissue (Granger et al. 1981). Since that time much work has been done to substantiate this hypothesis and to further expand on the pathophysiological alterations associated with ischemia reperfusion (I/R). Figure 1 illustrates that during ischemia, cellular ATP is converted to the catabolic substrate hypoxanthine while the enzyme xanthine dehydrogenase is converted to xanthine oxidase. Following the reintroduction of oxygen, this molecule reacts with hypoxanthine and xanthine oxidase to produce superoxide and hydrogen peroxide. These reactive oxygen metabolites may then be converted to the highly cytotoxic hydroxyl radical by the iron catalyzed Haber-Weiss reaction. This initiates the process of lipid peroxidation which may stimulate the release of chemoattractants and the subsequent activation and recruitment of granulocytes. The objective of this chapter is to summarize supportive evidence and identify areas of controversy and uncertainty, regarding each component of the scheme presented in Fig. 1.

* The work summarized in this chapter was supported by a grant from the National Institutes of Health (DK 33594)

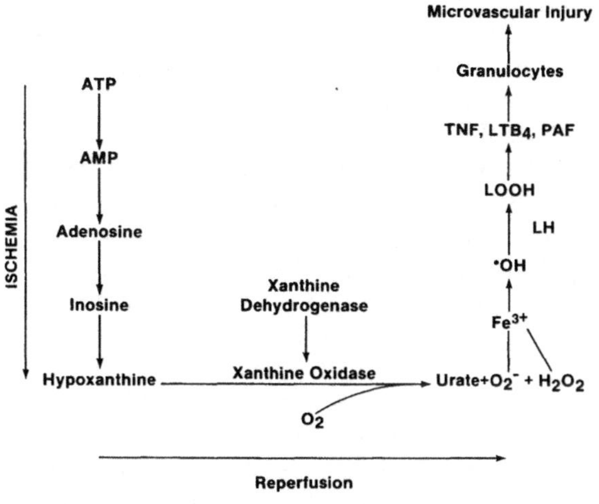

Fig. 1. Mechanism proposed to explain the involvement of xanthine oxidase-derived oxidants and granulocytes in ischemia/reperfusion-induced microvascular injury. (Modified from Granger 1988)

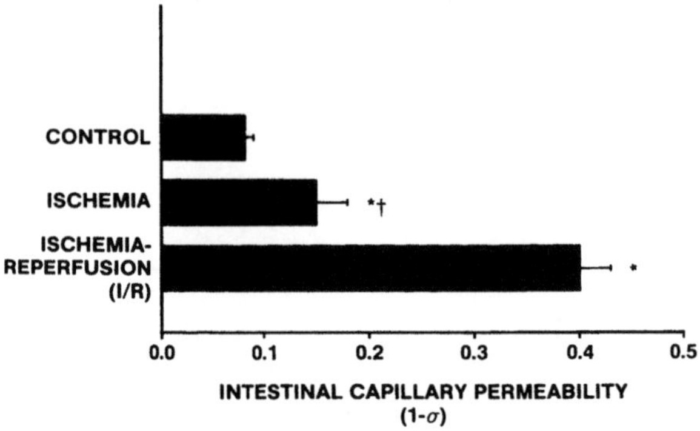

Fig. 2. Effects of 1 h ischemia and 1 h ischemia/reperfusion (I/R) on intestinal microvascular permeability (Granger et al. 1980). σ, osmotic reflection coefficient of intestinal capillaries to total plasma proteins. $*P<0.05$ relative to control; $\dagger P<0.05$ relative to I/R

The mechanisms underlying I/R related tissue injury have been studied in many organ systems, however the focus of this discussion will largely be confined to the small intestine. In our intestine model, microvascular permeability to plasma proteins has been a useful index for the assessment of the microvascular alterations produced by brief (1 h) periods of ischemia (Granger et al. 1980) whereas morphological alterations in the mucosal region of the small intestine serve as an index of the tissue injury produced by prolonged (3 h) periods of ischemia (Parks and Granger 1986a). Of particular interest has been the observation that if the blood flow is reduced to approximately 20% of control for 1 h (ischemia) and microvascualr permeability is measured at this time, a twofold increase (0.08 ± 0.01 vs 0.15 ± 0.03) is noted (Fig. 2). However, if 1 h of reperfusion follows the ischemia, microvascular permeability is greatly increased (0.40 ± 0.03). It is clearly during the reperfusion phase rather than the ischemic phase of I/R that the largest increment in permeability occurs. This view is further substantiated by the observation that the mucosal injury produced by 3 h of ischemia and 1 h of reperfusion is significantly greater than that produced by 4 h of ischemia alone (Parks and Granger 1986a).

The oxygen radical hypothesis of I/R is based on the premise that the tissue injury observed during reperfusion is dependent on the reintroduction of oxygen, resulting in the production of oxyradicals, rather than a delayed manifestation of injury incurred during the ischemic period. Although it is conceivable that the sudden surge in blood flow and pressure during reperfusion may lead to the obliteration of the villus layer, there are several lines of evidence to support the idea that I/R injury is oxygen dependent. Primarily, reperfusion with a nitrogenated electrolyte solution after 3 h of ischemia produced significantly less injury than that observed with whole blood (Parks and Granger 1986a). Furthermore, Korthuis et al. (1989) demonstrated that the increased microvascular permeability and injury associated with I/R was greatly attenuated in skeletal muscle if it is reperfused with anoxic rather than oxygenated blood. Finally, antioxidants and inhibitors of oxyradical formation offer protection against mucosal injury as effectively if given just prior to reperfusion as when the agents are administered before ischemia (Morris et al. 1987). Therefore the overall pattern and time course of injury in these studies is consistent with the view that the reintroduction of oxygen during reperfusion is largely responsible for the I/R model of injury.

Accumulation and Oxidation of Hypoxanthine During Ischemia

The first component of our working hypothesis is based on the assumption that during ischemia, adenosine triphosphate is catalyzed to the endogenous substrate hypoxanthine. Using magnetic resonance spectroscopy (MRS), Blum and his colleagues (1986) demonstrated that ATP levels in rat small bowel were completely depleted within 20 min of ischemia. Furthermore, Younes et al. (1984) demonstrated a reduction in ATP levels to 40% of the control value during ischemia in the cat small intestine but its catabolic substrate increased 20-fold. This indicates that ATP is degraded in the ischemic intestine while hypoxanthine accumulates.

Xanthine oxidase (XO) is a versatile enzyme most recognized for its rate-limiting role in nucleic acid degradation through which all purines are channelled for terminal oxidation. There is growing interest in the ability of this enzyme to serve as a source of oxidizing agents such as hydrogen peroxide and superoxide radical. It is widely distributed among tissues, the small intestine being the richest source (Krenitsky et al. 1974; Batelli et al. 1972). Its activity is found mainly in the mucosal layer with an increasing gradient from villus base to tip where levels of XO have been reported to exceed 100 mU/g wet wt of tissue (Parks and Granger 1986b). This finding is consistent with reports that the villus tip is most susceptible to ischemic injury. The cytotoxic potential of this xanthine oxidase activity in intestinal mucosa is exemplified by the observation in vitro that isolated cells are injured when exposed to XO levels as low as 2 mU/ml (Simon et al. 1981).

Under normal conditions XO exists in the cell as an NAD^+-reducing xanthine dehydrogenase (XD) and not the oxyradical producing oxidase (XO). However, conversion of XD to XO (D-to-O) can be induced by a number of conditions. Ischemia is one such condition which initiates this reaction (Roy and McCord 1983). McCord and Roy (1982) reported that D-to-O conversion was essentially complete in less than 1 min of ischemia. This finding was troubling, however, from a physiological viewpoint. If D-to-O conversion in ischemic tissue was truly this rapid and if injury was dependent on the conversion process, then one would predict that 1 min of ischemia would produce as severe an injury response as that observed following 1 h or 3 h of ischemia. Clearly, this is not the case as there is a distinct difference in the level of injury produced by reperfusion following even prolonged periods of ischemia i.e., 1 h and 3 h. Massive epithelial lifting, denudation, and disintegration of the lamina propria is present only after prolonged (3 h) ischemia. This would either suggest that XO was not the primary source of tissue damage following ischemia, or some other substrate in our scheme (Fig. 1) was rate limiting. However, it has previously been shown that hypoxanthine concentrations are typically 20–40 μ*M* (Mousson et al. 1983) in nonischemic tissue, well above the 11 μ*M* XO and XD. Since hypoxanthine levels rise during ischemia this substrate could not be rate limiting in either normal or ischemic small bowel. Furthermore, since the oxyradicals are produced during reperfusion there is an abundance of the remaining substrate, O_2.

Therefore, one would expect D-to-O conversion to be the rate-limiting step in oxyradical production. Parks et al. (1988) have recently shed some light on this query as they found that D-to-O conversion could occur during the homogenization and processing of tissue. This could be misinterpreted as in vivo conversion. Using extensive controls and careful maintenance of temperature during ischemia they reported that D-to-O conversion was a relatively constant and slow process (13% per h) over the 3 h of ischemia in the rat intestine. Furthermore, they alluded to the possibility that D-to-O conversion in the cat small bowel may be even slower. The latter findings are more consistent with physiological and morphological evidence of ischemic injury and provide further support for involvement of XO in intestinal injury associated with ischemia.

Xanthine Oxidase Inhibitors

The contention that xanthine oxidase is the primary source of oxygen radicals in ischemic tissues was for sometime based solely on the observation that allopurinol, a competitive inhibitor of this enzyme greatly reduced the injury observed following I/R (Fig. 3). Although allopurinol is a fairly specific XO inhibitor it does produce metabolic and physiologic responses beyond its inhibition of XO (Gilman et al. 1980). The possibility therefore exists that its *modus operandi* may be through other protective mechanisms. Direct free radical scavenging properties have been implicated in this drug's ability to protect against I/R injury in vitro (Moorhouse et al. 1987). However, in this study, concentrations well above those that afforded protection were required to induce radical scavenging. Nevertheless, to address this notion, other XO inhibitors were tested for their ability to protect against microvascular injury associated with reperfusion of the ischemic small intestine. Commercially prepared folic acid and its photolytic breakdown product pterin aldehyde (a potent inhibitor of intestinal xanthine oxidase) both attenuated the increased vascular permeability produced by reperfusion of the ischemic small bowel (Fig. 3). In fact, it has been suggested that the protective effect of folic acid may be entirely or in part due to the presence of pterin aldehyde as an impurity (Spector and Ferone 1984; Granger et al. 1986b). XO can also be inactivated if molybdenum replaces tungsten at the active site of the enzyme. It has been demonstrated that a molybdenum-deficient, tungsten-supplemented diet decreased xanthine oxidase activity to approximately 10% of control in rat small intes-

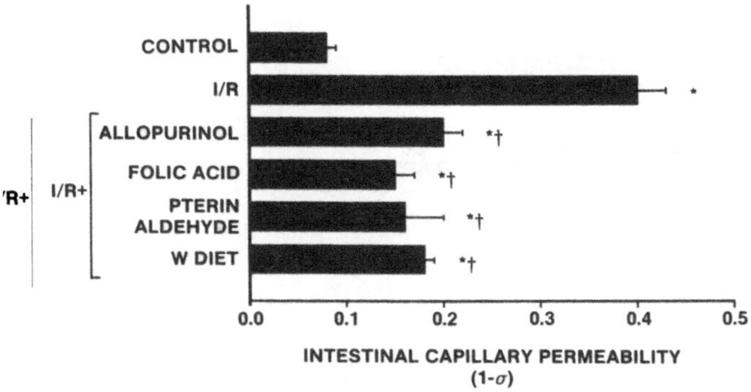

ʼig. 3. Effects of allopurinol, folic acid, pterin aldehyde, and tungsten (*W*) diet on the ncreased intestinal capillary permeability induced by I/R (Parks and Granger 1983; Granger et al. 1986b; Parks et al. 1986). σ, osmotic reflection coefficient of intestinal apillaries to total plasma proteins. $^*P<0.05$ relative to control; $^\dagger P<0.05$ relative to /R

ine (Topham et al. 1982). This regimen in cats greatly attenuated the increase n vascular permeability associated with I/R as presented in Fig. 3 (Parks et al. 986). In addition, conversion of xanthine dehydrogenase to xanthine oxidase an be prevented by the administration of protease inhibitors such as soybean rypsin inhibitor (Roy and McCord 1983). The ischemia-induced increase in ascular permeability (1 h I/R) and mucosal lesion formation (3 h I/R) were argely prevented in soybean trypsin inhibitor treated animals (Parks et al. 985). There has been some concern regarding the potential inhibitory effect of soybean trypsin inhibitor on neutrophil superoxide radical production. This ssue still remains to be resolved. However, taken as a whole, these results support the claim that XO is the major source of oxyradicals in the ischemic small ntestine.

Role of the Superoxide Radical

Having established that I/R increases vascular permeability in the small intestine, attention was focused on factors that may mediate this response. Since xanthine oxidase was implicated in our model of I/R, oxygen radicals were considered as strong candidates for the mediator of the I/R-induced increase n vascular permeability. However, numerous vasoactive substances including histamine, prostaglandins, and lysosomal enzymes have also been proposed as potential mediators in the pathogenesis of intestinal ischemia. This contention s based on indirect evidence that these substances are released from the ischemic small bowel and increase microvascular permeability when infused into the normally-perfused small intestine (Kobold and Thal 1963; Haglund et al. 977). Pretreatment with either antihistamines (benadryl + cimetidine), indomethacin, or methylprednisolone did not significantly alter the permeability ncrease induced by regional ischemia, suggesting that neither histamine, lyso-

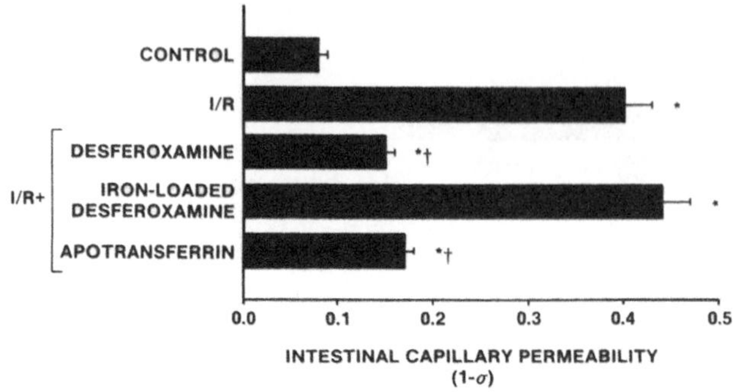

Fig. 4. Effects of desferoxamine, iron-loaded desferoxamine and apotransferrin pretreatment on intestinal capillary permeability induced by I/R (Hernandez et al. 1987a). σ, osmotic reflection coefficient of intestinal capillaries to total plasma proteins. $^*P<0.05$ relative to control; $^\dagger P<0.05$ relative to I/R

somal enzymes, nor prostaglandins are involved in the increased capillary permeability. Another possible mediator, bacterial endotoxin, was shown to increase capillary permeability (Ballin and Meyer 1960). However, since lethal doses of this substance are required to increase permeability and the magnitude of the increase in permeability produced by the endotoxin is small relative to I/R, it appears unlikely that endotoxins play a role in the I/R-induced vascular permeability changes (Granger et al. 1981).

Pretreatment with superoxide dismutase (SOD), a superoxide radical scavenging enzyme, significantly attenuated the permeability changes induced by regional ischemia (Fig. 4). Furthermore, a small lipophilic compound that is known to have SOD-like activity, Cu(II)-3,5-diisopropylsalicylic acid (Cu-DIPS) also attenuates the I/R-induced increase in capillary permeability noted in Fig. 4 (Hernandez et al. 1987b). Finally, when oxygen radicals are generated experimentally, by infusing xanthine oxidase and hypoxanthine into nonischemic intestine, the resulting increase in microvascular permeability mimics that observed following I/R. This permeability increase is largely prevented if SOD is infused along with xanthine oxidase and hypoxanthine (Parks et al. 1984). Although indirect, the bulk of this data implicates superoxide in the I/R-induced increase in microvascular permeability.

Until recently, the only available measure of radical production was the effect of radical scavengers on physiological or morphological parameters. The reason for the lack of oxyradical measurements prior to and during I/R is that it is very difficult to measure the superoxide anion radical because it is unstable, with a lifetime of milliseconds. Recently, two new techniques, chemiluminescence (Roldan et al. 1989) and electron-spin resonance spectroscopy (Nilsson et al. 1987) were used to demonstrate elevated levels of oxyradicals following reperfusion of the ischemic bowel. However, both of these studies have some incongruities with work reported using SOD. Nilsson et al. (1987) reported a transient increase in oxidant formation following 2 h of ischemia but the activity returned to preischemic control values by 10 min of reoxygenation. In contrast, Suzuki et al. (1989) reported that SOD administration following even 1 h of reperfusion was still effective in attenuating certain oxyradical-mediated responses, suggesting that oxyradicals still play a role at this time. In the chemiluminescence study, Roldan et al. (1989) observed a 40% increase in the emission of chemiluminescence following 3–5 min of ischemia in the rat small bowel, supporting the notion of McCord and Roy (1982) that oxyradical production can occur within a short ischemic period. One point of concern regarding this study was the absence of an increase in XO activity over the short interval of ischemia. Since hypoxanthine and O_2 are not limiting factors after reperfusion and xanthine oxidase activity did not increase following 5 min of ischemia, one would not expect enhanced oxyradical formation as predicted by the chemiluminescence response. Therefore, there are still a number of unanswered questions in this area that must await the development of new and more sensitive techniques for monitoring oxidant production.

Role of Hydrogen Peroxide and the Hydroxyl Radical

Although the SOD studies provided strong evidence for the involvement of oxygen radicals in I/R-induced microvascular injury, the superoxide anion per se is a relatively weak oxidant. The low reactivity of this compound suggests that it is unlikely to be the final mediator of I/R injury but it may be a precursor to a more potent oxidant that eventually mediates reperfusion damage. While superoxide is formed by xanthine oxidase, nearly 80% of the O_2 consumed by the enzyme is divalently reduced to H_2O_2. Furthermore, the superoxide generated by xanthine oxidase spontaneously and rapidly dismutates to produce hydrogen peroxide and O_2. Although H_2O_2 is stable in the absence of trace metals and a sluggish oxidant in its reactivity towards biological compounds, in the presence of certain transition metals, particularly iron, it yields (Haber-Weiss reaction) the hydroxyl radical (OH), a potent oxidizing agent. Normally, iron is stored in enterocytes in the form of ferritin micelles. However, superoxide can react with Fe^{3+} in ferritin to liberate Fe^{2+} (Thomas et al. 1985). Thus, xanthine oxidase-generated superoxide provides ferrous iron which would then react with H_2O_2 to form OH in the postischemic intestine.

To evaluate the role of iron in I/R-induced hydroxyl radical production an iron chelator (desferoxamine) and an iron-binding protein (apotransferrin) were tested to determine whether they afford protection against the increased intestinal microvascular permeability produced by I/R (Hernandez et al. 1987a). Figure 4 clearly demonstrates that both deferoxamine and apotransferrin provided significant protection in our I/R model. However, if desferoxamine or apotransferrin were iron-loaded prior to administration, then no protection was observed (Fig. 4), suggesting that iron binding accounts for the beneficial effects of these substances.

The hydroxyl radical, considered to be the most reactive free radical produced in vivo, is capable of damaging many biological compounds (Bielski and Shiue 1979; Jennings et al. 1981) including proteins, lipids, carbohydrates, and

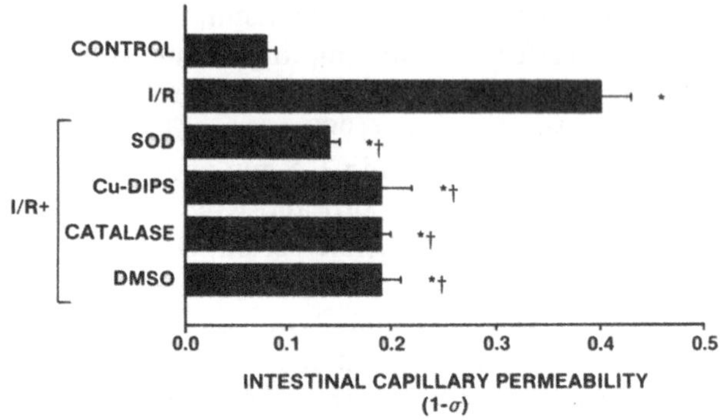

Fig. 5. Effects of superoxide dismutase (SOD), copper diisopropylsalicylate (Cu-DIPS), catalase and dimethylsulfoxide (DMSO) pretreatment on the increased capillary permeability induced by I/R (Granger et al. 1981, 1986a; Hernandez et al. 1987b; Parks and Granger 1983). σ, osmotic reflection coefficient of intestinal capillaries to total plasma proteins. $*P<0.05$ relative to control; $\dagger P<0.05$ relative to I/R

nucleotides (Buege and Aust 1976). The principal mechanism proposed to explain radical-mediated increases in permeability involves peroxidation of lipid components of cellular membranes. The formation of lipid-derived free radicals such as conjugated dienes, lipid hydroperoxide radicals, and fragmentation products (e.g., malondialdehydes), alters the structural integrity and biological function of cell membranes (Freeman and Crapo 1982). Evidence for reperfusion-induced lipid peroxidation in the intestinal mucosa was reported by Younes et al. (1987) who observed a 100% increase in the tissue levels of conjugated dienes, 10 min following reperfusion of the ischemic bowel. Furthermore, the assumption that the hydroxyl radical plays a critical role in I/R injury is supported by studies in which cats were treated with dimethylsulfoxide (DMSO) a hydroxyl radical scavenger (Fig. 5). Microvascular permeability was greatly attenuated in these animals. Similar results are obtained if the precursor molecule hydrogen peroxide is detoxified with catalase as noted in Fig. 5 (Granger et al. 1986a). Therefore, the protective effects of DMSO, catalase, deferoxamine, and apotransferrin, and elevated levels of conjugated dienes are consistent with the view that the cytotoxic hydroxyl radical is formed during reperfusion by the Haber-Weiss reaction, and it plays a role in the injury to intestinal cells induced by I/R.

The ubiquity and reactivity of radical-generating systems in cells has resulted in the evolution of defence mechanisms (endogenous antioxidants) against the deleterious effects of powerful oxidizing agents. For example, despite the continuous exposure to potentially harmful oxidants produced by particular food, bacteria, desquamated cells, saliva, and cigarette smoke (Cross et al. 1984; Grisham et al. 1986; Nayfield et al. 1976), the healthy intestinal epithelium appears to be unaffected by the presence of these reactive species. This would suggest that the gastrointestinal mucosa is endowed with efficient mechanisms to protect or scavenge these oxidants. Grisham et al. (1987)

suggested that mucin may provide protection to the surface epithelium of the gastrointestinal tract by scavenging luminally generated oxidants. The mucin fragments may then signal the cells to produce more glycoprotein for further protection. Such a feedback mechanism is supported by in vitro studies which demonstrate that exposure of gall bladder explants to xanthine oxidase generated radicals results in enhanced synthesis of mucin (Hale et al. 1986). Another naturally occurring scavenging enzyme, glutathione peroxidase (GPO), converts H_2O_2 to O_2 and H_2O with the formation of oxidized glutathione from reduced glutathione. Increased concentrations of oxidized glutathione have been observed during reperfusion of the ischemic bowel (Schoenberg et al. 1984), indicating that H_2O_2 is produced in the postischemic bowel. In this regard it is interesting to note that exogenous glutathione can protect intestinal cells against oxidative injury (Lash et al. 1986).

Role of Neutrophils

A role for neutrophils in oxyradical production after I/R was first proposed by Romson and coworkers (1983) in studies of the myocardium. Neutrophil depletion was observed to reduce infarct size to the same extent as pretreatment with oxyradical scavengers. Recent work in our laboratory indicates that neutrophils accumulate in the mucosa during reperfusion of the ischemic bowel (Grisham et al. 1986). Furthermore, this phenomenon can be prevented by pretreating animals with either allopurinol or SOD. This observation provides the foundation for the hypothesis that XO-derived oxyradicals play an important role in eliciting I/R-induced neutrophil infiltration. These findings raised the important question of whether neutrophils are a cause or an effect of the I/R-induced increase in microvascular permeability. Two approaches were used to assess the role of neutrophils in the I/R-induced increase in intestinal capillary permeability, i.e., neutrophil depletion and prevention of neutrophil adherence with monoclonal antibodies (MoAb 60.3 and IB_4) directed against specific membrane-associated glycoproteins that modulate adherence to endothelium. Figure 6 illustrates the ability of these immunologic technique to attenuate the I/R-induced permeability increases in the small intestine. These results indicate that neutrophils are the major mediators of I/R-induced microvascular injury. The observation that neutrophil depletion and prevention of neutrophil adherence are equally effective in attenuating the microvascular injury suggests that neutrophil adherence is the rate-limiting step in reperfusion-induced, neutrophil-mediated microvascular injury.

Although the results provide strong evidence that neutrophil infiltration is necessary for I/R-induced microvascular damage, the mechanism by which damage occurs is not fully understood. Neutrophils are capable of producing superoxide by the membrane-associated enzyme NADPH oxidase (Rossi 1986). Activated neutrophils also secrete myloperoxidase (MPO), an enzyme which catalyzes the formation of hypochlorous acid (HOCl) from H_2O_2 and chloride ions. The hydrogen peroxide which fuels this reaction is derived from the spontaneous dismutation of neutrophil-derived superoxide. HOCl is a po-

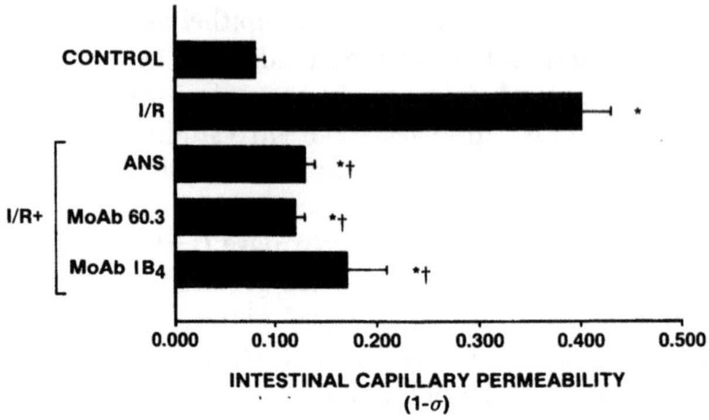

Fig. 6. Effects of antineutrophil serum (ANS) and monoclonal antibodies against leukocyte adhesion molecules (MoAb 60.3 and MoAb IB_4) on the increased intestinal capillary permeability induced by I/R (Hernandez et al. 1987c and unpublished observations). σ, osmotic reflection coefficient of intestinal capillaries to total plasma proteins. $^*P<0.05$ relative to control; $^\dagger P<0.05$ relative to I/R

tent oxidizing and chlorinating agent which can react with primary amines to yield N-chloramines. These substances cause extensive damage to a variety of proteins including hemeproteins, cytochromes, and DNA. Activated neutrophils can also release and spontaneously activate latent proteases, such as collagenase or gelatinase (Weiss 1986; Weiss et al. 1986). It is becoming apparent that the activation of these enzymes is also coupled to an oxidative process that requires the generation of HOCl (Weiss et al. 1985).

Studies in the small bowel have demonstrated that the neutrophil accumulation produced by reperfusion can be effectively attenuated by pretreatment with SOD, catalase, dimethylthiourea, or deferoxamine (Grisham et al. 1986; Zimmerman and Granger 1988). From these results there are a number of possible mechanisms to explain the granulocyte infiltration associated with reperfusion of ischemic tissues. First, the oxygen radicals per se or in combination with some plasmogen cause the recruitment of neutrophils. Second, the oxidants may interact with cell membranes (e.g., lipid peroxidation) and consequently initiate the formation and release of substances that have chemotactic potential for neutrophils. Finally, the interaction between oxidants and endothelial cell membranes may induce a conformational change or a change in the primary structure of surface proteins, thereby enhancing the adhesiveness of the endothelial cell surface to neutrophils.

We examined the chemotactic potential of feline plasma when exposed to oxyradical-producing substrates. The results from both in vivo and in vitro studies indicated that the chemotactic potential of feline extracellular fluid was not enhanced by exposure to hypoxanthine and xanthine oxidase (Zimmerman et al. 1987). Therefore, we were unable to obtain evidence in cats implicating plasma based superoxide-dependent chemoattractants in I/R injury. In contrast, other investigators have reported that human plasma exposed to these superoxide-generating substrates becomes potently chemotactic to human neutrophils in vitro (Petrone et al. 1980; Perez et al. 1980). Furthermore, intradermal injection of this plasma caused heavy infiltration of neutrophils at the injection site (Petrone et al. 1980). In both studies SOD was able to inhibit the neutrophil migration, suggesting that oxyradicals react with certain molecules in the extracellular fluid to produce a potent chemoattractant. It remains unclear whether hydrogen peroxide can interact with extracellular fluid to form a chemoattractant.

There is some evidence which supports the possibility that xanthine oxidase-derived oxidants produced at the time of reperfusion may initiate the formation and release of proinflammatory agents from endothelial cells which subsequently attract and activate leukocytes. It has been suggested that LTB_4, a product of arachidonic acid metabolism, may be released from endothelial and epithelial cells subjected to I/R and consequently promote leukocyte infiltration into the mucosa. First, LTB_4 has been shown to be a chemoattractant that promotes neutrophil adherence in the rat intestinal microcirculation (Sekizuka et al. 1989). Second, LTB_4 production has been shown to increase more than twofold following reperfusion of the feline ischemic bowel (Zimmerman and Granger 1989). Pretreatment of cats with the lipoxygenase inhibitor nordihydroguaiacetic acid (NDGA) significantly attenuated the I/R-induced increase in LTB_4 production and subsequent neutrophil infiltration. The results of this study indicate that LTB_4 plays an important role in mediating the granulocyte accumulation elicited by reperfusion of the ischemic bowel. One criticism of these techniques is that NDGA, like many other lipoxygenase inhibitors, may be an oxyradical scavenger. NDGA may therefore attenuate neutrophil infiltration by the same mechanism as SOD. It will be important to determine the effect of nonscavenging lipoxygenase inhibitors on I/R-induced neutrophil infiltration.

There is accumulating evidence supporting a role for platelet-activating factor (PAF) in ischemia-induced damage in the gastrointestinal tract. First, it has recently been reported that the concentration of PAF increases 14-fold and 4-fold at 5 and 60 min after reperfusion of the canine intestine, following 2 h of complete superior mesenteric artery occlusion (Filep et al. 1989). In that study, pretreatment of animals with the PAF antagonist BN 52021 prevented the functional impairments induced by the ischemia, indicating a major role for PAF in this system. Tagesson et al. (1988) have shown that the increase in lysosomal enzyme release, intestinal permeability, and lipid peroxidation following I/R of the rat distal ileum were all significantly reduced with BN 52021. Interestingly, in that study, BN 52021 had no effect on reperfusion-induced infiltration of neutrophils in the intestinal mucosa. These findings suggest that PAF plays a role in the activation, but not the attraction, of neutrophils in the postischemic intestine. In another study, SOD, allopurinol, and PAF antagonists were equally effective in protecting against postischemic mucosal damage in the rat stomach (Droy-Lefaix et al. 1988). These investigators proposed a possible pathologic role of oxyradicals and PAF in I/R-induced gastric mucosal ulcerations. The role that PAF plays in mediating damage following reperfusion of the ischemic small bowel is as yet unclear and requires further investigation.

Like PAF, tumor necrosis factor (TNF) has been shown to enhance neutrophil superoxide production and adherence (Berkaw et al. 1986). While it appears that TNF per se possesses proinflammatory properties, recent studies suggest that the relationship between TNF and PAF is very important, particularly in mediating endothelial cell damage (Braquet et al. 1989b). TNF can prime PAF-induced superoxide generation by human neutrophils and this effect is completely abolished by a number of structurally different PAF antagonists (Paubert-Braquet et al. 1988; Braquet et al. 1989a). Apart from inducing vascular damage via infiltration and degranulation of neutrophils, both TNF and PAF exert a direct effect on endothelial cells causing them to retract in vitro (Braquet et al. 1989b). It has recently been shown that TNF induces cultured endothelial cells to synthesize PAF, but the majority of the phospholipid remains associated with the endothelial cell membrane (Bussolino et al. 1988). In fact, Lewis et al. (1988) postulated that PAF synthesized by endothelial cells remains in contact with these cells and mediates the adhesive interaction to neutrophils. The in vitro data as a whole suggest that there is a complex multicomponent system involved in the neutrophil-mediated injury observed during I/R.

Clearly there are many questions that remain unanswered regarding the hypothesis proposed in Fig. 1. The complexity of our scheme continues to grow particularly in the area of neutrophil recruitment and activation. Future progress in this field, particularly from a therapeutic viewpoint, will depend on the development of new techniques for monitoring granulocyte function in vivo and the identification of new compounds that selectively interfere with one or more of the many granulocyte processes.

References

Ballin HM, Meyer MW (1960) Intestinal lymph flow in dogs after endotoxin. Proc Soc Exp Biol Med 103:93–95

Batelli MG, Dellacorte E, Stirpe F (1972) Xanthine oxidase type D (dehydrogenase) in the intestine and other organs of the rat. Biochem J 126:747–749

Berkaw RL, Wang D, Larrich JW, Howard TH (1986) Recombinant necrosis factor augments human neutrophil superoxide production. Blood 68:80 (abstr)

Bielski BHJ, Shiue GG (1979) Reaction rates of superoxide radicals with the essential amino acids. In: Ciba Found (ed) Oxygen free radicals and tissue damage. Elsevier, New York, pp 43–56

Blum H, Summers JJ, Schnall MD, Barlow C, Leigh JS, Chance B, Buzby GP (1986) Acute intestinal ischemia studies by phosphorous nuclear magnetic resonance spectroscopy. Ann Surg 204:83–88

Braquet P, Hosford D, Braquet M, Bourgain R, Bussolino F (1989a) Role of cytokines and platelet activating factor in microvascular immune injury. Int Arch Allergy Appl Immunol 88:88–100

Braquet P, Paubert-Braquet M, Koltai M, Bourgain R, Bussolino F, Hosford D (1989b) Is there a case for PAF antagonists in the treatment of ischemic states? Trendo Pharmacol Sci 10:23–30

Buege JA, Aust SD (1976) Lactoperoxidase-catalyzed lipid peroxidation of microsomal and artificial membranes. Biochim Biophys Acta 444:192–201
Bussolino F, Camussi G, Baglioni C (1988) Synthesis and release of platelet activating factor by human vascular endothelial cells treated with tumor necrosis factor or interleukin 1α. J Biol Chem 263:11856–11861
Cross CE, Halliwell B, Allen A (1984) Antioxidant protection: a function of tracheobronchial and gastrointestinal mucus. Lancet I:1328–1330
Droy-Lefaix M, Drouet Y, Geraud G, Braquet P (1988) Involvement of platelet activating factor in rat ischemia reperfusion gastric damage. In: Braquet P (ed) Ginkgolides: chemistry, biology, pharmacology and clinical perspectives. Prous, Barcelona, pp 563–574
Filep J, Herman F, Braquet P, Mozes T (1989) Incrased levels of platelet activating factor in blood following intestinal ischemia in the dog. Biochem Biophys Res Commun 158:353–359
Freeman BA, Crapo JD (1982) Free radicals and tissue injury. Lab Invest 47:412–426
Gilman AG, Goodman LS, Gilman A (1980) The pharmacological basis of therapeutics, 6th edn. MacMillan, New York
Granger DN (1988) Role of xanthine oxidase and granulocytes in ischemia-reperfusion injury. Am J Physiol 255:H1269–H1275
Granger DN, Sennett M, McElearney PM, Taylor AE (1980) Effect of local arterial hypotension on cat intestinal capillary permeability. Gastroenterology 79:474–480
Granger DN, Rutili G, McCord JM (1981) Superoxide radicals in feline intestinal ischemia. Gastroenterology 81:22–29
Granger DN, Hollwarth ME, Parks DA (1986a) Ischemia-reperfusion injury: role of oxygen-derived free radicals. Acta Physiol Scand [Suppl] 548:47–64
Granger DN, McCord JM, Parks DA, Hollwarth ME (1986b) Xanthine oxidase inhibitors attenuate ischemia-induced vascular permeability changes in the cat intestine. Gastroenterology 90:80–84
Grisham MB, Hernandez LA, Granger DN (1986) Xanthine oxidase and neutrophil infiltration in intestinal ischemia. Am J Physiol 251:G567–G574
Grisham MB, Van Ritter C, Smith BF, Lamont JT, Granger DN (1987) Interaction between oxygen radicals and gastric mucin. Am J Physiol 253:G93–G96
Haglund U, Lundholm K, Lundgren O et al. (1977) Intestinal lysosomal enzyme activity in regional simulated shock: influence of methylprednisolone and albumin. Circ Shock 4:27–27
Hale WB, Turner B, Lamont JT (1986) Superoxide radicals stimulate gall bladder mucin hypersecretion. Gastroenterology 90:1731 (abstr)
Hernandez LA, Grisham MB, Granger DN (1987a) A role for iron in oxidant-mediated ischemic injury to intestinal microvasculature. Am J Physiol 253:G49–G53
Hernandez LA, Grisham MB, Granger DN (1987b) Effects of Cu-DIPS on ischemia-reperfusion injury. In: Sorenson JRJ (ed) Biology of copper complexes. Humana, Clifton Nj, pp 201–210
Hernandez LA, Grisham MB, Twohig B, Arfors KE, Harlan JM, Granger DN (1987c) Role of neutrophils in ischemia-reperfusion induced microvascular injury. Am J Physiol 253:H699–H703
Jennings RB, Reimer KA, Hill ML, Mayer SE (1981) Total ischemia in dog hearts in vitro. Circ Res 49:892–899
Kobold EE, Thal AP (1963) Quantitation and identification of vasocactive substances liberated during various types of experimental and clinical intestinal ischemia. Surg Gynecol Obstet 117:315–322
Korthuis RJ, Smith JK, Carden DL (1989) Hypoxic reperfusion attenuates postischemic microvascular injury. Am J Physiol 256:H315–H319
Krenitsky TA, Tuttle JV, Cattau EL, Wang PA (1974) A comparison of the distribution and electron acceptor specificities of xanthine oxidase and aldehyde oxidase. Comp Biochem Physiol 181:177–182

Lash LH, Hagen TM, Jones DP (1986) Exogenous glutathione protects intestinal epithelial cells from oxidative injury. Proc Natl Acad Sci USA 83:4641–4645

Lewis MS, Whatley RE, Cain P, McIntyre TM, Prescott SM, Zimmerman GA (1988) Hydrogen peroxide stimulates the synthesis of platelet activating factor by endothelium and induces endothelial cell-dependent neutrophil adhesion. J Clin Invest 82:2045–2055

McCord JM, Roy RS (1982) The pathophysiology of superoxide: roles in inflammation and ischemia. Can J Physiol Pharmacol 60:1346–1352

Moorhouse PC, Grootveld M, Halliwell B, Quinlan JG, Gutteridge JMC (1987) Allopurinol and oxypurinol are hydroxy radical scavengers. FEBS Lett 213:23–28

Morris JB, Bulkley GB, Haglund U, Cadenas E, Sies H (1987) The direct, real-time demonstration of oxygen free radical generation at reperfusion following ischemia in rat small intestine. Gastroenterology 92:1541

Mousson B, Desjacques P, Baltassat P (1983) Measurement of xanthine oxidase activity in some human tissues. Enzyme 29:32–43

Nayfield SG, Kent TH, Rodman NF (1976) Gastrointestinal effects of acute ferrous sulfate poisoning in rats. Arch Pathol Lab Med 100:325–328

Nilsson UA, Lundgren O, Haglind E, Bylund-Fellienius AC (1987) Radical production during intestinal ischemia and reperfusion in vivo in the cat – an ESR study. In: Simic M (ed) Proceedings of the 4th International Congress on Oxygen Radicals, June 27–July 3, University of California, AT San Diego, La Jolla, California, USA pp 150–152

Parks DA, Granger DN (1983) Ischemia-induced vascular changes: role of xanthine oxidase and hydroxyl radicals. Am J Physiol 245:G285–G289

Parker DA, Granger DN (1986a) Contributions of ischemia and reperfusion to mucosal lesion formation. Am J Physiol 250:G749–G753

Parks DA, Granger DN (1986b) Xanthine oxidase: biochemistry, distribution and physiology. Acta Physiol Scand [Suppl] 548:87–99

Parks DA, Granger DN, Bulkley GB, Shah AK (1985) Soybean trypsin inhibitor attenuates ischemic injury to the feline small intestine. Gastroenterology 89:6–12

Parks DA, Shah AK, Granger DN (1984) Oxygen radicals: effects on intestinal vascular permeability. Am J Physiol 247:G167–G170

Parks DA, Henson JL, Granger DN (1986) Effect of xanthine oxidase inactivation on ischemic injury to the small intestine. Physiologist 29:101 (abstr)

Parks DA, Williams TK, Beckman JS (1988) Conversion of xanthine dehydrogenase to oxidase in ischemic rat intestine: a reevaluation. Am J Physiol 254:G768–G774

Paubert-Braquet M, Longchampt MO, Koltz P, Guilbund J (1988) Tumor necrosis factor (TNF) primes human neutrophils (PMN) platelet activating factor (PAD)-induced superoxide generation. Consequences in promoting PMN-mediated endothelial cell (EC) damages. Prostaglandins 35:803 (abstr)

Perez HD, Weksler BB, Goldstein IM (1980) Generation of a chemotactic lipid from arachidonic acid by exposure to a superoxide-generating system. Inflammation 4:313

Petrone WF, English DK, Wong K, McCord JM (1980) Free radicals and inflammation: superoxide dependent activation of a neutrophil chemotactic factor in plasma. Proc Natl Acad Sci USA 77:1159

Roldan EJA, Pinus CR, Turrens JF, Boveris A (1989) Chemiluminescence of ischaemic and reperfused intestine in vivo. GUT 30:184–187

Romson JL, Hook BG, Kunkel SL, Abrams GD, Schork A, Lucchesi BR (1983) Reduction of the extent of ischemic myocardial injury by neutrophil depletion in the dog. Circulation 67:1016–1023

Rossi F (1986) The superoxide forming NADPH oxidase of phagocytes: nature, mechanisms of activation and function. Biochim Biophys Acta 853:65–89

Roy RS, McCord JM (1983) Superoxide and ischemia: conversion of xanthine dehydrogenase to xanthine oxidase. In: Greenwald RA, Cohen G (eds) Oxy radicals and their scavenger system, vol 2: cellular and medical aspects. Elsevier/North-Holland, New York, pp 143–153 ekizuka E, Benoit JN, Grisham MB, Granger DN (1989) Dimethylsulfoxide prevents chemoattractant induced leukocyte adherence. Am J Physiol 256:H594–H597

choenberg MH, Muhl E, Sellin D, Younes M, Schildberg FW, Haglund U (1984) Posthypotensive generation of superoxide free radicals – possible role in the pathogenesis of the intestinal mucosal damage. Acta Chir Scand 150:301–309

imon RH, Scoggin CH, Patterson D (1981) Hydrogen peroxide causes the fatal injury to human fibroblasts exposed to oxygen radicals. J Biol Chem 256:7181–7186

pector T, Ferone R (1984) Folic acid does not inactivate xanthine oxidase. J Biol Chem 259:10784–10786

uzuki M, Grisham MB, Granger DN (1989) Superoxide plays a role in reperfusion-induced leukocyte adherence to microvascular endothelium. Gastroenterology (abstr) 96:A497

'agesson C, Lindahl M, Otamiri T (1988) BN 52021 ameliorates mucosal damage associated with small intestinal ischaemia in rats. In: Braquet P (ed) Ginkgolides: chemistry, biology, pharmacology and clinical perspectives. Prous JR, Barcelona, pp 553–561

'homas CE, Morehouse LA, Aust SD (1985) Ferritin and superoxide-dependent lipid peroxidation. J Biol Chem 260:3275–3280

'opham RW, Walker MC, Calisch MP, Williams RW (1982) Evidence for the participation of intestinal xanthine oxidase in the mucosal processing of iron. Biochemistry 21:4529–4535

Veiss SJ (1986) Oxygen, ischemia, and inflammation. Acta Physiol Scand [Suppl] 548:9–38

Veiss SJ, Peppin G, Oritz X, Ragsdale C, Test ST (1985) Oxidative autoactivation of latent collagenase by human neutrophils. Science 227:747–749

'ounes M, Schoenberg MH, Jung H, Fredholm BB, Haglund U, Schildberg FW (1984) Oxidative tissue damage following regional intestinal ischemia and reperfusion in the cat. Res Exp Med (Berl) 184:259–264

'ounes M, Mohr A, Schoenberg MH, Schildberg FW (1987) Inhibition of lipid peroxidation by superoxide dismutase following regional intestinal ischemia and reperfusion. Res Exp Med (Berl) 187:9–17

;immerman BJ, Granger DN (1988) Role of hydrogen peroxide, iron and hydroxyl radicals in ischemia/reperfused-induced neutrophil infiltration. Physiologist 31:A229 (abstr)

;immerman BJ, Granger DN (1989) Role of leukotriene B4 in ischemia/reperfusion-induced granulocyte infiltration. Gastroenterology 96:A697

;immerman BJ, Grisham MB, Granger DN (1987) Role of superoxide-dependent chemoattractants in ischemia-reperfusion induced neutrophil infiltration. Fed Proc 46:1124 (abstr)

Monitoring

Preoperative Assessment and Monitoring of High-Risk Patients

). Mayr and L. Hannemann

Mortality statistics of the past 30 years show that the total perioperative mortality has not changed [1]. However, this does not mean that no advances have been made in anesthesiology and surgery. Rather, dynamics and changes in the clinical pictures have to be considered, as well as the fact that severe functional disorders of vital systems already exist prior to surgery. These are the factors that ultimately determine the outcome at the usual level.

It is a characteristic of our time that the general public becomes more and more aware of risk analyses. "Public opinion" [21, 36] plays an important role in the individual's awareness of the problems of our time, and everybody who wants to does know about the health risks associated with smoking, alcohol, and malnutrition, and the hazards to which we all are exposed through the uncritical use of the possibilities made available by technical progress.

Within in the last 20 years, considerations in connection with assessing the perioperative risk have been focussed on the cardiocirculatory system. This can be explained, in part, by medical history, and, in part, by irrational reasons, but also by the fact that access to this system is relatively easy and that it is possible to measure and calculate pressures and flow phenomena.

In the attempt to assess the functional situation or the range of functions of other organs and organ systems, such as the immune system, we lag far behind in the development of a comparable monitoring. It therefore continues to be difficult to assess the risk in the perioperative phase, during which all organs and organ systems are exposed to extreme strain. This is one of the reasons why the clinical assessment of the patient's general condition, which was developed by Saklad [79] as early as 1941, is still an accepted form of risk assessment all over the world. It was modified in 1963 [5, 53], and this version, known as the ASA classification, is still valid today. It was not even Saklad's primary intention to predict the effect of a surgical intervention on a patient in a certain general physical condition, but rather to obtain a better definition of patients by a description of their general condition for statistical assessment.

Marx [61], who correlated the preoperative ASA classification with perioperative mortality, demonstrated that higher ASA classes are associated with an increased mortality. It has since been shown by several investigators that the ASA classes are an excellent indicator of the perioperative risk [29, 44, 61, 90].

The Goldmann index [40], which is used for assessing the perioperative risk especially in patients with a high cardiac risk, is based on a system of nine risk factors and assigns a high score to recent cardiac infarction and congested jugular veins. This is done in an attempt to predict the probability of perioperatively occurring circulatory complications as precisely as possible. It is noteworthy that, according to Goldmann [41], stable angina pectoris does not increase the risk, even if the patients undergo major surgery. Nevertheless, the role of coronary heart disease with its multiple forms of clinical manifestitations is discussed controversially. According to Davis and Nemay [24, 71], in patients with a stable form of exertion-induced angina, the combined risk associated with coronary angiography and bypass surgery is higher than that associated with an elective noncardiac intervention. On the other hand, it is known that the cardiac risk associated with noncardiac interventions is markedly lowered following aortocoronary bypass surgery [10, 45, 50, 60], though this opinion is not shared by all authors [20]. But in cases of unstable angina pectoris, Diehl and coworkers [27] strictly recommend to define a patient's cardiac exertion range on the basis of a carefully established case history and additional diagnostic measures such as ergometry or coronary angiography before he or she can undergo elective surgery. If necessary, aortocoronary bypass surgery is to be preferred. In this connection, the risk of patients with a previous cardiac infarction is frequently discussed. Arkins and Hertzer [4, 46] report a reinfarction rate of about 6% in patients with a history of recent infarction. We can, however, not ignore investigations by Steen and Tharan [82, 85], who report a reinfarction rate of 27% for patients with a history of infarction within the 3 months beforehand, a rate of 11% for infarction within 3 to 6 months, and a rate of 6% only for patients in whom cardiac infarction occurred more than 6 months previously.

These very serious results have been somewhat qualified by more recent investigations. Rao and coworkers [77] presented a study in 1983, in which 1097 patients with a history of cardiac infarction were investigated. One group included patients from 1973–1976, a period, during which invasive monitoring and the use of vasoactive substances had not been established. The second group (1977–1982) comprised patients who benefitted from invasive cardiovascular monitoring and the resulting possibilities of immediately correcting hemodynamic changes.

Though the pros and cons as well as risks and benefits of invasive hemodynamic monitoring will continue to be discussed for a long time [11], I would like to conclude my discussion of this problem by pointing out the paper by Barron [7], in which the value of routine right-heart catheterization of patients undergoing angiography for anginose complaints is questioned. The study included 2178 patients, in whom the degree of complaints was assessed according to the classification of the Canadian Cardiocirculatory Society for Angina pectoris [15]. Of the patients 4.8% had a wedge pressure of >18 mmHg and 6% a cardiac index of <2 l/min·m^2, a finding, which, at least subclinically, suggests a left-ventricular insuffiency. Altogether, 14.5% or approximately 300 of the 2178 patients showed pathological changes in hemodynamic paramters, which could be additionally objectified by right-heart catheterization. The knowledge of these cardiac limitations could be taken into consideration during the perioperative phase for the benefit of the patients.

Besides routine procedures, such as case history, clinical examination, ECG, chest X-ray, pulmonary function, and laboratory parameters, exercise tests and determination of the ejection fraction have been established as useful tools in assessing the range of cardiac function.

A number of outhors advocate mandatory ergometry tests prior to a surgical intervention for patients with manifest coronary heart disease [34, 35]. In case of positive findings they recommend to perform a coronary angiography with a subsequent aortocoronary bypass operation prior to the elective intervention in order to lower the risk of perioperative myocardial ischemia. It is known [22, 58, 62] that, during the perioperative phase, cardiac-induced complications occur in 30%–90% of the patients with pronounced ischemic ST-segment reactions to ergometric exercise. However, one must keep in mind the disadvantages of this method, like the relatively low sensitivity, and individual factors, such as circulatory disturbances, joint arthrosis, dyspnea, and fear, which frequently make it necessary to discontinue the test before maximal cardiac performance is reached and, thus, reduce the informational value of exercise tests.

In this connection, we would like to call attention to the study by Gerson and coworkers [38], who submitted all patients over 65 years to an exercise test prior to major surgery. The authors demonstrated that only the inability to reach a heart rate of 100/min or to endure the ergometric exercise for at least 2 min in an upright sitting posture could be correlated with the survival rate. This considerably limits the value of ST-segment analysis during exercise for predicting the perioperative risk.

The value of conventional exercise testing can be improved by spiroergometry [8, 28, 32, 33, 37, 48, 91, 92]. Electrochemical gas analyzers, which meanwhile have a response time of milliseconds, facilitate the measurement of O_2 consumption and CO_2 production during rest and exercise. Maximal exercise tolerance is defined as maximal oxygen consumption and is reached when – after the anaerobic threshold is reached – oxygen consumption remains constant for at least 30 s to 2 min while the subject is exposed to increasing strain [6, 9, 49, 64]. At this point, oxygen extraction in the tissue and cardiac output have reached their maximum and cannot be increased further. This cardiocirculatory reserve is dependent upon age, sex, and training condition, and is subject to the discontinuation criteria usually applied for exercise tests.

According to Weber and Janicki [93], values of about 20 ml/kg/min for maximal oxygen consumption as a measure of individual exercise tolerance are considered normal for patients with chronic left-heart insufficiency, while values of 10 ml/kg/min during maximal exercise must be regarded as hazardous. This finding is in good agreement with clinical examinations as well as hemodynamic parameters. All patients with reduced oxygen consumption during exercise are characterized by pronounced systolic weakness, wedge pressures of >20 mmHg at rest, and maximal oxygen extraction in tissue. Under these conditions, the O_2 supply to the tissue can only be increased by the heart rate. It is precisely these patients, in whom it would be very important to determine the range of cardiac function, who frequently fail to reach the anaerobic threshold or maximal O_2 consumption, because other criteria render it necessary to discontinue the exercise test. Because of this fact and also according to our experience, spiroergometry, like all other exercise tests, is of limited value in predicting the perioperative risk of critically ill patients, although it is a simple, elegant, and noninvasive procedure.

Radionuclide ventriculography has proven its effectiveness as a noninvasive procedure in the assessment of left-ventricular function [80]. It is a procedure to which a patient can be submitted any time because it involves little discomfort; and the determination of the regional and global ejection fraction as well as of the end-systolic and end-diastolic volumes allow a precise description of the left ventricle, which is comparable to that obtained by contrast ventriculography [81]. A markedly lowered ejection fraction of <0.36 already before the operation is associated with a high complication rate in patients undergoing reconstructive vascular surgery of the distal abdominal aorta [65, 74]. Lazor and coworkers [31] report a mortality rate of noncardiac interventions of about 20% in patients with a markedly lower ejection fraction.

Foster and coworkers [31] showed that radionuclide ventriculography is also suitable for assessing the risk associated with noncardiac surgery in patients with coronary heart disease. These authors investigated 1600 patients with preexisting coronary heart disease who had to undergo noncardiac surgery. They demonstrated that only angiographically confirmed left-heart insufficiency correlated with perioperative mortality, while the extent of the disease and the number of affected coronary vessels did not. Since the important question as to the presence of left-ventricular insufficiency can be answered by RNV just as well or even better, the latter is an optimal method for assessing left-ventricular insufficiency prior to noncardiac interventions.

The detection of impaired pulmonary function is just as important as the assessment of cardiac risks. Pulmonary risk factors can best be assessed by carefully establishing the patient's history of previous pulmonary disease, supplemented by spirometry and blood gas analysis. The incidence and severity of perioperative pulmonary complications is closely correlated with perioperative pulmonary function [26]. Chronic-obstructive respiratory tract disease is the most frequent underlying pulmonary disease and is associated with a fourfold higher complications rate [89]. Kawakami [52] demonstrated that patients suffering from chronic-obstructive lung disease with low arterial oxygen tension and mixed venous saturation in addition to increased CO_2 tension in arterial and mixed venous blood have a markedly life expectancy than patients with obstructive lung disease who do not have this constellation of findings. Postoperative complications and mortality through already preoperatively detectable bronchopulmonary disorders were ranked first and second, respectively, by the study group associated with Ahnefeld, Lutz, and Striebel [2, 59, 83]. Thus, it seems all the more important to recommend that pulmonary deficits that are clearly recognizable by screening methods be corrected already ıreoperatively, if possible. In case of elective surgery, we consider it necessary nd useful that patients with objectified bronchopulmonary disease which may ıe improved by conservative therapy be treated until the therapeutic goal is eached. For economic reasons we are in favor of discharging these patients rom hospital and have them continue treatment on an outpatient basis. The ıatients are again hospitalized after control of the ambulatory therapy and it ; only then that he or she may undergo elective surgery.

The correct type of hemodynamic monitoring can always be determined or a patient who can be clearly assigned to a risk group. However, it is difficult o correctly assess an asymptomatic high-risk patient, choose the right type of ıonitoring, and get him safely through the perioperative phase. A careful anmnesis and sufficient experience in the treatment of high-risk patients are necssary in addition to theoretical knowledge. There are a number of strategies /hich can be applied to reduce the risk during routine work:

Indication and type and time of the surgical intervention play an important ole. If possible, the intervention which puts the least strain on the patient hould be chose, although even then there still remains a considerable risk. If outine examination procedures confirm a high cardial risk and there is no alernative to the scheduled surgical intervention, apply invasive hemodynamic nonitoring with the Swan-Ganz catheter and direct arterial pressure measurenent according to Rao et al. [77]. Also, immediately prior to the intervention, letermine the filling pressure at which the highest CI can be obtained by means ıf a step-by-step volume loading in order to create the best hemodynamic tarting position for that patient. We consider it important that a high-risk paient is cared for perioperatively by an experienced anesthetist and a surgeon nd monitored for an extended period of time in the intensive care unit.

Not only the treatment principles but also the monitoring and management pplied in connection with these clinical pictures have to be reevaluated and orrected on the basis of mortality statistics. It starts with the preoperative risk ssessment because it is here that the course is set and the decisions are made /hich later play a decisive role in determining the outcome. It must be considred whether substantial risk factors were recognized as such already preopertively or were overlooked and if they could have been minimized or even elimnated. It should also be checked if the monitoring system chosen by us was pplied in such a way that the areas with the highest number of complications ır lethal courses were monitored most closely.

We have investigated this problem for the year 1988 on the basis of our own nortality statistics in general surgery and intensive care patients: 348 of a total ıf 1088 patients came from the department of general, thoracic, and vascular urgery; 53 of these patients, or 15.3%, died on the intensive care unit. Two ıatients died from acute cardiac infarction, 1 from malignant dysrhythmia, 11 ıatients died in hemorrhagic shock. Thirty-two patients died of sepsis with nultiple organ failure, lungs and abdomen being the most frequent focus of nfections. Seven patients died of other causes. It should be stated that lethal ıemodynamic complications now occur less frequently due to excellent carliovascular monitoring and management. However, severe infections ending in septic shock with multiple organ failure still have a high mortality rate. It is thus necessary to develop an immunological or infectiological monitoring system that is as efficient as the one already existing in hemodynamics. Immunologically, the following aims should be fulfilled:

1. Assess the actual immune status
2. Favorably influence the patients perioperative risk via a modification of the immune system, if necessary

The immune system can be stimulated directly via interferon, BCG, steroids, interleukin I, etc., or indirectly via alimentary therapeutics, resection of malignant growths, or removal of chronic inflammatory processes.

To what extent is it possible today to record the immune status in such a manner that in allows reliable conclusions with regard to the actual state of the immune reaction and can it be applied in a reliable, easy, and economical routine procedure? There are no quantitative or qualitative measurements or methods which come even close to meeting these requirements. Nevertheless, there is no doubt nowadays that both static and functional measurements of the immune response are in a statistically confirmed correlation to the probability of postoperative complications [3, 17, 43, 54, 68]. Static measurements include, for example, immunoglobulin in serum, absolute lymphocyte count, and distribution of lymphocytes among cells with helper or suppressor function by means of monoclonal antibodies. Functional measurements comprise the intracutaneous test of retarded immunity, phagocytosis, vaccine-stimulated antibody production, etc. Sensitivity and specificity of the parameters studied so far are, however, too negligible to be considered a decisive criterion for the individual patient during a treatment phase. Among the large number of parameters, the intracutaneous test of retarded immunity and the absolute lymphocyte count have only distinguished themselves insofar as they are at best suited to remain integrated as links in complex risk formulas.

What is, at this point, an established therapeutic approach?

1. Surgical interventions like removal of foci or tumors may contribute to restoring immunity [18, 30, 76, 88].
2. Surgery itself can lead to severe disturbances of the immune status: sustained disorder of lymphocytes or increase of suppressor cells, e.g., pneumococcus sepsis after splenectomy in children [87].
3. Improving the nutritional status is the only reliable therapeutic measure in confirmed immune deficiency.
4. Not only the usefulness but also the harmlessness of immunomodulators have yet to be proved [19, 63, 66, 75, 86].

The nutritional status is of great importance in the evaluation of the perioperative risk of infection [3, 17, 43, 54, 68]. As early as 1936, Studley [84] observed that the mortality rate of gastrectomy patients who lost more than 20% of body weight preoperatively was much higher than that of patients without substantial weight loss. In 1944, Cannon [16] described an increased risk of infection in hypoproteinemic patients; in 1955, Rhoads and Alexander [78] reported a higher rate of postoperative complications in hyperproteinemia <63 g/l, and Neumann [73], in 1975, was one of the first to observe a reduced cellular immune reaction with an increased infection rate in children suffering from malnutrition.

We know now that there is an inverse correlation between serum albumin level and hospital mortality in surgical patients [39]. In addition, proteins with a shorter half-life than albumin, like prealbumin, transferrin, retinol-binding protein, and a reduced iron-binding capacity in serum are valid indications of nutritional deficiency [14, 51, 56]. A reflection of the "inner parameters" just described are antropometric measurements like weight behavior, triceps skinfold thickness, or brachial muscle circumference [23, 47, 71].

The correlation between nutritional state and immunological capacity is well known [23, 42]. A number of studies have been published on this problem in recent years which found it difficult to quantify the close correlation. One possible explanation may be that, besides the nutritional status, the low sensitivity of the retarded intracutaneous test may be influenced by a number of other factors such as tumor stage, sensitization by the corresponding antigen, etc.

An evaluation of the preoperative risk must obviously take into account the parameters briefly discussed by us. Deficits of other organs, e.g., liver or kidney or a combination of clinical pictures, play a similarly decisive role. In this connection it is absolutely necessary to collaborate with other disciplines to determine the importance of different clinical pictures for the perioperative period. At the same time, no discipline should be required to "agree that a patient undergo surgery" in medically doubtful and legally contestable cases. Rather, it is necessary to find out whether the individual clinical picture can be improved preoperatively by conservative treatment, whether a surgical intervention can be chosen which puts less strain on the patient, and, if not, how the patient can pass through the perioperative phase with as little discomfort as possible.

The so-called routine problems, such as structure of the clinic, professional qualificatioins, duration of the intervention, intraoperative risks, personal monitoring, etc. should not be neglected as they are by no means an insignificant in the causes of perioperative mortality.

References

1. Ahnefeld FW, Heinrich H (1983) Hat sich in der Routine des Anästhesisten die Berücksichtigung von Risikofaktoren bewährt? Langenbeck's Arch Chir 361:263–267
2. Ahnefeld FW, Bergmann H, Burri C, Dick W, Halmagyi M, Rügheimer E (eds) (1976) Vorwort (Preface). In: Der Risikopatient in der Anaesthesie, vol 2. Respiratorische Störungen. Springer, Berlin Heidelberg New York, S 12
3. Allgöver M, Dürig M, Heberer M (1985) Two techniques of measurement of the delayed type hypersensitivity skin test response for the assessment of bacterial host resistance. Invited commentary. World J Surg 9:805–806
4. Arkins R, Smessaert AA, Hicks RG (1964) Mortality and morbidity in surgical patients with coronary artery disease. JAMA 190:485–488

5. ASA (1963) New classification on physical status. Anesthesiology 24:111
6. Astrand P-O (1976) Quantification of exercise capability and evaluation of physical capacity in man. Prod Cardiovasc Dis 19:51–67
7. Barron JT, Ruggie N, Uretz E, Messer JV (1988) Findings on routine right heart catheterization in patients with suspected coronary artery disease. Am Heart J 6:1193–1198
8. Benje W, Litchfield RL, Marcus ML (1980) Exercise capacity in patients with severe left ventricular dysfunction. Circulation 61:955–959
9. Bergh U, Kanstrup I-L, Ekblom B (1976) Maximal oxygen uptake during exercise with various combinations of arm and leg work. J Appl Physiol 41:191–196
10. Bernhard VM, Johnson WD, Peterson JJ (1972) Carotid artery stenosis – association with surgery for coronary artery disease. Arch Surg 105:837–840
11. Bille-Brahe NE, Eickhoff JH (1980) Measurement of central haemodynamic parameters during preoperative exercise testing in patients suspected of arteriosclerotic heart disease: value in predicting postoperative cardiac complications. Acta Chir Scand 502:38–45
12. Bistrian BR, Blackburn GL, Vitale J et al. (1976) Prevalence of malnutrition in general medical patients. JAMA 235:1567–1570
13. Bistrian BR, Blackburn GL, Hallowell E et al. (1974) Protein status of general surgical patients. JAMA 230:858–860
14. Blackburn GL, Bistrian BR, Harvey K (1981) Indicies of protein-calorie malnutrition as predictors of survival. In: Levensoen SM (ed) Nutritional assessment – present status. Ross Laboratories, Columbus, pp 131–137
15. Campeau L (1976) Grading of angina pectoris. Circulation 54:522–523
16. Cannon PR, Wissler RV, Woolridge RL et al. (1944) The relationship of protein deficiency to surgical infection. Ann Surg 120:514–525
17. Christou NV, Boisvert G, Broadhead M, Meakins JL (1985) Two techniques of measurement of the delayed type hypersensitivity skin test response for the assessment of bacterial host resistance. World J Surg 9:805–806
18. Christou NV, Meakins JL (1979) Neutrophil function in surgical patients: two inhibitors of granulocyte chemotaxis associated with sepsis. J Surg Res 26:355–364
19. Christou NV, Meakins JL (1979) Neutrophil function in surgical patients: in vitro correction of abnormal neutrophil chemotaxis by levamisole. Surgery 85:543–548
20. Crawford ES, Morris GC, Howell JF, Flynn WF, Moorhead DT (1978) Operative risk in patients with previous coronary artery bypass. Ann Thorac Surg 26:215–221
21. Cumming RB (1982) Myocardial infarction as a postoperativ complication of major surgery. Risk Anal 1–3:47–54
22. Cutler BS, Wheeler HB, Paraskos JA, Cardullo PA (1981) Applicability and interpretation of electrocardiographic stress testing in patients with peripheral vascular disease. Am J Surg 141:501–506
23. Daly JM, Dudrick SJ, Copeland EM (1978) Effects of protein depletion and repletion on cell mediated immunity inexperimental animals. Ann Surg 188:791–796
24. Davis K, Kennedy JW, Kemp HG Jr, Judkins MP, Gosselin AJ, Killip T (1979) Complications of coronary arteriography from the collaborative study of coronary artery surgery (CASS). Circulation 59:1105–1111
25. Dempsey DT, Mullen JL, Buzby GP (1988) The link between nutritional status and clinical autcome. Can nutritional intervention modify it? Am J Clin Nutr 47:352–356
26. Deutsches Ärzteblatt (1985) Praeoperative Lungenfunktionsdiagnostik. Empfehlungen der Deutschen Gesellschaft für Pneumologie und Tuberkulose, Heft 20, Ausgabe B
27. Diehl JT, Cali RF, Hertzer NR, Beven MD (1983) Complications of abdominal aortic reconstruction. Ann Surg 197:49–56
28. Engler R, Ray R, Higgins C, McNally C, Buxton WH, Bhargava V, Shabetal R (1982) Clinical assessment and follow-up of functional capacity in patients with chronic congestive cardiomyopathy. Am J Cardiol 49:1832–1937

29. Filzwieser G, List WF (1983) Morbidity and mortality in elective geriatric surgery. In: Vickers MD, Lunn JN (eds) Mortality in anaesthesia. Springer, Berlin Heidelberg New York Tokyo, p 75
30. Flad HD, Betzler M, Herthart CH (1979) Zum heutigen Stand der Immuntherapie maligner Tumoren. Chirurg 50:11–15
31. Foster ED, Davis KB, Carpenter JA, Abele S, Fray D (1986) Principal investigators of CASS and their associates. Risk of noncardiac operation in patients with defined coronary disease: the coronary artery surgery study (CASS) registry experience. Ann Thorac Surg 41:42–50
32. Franciosa JA, Ziesche S, Wilen M (1979) Functional capacity of patients with chronic left ventricular failure. Am J Med 67:460–466
33. Franciosa JA, Park M, Levine B (1981) Lack of correlation between exercise capacity and indices of left ventricular performance in heart failure. Am J Cardiol 47:33–39
34. Fudge TL, McKinnon WMP, Schoettle GP, Ochsner JL, Mills NL (1981) Improved operative risk after myocardial revascularization. South Med J 74:799–801
35. Gage AA, Bhayana JN, Balu V, Hook N (1977) Assessment of cardiac risk in surgical patients. Arch Surg 112:1488–1492
36. Garfield E (1982) Risk Anal. Current Contents 35:5
37. Gelberg HJ, Rubin SA, Ports TA, Brundge H, Pamley WW, Chatterjee K (1979) Detectioin of left ventricular functional reserve by supine exercise hemodynamics in patients with severe, chronic heart failure. Am J Cardiol 44:1062–1067
38. Gerson MC, Hurst JM, Hertzberg VS et al. (1985) Cardiac prognosis in noncardiac geriatric surgery. Ann Int Med 103:832–837
39. Golden MHN (1982) Transport proteins as indices of protein status. Am J CLin Nutr 35:1159–1165
40. Goldmann L, Caldera D, Nussbaum SR, Southwick FS, Derba RN, Krogstad D, Murray B, Burke DS, O'Malley TA, Goroll AH, Caplan AH, Caplan SH, Nolan J, Carabello B, Slater EE (1977) Multifactorial index of cardiac risk in noncardiac surgical procedures. N Engl J Med 197:845
41. Goldmann L (1983) Cardiac risk and complications of noncardiac surgery. Ann Int Med 98:504–513
42. Haffejee HH, Angorn IB (1979) Nutritional status and the nonspecific cellular and humoral immune response in esophageal carcinoma. Ann Surg 189:475–479
43. Heberer M, Dürig M, Harder F (1984) Die oropharyngo-oesophagealen Carcinome. Aspekte des Ernährungszustandes und der Immunabwehr. Helv Chir Acta 51:283–286
44. Heinrich H, Ahnefeld FW, Bisio E, Erdle HP, Winter H (1985) Zusammenhänge zwischen präoperativer Risikobeurteilung und intraoperativer Rate kardiozirkulatorischer Komplikationen. Herz/Kreislauf 3:122
45. Hertzer NR, Young JR, Kramer JR et al. (1979) Routine coronary angiography prior to elective aortic reconstruction: results of selective myocardial revascularization in patients with peripheral vascular disease. Arch Surg 114:1336–1344
46. Hertzer NR (1983) Management of coronary artery disease in patients undergoing surgery for aortic and distal occlusive disease. Presented at the Tenth Annual Symposium on Current Critical Problems in Vascular Surgery. 10–12 November, New York
47. Hickman DM, Miller RA, Rombeau JL et al. (1980) Serum albumin and body weight as predictors of postoperative course in colorectal cancer. JPEN 4:314–316
48. Higginbotham MD, Morris KG, Conn EH, Coleman RE, Cobb FR (1983) Determinants of variable exercise performance among patients with severe left ventricular dysfunction. Am J Cardiol 5:51–60
49. Jones NL, Campbell EJM, Edwards RHT, Robertson DG (1975) Clinical exercise testing. Saunders, Philadelphia, pp 25–29

50. Kaklan JA, Dunbar RW (1979) Anesthesia for noncardiac surgery in patients with cardiac disease. In: Kaplan JA (ed) Cardiac anesthesia. Grune & Stratton, New York
51. Kaminski MV, Fitzgerald MJ, Murphy RJ et al. (1977) Correlation of mortality with serum transferrin and anergy. JPEN 1:27
52. Kawakami Y, Kishi F, Yamamoto H, Miyamoto K (1983) Relation of oxygen delivery, mixed venous oxygenation, and pulmonary hemodynamics to prognosis in chronic obstructive pulmonary disease. N Engl J Med 308:1045–1049
53. Keats AS (1978) The ASA classification of physical status – a recapitulation. Anesthesiology 49:233
54. Kremer B, Früh C, Homann NP, Reuter K, Bornholdt D (1983) Immunreaktivität, ein präoperativ faßbarer Parameter? Langenbeck's Arch Chir 361:269–275
56. Lahey ME, Behar M, Viteri F, Scrimshaw NS (1958) Values for copper, iron, and iron-binding capacity in the serum of kwashiorkor. Pediatrics 22:72–78
57. Lazor L, Russell JC, DaSilva J, Radford M (1988) Use of the multiple uptake gated acquisition scan for the preoperative assessment of cardiac risc. Surg Gynecol Obstet 167:234–238
58. Leppo J, Joaquin P, Gionet M, Tumulo J, Paraskos JA, Cutler BS (1987) Noninvasive evaluation of cardiac risk before elective vascular surgery. J Am Coll Cardiol: 269–276
59. Lutz H, Klose R, Peter K (1976) Die Problematik der präoperativen Risikoeinstufung. Anästh Forum 17:342
60. Mahar LJ, Steen PA, Tinker JH, Vlietstra RE, Smith HC, Pluth JR (1978) Preoperative myocardial infarction in patients with coronary artery disease with and without aorta-coronary bypass grafts. J Thorac Cardiovasc Surg 76:533–537
61. Marx G, Mateo CV, Orkin LR (1973) Computer analysis of postanaesthetic deaths. Anesthesiology 39:54
62. McCabe CJ, Reidy NC, Abbott WM, Fulchino DM, Brewster DC (1981) The value of electrocardiogram monitoring during treadmill testing for peripheral vascular disease. Surgery 89:183–186
63. Meakins JL, Christou NV, Shizgal HM, MacLean LD (1979) Therapeutic approaches to anergy in surgical patients. Ann Surg 190:286–296
64. Mitchell JD, Sproule BJ, Chapman CB (1958) The physiological meaning of the maximal oxygen intake test. J Clin Invest 37:538
65. Mosley JG, Clarke JMF, Ell PJ, Marston A (1985) Assessment of myocardial function before aortic surgery by radionuclide angiocardiography. Br J Surg 72:886–887
66. Müller J, Botzenhardt U, Alföldi P, Lemmel EM (1982) Studies on the mechanism of PMN-activation I by dextran sulfates. Blut 44:371–378
67. Müller JM, Brenner U, Dienst C, Pichlmayer H (1982) Preoperative parenteral feeding in patients with gastrointestinal carcinoma. Lancet I:68
68. Mullen JL (1981) Consequences of malnutrition in the surgical patient. Surg Clin North Am 61:465–488
69. Mullen JL, Buzby GP, Waldman MP, Gertner MH, Hobbs ChL, Rosato EF (1979) Prediction of operative morbidity and mortality by preoperative nutritional assessment. Surg Forum 30:80
70. Mullen JL, Buzby GP, Matthews DC, Smale BF, Rosato EF (1980) Reduction of operative morbidity and mortality by combined preoperative nutritional support. Ann Surg 192:604
71. Moghissi K, Teasdale PR (1980) Parenteral feeding in patients with carcinoma of the esophagus treated by surgery: energy and nitrogen requirements. JPEN 4:371–375
72. Namay DL, Hammermeister KE, Zia MS, DeRouen TA, Dodge HT, Namay K (1982) Effect of perioperative myocardial infarction on late survival in patients undergoing coronary artery bypass surgery. Circulation 65:1066–1071

73. Neumann CG, Lawlor GL, Stiehm ER et al. (1975) Immunologic responses in malnourished children. Am J Clin Nutr 28:89–104
74. Pasternack PF, Imperato AM, Bear G (1984) The value of radionuclide angiography as a predictor of preoperative myocardial infarction in patients undergoing abdominal aortic aneurism resection. J Vasc Surg 1:320–325
75. Pietsch JB, Meakins JL, McLean LD (1977) The delayed hypersensitivity response: application in clinical surgery. Surgery 82:349–355
76. Quentmeier A, Betzler M, Flad HD, Geisenhainer U, Herfarth CH (1981) Postoperative individuelle Verlaufskontrollen der natürlichen Killerzell-Aktivität und der CEA-Werte bei Patienten mit gastrointestinalen Carcinomen. Langenbeck's Arch Chir Suppl Chir Forum: 229–233
77. Rao TLK, Jacobs KJH, El-Etr AA (1983) Reinfarction following anesthesia in patients with myocardial infarction. Anesthesiology 59:499–505
78. Rhoads JE, Alexander CE (1955) Nutritional problems of surgical patients. Ann NY Acad Sci 63:268–275
79. Saklad M (1941) Grading of patients for surgical procedures. Anesthesiology 2:281
80. Sanz G, Castaner A, Bertriu A, Magrina J, Roig E, Coll S, Pare JC, Navarro-Lopez F (1982) Determinants of prognosis in survivors of myocardial infarction. A prospective clinical Angiographic Study. N Engl J Med 306:1065–1070
81. Silber S, Schwaiger M, Klein U, Rudolph W (1980) Quantitative Beurteilung der linksventrikulären Funktion mit der Radionuklid-Ventrikulographie. Herz 5:146–158
82. Steen PA, Tinker JH, Tarhan S (1978) Myocardial reinfarction after anesthesia and surgery. JAMA 239:2566–2570
83. Striebel JP, Scherrer R, Stähler-Hambrecht I, Lutz H (1981) Wertigkeiten verschiedener Parameter bei der präoperativen Beurteilung des Anästhesierisikos. In: Haid B, Mitterschiffthaler G (eds) Zentraleuropäischer Anaesthesiekongress, vol 1. Springer, Berlin Heidelberg New York 139:50–60
84. Studley HO (1936) Percentage of weight loss: a basic indicator of surgical risk in patients with chronic peptic ulcer. JAMA 106:458–460
85. Tarhan S, Moffit EA, Taylor WF et al. (1972) Myocardial infarction after general anesthesia. JAMA 220:1451–1454
86. Tilden AB, Balch CM (1981) Indomethacin enhancement of immunocompetence in melanoma patients. Surgery 90:77–84
87. Trigg ME (1979) Immune function of the spleen. South Med J 72:593–599
88. Tripodi D, Parks LC, Brugmans J (1973) Drug-induced restoration of cutaneous delayed hypersensitivity in anergic patients with cancer. N Engl J Med 16:354–357
89. Unertl H, Wroblewski A, Glükler S, Heinrich G, Hauck M, Peter K (1985) Das Risiko in der Anästhesie. Münch Med Wochenschr 127:609–612
90. Vacanti CJ, Van Houten RJ, Hill RC (1970) A statistical analysis of the relationship of physical status to postoperative mortality in 68388 cases. Anesth Analg Cleve 49:564
91. Weber KT, Kinasewitz GT, Janicki JS, Fishman AP (1982) Oxygen utilization and ventilation during exercise in patients with chronic cardiac failure. Circulation 65:1213–1223
92. Weber KT, Janicki JS, Likoff MJ (1984) Exercise testing in the evaluation of cardiopulmonary disease. Clin Chest Med 5:173–180
93. Weber KT, Janicki JS (1985) Cardiopneumonary exercise testing for evaluation of chronic cardiac failure. Am J Cardiol 55:22A–31A

Diagnosis, Causes, and Treatment of Myocardial Ischemia in the Operating Room *

S. Reiz

Perioperative myocardial ischemia is common in patients with coronary artery disease (CAD) subjected to cardiac and major noncardiac surgical procedures [1–7]. As outlined in Tables 1 and 2, its incidence varies widely. Differences in populations studied and, in particular, in techniques employed to detect ischemia are the most obvious reasons for this variable incidence.

From studies performed in patients undergoing coronary artery bypass surgery (CABG) it appears as if the frequency of postoperative myocardial infarction is directly proportional to the incidence and severity of pre-bypass

* Supported in part by grants from the Swedish National Heart and Lung Foundation

Table 1. Incidence of pre-bypass myocardial ichemia in CABG

	(*n*)	Incidence (%)		Mode of detection
		Pre-induction	Total	
Wilkinson et al. (1981)	26	27	62	2-lead ECG, lactate
Lieberman et al. (1983)	30	NA	67	2-lead ECG
Slogoff and Keats (1985)	1023	18	37	2-lead ECG
Slogoff and Keats (1986)	495	26	55	2-lead ECG

NA, not available

Table 2. Incidence of myocardial ischemia in vascular and other noncardiac surgery

	(*n*)	Incidence (%)		Mode of detection
		Pre-induction	Total	
Roy et al. (1979)	29	NA	38	Multilead ECG
Coriat et al. (1982)	50	NA	39	V5 ECG
Reiz et al. (1989)	112	18	86	12-lead ECG, lactate, wall function

NA, not available

myocardial ischemia [3, 4]. Tachycardia but not hypotension or hypertension correlated positively with ischemia. Interestingly, almost 50% of all ischemic events were not accompanied by any hemodynamic aberrations. In these studies, other important factors contributing to postoperative infarction were the time on bypass and the surgeon's judgment of the quality of the distal graft anastomosis. Corresponding data from patients with CAD subjected to noncardiac surgery are largely lacking.

Although all logic dictates that treatment of perioperative myocardial ischemia would reduce postoperative cardiac risk, neither prospective, nor retrospective studies have, as yet, addressed this important question.

The aims of this chapter are (a) to discuss the diagnosis of myocardial ischemia in the operating room, (b) to outline the mechanisms by which ischemia may be caused during anesthesia and surgery, (c) to analyze the relationship between intraoperative ischemia and postoperative myocardial ischemia/infarction, and (d) to suggest therapy by which ischemia could be prevented and/or treated.

Diagnosis of Myocardial Ischemia

The Awake Patient

Many anesthesiologists and surgeons still maintain that the awake patient is the best monitor of her myocardial oxygenation, therefore, if possible, surgery in patients at risk for ischemic events should be performed under local or regional anesthesia. However, besides the fact that patients under the influence of premedication and additional sedatives and analgesics may fail to report angina pectoris, it appears that the incidence of ischemia might be higher in the awake state than during general anesthesia.

Two studies from the same group of investigators in patients subjected to CABG [8] and major abdominal surgery [9] using the two-lead Holter technique demonstrated a 42% and 19% incidence of ischemia respectively during the 24 h preceding the operation. In comparison, the intraoperative incidence of ischemia was 18% and 14% respectively. Other studies performed during daily life activities have discovered that a majority of ischemic events are silent, e.g., unaccompanied by angina pectoris [10, 11]. In addition, it was also evident from these studies that many of the ischemic events were unrelated to hemodynamic changes such as tachycardia (Fig. 1). Similar results were reported in the studies of perioperative ischemia related to angina pectoris and hemodynamic changes cited above [8, 9]. For instance, in the study by Fegert and colleagues [9], not a single ischemic event among the 50 patients studied in the pre- and postoperative periods was accompanied by chest pain. Only 24% of the events were associated with an increase in heart rate by more than 20% from control. The use of the Holter technique allows retrospective diagnosis of ischemia only. Difficulties therefore exist in relating ischemia to changes in systemic hemodynamics other than heart rate.

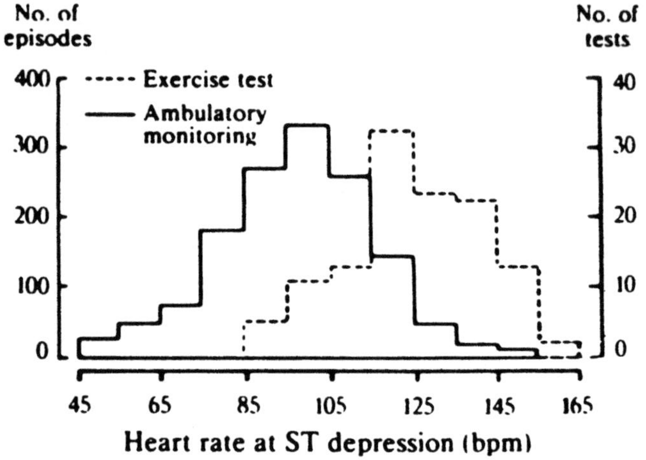

Fig. 1. Distribution of heart rates at onset of ST-segment depression during ambulatory monitoring and exercise testing in patients with stable angina pectoris. In 73% of episodes, heart rate was 20 beats per minute or more below that at ST depression during exercise. (Reproduced from [10] with permission)

Our group studied 95 patients with CAD scheduled for abdominal aortic reconstructive surgery using intermittent 12-lead ECG and myocardial metabolic studies to secure the diagnosis of myocardial ischemia. We found six patients with new ST-segment depression, six with myocardial lactate production, and another patient with both these indices of ischemia prior to induction of anesthesia. Although all patients were carefully questioned with regard to symptoms of ischemia, only one of 13 reported angina or chest discomfort while displaying ECG and/or lactate abnormalities.

In summary, all these data suggest that the awake patient cannot reliably "monitor" her myocardial oxygenation. Furthermore, staying awake during surgery might indeed contribute to an increased incidence of myocardial ischemia due to higher myocardial oxygen requirements compared with general anesthesia.

Metabolic Diagnosis of Ischemia

Production of lactate in a territory of the myocardium deprived of oxygen is the gold standard for identifying myocardial ischemia. More infrequently, myocardial release of inosine [12] or hypoxanthine [12] have been used to indicate ischemia. These are techniques which require cannulations of an artery and the coronary sinus with subsequent sampling of blood at the time of suspected ischemia. Latate can be analyzed in the operating room [13] and may therefore be regarded as an off-line tool to diagnose ischemia. In contrast, inosine and hypoxanthine require sophisticated instrumentation and meticulous preparation of the blood samples and, thus, allow for retrospective analysis only. Since very limited information on the use of these two techniques in anesthesia is available [14, 15] they will not be further discussed.

Lactate is utilized as a substrate by the heart. In case of insufficient oxygenation it will be produced by the myocytes. This may result in higher concentrations of lactate in coronary venous compared with arterial blood, i.e., a negative lactate extraction (lactate production). Several factors may explain why lactate production is not necessarily recorded despite obvious ischemia detected by other methods [16]. First, the ischemic territory may be too small to offset sufficient increase in coronary venous concentration of lactate. Second, flow through the ischemic territory may be so low that the wash-out of lactate dose not contribute to a significant rise in coronary venous concentration. Finally, the coronary venous sampling catheter may be positioned distally to the outflow of the vein draining the ischemic territory. The latter phenomenon is particularly common in ischemia of the right ventricle, which has its main venous drainage close to the coronary sinus orifice and/or in the right atrium. Our estimate from studies comparing different techniques is that only 1/4 to 1/3 of regional ischemic events are associated with myocardial lactate production [7]. The relationship between myocardial lactate production and other indices of myocardial ischemia will be discussed further later in this chapter.

The Electrocardiogram

Electrocardiography is by far the most commonly employed technique to detect myocardial ischemia in the operating room. Although the specificity of ST-segment deviations for myocardial ischemia is high, the sensitivity is very variable and related to a number of important factors. In most operating rooms, a single-lead ECG displayed on an oscilloscope is the only available monitor for myocardial ischemia. If an extremity lead is observed for new ST-segment changes, the sensitivity is probably in the order of 2% to 10% only. Sensitivity is affected by the level of attention and the degree of preexisting ST-segment abnormality. Modification of the electrode placement so as to display a lateral chest lead monitoring the anterior left ventricular wall markedly improves the sensitivity of the single-lead ECG [17] and detects about 85% of ST-segment abnormalities displayed on a 12-lead ECG [18].

Standard oscilloscopes always incorporate a low-frequency filter to minimize the influence of the electrocautery and other electrical interference. Too frequently, the ECG signal has not been calibrated. Therefore, changes in the raw ECG signal ST-segments around the diagnostic deviation level of 0.1 to 0.2 mV may be distorted or blunted and, thus, go by undetected. Display of the calibrated ECG signal on paper via amplifiers with high bandwidth markedly improves the sensitivity of the ECG compared with standard operating room oscilloscopes.

The use of multiple ECG leads increases the level of detection of ischemia. If leads II, V4, and V5 are monitored, almost 100% of changes detected by the 12-lead ECG will be obvious [19]. In recent years, computerized analysis of multiple ECG leads has been developed in order to reduce the need for continuously running recorders and eliminate the low sensitivity resulting from inattention to the ECG and difficulty in remembering the degree of preexisting

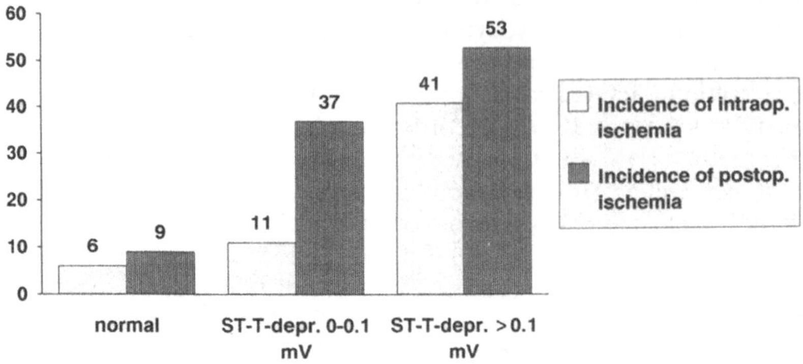

Fig. 2. Intra- and postoperative myocardial ischemia by ECG (incidence in %) in relation to preoperative ST-T segment

abnormality [20]. These systems provide a readout of the degree of ST-segment deviation in each of the leads monitored at the same time as the mean complexes of the selected leads are displayed in versions updated every minute. In addition, each lead can be displayed in a trend mode. Although multiple filters are available to reduce the problem of low bandwidths, the sensitivity of this type of equipment in relation to a high bandwidth 12-lead ECG displayed on paper remains to be evaluated.

It appears as if the degree of ST-segment deviation on the preoperative ECG is a useful predictor of intra- and postoperative ischemia as diagnosed by the 12-lead ECG (Fig. 2). Nevertheless, several problems have to be addressed in future research aimed at defining the importance of new ST-segment and other ECG abnormalities occurring during anesthesia. First, is the degree of ST-segment deviation proportional to the magnitude of ischemic territory? Second, what is the prognostic value of an ST-segment deviation in the face of a preexisting ST-segment abnormality? Is, for instance, a 0.1 mV depression from the isoelectric line in a patient with a previously normal ECG equally important as a comparable change in a patient with preexisting ST-segment depression due to left ventricular hypertrophy, ischemic heart disease, digitalis medication, or other cause? Third, has the degree of ST-segment deviation, its duration, or the product of these two variables any prognostic value for postoperative cardiac risk? Finally, the prognostic importance of other ECG abnormalities, hitherto not regarded as diagnostic for ischemia, such as new T-wave inversions, nodal rhythm, and multiple premature ventricular contractions has to be considered.

Ventricular Wall Function

Experimentally, there is strong evidence that myocardial ischemia leads to abnormal wall function and stunning of the ischemic territory [21, 22]. Such changes usually occur before or in the absence of other abnormalities indicating ischemia [23]. It does not, however, imply that all new wall motion abnormality is the consequence of ischemia. Interestingly, there is only one study reporting the incidence of new wall motion abnormality during anesthesia in patients without CAD [24]. In this study, one of 25 ASA I patients demonstrated new anterior wall motion abnormality during induction and endotracheal intubation. Since there is no gold standard for ischemia which can be used clinically, the specificity of new wall motion abnormality for ischemia has yet to be defined. There are several reasons why new wall motion abnormality could occur without any relation to ischemia in the territory contracting abnormally. For instance, an area of the myocardium which has suffered a previous nontransmural infarction or a myocarditis may contract normally at normal hemodynamics. When load increases on the ventricle and/or heart rate rises, this territory might display an abnormal contraction pattern without being ischemic. Videcoq et al. [25] found wall motion abnormalities in the presumed absence of myocardial ischemia when a calcium channel blocker was administered to dogs receiving isoflurane. They attributed this to a delayed onset of cardiac contraction. Similar results have been reported after intracoronary injection of nifedipine in man [26]. It is possible that any technique using ventricular wall motion as a gold standard for ischemia may overestimate its true incidence. Two techniques for detection of abnormal wall function have been applied to patients in the operating room. These are echocardiography and cardiokymography.

Echocardiography

M-mode echocardiography was introduced over 10 years ago as a simple technique to document changes in left ventricular contraction pattern during anesthesia [27]. The development of transesophageal two-dimensional echocardiography (TEE) has markedly increased the ability to assess left ventricular (LV) contraction patterns compared with the M-mode technique. For the purpose of studying regional LV function, the TEE transducer is placed in the distal part of the esophagus, thus displaying a cross section of the left ventricle at the level of the insertion of the papillary muscles. This position of the probe allows recording of the regional contraction pattern and the degree of systolic wall thickening of the anterior, lateral, and posterior LV walls, as well as of the interventricular septum. Akinesia and dyskinesia are easily detected and both intra- and interobserver variability as regards these abnormalities are low [28]. Hypokinesia and, in particular, impairment of systolic wall thickening are not as easily detected and are subject to major disagreement between independent observers [28]. A stand-alone system for display of several cine-loops simultaneously is essential for the use of the TEE technique for on-line diagnosis of hypokinesia and wall thinning. Such a system allows comparison of suspected abnormalities with a control loop and also improved accuracy of assessment of the degree of abnormal contraction within each cardiac cycle. In addition to the previously mentioned factors, a change of the position of the heart within the thoracic cavity using various maneuvers such as sternotomy, opening of the pericardium, and positive pressure ventilation, or an altered position of the transducer in the esophagus, may affect the ability to reliably diagnose myocardial ischemia by this technique.

It is evident that new hypokinesia and abnormal systolic wall thickening is usually detected during retrospective analysis of the TEE tapes. Such changes are more common than akinesia and dyskinesia [28]. This indicates that the high sensitivity of TEE in detecting myocardial ischemia hitherto reported is of little importance for the anesthesiologist in the operating room who needs on-line information for his decision-making. It is possible that future computerized systems with automated on-line analysis of several cine-loops will provide instant information when new regional wall function impairment occurs. In this context, it is indeed interesting that the lack of treatment of patients with intraoperative ischemia diagnosed retrospectively as new wall motion abnormality by TEE has not resulted in increased cardiac morbidity [29].

Cardiokymography

Cardiokymography (CKG) was originally developed to improve the sensitivity of the exercise test for the diagnosis of CAD [30–32]. It uses a 5-cm diameter transducer strapped to the chest over the anterior LV wall. The transducer induces an electromagnetic field which can penetrate totally through the body. Motion within this field causes a change in effective capacitance and frequency of oscillation. The change in frequency is converted into a change in voltage proportional to the original motion. It is displayed with the ECG signal on a recorder to allow estimation of the ventricular ejection period. The CKG is highly focal and therefore ignores motions which are not perpendicular to and directly under the coil. It is evident that respiration interferes with the recording of the LV contractions. Samples therefore have to be taken during apnea at end-expiration. Surgical manipulation is another obvious cause of baseline drift and signal interference.

The validation of the ability of the CKG to record anterior LV wall motion has been performed under numerous experimental and clinical conditions [30–34]. The combination of 12-lead ECG and CKG during exercise has the same sensitivity and specificity as the nonquantitative thallium scintigraphic stress test for the diagnosis of CAD verified by coronary angiography [35, 36]. Compared with the normal, systolic inward motion (type I), CKG abnormality is graded as type II (partial systolic outward motion) or type III (total systolic outward motion) [32] (Fig. 3).

There are only a few studies which have documented the incidence of new wall motion abnormality during anesthesia by CKG. Bellows and coworkers [24] studied patients during induction of anesthesia for CABG. Their CKGs were compared with those recorded in a control group of ASA class I patients anesthetized for dental extractions. In the latter group, one of the 25 patients displayed a new CKG abnormality. In comparison, eight of 25 patients with CAD had evidence of new wall motion abnormality during the induction.

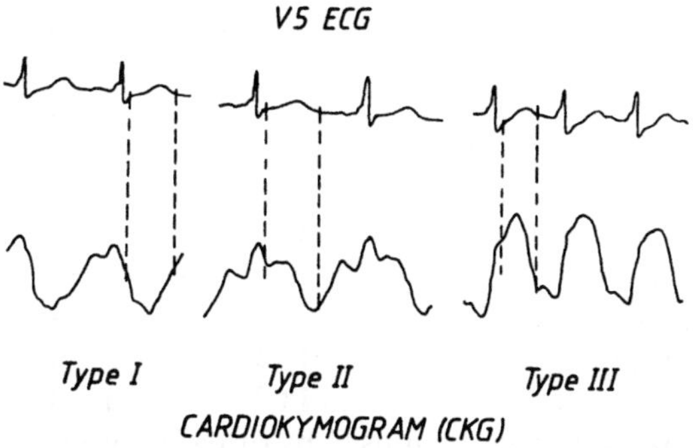

Fig. 3. V_5 ECG (top) and CKG (bottom) recorded simultaneously during tracheal intubation of one study patient. Before intubation there is a normal systolic inward motion (Type I). Within seconds of insertion of the laryngoscope, a partial early systolic outward motion (Type II) is recorded without ECG changes. Two minutes later the CKG demonstrates total outward motion during systole (Type III). At this time the ECG is still not diagnostic of ischemia. *Hatched lines* denote the ejection period. (From [7])

Only one of these patients had simultaneous ST-segment depression exceeding 0.1 mV on the ECG.

Häggmark and associates [7] recorded the CKG in 53 vascular surgical patients at defined perioperative intervals; preinduction, periinduction, prior to skin incision and 10 and 30 min after the start of abdominal surgery. They documented 89 ischemic episodes in 39 of the 53 patients. Seventy-four episodes were diagnosed by a new abnormal CKG. They also recorded the V5 ECG and measured myocardial lactate extraction at the same intervals. In this study, CKG abnormality was significantly more common than ischemia, as indicated by the other two techniques.

Despite the obvious advantage of high "sensitivity" and low cost, the CKG technique has several drawbacks compared with the TEE. It only allows analysis of the contraction pattern in the anterior LV wall, it is subjected to interference from respiratory movements and surgical manipulations, and it cannot be used during cardiothoracic surgery. Finally, as with TEE, new wall motion abnormalities diagnosed retrospectively and, thus untreated at the time they occurred, have not been shown to lead to increased postoperative cardiac morbidity.

Hemodynamic Indices of Myocardial Ischemia

It has been suggested that the rate-pressure product (RPP = SAP × HR) should be a valid index for myocardial ischemia. RPP correlates with myocardial oxygen consumption in the exercising patient [37], whereas these variables agree poorly during anesthesia [14, 38]. In addition, the worst possible combination of hemodynamic aberrations, hypotension and tachycardia [2] (see below) results in a normal RPP. A hemodynamic ischemia risk index, the pressure-rate ratio (P/R = MAP/HR), which would be more logical during anesthesia, has been proposed by Buffington [39]. In experimental studies in dogs with a fixed coronary artery stenosis, he was able to demonstrate a close correlation between ischemia in the territory supplied by the stenosed artery and a P/R < 1. Since a majority of coronary artery stenoses in humans are eccentric, incorporating an elastic vascular wall element, it is possible that this ischemia risk index does not always have the same high preditive value.

Kaplan and Wells [40] suggested that an elevation of the pulmonary capillary wedge pressure (PCWP) associated with abnormal wave form (A-C or v-waves) was a more sensitive index of myocardial ischemia than the V5 ECG ST-segment depression. The agreement between an elevated PCWP combined with abnormal pressure wave form and ischemia diagnosed by other methods was confirmed in vascular surgical patients by Häggmark and coworkers [7]. However, it did not appear as if the hemodynamic index of ischemia was more sensitive than the ECG. An increase of PCWP by 8 mmHg or more in the absence of an abnormal wave form coincided with ischemia, as detected by any of the other techniques (ECG, lactate metabolism, and wall function), alone or in combination, in about 50% of observations. A similar inability of an isolated elevation of the PCWP to predict ischemia was demonstrated by Lieberman et al. [2] in patients undergoing CABG. In comparison, vascular patients who demonstrated an increase of PCWP by 8 mmHg or more, associated with abnormal PCWP wave form, had a 92% likelihood of being ischemic [7]. However, only 13% of all PCWP measurements and 21% of all ischemic events were associated with an abnormal wave form. Thus, the value of the pulmonary artery catheter for the diagnosis of ischemia is limited. Häggmark et al. [7] also analyzed changes in stroke volume in relation to myocardial ischemia and could not find that this index of ventricular pump function sensitively could discriminate between ischemic and nonischemic events.

Comparison of Different Techniques Used to Diagnose Ischemia

Only a few research groups have performed studies aimed at comparing the "sensitivity" of various techniques used to detect myocardial ischemia in the operating room. As may be realized from the above discussion, there is no gold standard for ischemia that can be used clinically. Consequently, these studies do not give us an indication as to the degree of sensitivity of these techniques, but rather the frequency by which they demonstrate abnormalities suggestive of ischemia when applied simultaneously in the same patient.

Wilkinson and coworkers [1] studied the patterns of ischemia during halothane or morphine anesthesia for CABG. They found that ST-segment depressions were not statistically more common than simultaneously measured myocardial lactate production. In contrast, Reiz et al. [41], who studied vascular surgical patients subjected to isoflurane anesthesia found only one of 21 patients with lactate production compared with 11 with simultaneous ECG abnormalities suggesting ischemia.

Lowenstein and Reiz [42] compared the V5 ECG with myocardial lactate extraction in vascular surgical patients with CAD and in patients without

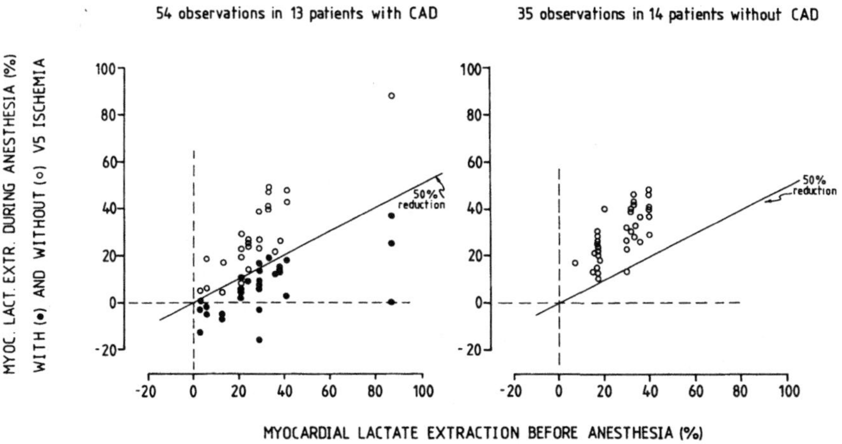

Fig. 4. Relationship of coronary sinus lactate extraction before anesthesia to lactate extraction during anesthesia in 13 patients with coronary artery disease (CAD) who demonstrated ischemia at least once during anesthesia, and in 14 patients without CAD. Presence of ischemia was defined as depression of 1.0 mm in the ST segment of ECG lead V_5. ECG depression occurred only in patients with CAD. In only one instance did lactate extraction decrease by more than 50% in normal patients. In contrast, ECG depression was evident in about one-half of the measurements in patients with CAD. Virtually all of these ECG changes were associated with reduction of greater than 50% in lactate extraction, though less than one-third were associated with lactate production. These data emphasize the insensitivity of lactate production as an index of ischemia when coronary sinus blood is sampled, and the desirability of regional blood sampling for estimation of ischemia in the heart with CAD. They suggest that large decreases of lactate extraction may be indicative of regional ischemia during anesthesia

CAD. Only one of 35 intraoperative samples from patients without CAD demonstrated a greater than 50% decline in myocardial lactate extraction from awake values and none were associated with new ECG abnormalities. Compared with the awake control measurements, mean myocardial lactate extraction for the group was not altered by anesthesia. At the time when patients with CAD displayed new perioperative ST-segment depressions, myocardial lactate extraction had decreased by 50% or more in 92% of measurements. Lactate production was, however, present in only 29% of the ischemic events as displayed by the ECG (Fig. 4). When ischemia was not evident from the ECG, myocardial lactate extractions were not different from the awake values or from those measured in patients without CAD (Fig. 4).

In another set of experiments, Reiz and coworkers analyzed the 12-lead ECG when lactate production was first observed in 26 patients subjected to anesthesia for major vascular surgery. Only 12 patients (45%) demonstrated diagnostic ST-segment depressions (>0.1 mV) at the time of lactate production. However, all the remaining 14 patients had some kind of new ECG abnormality, most commonly an ST-segment depression which was less than 0.1 mV in one or more leads. Other abnormalities included new inverted T-waves, sudden onset of nodal or ectopic atrial rhythm and appearance of multiple premature ventricular contractions. Our approach in clinical practice is therefore to regard all new ECG abnormalities observed during anesthesia in patients with CAD as the result of myocardial ischemia until proven otherwise.

Using M-mode echocardiography, Elliot and coworkers [27] demonstrated periinduction LV wall dysfunction, interpreted to be ischemia in 10 of 24 patients with CAD. In comparison, the ECG was indicative of ischemia in one patient only. Strikingly similar results in comparable patients were obtained by Bellows et al. [24], who found eight of 24 patients with new periinduction CKG abnormalities, whereas the ECG indicated ischemia in only one.

Smith et al. [29], using TEE, documented new systolic wall motion abnormalities at some time during anesthesia and surgery in 24 of 50 patients with previous myocardial infarction undergoing either vascular surgery or CABG. Only six patients experienced ST-segment changes indicative of ischemia. Furthermore, all patients demonstrating an ECG abnormality also had abnormal wall motion. Häggmark et al. [7] could not find that all instances of ECG abnormality were accompanied by wall motion abnormality as detected by the CKG. It is, however, possible that wall motion abnormalities were present in

Table 3. Incidence of myocardial ischemia in vascular surgery in relation to mode of detection. (Data from Häggmark et al. [7])

Mode of detection	Incidence of ischemia (%)
Cardiokymography (wall function)	53
12-lead ECG	41
Myocardial lactate production	20
Elevated PCWP with abnormal wave form	17
All modalities	86

Table 4. Mode of detection of preinduction myocardial ischemia in 12 of 68 vascular surgical patients without chest pain at this time

Patient no.	12-lead ECG	Cardiokymography	Lactate production
2			Yes
22		Yes	
25		Yes	
27			Yes
28		Yes	Yes
31	Yes	Yes	Yes
34			Yes
50		Yes	
54		Yes	
59			Yes
62			Yes
68			Yes

areas not sampled by the CKG, or that wall motion abnormality was too slight to be detected by this technique.

The study by Häggmark et al. [7] also indicated that wall motion abnormalities are far more common than ischemic ECG changes, myocardial lactate production, or elevated PCWP with an abnormal pressure wave form (Table 3). Furthermore, it was evident that the concurrance between the various techniques was poor. This is further demonstrated in Table 4, in which the distribution of preinduction ischemic abnormalities as detected by 12-lead ECG, lactate production, and/or CKG in patients scheduled for major vascular surgery is outlined.

From all these data, it appears that multiple modalities are needed to increase the level of detection of myocardial ischemia by conventional ECG. However, the ability of interventions guided by these techniques to alter cardiac outcome should be assessed before they are included in everyday clinical practice.

Causes of Perioperative Myocardial Ischemia

Ischemia Associated with Hemodynamic Abnormalities

It is generally accepted that hemodynamic aberrations may lead to myocardial ischemia. Only a few studies have, however, systematically investigated the degree of abnormality of single variables needed to produce ischemia. Lieberman et al. [2] studied patients subjected to coronary artery bypass surgery. Of single variables, they found that tachycardia, defined as heart rate above bpm and hypotension, defined as a systolic blood pressure below 80 mmHg or more than 20% above resting values correlated with ischemia. A PCWP greater than 15 mmHg had only a 55% chance of being associated with ischemia. Of all combinations of abnormalities tested, tachycardia and hypotension were those that correlated most closely with myocardial ischemia.

In comparison, the studies by Slogoff and Keats [3, 4], performed in similar patients, demonstrated that tachycardia but not hypotension or hypertension correlated with ischemia. Since these studies retrospectively analyzed ischemia from Holter tapes, it is possible that hemodynamic aberrations other than tachycardia could have been missed.

There are no systematic studies addressing the corresponding questions in noncardiac surgical patients with CAD. However, all logic dictates that such patients should not be different from those subjected to CABG as regards hemodynamic correlates of myocardial ischemia.

Ischemia Without Associated Hemodynamic Abnormalities

Coronary Vasospasm

In the studies by Slogoff and Keats [3, 4], almost 50% of ischemic episodes recorded in the operating room did not coincide with hemodynamic abnormalities. It has been suggested that coronary vasospasm could be a probable cause [43]. Kleinman and coworkers [44] studied patients during induction of anesthesia with either halothane or high dose fentanyl. They recorded myocardial perfusion by thallium scintigraphy and found that approximately 45% of their patients, regardless of anesthetic technique used, had evidence of regional perfusion defects following endotracheal intubation. Although the scintigraphic technique does not allow absolute measurement of regional myocardial blood flow, these data suggest that flow distribution was not uniform. One possible mechanism would be coronary vasospasm. However, the results might also indicate an inability to increase flow to areas distal to significant coronary stenoses, whereas territories supplied by nonstenosed coronary arteries would have an increase of flow.

Lowenstein and Reiz [42] reported the coronary flow changes that occur during laryngoscopy and intubation in vascular surgical patients with coronary artery disease. Patients who demonstrated ischemia as diagnosed by lactate production and ECG or CKG abnormalities had a decrease in coronary blood flow despite unaltered myocardial oxygen requirements (Fig. 5). Patients who did not become ischemic did not demonstrate any change in coronary blood flow. The decrease in flow occurred within a few heart beats, suggesting a neurogenic rather than humoral mechanism for the flow reduction. Moffitt and coworkers [45] studied patients scheduled for CABG during endotracheal intubation. They did not record any changes in systemic hemodynamics or coronary blood flow. However, myocardial oxygen extraction increased, suggesting some coronary vasoconstriction.

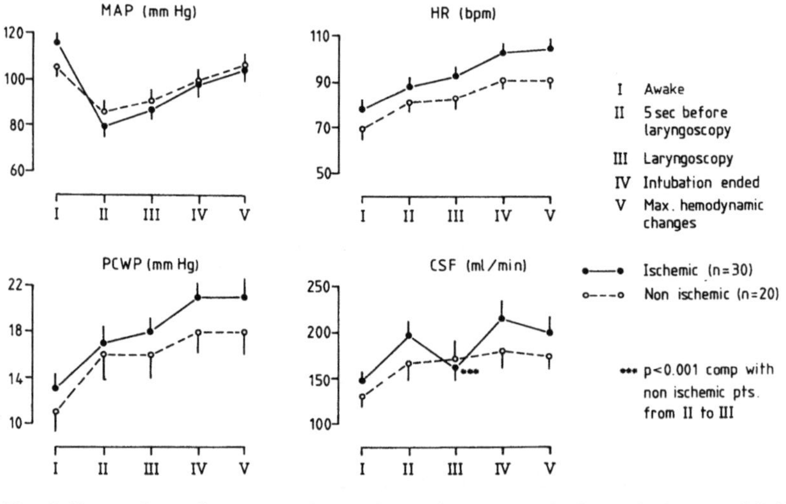

Fig. 5. Systemic and coronary hemodynamic changes before, during, and following laryngoscopy and tracheal intubation in 30 patients who became ischemic and 20 matched patients who did not. Coronary blood flow decreased rapidly and transiently with laryngoscopy in patients who developed ischemia, suggesting a neurogenic mechanism. For further discussion see text. (Data from [42])

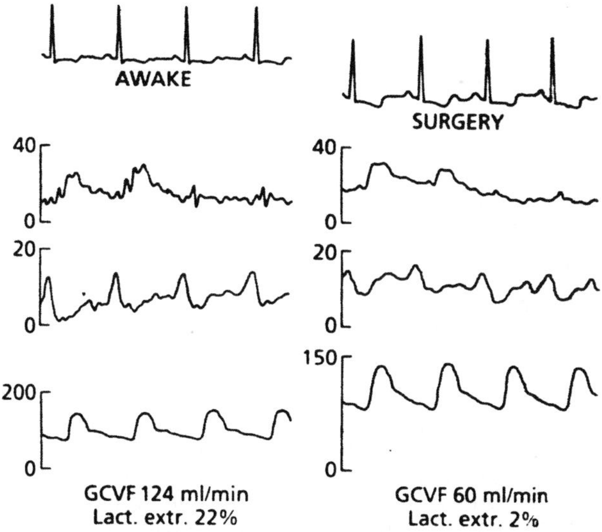

Fig. 6. The V_5 ECG, pulmonary artery, central venous, and arterial pressures *(top* to *bottom)*, awake *(left panel)* and during abdominal surgery *(right panel)* in a patient with coronary artery disease. ST-segment depression and metabolic changes suggestive of ischemia developed despite comparable heart rate, pulmonary artery-occluded pressure, and system blood pressure. The pronounced decline in blood flow through the territory perfused by the left anterior descending coronary artery (GCVF) suggests coronary vasospasm as the mechanism for ischemia

Thus, there is evidence that coronary vasoconstriction with a reduction in flow but without a parallel decline in myocardial oxygen requirements may occur during anesthesia. In some patients, this decrease in flow may be associated with myocardial ischemia. Vasospasm seems to be most common during laryngoscopy and endotracheal intubation, but has also been observed during surgical stimulation (Fig. 6).

Coronary Blood Flow Maldistribution

In 1983, Reiz and coworkers [41] suggested that the coronary vasodilatory action of isoflurane might contribute to redistribution of myocardial blood flow and subsequent myocardial ischemia in the territory deprived of oxygenated blood. Recently, two large studies in patients undergoing CABG have, however, failed to demonstrate that isoflurane given as an adjunct to opioid anesthesia is associated with greater postoperative cardiac morbidity than other anesthetic agents [46, 47].

Isoflurane dilates coronary resistance vessels [48] and is in this respect considerably more powerful than the other inhalational agents [49]. Recent animal experiments have demonstrated that the coronary vasodilatation is dose dependent and that high doses of isoflurane severely impair coronary vasodilator reserve [50]. Isoflurane causes a dose-dependent coronary vasodilatation in patients with CAD as well [51]. Several animal experiments demonstrate that iso-

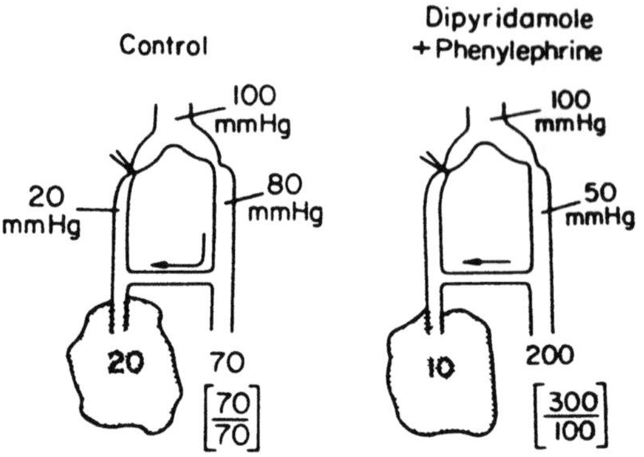

Fig. 7. Schematic diagram of the coronary circulation showing proposed mechanism for a vasodilator-induced coronary steal. The coronary artery divides into two branches, one completely occluded, and the other stenosed but providing collaterals to the first. In the control situation on the left, distal pressure is low in the occluded arterial bed and there is a small gradient in mean pressure across the stenosis. Flow in the ischemic region *(dotted area)* is 20 ml/min/100 g and is determined by the collateral driving pressure, or the difference between distal pressures in the bed supplying collaterals (80 mmHg) and the ischemic bed (20 mmHg). Flow in the distribution of the stenotic vessel is normal at 70 ml/min/100 g and is evenly distributed between subendocardium (lower value in bracket) and subepicardium (upper value). During dipyridamole administration, with blood pressure maintained constant by phenylephrine, flow increases in the nonischemic bed to 200 ml/min/100 g, but becomes maldistributed between subendocardium and subepicardium. In addition, pressure distal to the stenosis falls to 50 mmHg, causing a reduction in collateral driving pressure. As a result, flow to the ischemic region decreases to 10 ml/min/100 g, interpreted as a coronary steal. (Reproduced from [56] with permission)

flurane but not halothane can produce regional as well as transmural flow maldistribution [52–55]. The question as to whether or not the flow maldistribution may cause myocardial ischemia in the territory or layer deprived of flow is more controversial.

A number of prerequisites are needed for ischemia to be caused by isoflurane. First, an anatomical basis for flow maldistribution has to be present. Second, vasodilation has to occur at the level of the resistance vessels rather than large coronary arteries. As demonstrated by Becker [56], a territory distal to a complete coronary occlusion, perfused via collaterals supplied by a stenosed artery can be deprived of flow if the poststenotic pressure is reduced by a small vessel dilator such as dipyridamole (Fig. 7). This type of coronary anatomy is found in around 23% of patients evaluated for CABG [57]. In a similar model, isoflurane as well as adenosine were demonstrated to produce both regional and transmural flow maldistribution [52]. Third, systemic hemodynamic alterations limiting coronary flow reserve, like a decrease in coronary perfusion pressure and/or an increase in heart rate, reduce the tolerance to pharmacologically induced coronary vasodilatation. These are common hemodynamic changes observed during isoflurane anesthesia. The negative inotropic effect of isoflurane does, however, counterbalance the risk of blood flow maldistribution by increasing coronary dilator reserve, provided coronary back pressure is not increased. Since most elderly patients with suspected CAD presenting for noncardiac surgery do not have coronary angiograms, the assessment of risk for isoflurane-induced ischemia becomes complex.

However, since isoflurane causes a dose-dependent coronary vasodilatation, which is clinically insignificant in inhaled concentrations below 1.5% [51], moderate doses of the drug, administered as an adjunct to other anesthetics, such as opioids or regional anesthesia, can most probably be tolerated in any patient with CAD, provided hemodynamic alterations which limit coronary vasodilator reserve are avoided.

Relationship Between Perioperative Myocardial Ischemia and Infarction

In CABG patients, there seems to be a close correlation between pre-bypass myocardial ischemia and postoperative myocardial infarction [3, 4]. Other important determinants for postoperative myocardial infarction in such patients were the time on bypass and the surgeon's judgment of the quality of the distal graft anastomosis. As yet, there are no published studies which have prospectively evaluated the relationship between postoperative myocardial infarction and perioperative myocardial ischemia in noncardiac surgical patients. In the preliminary study by Fegert et al. [9], adverse cardiac outcome, defined as death, myocardial infarction, and/or LV failure, occurred in seven of their 50 patients (14%) with only 2/7 having intraoperative ischemia. In our series of 95 patients, there were five patients who infarcted but no cardiac deaths within the first 3 postoperative weeks. Two infarcts were transmural. Three of the five patients had had previous myocardial infarction, only two displayed intraoperative ischemia but postoperatively all five had ischemia (ST-T changes in one or more ECG recordings) before infarcting. Hemodynamic abnormalities (tachycardia with or without hypotension but never hypertension) were present in all five patients for prolonged periods despite aggressive therapy to restore hemodynamic normality. None of these infarcts were regarded as the consequence of intraoperative events.

Treatment of Myocardial Ischemia in the Operating Room

It appears as if several preventive measures could be taken to reduce the risk of perioperative myocardial ischemia. Adequate premedication and oxygen administration before induction as well as maintenance of cardiac drugs which reduce the risk for tachycardia or coronary vasospasm are indicated. As recently demonstrated by Stone et al. [58], a single dose of an oral beta-blocker administered preoperatively to hypertensive patients scheduled for noncardiac surgery results in a reduced incidence of intraoperative ischemia compared with untreated patients. In a placebo-controlled study [59], the calcium channel blocker diltiazem also reduced the incidence of myocardial ischemia during noncardiac surgery. Patients undergoing CABG who were administered beta-blockers preoperatively had a lower incidence of intraoperative ischemia compared with those not on beta-blockers. Interestingly, CABG patients on chronic calcium channel blocker medication had a significantly higher incidence of intraoperative ischemia than those on beta-blockers alone or those taking a combination of the two [60, 61]. These results are not surprising, since the dominating calcium channel blocker in these studies was nifedipine, known to be able to cause tachycardia. In addition, patients were grouped according to their preoperative chronic drug therapy instead of being assigned to a prevention drug or placebo according to randomized, double-blind, protocol.

Intravenous nitroglycerin reduces coronary back pressure by dilatation of capacitance vessels, dilates large coronary arteries, and prevents spasm of elastic coronary stenoses. It had also been shown to reduce the incidence of intraoperative ischemia in patients undergoing noncardiac surgical procedures [62]. Which of the above mechanisms is most important in the prevention of ischemia is, however, unclear.

Thus, there are, as yet, only a few controlled studies of pharmacological therapies aimed at reducing the incidence of intraoperative myocardial ischemia and their effects on outcome. More importantly, we do not know if meticulous control of the circulation will reduce the number and/or severity of perioperative cardiac complications. Nevertheless, it appears logical to attenuate major hemodynamic changes which may cause myocardial ischemia. Adequate anesthetic depth during induction and surgical stimulation, avoidance of drugs which cause tachycardia, such as atropine and pancuronium bromide [63, 64], and adequate volume and blood replacement are strategies which should result in reduced cardiac morbidity. If drugs have to be used to control the circulation, they should be receptor specific rather than having mixed actions. An easily titratable volatile anesthetic agent with a vasodilator action, a short-acting beta-1 antagonist, a short-acting alpha-adrenergic agonist, nitroglycerin, and a short-acting beta-1 agonist should belong to the armamentarium of the anesthesiologist dealing with patients with CAD undergoing major surgical procedures. Nevertheless, it is likely that ischemia may occur without associated hemodynamic abnormalities. In this situation calcium channel blockers or nitroglycerin should be used if coronary vasospasm is suspected. If isoflurane is used, the possibility of coronary blood flow maldistribution should be considered. Under these circumstances isoflurane should be replaced temporarily while systemic hemodynamics are maintained at close to normal levels in an effort to establish the mechanism of ischemia.

References

1. Wilkinson PL, Hamilton WK, Moyers JR et al. (1981) Halothane and morphine-nitrous oxide anesthesia in patients undergoing coronary artery bypass operations – patterns of intraoperative ischemia. J Thorac Cardiovasc Surg 82:372–378
2. Lieberman RW, Orkin FK, Jobes DR, Schwartz AJ (1983) Hemodynamic predictors of myocardial ischemia during halothane anesthesia for coronary-artery revascularization. Anesthesiology 59:36–41

3. Slogoff S, Keats A (1985) Does perioperative myocardial ischemia lead to postoperative myocardial infarction? Anesthesiology 62:107–114
4. Slogoff S, Keats A (1986) Further observations on perioperative myocardial ischemia. Anesthesiology 65:539–542
5. Coriat P, Harari A, Daloz M, Viars P (1982) Clinical predictors of intraoperative myocardial ischemia in patients with coronary artery disease undergoing non-cardiac surgery. Acta Anaesthesiol Scand 26:287–290
6. Roy WL, Edelist G, Gilbert B (1979) Myocardial ischemia during non-cardiac surgical procedures in patients with coronary-artery disease. Anesthesiology 51:393–397
7. Häggmark S, Hohner P, Östman M et al. (1988) Comparison of hemodynamic, electrocardiographic, mechanical and metabolic indicators of intraoperative myocardial ischemia in vascular surgical patients with coronary artery disease. Anesthesiology 70:19–25
8. Knight AA, Hollenberg M, London MJ et al. (1988) Perioperative myocardial ischemia: importance of the preoperative ischemic pattern. Anesthesiology 68:681–688
9. Fegert G, Hollenberg M, Browner W et al. (1988) Perioperative myocardial ischemia in the noncardiac surgical patient. Anesthesiology 69:A49
10. Deanfield JE, Maseri A, Selwyn AP et al. (1983) Myocardial ischemia during daily life in patients with stable angina: its relation to symptoms and heart rate changes. Lancet II:753–758
11. Maseri A, Chierchia S, Davies G, Glazier J (1985) Mechanisms of ischemic cardiac pain and silent myocardial ischemia. Am J Med 79:7–11
12. Kugler G (1979) Myocardial release of lactate, inosine and hypoxanthine during atrial pacing and exercise-induced angina. Circulation 59:43–49
13. Soutter WP, Sharp F, Clark DM (1978) Bedside estimation of whole blood lactate. Br J Anaesth 50:445–450
14. Reiz S, Häggmark S, Östman M (1981) Invasive analysis of non-invasive indicators of myocardial work and ischemia during anaesthesia soon after myocardial infarction. Acta Anaesthesiol Scand 25:303–311
15. Reiz S, Bålfors E, Gustavsson B et al. (1982) Effects of halothane on coronary haemodynamics and myocardial metabolism in patients with ischemic heart disease and heart failure. Acta Anaesthesiol Scand 26:133–138
16. Apstein CS, Gravino F, Hood WB Jr (1979) Limitations of lactate production as an index of myocardial ischemia. Circulation 60:877–887
17. Kaplan JA, King SB (1976) The precordial electrocardiographic lead (V5) in patients who have coronary-artery disease. Anesthesiology 45:570–574
18. Blackburn H, Katigbak R (1964) What electrocardiographic leads to take after exercise. Am Heart J 67:184–185
19. London MJ, Hollenberg M, Wong MG et al. (1988) Intraoperative myocardial ischemia: localization by continuous 12-lead electrocardiography. Anesthesiology 69:232–241
20. Kotrly KJ, Kotter GS, Mortara D, Kampine JP (1984) Intraoperative detection of myocardial ischemia with an ST segment trend monitoring system. Anesth Analg 63:393–397
21. Forrester JS, Wyatt HL, Tyberg JV et al. (1976) Functional significance of regional ischemic contraction abnormalities. Circulation 54:64–70
22. Waters HL, daLuz PL, Wyatt HL et al. (1977) Early changes in regional and global left ventricular function induced by graded reduction in regional coronary perfusion. Am J Cardiol 39:537–543
23. Lowenstein E, Foex P, Francis CM et al. (1981) Regional ischemic ventricular dysfunction in myocardium supplied by a narrowed coronary artery with increasing halothane concentration in the dog. Anesthesiology 55:349–359
24. Bellows WH, Bode RH, Levy JH et al. (1984) Noninvasive detection of periinduction ischemic ventricular dysfunction by cardiokymography in humans: preliminary experience. Anesthesiology 60:155–158

25. Videcoq M, Arvieux CC, Ramsay JG et al. (1987) The association isoflurane-verapamil causes regional left ventricular dyssynchrony in the dog. Anesthesiology 67:635–641
26. Serruyus BN, Hooghoudt TEH, Reiber JHC et al. (1983) Influence of intracoronary nifedipine on left ventricular function, coronary vasomotility, and myocardial oxygen consumption. Br Heart J 49:427–441
27. Elliott PL, Schauble JF, Weiss J et al. (1980) Echocardiography and LV function during anesthesia. Anesthesiology 53:S105
28. Abel MD, Nishimura RA, Callahan MJ et al. (1987) Evaluation of intraoperative transesophageal two-dimensional echocardiography. Anesthesiology 66:64–68
29. Smith JS, Cahalan MK, Benefield DJ et al. (1985) Intraoperative detection of myocardial ischemia in high-risk patients: electrocardiography versus two-dimensional transesophageal echocardiography. Circulation 72:1015–1021
30. Diamond GA, Chag M, Vas R, Forrester JS (1978) Cardiokymography: quantitative analysis of regional ischemic left ventricular dysfunction. Am J Cardiol 41:1249–1257
31. Vas R, Diamond GA, Silverberg RA et al. (1979) Assessment of the functional significance of coronary artery disease with atrial pacing and cardiokymography. Am J Cardiol 44:1283–1289
32. Silverberg RA, Diamond GA, Vas R et al. (1980) Noninvasive diagnosis of coronary artery disease: the cardiokymographic stress test. Circulation 61:579–589
33. Vas R (1967) Electronic device for physiologic kinetic measurements and detection of extraneous bodies. IEEE Trans Biomed Eng 14:2–10
34. Vas R, Diamond GA, Wyatt HL et al. (1977) Noninvasive analysis of regional wall motion: cardiokymography. Am J Physiol 233:H700
35. Burke JF, Morganroth J, Soffer J et al. (1984) The cardiokymographic stress test compared to the thallium-201 perfusion exercise test in the diagnosis of coronary artery disease. Am Heart J 107:718–725
36. Weiner DA, Principal Investigators (1985) Accuracy of cardiokymography during exercise testing: results of a multicenter study. J Am Coll Cardiol 6:502–509
37. Gobel FL, Nordstrom LA, Nelson RR et al. (1978) The rate-pressure product as an index of myocardial oxygen consumption during exercise in patients with angina pectoris. Circulation 57:549–556
38. Moffitt EA, Sethna DH, Gray RJ et al. (1984) Rate-pressure product correlates poorly with myocardial oxygen consumption during anaesthesia in coronary patients. Can Anaesth Soc J 31:5–12
39. Buffington CW, Bashein G, Sivarajan M (1987) Blood pressure and heart rate predict ischemia in collateral-dependent myocardium. Anesthesiology A5
40. Kaplan JA, Wells PH (1981) Early diagnosis of myocardial ischemia using the pulmonary artery catheter. Anesth Analg 60:789–793
41. Reiz S, Bålfors E, Sorensen MB et al. (1983) Isoflurane – a powerful coronary vasodilator in patients with coronary artery disease. Anesthesiology 59:91–99
42. Lowenstein E, Reiz S (1987) Effects of inhalation anesthetics on systemic hemodynamics and the coronary circulation. In: Kaplan JA (ed) Cardiac anesthesia. Grune and Stratton, New York, pp 3–35
43. Lowenstein E (1985) Perianesthetic ischemic episodes cause myocardial infarction in humans – a hypothesis confirmed. Anesthesiology 62:103–106
44. Kleinmann F, Henkin RE, Glisson SN et al. (1986) Qualitative evaluation of coronary flow during anesthetic induction using thallium-201 perfusion scans. Anesthesiology 64:157–164
45. Moffitt EA, Sethna DH, Bussell JA et al. (1985) Effects of intubation on coronary blood flow and myocardial oxygenation. Can Anaesth Soc J 32:105–111
46. Slogoff S, Keats AS (1989) Randomized trial of primary anesthetic agents on outcome of coronary bypass operations. Anesthesiology 70:179–188
47. Tuman KJ, McCarthy RJ, Spiess BD et al. (1989) Does choice of anesthetic agent significantly affect outcome after coronary artery surgery. Anesthesiology 70:189–198

48. Sill JC, Boye AA, Nugent M et al. (1987) Effects of isoflurane on coronary arteries and coronary arterioles in the intact dog. Anesthesiology 66:273–279
49. Hickey RF, Sybert PE, Verrier ED, Cason BA (1988) Effects of halothane, enflurane and isoflurane on coronary blood flow, autoregulation and coronary vascular reserve in the canine heart. Anesthesiology 68, 21–30
50. Cutfield GR, Francis CM, Foex P et al. (1988) Isoflurane and large coronary artery haemodynamics. Br J Anaesth 60:784–790
51. Hohner P, Häggmark S, Johansson G et al. (1988) Dose-dependent coronary vasodilation by isoflurane in surgical patients with coronary artery disease. Proceedings of the European Association of Cardiothoracic Anaesthesiologists, p 10, Lyon 1988
52. Buffington CW, Romson JL, Levine NC et al. (1987) Isoflurane causes coronary steal in a canine model of chronic coronary occlusion. Anesthesiology 66:280–292
53. Priebe HJ, Foex P (1987) Isoflurane causes regional myocardial dysfunction in dogs with critical coronary artery stenoses. Anesthesiology 66:293–300
54. Priebe HJ (1988) Isoflurane causes more severe regional myocardial dysfunction than halothane in dogs with a critical coronary artery stenosis. Anesthesiology 69:72–80
55. Tatekawa S, Traber KB, Hantler CB et al. (1987) Effects of isoflurane on myocardial blood flow, function and oxygen consumption in the presence of critical coronary stenosis in the dog. Anesth Analg 66:1073–1082
56. Becker LC (1978) Conditions for vasodilator-induced coronary steal in experimental myocardial ischemia. Circulation 57:1103–1110
57. Buffington CW, Davis KB, Gillispie S, Pettinger M (1988) The prevalence of steal-prone coronary anatomy in patients with coronary artery disease: an analysis of the Coronary Artery Surgery Study Registry. Anesthesiology 69:721–727
58. Stone JG, Foex P, Sear JW et al. (1988) Risk of myocardial ischaemia during anaesthesia in treated and untreated hypertensive patients. Br J Anaesth 61:675–679
59. Godet G, Coriat P, Baron JF et al. (1987) Prevention of intraoperative myocardial ischemia during noncardiac surgery with intravenous diltiazem: a randomized trial versus placebo. Anesthesiology 66:241–245
60. Slogoff S, Keats AS (1988) Does chronic treatment with calcium entry blocking drugs reduce perioperative myocardial ischemia? Anesthesiology 68:676–680
61. Chung F, Houston PL, Cheng DCH et al. (1988) Calcium channel blockade does not offer adequate protection from perioperative myocardial ischemia. Anesthesiology 69:343–347
62. Coriat P, Daloz M, Bousseau D et al. (1984) Prevention of intraoperative myocardial ischemia during noncardiac surgery with intravenous nitroglycerin. Anesthesiology 61:193–196
63. Thomson IR, Putnins CL (1985) Adverse effects of pancuronium during high-dose fentanyl anesthesia for coronary artery bypass grafting. Anesthesiology 62:708–713
64. O'Connor JP, Ramsay JG, Wynands JE et al. (1989) The incidence of myocardial ischemia during anesthesia for coronary artery bypass surgery in patients receiving pancuronium or vecuronium. Anesthesiology 70:230–236

Physiological and Biochemical Indicators of Impaired Tissue Oxygenation

D. R. Dantzker

The earliest life was formed in the anaerobic environment which characterized the first half of Earth's existence. The ability to use O_2 in the metabolic process evolved about 2 billion years ago and markedly improved the efficiency of energy extraction from foodstuffs. The oxidation reaction could now be carried to completion using O_2 as the terminal electron acceptor. This change in energy production required the evolution of the cytochrome chain and adenosine triphosphate (ATP) which permitted the controlled release of the energy contained in the food and its storage in the easily controllable small packets of the high energy phosphate bond. As life became more complex, the machinery required to deliver adequate amounts of O_2 required modification since, unlike very simple organisms, these life forms were no longer able to provide each cell with a continual supply of O_2 directly from the environment. The more complex the life form, the more likely the possibility that under certain circumstances sufficient O_2 would not be available everywhere in the body to maintain adequate energy supplies using aerobic metabolic pathways. This required the persistance of anaerobic means of energy generation to be available as backup.

Cells require a continuous supply of energy to maintain the integrity of the cell membrane and to allow for important functions such as protein synthesis, muscular contraction, and active transport. When adequate O_2 is present, energy is generated most efficiently through the combustion of carbohydrates, protein, and fat in the Krebs tricarboxylic acid (TCA) cycle (Fig. 1) [1]. The TCA cycle, which takes place in the mitochondria, is a series of oxidation-reduction reactions during which the energy released from the transfer of electrons is captured. This involves the reduction of NAD^+ to NADH, a transfer of the electrons along a series of electron-carrier enzymes (the cytochrome chain), and the capture of the energy in ATP. Since oxygen is the terminal electron acceptor in this scheme adequate amounts are required if energy generation through this pathway is to continue.

When sufficient O_2 is not present, energy is generated, for the most part, through glycolysis (Fig. 2). In this process, glucose (or glycogen) is the substrate and pyruvate becomes the terminal electron acceptor. This is a much less efficient means of generating energy since 1 mol of glucose produces 2 mol of ATP through glycolysis and 36 mol of ATP when fully oxidized in the TCA cycle. The fate of the pyruvate produced as the end product of glycolysis depends on the presence of adequate amounts of necessary cofactors. It can be

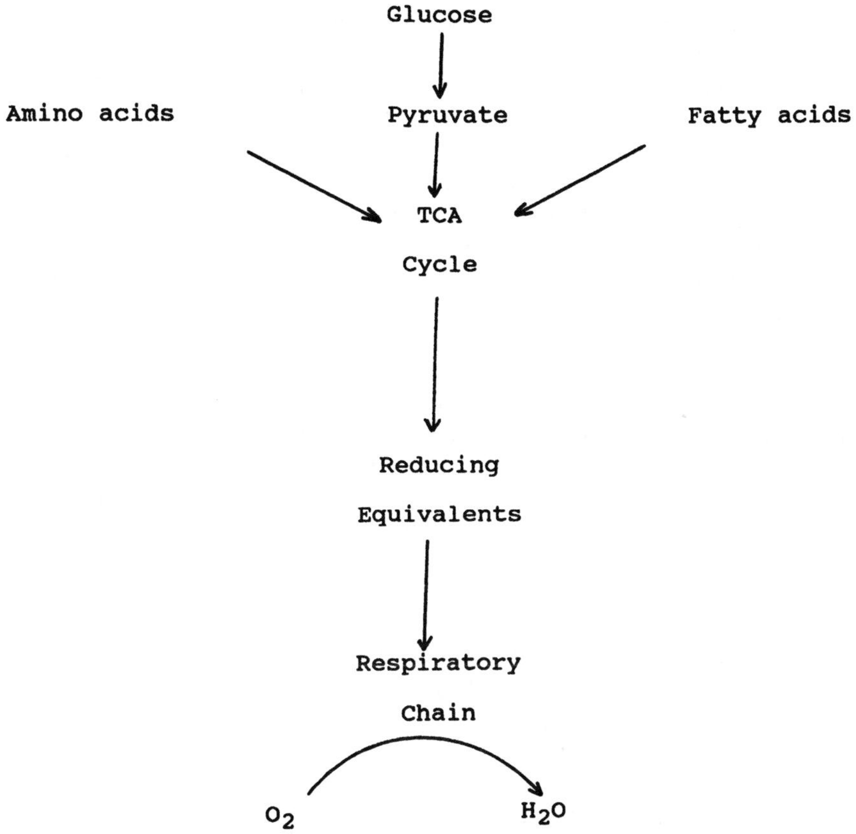

Fig. 1. Oxidative phosphorylation is the primary mechanism for the production of ATP. Oxygen is the terminal electron acceptor

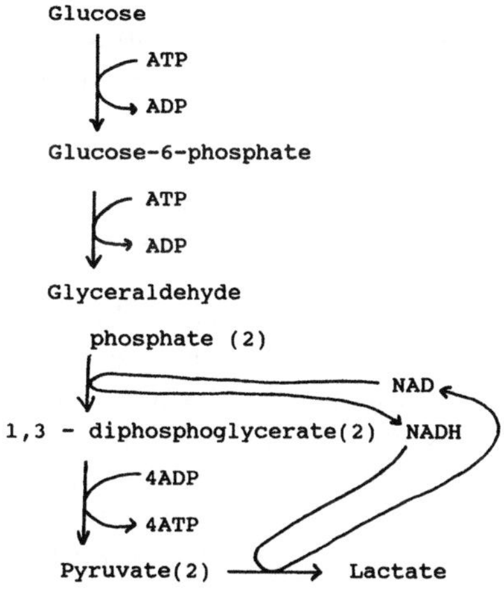

Fig. 2. Glycolysis allows for the production of ATP under anaerobic conditions with pyruvate the terminal electron acceptor. The reduction of pyruvate to lactate regenerates NAD which is necessary for glycolysis to continue

further oxidized to acetyl-CoA and be carried through the TCA cycle. However, this requires the presence of NAD^+. Alternatively, pyruvate can be used as substrate for gluconeogenesis which requires the expenditure of ATP. When both of these are in short supply, as with inadequate tissue oxygenation, the pyruvate is instead reduced to lactate, regenerating NAD^+ in the process, which is required in order for glycolysis to continue. The acidosis associated with anaerobic glycolysis does not come, as is commonly assumed, from the reduction of the lactate to pyruvate since there is no net H^+ production during the conversion of glucose to lactate. The H^+ comes instead from the hydrolysis of ATP as the stored energy is released for utilization:

$$ATP \rightarrow ADP + Pi + H^+$$

where Pi is inorganic phosphate [2]. Since the rephosphorylation of ADP under anaerobic conditions (one of the means of reusing the protons generated from ATP hydrolysis) is inefficient and the other ways of utilizing the protons, namely gluconeogenesis and oxidative phosphorylation, are also not functioning optimally under anaerobic conditions, the protons accumulate and metabolic acidosis results.

An alternative pathway to glycolysis for the anaerobic production of ATP, at least in skeletal muscle, heart, and brain, is through the creatine kinase reaction [3]. This allows the transfer of a high-energy phosphate bond from the storage compound phosphocreatine (PCr) to ADP to produce ATP:

$$PCr + ADP + H^+ \rightleftharpoons ATP + Cr + Pi.$$

An additional advantage of this method of anaerobic ATP generation is that it consumes hydrogen ions and thus limits the metabolic acidosis produced by glycolysis. While the creatine kinase reaction constitutes a ready source of energy, its usefulness is limited by the PCr stores.

Given this brief introduction, we can now look at parameters which are available to access the adequacy of tissue oxygenation. The ideal parameter would be easy to obtain and interpret, bearing some clear-cut relationship to tissue oxygenation during all kinds of physiologic and pathologic stresses. Potential candidates would include those variables which monitor the level of oxygen available, those that provide an index of how the foodstuffs are being metabolized i.e., aerobically versus anaerobically, and those that provide some direct measure of the energy balance sheet of the cells.

The PO_2 required to guarantee sufficient energy production from oxidative phosphorylation in man is unknown. However, isolated mitochondria are able to function maximally at a PO_2 of far less than 1.0 torr [4]. Similar low PO_2 requirements have been demonstrated in isolated whole organs [5] and in situ working skeletal muscle [6]. This high affinity for oxygen would suggest that man can tolerate significant hypoxemia. In fact, in young normal subjects an arterial partial pressure of O_2 (PaO_2) in the mid-20s will be tolerated without evidence of compromised tissue function [7].

In critically ill patients, however, evidence of presumed tissue hypoxia is often found at levels of PaO_2 considerably higher than the values achievable, without any apparent tissue dysfunction in the young, otherwise healthy, individuals. To a minor degree, this may reflect the influence of important oxygen-dependent, extramitochondrial processes which have a much lower oxygen affinity and thus presumably a higher critical PO_2 than that necessary for oxidative phosphorylation [8]. More likely, it is because the PaO_2 is a poor index of the significant variables which limit O_2 flux into the tissues.

For any tissue, the O_2 flux can be thought of in the following simplified way:

$$\text{Tissue } O_2 \text{ Flux} = D \times (PcapO_2 - PmitoO_2)$$

where D represents the diffusing capacity for O_2 in the tissue and Pcap and Pmito are the partial pressures in the capillary and mitochondria. The factors which regulate D are predominantly those that relate to the control of the microvasculature and are discussed elsewhere in this volume. We will concern ourselves here with the Pcap, to see if any of the commonly measured variables allow us to monitor the driving pressure for O_2 into the tissues, a key factor determining the adequacy of tissue oxygenation.

The Pcap at any point along the capillary is determined by a complex interaction of bulk O_2 delivery, tissue O_2 utilization, and the kinetics of oxygen-hemoglobin binding. At the beginning of the capillary, the Pcap is equal to the PaO_2, but as oxygen is extracted by the tissues, there is a fall in the Pcap as we progress towards the venous end. Traditional concepts of the capillary PO_2 profile are based on the Krogh tissue cylinder model and suggest that the blood exits from the capillary with a $PcapO_2$ equal to the venous value [9] (Fig. 3). Using this model it has been suggested that there is a gradient of tissue PO_2 which varies from the PaO_2 (near the capillary wall at the arterial end of the capillary) to less than the venous PO_2 (at the edge of the cylinder on the venous end, the "lethal corner"), and that under certain conditions the venous PO_2 serves as a good approximation of the mean tissue PO_2 [10]. However, as pointed out by Tenney [10], this assumption would only hold under conditions of normal oxygenation and when capillary density resulted in normal diffusion distances from red cell to tissue. When these normal conditions are perturbed, however, he pointed out that the venous PO_2 might over- or underestimate the tissue PO_2.

The applicability of this theoretical model to the clinical situation in man has been challenged on a number of grounds. First, and perhaps most importantly, the Krogh model ignores the kinetics of the oxygen-hemoglobin dissociation reaction when calculating the capillary PO_2 profile, assuming instead an instantaneous release of O_2 from hemoglobin. Theoretical computations, however, suggest that the time required for the O_2 bound in the red blood cell to dissociate from hemoglobin, diffuse into the plasma, and thus become available for diffusion into the tissues, may be rate limiting [11]. As a consequence, the actual $PcapO_2$ at any point in the capillary, and thus the true driving pressure for O_2 diffusion, may be less than expected from calculations based on the Krogh model (Fig. 3). The more the true Pcap diverges from that predicted from the Krogh model, the more the venous PO_2 will differ from the end capil-

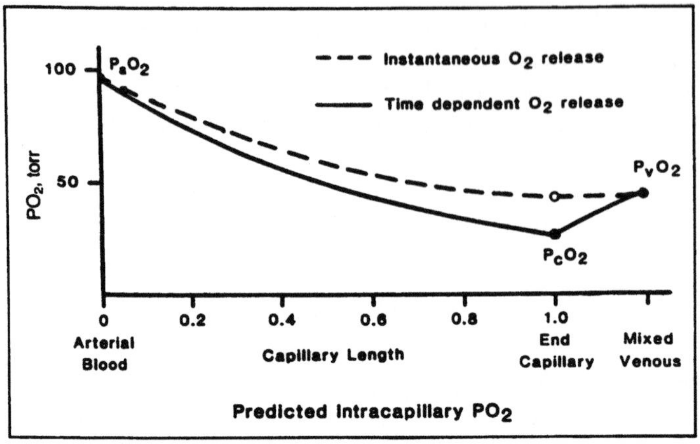

Fig. 3. The capillary oxygen profiles calculated assuming instantaneous oxygen release from hemoglobin and taking into account the actual kinetics of the oxyhemoglobin dissociation. The time-dependent model would predict a lower PO_2 driving pressure along the length of the capillary as well as a difference between the PO_2 in the end-capillary and venous blood. (From [11], with permission)

lary PO_2, and thus the less likely that it will represent mean tissue PO_2 even under the most ideal circumstances. This divergence is exaggerated in situations of low O_2 transport to the tissues, especially in the presence of anemia, and when the transit time is very short, reducing the time available for diffusion.

Factors that would increase the end-capillary venous oxygen difference include:

1. Decreased oxygen delivery
2. Increased oxygen uptake
3. Increased oxygen affinity of the blood
4. Anemia
5. Decreased cardiac output
6. Decreased capillary transit time

It has also been hypothesized that because arteries and veins run together, oxygen may diffuse directly from the artery to the vein creating, in effect, a diffusion shunt for O_2 [12]. This would result in a progressive fall in the arterial PO_2 as the blood moves towards the capillary bed and once again result in a venous PO_2 that is higher than that in the venous end of the capillary. Regardless of which tissue model is used to calculate the capillary PO_2 profile, the presence of this type of counter-current mechanism would result in a capillary PO_2 that is lower than might be assumed based upon either the arterial or venous values.

Based upon this brief summary, what can we deduce about the utility of arterial or mixed venous PO_2 (PvO_2) measurements as an index of adequate tissue oxygenation? The first thing to emphasize is that while the PaO_2 measures the input to all of the tissues, the PvO_2 is a blood flow weighted mean of the venous effluent from each of the tissue beds and is equal to none of them. Thus, the PvO_2 is influenced by the relative contributions from organs with high and low metabolic rates, and changes in the PvO_2 may reflect only an alteration in blood flow distribution. More importantly, neither the PaO_2 nor the PvO_2 can be looked on, necessarily, as an estimate of either the effective Pcap, or the tissue PO_2, even if we knew what those values needed to be in order to ensure adequate oxygenation. Clinical studies have suggested, for example, that values of PvO_2 below 28 torr were associated with a poor prognosis [13] and yet values of PvO_2 much lower than that are found in situations in which normal tissue function is present. Perhaps the prognostic information inherent in marked abnormalities in either the PaO_2 or PvO_2 is due more to their association with other physiological abnormalities (abnormal lung function, low cardiac output, etc.) than to their ability to predict the adequacy of tissue oxygenation.

Since the capillary driving pressure for O_2 is not definable by either the arterial or venous PO_2 and is dependent on the amount of O_2 delivered to the capillaries as well as on the partial pressure, it is worth considering the use of total O_2 transport as a useful index of adequate tissue oxygenation. O_2 transport (TO_2) is defined as:

$$TO_2 = \text{cardiac output} \times \text{arterial } O_2 \text{ content.}$$

In normal subjects, TO_2 is determined by metabolic requirements of the tissues with prompt increases in response to any increases in VO_2 [14]. The importance of an adequate TO_2 to normal tissue function was first emphasized by Cain, who found that a critical TO_2 (TO_2crit) existed in anesthetized dogs, below which basal levels of O_2 consumption (VO_2) could not be maintained (Fig. 4) [15]. The TO_2crit in the dogs was approximately 10 ml/kg/min and was independent of the arterial or mixed venous PO_2. With hypoxemia the critical TO_2 was reached at a PaO_2 of 25 torr and PvO_2 of 17 torr, while with anemic hypoxia the values were 90 and 45 torr. This was initially taken as evidence for the primacy of volume delivery over capillary driving pressure in limiting tissue O_2 delivery. However, it should be apparent from the prior discussion that the true $PcapO_2$ could not be derived in either case from the variables which were measured. In fact, it has been suggested that when the kinetics of the oxyhemoglobin dissociation reaction are taken into account, similar Pcap may have been present in both situations despite the marked differences in PaO_2 and PvO_2 [11]. This does not detract from the importance of the observation that when TO_2 is reduced to below normal it is an important limiting variable regardless of the mechanism.

While a similar study in normal man has not been carried out, observations in patients about to undergo surgery seem to demonstrate a comparable biphasic TO_2-VO_2 relationship and similar TO_2crit [16]. Based on this experimental data, one could argue that tracking the relationship between VO_2 and TO_2 could provide a useful index of adequate tissue oxygenation. Main-

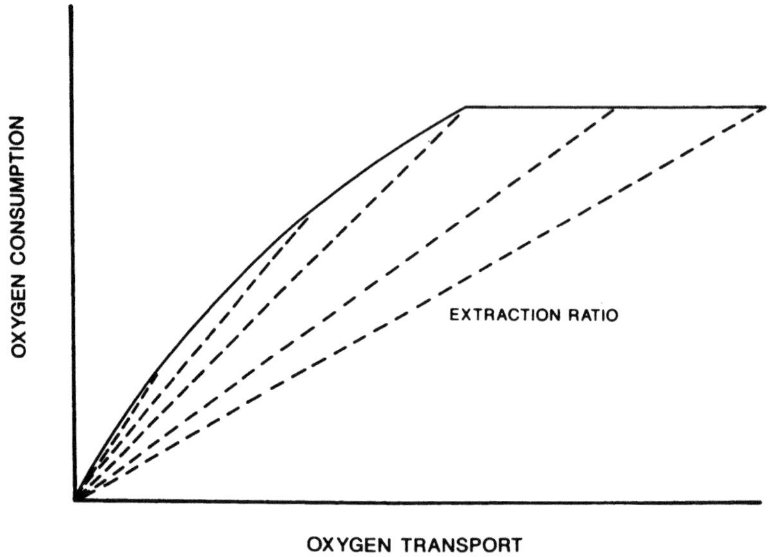

Fig. 4. The relationship between oxygen transport (TO_2), oxygen consumption (VO_2) and the oxygen extraction ratio (ER). When TO_2 is more than adequate, VO_2 can be maintained as TO_2 is decreased by increasing the ER. Below the critical TO_2, VO_2 falls despite a continuing increase in ER

taining TO_2 above the critical point should insure optimal tissue oxygenation.

Unfortunately when this relationship has been studied in the clinical setting, in patients with both acute and chronic abnormalities of tissue oxygenation, a clear biphasic relationship is usually not found. In many of the patients studied, however, the relationship has been looked at only over a very narrow range of TO_2, confined mainly to levels which varied from the normal TO_2 to slightly below the TO_2crit reported in the normal anesthetized subjects. In patients with ARDS, a linear relationship between TO_2 and VO_2 has been described over a much wider range of TO_2, with no evidence of a TO_2crit or a plateau phase, despite levels of TO_2 well above normal (Fig. 5) [17]. This has been termed "pathological supply dependency" and its pathophysiological basis has yet to be clearly defined. Since there are no studies to date which have demonstrated that reaching the plateau of the TO_2-VO_2 relationship is even possible, no less beneficial, monitoring the TO_2-VO_2 relationship will need to be more completely understood before it can be recommended as a good tool for accessing the adequacy of tissue oxygenation.

In addition to altering TO_2 in response to changing metabolic needs, the tissues can alter the percent of the delivered oxygen that it extracts, the extraction ratio ($ER = VO_2/TO_2$; Fig. 4). In normal subjects in whom VO_2 is increasing due to increasing metabolic demands, such as during exercise, the ER increases along with the increase in TO_2. The increase in ER is necessary to allow the desired increases in VO_2 since TO_2 can only be increased by about four to five times while VO_2 may go up by ten times or more in highly conditioned athletes. An ER of 0.80 or even 0.90 can be seen at maximal VO_2 [14]. As VO_2 increases, a point is reached, usually about 40% to 50% of maximal VO_2 in normal sedentary individuals, where aerobic metabolism is no longer able to provide all of the required energy and anaerobic pathways are needed in addition (the anaerobic threshold) [18]. The ER at the anaerobic threshold is about 0.60. Since increases in ER are accomplished by microvascular adjustments which optimize the conditions for O_2 diffusion, the ER at anaerobic threshold must represent the limit that these microvascular alterations are capable of compensating for an imbalance between TO_2 and VO_2.

Under the conditions that are of greater concern in critically ill patients, where TO_2 is falling, data in normal subjects with respect to the ability to increase ER are less clear. In animal studies, TO_2crit is achieved at an ER that is usually greater than 45% [19]. However, in the only study in relatively normal man, VO_2 began to fall at an ER of about 0.3 very close to the normal ER at basal levels [16]. If this is true, it would suggest a very poor diffusion reserve in the setting of reduced TO_2. To further complicate the problem, many sick patients have a very low and fixed ER even at low levels of TO_2, suggesting a primary defect in microvascular control. Additional information will clearly be necessary in order to define what the real critical ER is in various states before it can be used as a basis for therapeutic decision-making.

Regardless of the physiological interpretation of pathological supply dependency or our present ability to use TO_2 or ER as a monitor of adequate tissue oxygenation, it is of great concern when a linear TO_2-VO_2 relationship

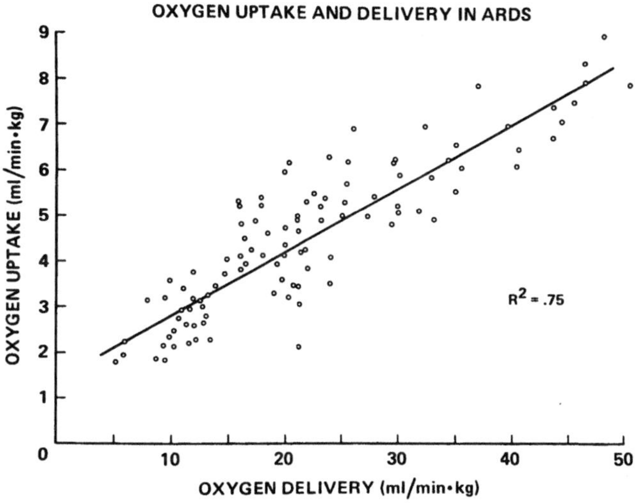

Fig. 5. The relationship between oxygen consumption and transport in a series of patients with the adult respiratory distress syndrome. There appears to be no critical level of oxygen delivery despite levels of oxygen delivery well above normal. This is an example of pathological supply dependency. (From [17], with permission)

is accompanied by low, fixed extraction ratios. In two clinical studies, it has now been shown that patients with this pattern have a poor prognosis when compared with other critically ill patients who do not demonstrate the phenomenon [20, 21].

Trying to judge tissue oxygenation by estimating the adequacy of factors which bear on the limits of aerobic metabolism is a relatively recent innovation. Looking for evidence of anaerobic metabolism as an index of deficient tissue oxygenation, however, is standard practice. The energy stored in PCr is quite limited, even in those tissues which contain the largest amounts: brain, heart, and skeletal muscle. As already discussed, when there is insufficient oxygen to maintain energy requirements through oxidative phosphorylation, the cells depend on glycolysis as the major synthetic pathway for ATP. Increasing lactate levels are a marker of increased glycolysis and are often considered as de facto evidence of inadequate tissue oxygenation.

The lactate level is the balance between production and utilization [22, 23]. Some tissues, such as the erythrocyte, renal medulla, and portions of the eye depend routinely on glycolysis for their energy needs. Their overall contribution to the lactate pool, however, is small, about 40 g/day. Some tissues such as skeletal muscle, brain, intestine, and skin, may also produce small additional amounts of lactate even when there is adequate tissue oxygenation. These tissues will produce much larger amounts, however, when their oxygenation is insufficient to support the necessary ATP production through oxidative phosphorylation. In addition to tissue hypoxia, increased lactate production may be induced by factors which increase the rate of glycolysis in excess of the ability of pyruvate to be utilized in the TCA cycle. These include alkalosis, excess insulin or catecholamine release, as well as factors which reduce the levels of acetyl-CoA, such as starvation and diabetes. Finally, drugs and chemicals such as ethanol, methanol, ethylene glycol, salicylates, and phenformin can elevate lactate levels by interfering with gluconeogenesis.

On the other side of the balance sheet, lactate is removed from the circulation predominantly by the liver. The liver's capacity to remove lactate is thought to be several-fold greater than the ability of the peripheral tissues to produce it. Thus, any compromise of hepatic function can have a rather dramatic influence on the lactate level which is present for any rate of accelerated glycolysis. Lactate produced in one organ may also be used for substrate by another, in particular, the heart and skeletal muscle. Finally, the production of lactate may be inhibited even in the presence of inadequate oxygenation by factors which interfere with glycolysis. In malnutrition, glucose stores may be inadequate to sustain glycolysis at required levels. Increasing H^+ concentration inhibits phosphofructokinase and therefore reduces glycolytic flux. Thus, the acidosis usually associated with increased lactate production can serve as a sort of negative feedback control on glycolysis.

Factors which determine the balance of lactate production and utilization, therefore, may be independent of the adequacy of tissue oxygenation and not uniformly associated with tissue hypoxia. Even if associated with the presence of hypoxia, the level is not necessarily a direct quantitative measure of the severity of the oxygen lack and individual organ hypoxia may be masked by mechanisms available for lactate removal. In many settings, therefore, lactate may be an insensitive and not very specific index of inadequate tissue oxygenation.

All of the monitoring techniques described thus far have been only indirect reflections of what is going on at the level of the tissues. Because of this there is great interest in developing methods for actually measuring the bioenergetic balance within the cell to determine the adequacy of oxidative metabolism. Nuclear magnetic resonance spectroscopy (MRS) provides a well-characterized, noninvasive means of measuring the key biological molecules involved in the energy balance sheet [24, 25]. When tissue is placed in a strong magnetic field and subjected to radio-frequency waves, certain isotopic species will adsorb and then emit some of the energy in the form of a radio-frequency signal which can be characterized and quantitated. Phosphorus 31 is a stable isotope which forms a part of several of the molecules which we have already discussed as playing a central role in the storage and transfer of energy in the cell. These include ATP, ADP, PCr, and inorganic phosphate (Pi). The ratio of PCr/Pi is the equivalent of the cellular phosphate potential, ATP/[ADP] [Pi], the energy charge of the cell (Fig. 6).

When TO_2 is reduced, either by hypoxemia or hypoperfusion, a level is eventually reached where the PCr/Pi begins to fall. In skeletal muscle this point has been shown to correlate with TO_2crit [26]. In the brain, the PCr/Pi falls at a PO_2 below 40 torr while skeletal muscle appears to be more resistant [27]. At this point, the level of ATP is normal, supplemented in part by the creatine kinase reaction. Whether or not glycolysis is induced at this stage as an additional source of ATP production or is only invoked when the PCr is exhausted is unclear. In the brain, the use of PCr appears to be the preferred source of anaerobically generated ATP, perhaps to decrease the generation of H^+ which is detrimental to neuronal function. In the skeletal muscle this is less clear since a fall in pH is seen to coincide with the fall in PCr/Pi, suggesting that glycolysis begins concomitantly with the usage of the creatine kinase reaction.

As tissue oxygenation becomes increasingly impaired, the PCr/Pi continues to fall and the intracellular pH (also measurable by MRS) falls along with it. The ATP levels, however, remain normal until very severe hypoxia (PaO_2 < 18 torr in the brain), when the PCr is almost entirely depleted and only then begins to fall. In experimental preparations, decreases in ATP appear to be irreversible and thus below this level of hypoxia, cell death may be inevitable.

Since energy levels may remain normal until the ATP-generating ability of the cell is severely taxed, organ function may remain adequate almost until cell death intervenes, which emphasizes that monitoring the changes which take place prior to a fall in ATP would be very useful. At the moment, unfortunately, MRS as a clinical tool, is impractical because of the expense and complexity of the equipment and the logistical problems of bringing patients to the magnet on a regular basis or placing a strong magnetic field in the complicated world of the intensive care unit. However, new technology involving miniaturization and shielding may well make it practical in the near future.

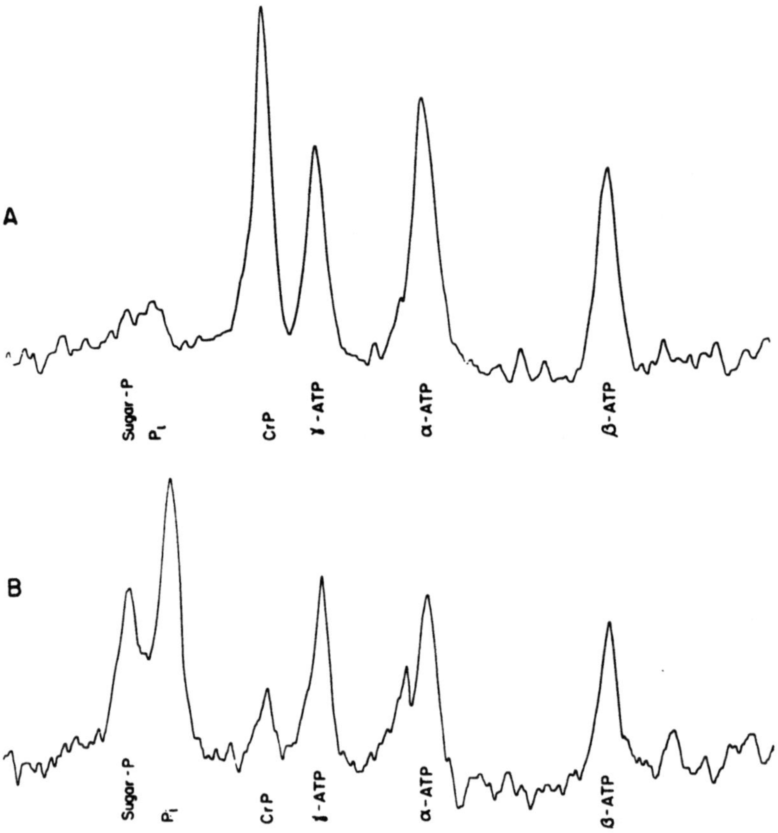

Fig. 6 A, B. The magnetic resonance spectrum from a normal and ischemic heart. (From [29])

Another technique for direct quantitation of cellular bioenergetics that may be closer to practical use is the optical monitoring of the reduction/oxidation status of the mitochondrial energy chain, in particular cytochrome aa^3 [27]. In the brain, where much of this work has been done, reduction of cyto aa^3 occurs with much more modest hypoxia than is necessary to achieve a fall in PCr/Pi. It has been suggested that the reduction of cyto-aa^3 could therefore be used as an early warning sign of impending tissue hypoxia. However, because it is very difficult to calibrate the optical techniques, they may be useful only as a way of following trends and not as a measure of any absolute level of tissue oxygenation.

Both of these techniques, while sensitive and specific markers of the energy status of the cell, suffer from being representative only of the tissue being actively monitored. In situations of hypovolemia or generalized hypoxemia, it may indeed be possible to utilize a single tissue as a good window to the rest of the body. However, in situations such as sepsis or ARDS, where heterogeneity of TO_2 may be the norm, adequate oxygenation of one organ may not connote sufficient oxygenation of all organs. Some less organ specific monitor of insufficient cellular energy homeostasis would be useful.

If ATP utilization exceeds its production, AMP will accumulate and be hydrolysed through a series of steps to hypoxanthine. In tissues which contain xanthine oxidase, predominantly the liver, the hypoxanthine can be further oxidized to xanthine and then uric acid. This degradative pathway generates oxygen radicals and is thought to contribute to the tissue damage which occurs following reprofusion of a previously ischemic organ. Increased levels of adenine nucleotide degradation products have been reported in the blood of critically ill patients, suggesting some utility of these measurements as a more generalized screen for inadequate tissue oxygenation [28]. However, at the present time, these measurements are difficult to do accurately, and carefully done studies in critically ill patients must be done before their utility is proven.

In summary, the factors that determine the adequacy of tissue oxygenation are becoming better understood as the technology for making the important physiological measurements becomes available. At the present time, however, we are only at the point of knowing enough to begin asking the correct questions. These technological advances may also eventually provide us with the ability to actually monitor the adequacy of tissue oxygenation. However, at this time it is clear only that the we do not yet have any definitive answers to the monitoring question and for the moment must depend to a great deal on clinical skills. This early stage in our understanding as well as the present lack of definitive variables to monitor should be kept in mind whenever we are tempted to institutionalize protocols for patient management.

References

1. Newsholme EA, Leech AR (1983) Biochemistry for the medical sciences. Wiley, Chichester
2. Gevers W (1977) Generation of protons by metabolic processes in heart cells. J Mol Cell Cardiol 9:867–874
3. Saks VA, Rosenshtrautch LV, Smirnov VN, Chazov EI (1978) Role of creatine phosphokinase in cellular function and metabolism. Can J Physiol Pharmacol 56:691–706
4. Jobsis FF (1972) Oxidative metabolism at low PO_2. Fed Proc 31:1404–1413
5. Fisher AB, Dodia C (1981) Lung as a model for evaluation of critical intracellular PO_2 and PCO_2. Am J Physiol 241:E47–50
6. Gayeski TEJ, Honig CR (1986) O_2 gradients from sarcolemma to cell interior in red muscle at maximal VO_2. 251:H789–799
7. Sutton JR, Reeves JT, Wagner PD et al. (1988) Operation Everest II: oxygen transport during exercise at extreme simulated altitude. J Appl Physiol 64:1309–1321
8. Robin ED (1980) Of men and mitochondria: coping with hypoxic dysoxia. Am Rev Respir Dis 122:517–529
9. Krogh A (1919) The number and distribution of capillaries in muscles with calculations of the oxygen pressure head necessary for supplying the tissue. J Physiol (Lond) 52:409–415
10. Tenney SM (1974) A theoretical analysis of the relationship between venous blood and mean tissue oxygen pressures. Respir Physiol 20:283–296

11. Gutierrez G (1985) The rate of oxygen release and its effect on capillary O_2 tension: a mathematical analysis. Respir Physiol 63:79–96
12. Piiper J, Meyer M, Scheid P (1984) Dual role of diffusion in tissue gas exchange: blood-tissue equilibrium and diffusion shunt. Respir Physiol 56:131–144
13. Kasnitaz P, Druger GL, Yorra F, Simmons DH (1976) Mixed venous oxygen tension and hyperlactatemia. JAMA 236:570–574
14. Astrand P, Cuddy TE, Saltin B, Stenberg J (1964) Cardiac output during submaximal and maximal work. J Appl Physiol 19:268–274
15. Cain SM (1977) Oxygen delivery and uptake in dogs during anemic and hypoxic. J Appl Physiol 42:228–234
16. Shibutani K, Komatsu T, Kubal K et al. (1983) Critical level of oxygen delivery in anesthetized man. Crit Care Med 11:640–643
17. Danek SH, Lynch JP, Weg JG et al. (1980) The dependence of oxygen uptake on oxygen delivery in the adult respiratory distress syndrome. Am Rev Respir Dis 122:387–395
18. Wasserman K, Van Kessel AL, Burton GG (1967) Interactions of physiological mechanisms during exercise. J Appl Physiol 22:71–85
19. Gutierrez G, Warley AR, Dantzker DR (1986) Oxygen delivery and utilization in hypothermic dogs. J Appl Physiol 60:751–757
20. Bihari D, Smithies M, Gimson A et al. (1987) The effects of vasodilation with prostacyclin on oxygen delivery and uptake in critically ill patients. N Engl J Med 317:397–404
21. Gutierrez G, Pohil RJ (1986) Oxygen consumption is linearly related to O_2 supply in critically ill patients. J Crit Care 1:45–53
22. Kresiberg RA (1980) Lactate homeostasis and lactic acidosis. Ann Intern Med 92:227–237
23. Madias NE (1986) Lactic acidosis. Kidney Int 29:752–774
24. Gadian DG (1982) Nuclear magnetic resonance and its application to living systems. Oxford University Press, Oxford
25. Gutierrez G, Pohil RJ, Strong R et al. (1988) Bioenergetics of rabbit skeletal muscle during hypoxemia and ischemia. J Appl Physiol 65:608–616
26. Collaborative group on intracellular monitoring (1988) Intracellular monitoring of experimental respiratory failure. Am Rev Respir Dis 138:484–487
27. LaManna JC, Sick TJ, Pikarsky SM, Rosenthal M (1987) Detection of an oxidizable fraction of cytochrome oxidase in intact rat brain. Am J Physiol 253:C477–483
28. Grum CM, Simon RH, Dantzker DR, Fox IH (1985) Evidence for adenosine triphosphate degradation in critically ill patients. Chest 88:763–767
29. Ingwall JS (1982) Phosphorus nuclear magnetic resonance spectroscopy of cardiac and skeletal muscles. Am J Physiol 242:H729–H744

Monitoring O_2 Transport and Tissue Oxygenation in Critically Ill Patient

K. Reinhart

Introduction

Only a little more than 100 years ago, the German physiologist Pflüger was first to realize that the cardiorespiratory system fulfills its physiological task by guaranteeing the cellular O_2 supply and removing the waste products of cellular metabolism. He stated that everything else was secondary: "arterial oxygen content, arterial pressures, blood flow velocity, mode of cardiac work, and mode of respiration, all are incidental and subordinate; they all combine their actions only in service to the cells" [31]. But even today, with all that twentieth century technology has to offer, we are only able to monitor that which Pflüger called "incidental and subordinate."

Continuous measurements of the systemic blood pressure and heart rate are routinely done in critically ill patients, and pulmonary artery catheters are often used to determine right- and left-sided cardiac filling pressures and cardiac output and to obtain mixed venous blood samples. Noninvasive pulse oximetry is routinely applied during anesthesia and intensive care with increasing frequency. The basic question is to what extent the cardiorespiratory variables, measured directly or calculated from measurements, give the physician information on the adequacy of oxygen transport and, more importantly, on the quality of tissue oxygenation.

This chapter attempts to offer some answers to this question and to point out the problems arising from the fact that the cardiorespiratory system can fulfill its physiological task only at the level of the microcirculation, which in the critically ill is often disturbed.

There is no better monitor of the adequacy of oxygen transport and tissue oxygenation than organ function. But intensive-care patients already have compromised organ functions for various reasons. It would therefore be useful to know about cardiorespiratory status and the adequacy of tissue oxygenation before there is further loss or deterioriation of organ function and/or the appearance of biochemical indicators of tissue oxygen deficits, such as elevated blood lactate levels, which may already have an unfavorable impact on the prognosis [2, 9, 21, 53].

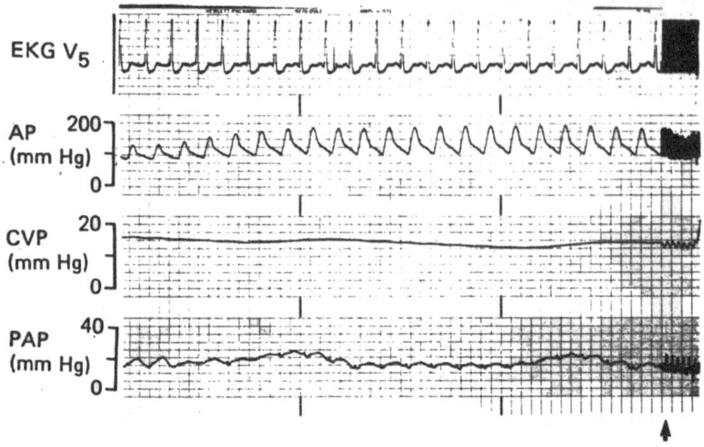

Fig. 1. Beat-to-beat increase in systemic blood pressure by better coordination of atrial and ventricular contraction; 65-year-old patient during aortobifemoral bypass surgery

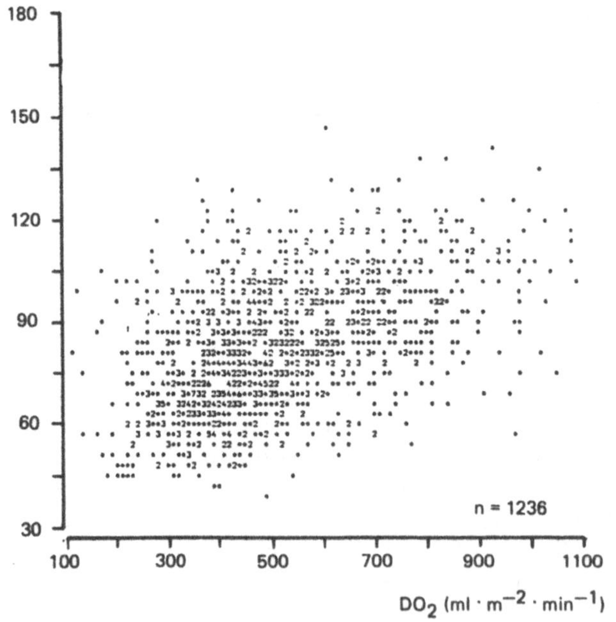

Fig. 2. Correlation between heart rate (HR) and oxygen delivery (DO_2) during the perioperative period in patients with major vascular surgery. (From Reinhart [35])

Basic Hemodynamic Variables and Convective Oxygen Transport

Convective oxygen transport or oxygen delivery (DO_2) to the tissues is defined as the product of the cardiac output (CO) and the arterial oxygen content (CaO_2) [33, 35]: $DO_2 = CO \times CaO_2$. This is the amount of oxygen that is pumped by the heart toward the periphery per minute. We will see later that although it is not identical to tissue oxygenation, DO_2 is nevertheless one major determinant of cellular O_2 supply.

ECG monitoring may not only be helpful in detecting myocardial ischemia and electrolyte imbalances; sudden changes of cardiac rhythm can also indicate alterations in oxygen transport. Figure 1 depicts a patient in whom intraoperatively an ectopic pacemaker was found, with desynchronization between atrial and ventricular contraction. The appearance of a P-wave was paralleled by a beat-to-beat improvement of cardiac output through better end-diastolic filling of the ventricle due to the atrial kick. Therefore, in cases where continuous blood-pressure monitoring is not available, every acute change in cardiac rhythm should be followed by a blood pressure check. Though heart rate, along with systemic blood pressure, is one of the cornerstones of hemodynamic monitoring, it is not a good indicator of oxygen delivery (Fig. 2). The same holds true for mean arterial blood pressure (MAP) (Fig. 3). An MAP of

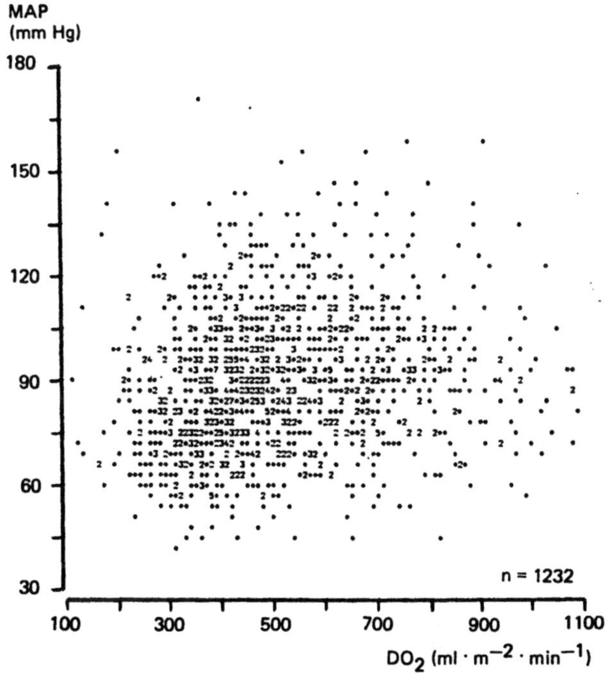

Fig. 3. Correlation between mean arterial pressure (MAP) and oxygen delivery (DO_2) during the perioperative period in patients with major vascular surgery. (From Reinhart [35])

50 can be accompanied by a DO_2 which may be well above normal in one patient but below the critical level under other circumstances or in another patient.

Cardiac Output and Oxygen Delivery

CO correlates closely with DO_2, since during anesthesia and intensive care the other determinant of DO_2 – arterial O_2 content – can usually be readily maintained with in the normal range (Fig. 4). The fact that cardiac output can be measured by thermodilution or even noninvasively, now, using doppler echocardiography [17, 43] or bioimpedance techniques [51], might lead us to assume that the problem of monitoring oxygen transport and tissue oxygenation has been solved. However, what we need to know about our patient is not primarily the absolute level of CO or DO_2 but the extent to which CO or DO_2 matches current metabolic needs, i.e., O_2 consumption (VO_2), in every situation.

VO_2 can change considerably in the critically ill, especially during the perioperative period [37]. Figure 5 shows the pre-, intra-, and postoperative undergoing aortobifemoral bypass surgery. The almost parallel traces indicate that the drop in CO with induction of anesthesia does not signify a deterioration of cardiac function due to the negative inotropic effects of the anesthetics,

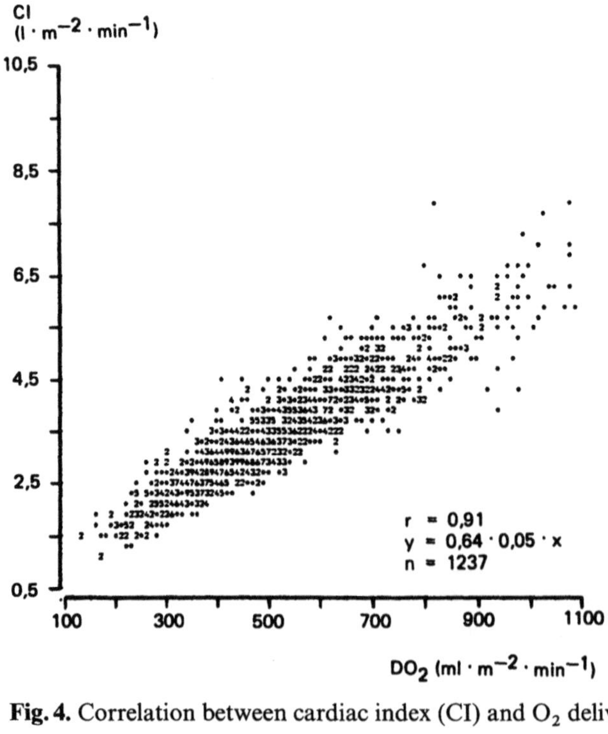

Fig. 4. Correlation between cardiac index (CI) and O_2 delivery (DO_2)

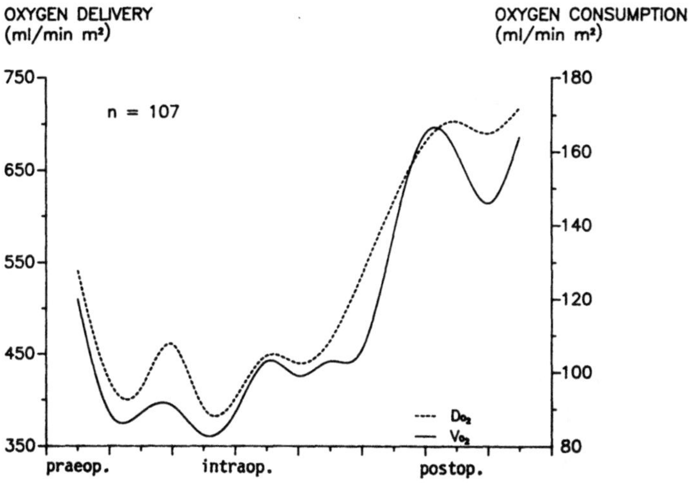

Fig. 5. Course of cardiac index (CI) and oxygen consumption (VO_2) during the perioperative period in patients with major vascular surgery

but only the physiologic adaptation of CO to the decrease in metabolic demands caused by the anesthetics and intraoperative cooling. If consideration were given only to the course of CO and not to that of the VO_2, the wrong conclusion might be drawn, namely that the cardiorespiratory status is worst intraoperatively and best postoperatively. In fact, the opposite is true: the stress is highest for the cardiorespiratory system in the immediately postoperative period, when CO is elevated. This can also be concluded from the O_2 supply/demand ratio (DO_2/VO_2), which is raised intraoperatively and drops postoperatively [37].

Oxygen Supply-to-Demand Ratio and Cardiac Output

Oxygen delivery measurements are not easily obtainable in the clinical setting, since they must be calculated from determinations of CO and arterial O_2 content. Oxygen consumption can be calculated either as the product of the CO and the arteriovenous oxygen content difference, according to the Fick principle, or noninvasively from the respiratory gases [13, 15, 35]. The latter method, however, has severe limitations when FiO_2 exceeds 0.6 [10] and is limited in its routine use owing to other methodological problems [13]. Because of these difficulties in determining VO_2 and DO_2 in the clinical setting, we examined to what extent the oxygen supply-to-demand ratio is reflected by the mixed venous O_2 saturation (SvO_2). Figure 6 shows that, over a wide range, DO_2/VO_2 is closely paralleled by SvO_2 [35]. Mixed venous O_2 saturation can now be monitored continuously via a fiberoptic device that is incorporated into conventional PA catheters [7, 33].

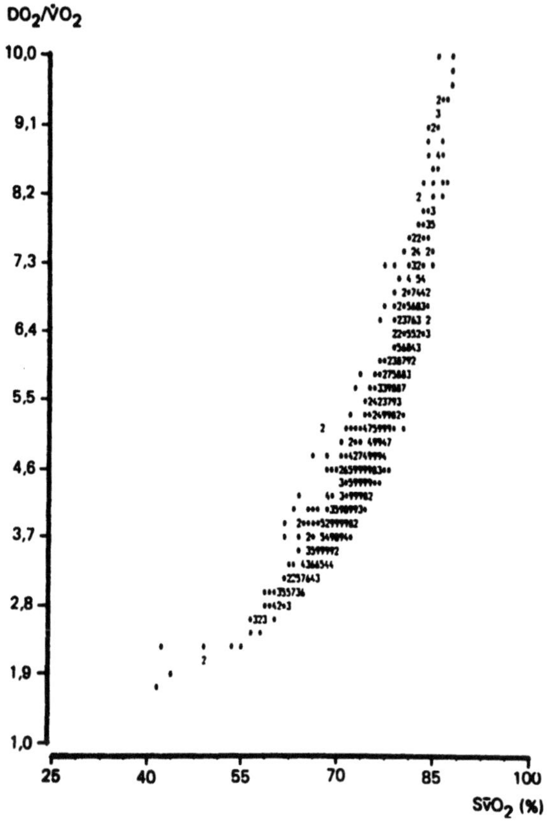

Fig. 6. Relationship between oxygen supply/demand (DO_2/VO_2) and SvO_2 during the perioperative period in patients with major vascular surgery. (From Reinhart [35])

Mixed Venous O_2 Saturation and Cardiac Output

There are numerous statements in the literature to the effect that changes of SvO_2 are good indicators of changes in CO:

> Our data suggest that there is a close relation between cardiac output and mixed venous oxygen saturations. (Muir et al. [30])

> The conclusion is therefore reached that for clinical purposes MvO_2 (SvO_2) provides a reliable first approximation of cardiac output ... (Krauss et al. [27])

> We believe that SvO_2 may predict within a matter of minutes a subsequent fall in CI to critical levels. (Rocha et al. [42])

> Our study documents a highly significant correlation between changes in SvO_2 values and changes in cardiac output ... (Waller et al. [52])

> In the absence of shivering, the in vivo oximetry capabilities (PAC-OX) offer the physician a continuous index of cardiac output ... (Sottile et al. [50])

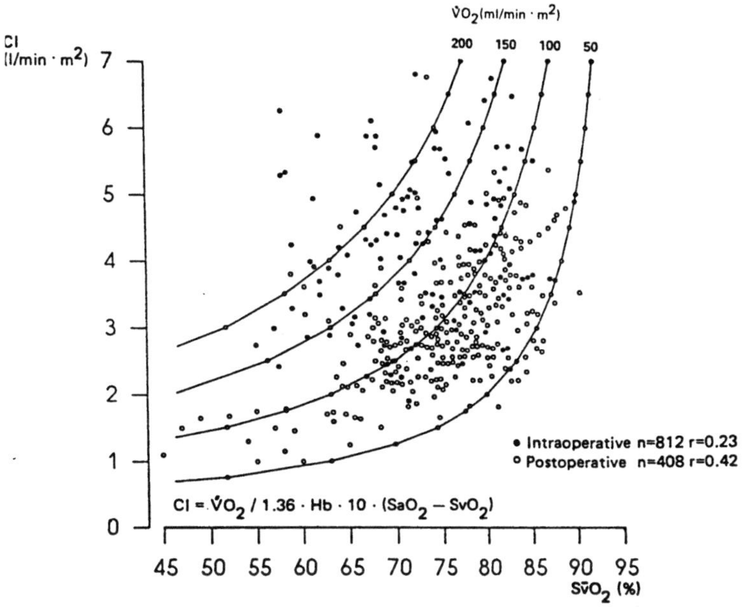

Fig. 7. Correlation between cardiac index (CI) and mixed venous O_2 saturation (SvO_2) with isolines for fixed O_2 consumptions

> Mixed venous oxygen saturation is a nonspecific indicator of the adequacy of cardiac output and tissue perfusion. (Jamieson et al. [22])

Unfortunately, this is not true. According to the Fick principle [15], the relationship between CO and SvO_2 is not linear but curvilinear; even more important is the fact that this is only true if VO_2 is unchanged. In Fig. 7 we have calculated this relationship for several values of VO_2. The tendency of VO_2 to change considerably in the perioperative period and also in intensive care patients is the reason for the frequent lack of correlation between the two variables in the clinical setting (Fig. 7). In our opinion, this does not limit the clinical usefulness of SvO_2 monitoring, since from a physiological point of view, knowledge about DO_2/VO_2 is of greater interest to the clinician than the absolute value of CO alone.

Mixed Venous O_2 Saturation and Tissue Oxygenation

Numerous statements have been made in the literature to the effect that mixed venous PO_2 or SvO_2 reflects tissue oxygenation [29]. Unfortunately, this does not hold true, for several reasons.

SvO_2 reflects only global O_2 extraction and is measured only after mixing of venous blood from all organs in the right heart [38] (Fig. 8). Therefore, normal or even higher-than-normal SvO_2 values cannot exclude tissue hypoxia in individual organs. SvO_2 is also severely limited as a mirror of tissue oxygen-

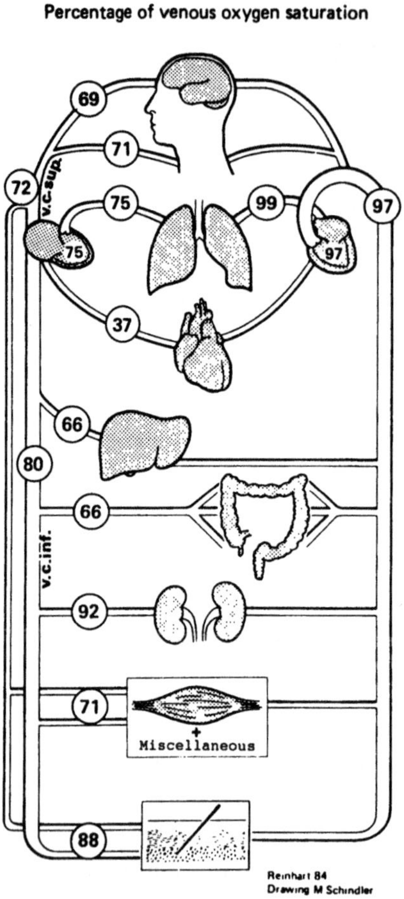

Fig. 8. Percentages of venous oxygen saturation in the various organ systems under physiological conditions. (From Reinhart [35])

ation in all diseases involving microcirculatory disturbances, like sepsis and ARDS, where maldistribution of nutritive blood flow with increased arteriovenous shunting and relative tissue hypoxia is known to occur [39, 48].

Elevated SvO_2 as a sign of decreased O_2 extraction is a common finding in hyperdynamic septic shock and can be accompanied by increased lactate levels indicating tissue hypoxia with anaerobic metabolism. These limitations do not imply that SvO_2 monitoring is useless in sepsis and ARDS; even under these circumstances, changes in SvO_2 reflect changes in the oxygen supply-to-demand ratio. Due to the pathologic O_2 supply dependency in these diseases, it is crucial to keep DO_2 optimally high [11, 39, 47]. A drop in SvO_2 in hyperdynamic septic patients indicates a fairly marked fall in DO_2 or CO, owing to the curvilinear relationship between SvO_2 and CO (Fig. 9).

The fact that SvO_2 does not necessarily reflect tissue oxygenation and that oxygen delivery to the tissues is not identical with tissue oxygenation can be concluded from our findings in two different groups of patients. Group 1 consisted of patients with hyperdynamic septic shock and group 2 of patients with

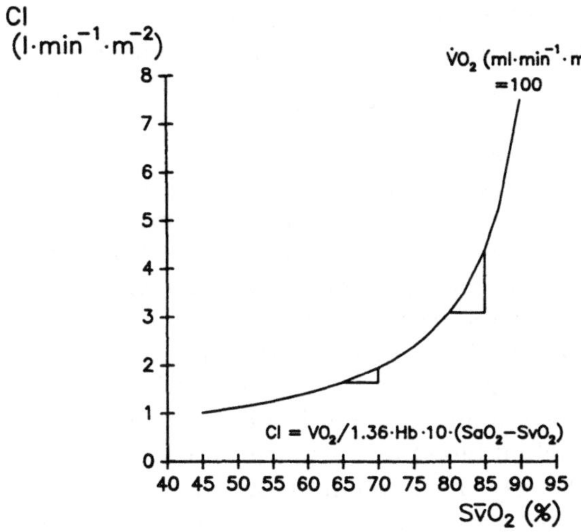

Fig. 9. Theoretical relationship between cardiac index (CI) and mixed venous O_2 saturation (SvO_2) under conditions of unchanging oxygen consumption

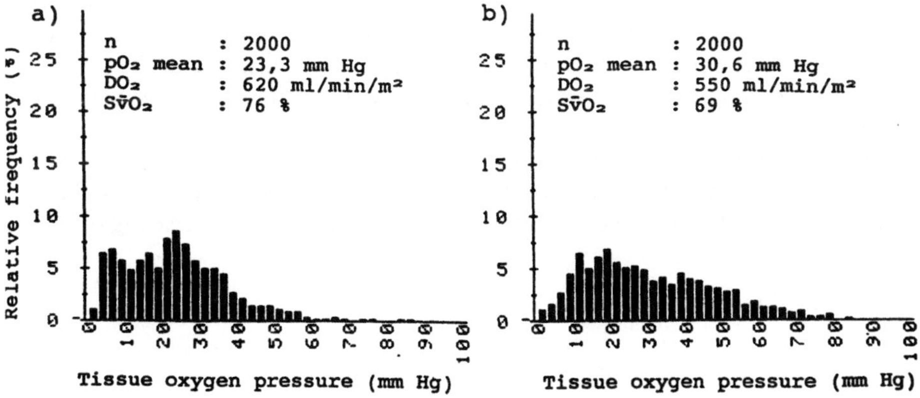

Fig. 10a, b. PO_2 histograms obtained from the musculus quadriceps femoris in patients with sepsis ($n=10$, group **a**) and patients with cardiorespiratory insufficiency without sepsis ($n=10$); *n*, number of PO_2 measurements, PO_2 mean, mean tissue PO_2; DO_2, oxygen delivery; SvO_2, mixed venous O_2 saturation

cardiorespiratory failure without shock. Group 1 patients showed a 7 mmHg lower tissue PO_2 (quadriceps femoris muscle) with a higher number of low tissue PO_2 classes in the PO_2 histograms despite a higher SvO_2 and DO_2 (Fig. 10).

Mixed Venous Versus Central Venous O_2 Saturation

Measurement of true mixed venous O_2 saturation requires pulmonary artery catheterization; its costs and risks limit it to high-risk patients [32, 41]. We were therefore interested in investigating to what extent the measurement of central venous O_2 saturation ($ScvO_2$) can replace that of mixed venous O_2 saturation. From a theoretical point of view, the difference between SvO_2 and $ScvO_2$ should increase in all situations involving changes in regional blood flow and regional oxygen consumption. This is known to occur in shock states and severe hypoxia [1], as well as under inhalation anesthetics [34].

During aortobifemoral bypass surgery, changes in the O_2 supply-to-demand ratio are paralleled by changes in central venous O_2 saturation [34]. Studies reveal that the difference between $ScvO_2$ and SvO_2 is increased by the specific influence of the anesthetics on regional blood flow and regional O_2 consumption. With halothane, the difference between these two parameters increases. $ScvO_2$ is up to 6% higher than SvO_2. Figure 11 shows the difference between the two values for three different anesthetic regimens. We found similar differences for enflurane and isoflurane (unpublished data). It is known that these anesthetics increase cerebral blood flow and decrease cerebral O_2 consumption. This results in higher O_2 saturation in the superior vena cava, where the venous blood is drained from the brain. Redistribution of blood flow is also known to occur in hemorrhagic shock, where relative blood flow to the vital organs, heart and brain, is increased at the expense of perfusion of the kidneys, gut, muscle, and skin [18]. Most of the latter organs drain into the inferior vena cava, which results in a more marked decrease of O_2 saturation in this region than in the superior vena cava. Thus, the difference between $ScvO_2$ and SvO_2 increases.

Human septic shock involves an up to 20% lower saturation in hepatic venous blood than in mixed venous blood, which was attributed to increased hepatic VO_2 [12]. This is in accordance with our findings of an increasing differ-

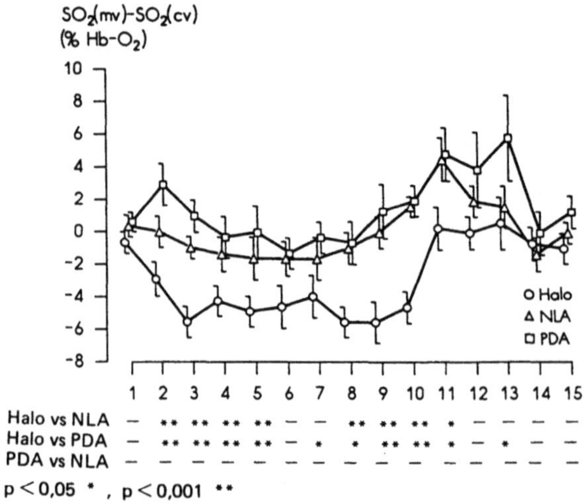

Fig. 11. Differences between mixed venous (SO_2(mv)) and central venous (SO_2(cv)) oxygen saturation in patients with major vascular surgery within the periods indicated. *1–2*, preoperative; *3–10*, intraoperative; *11–12*, postoperative. (From Reinhart et al. [34])

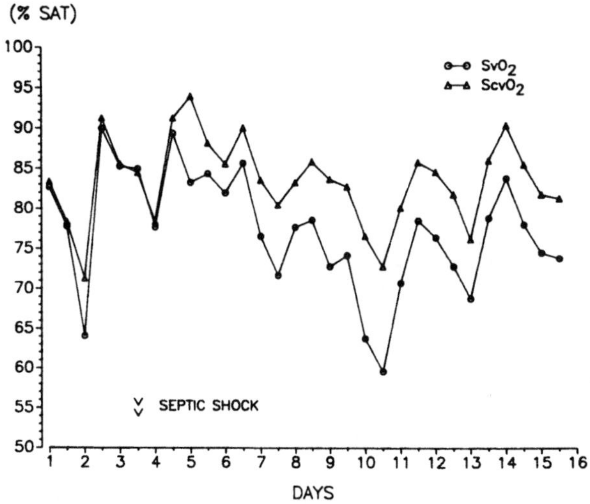

Fig. 12. Course of mixed venous (SvO_2) and central venous ($ScvO_2$) O_2 saturation over several days in septic patient who developed septic shock. (From Reinhart [35])

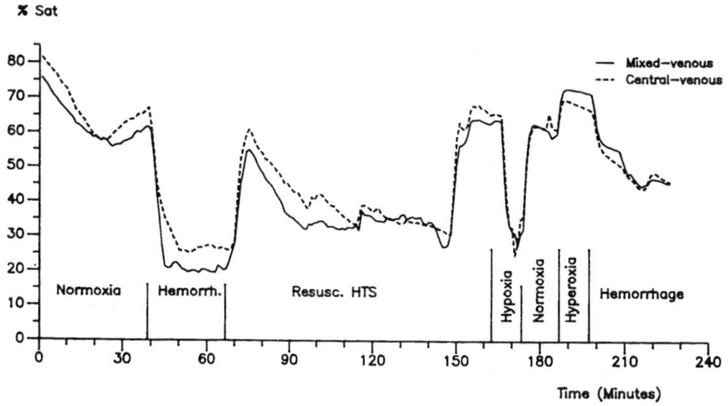

Fig. 13. Continuous in vivo monitoring of mixed venous (SvO_2) and central venous ($ScvO_2$) O_2 saturation during changes in oxygen supply/demand in dogs. Baxter Edwards Sat 1. (From Reinhart et al. [36])

ence between $ScvO_2$ and SvO_2 with the onset of septic shock [35]. The changes in $ScvO_2$, SvO_2, and hepatic venous O_2 saturation were unidirectional, however, when alterations occurred in the O_2 supply/demand ratio [12, 35] (Fig. 12).

In a study using dogs, we were able to measure $ScvO_2$ and SvO_2 continuously in vivo during marked changes in the oxygen supply/demand ratio induced by hemorrhage, hypoxia, hyperoxia, resuscitation, and catecholamines. Even in severe shock states, we found that SvO_2 was closely paralleled by $ScvO_2$ [36]. Figure 13 shows a typical original registration.

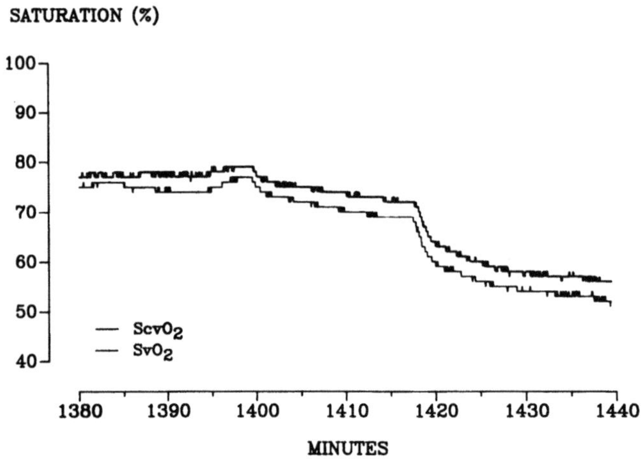

Fig. 14. Continuous in vivo monitoring of mixed venous (SvO_2) and central venous ($ScvO_2$) O_2 saturation in patients with multiple system organ failure after discontinuation of catecholamines. Baxter Edwards Sat 1

We have now developed a multilumen central venous catheter with a fiberoptic device that provides continuous in vivo monitoring of $ScvO_2$ in patients [40]. Parallel measurements of both parameters in septic shock or cardiorespiratory failure revealed that changes in SvO_2, even under these conditions, are closely reflected by similar changes in $ScvO_2$ (Fig. 14).

Central venous catheterization with multilumen central venous catheters is routinely performed in many ICU patients. Continuous control of the O_2 supply-to-demand ratio via a fiberoptic device incorporated into a central venous catheter would yield important additional information on the function of the patient's cardiorespiratory system. Although it cannot be trusted in the absolute values of $ScvO_2$, changes in the O_2 supply-to-demand ratio are similarly indicated by changes of both $ScvO_2$ and SvO_2. This method makes it possible to follow not only pathophysiological changes but also the effects of the ongoing therapy on the O_2 balance. Without any increase of invasiveness and only some limitations, the advantages of online SvO_2 monitoring can be extended to critically ill patients who do not need Swan-Ganz catheterization.

Further clinical studies with this new method are needed in order to determine the extent to which the indication for pulmonary artery catheters can be reduced by continuous $ScvO_2$ monitoring.

Arterial O_2 Saturation Via Pulse Oximetry

The major advantage of pulse oximetry is that it is noninvasive [54]. There are methodological limitations with this technique in very low saturation ranges [45, 46], in states of hypoperfusion, and with high levels of CO-Hb and Meth-Hb [3, 4]. However, new systems that promise improvement by eliminating these limitations are currently under clinical investigation.

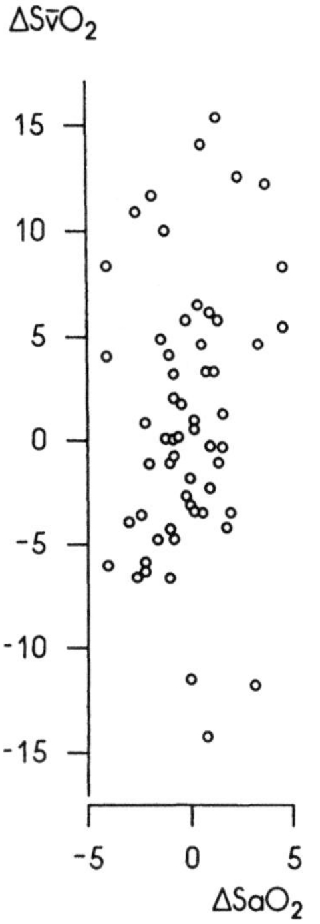

Fig. 15. Changes in arterial (SaO_2) versus changes in mixed venous (SvO_2) oxygen saturation during the postoperative period in patients with major vascular surgery

One fundamental drawback of pulse oximetry is that it only provides information on arterial O_2 saturation and this only reveals the quality of O_2 uptake by the lungs. Arterial oxygenation of the blood can be severely impaired in the critically ill or in the perioperative period; that is why this new monitoring technique has become so widely accepted in the United States and Europe. It is very helpful in the early detection of potentially life-threatening periods of hypoxia. As a rule, arterial oxygenation can be well maintained during anesthesia and intensive care [40]. The cellular O_2 supply, however, can be restricted or endangered not only by arterial hypoxia, but, even more commonly, by insufficient O_2 transport to the tissues due to a reduced O_2 transport capacity of the blood and/or an impaired cardiac output, or by maldistribution of nutritive blood flow and increased arteriovenous shunting, as in sepsis or ARDS [11, 39, 47]. Obviously, arterial O_2 saturation cannot indicate the quality of O_2 transport and tissue oxygenation or the O_2 supply-to-demand relationship.

Figure 15 shows that, in intensive care patients, changes of SvO_2 observed over several days are much greater than those of arterial O_2 saturation and reflect alterations in the whole-body O_2 balance.

Conclusions and Future Perspectives

What we have learned during the past decades is to better monitor and optimize O_2 uptake by the lung as well as O_2 transport *to* the tissues. I am convinced that this has had a great impact on patient outcome and morbidity. We are now able to perform major surgery in patients that no surgeon would have dared to operate on 30 years ago because the chance that such a patient would have survived the first 24 h after surgery then was minimal. On the other hand, we have new problems to deal with nowadays. Multiple-system organ failure (MSOF) is the main cause of death today in operative intensive care units. The incidence of this syndrome, which was first described only 20 years ago [5], is still increasing. It seems paradoxical that this may be due to better interdisciplinary treatment and especially to improved intensive care of high-risk patients. Some decades ago, however, many of these patients would not have survived the immediate postoperative period. But forms of tissue hypoxia may exist despite normal or even increased O_2 delivery, especially in sepsis and ARDS patients [8, 11, 20, 39].

Tissue hypoxia and bioenergetic cell status seem to play an important role in the pathogenesis of MSOF [47, 48]. The incidence and high mortality of MSOF can only be reduced by gaining a better understanding of how to guarantee the cellular O_2 supply in the critically ill endangered by MSOF.

Unfortunately, there is no hemodynamic or even oxygen-transport-related variable that is able to reflect directly the adequacy of tissue oxygenation and the cellular O_2 supply. What we can evaluate is the adequacy of the macrocirculation and of O_2 transport *to* the tissue, but we have to remember that the cardiorespiratory system can fulfill its physiological role only at the level of the microcirculation, which is the other major determinant of tissue oxygenation. The monitoring devices of the future should enable us to quantify the bioenergetic status of the cells; only then will we be able to judge directly whether our therapeutic interventions really improve the cellular O_2 supply or only result in useless or even harmful blood-pressure or other hemodynamic cosmetics.

Up to now, there have been only few techniques that provide indications of the cellular energy status. One of these is nuclear magnetic resonance (NMR) spectroscopy, which makes it possible to determine phosphocreatinine-to-phosphate ratios, ATP as well as ADP levels, and intracellular pH [14, 19, 49]. NMR spectroscopy, however, is limited to research and very difficult to apply in the critically ill. Near-infrared spectroscopy provides ratios not only for oxyhemoglobin and desoxyhemoglobin, but also for reduced and oxidized cytochrome aa_3 [23, 24]. Due to methodological problems, its use is mostly limited to newborns, but it may open up interesting perspectives for adults as well, especially in brain monitoring [24]. Direct tissue PO_2 measurements enable us to investigate the effects of different drugs and therapeutic interventions on tissue oxygenation [16, 26, 44], but still involve some methodological problems, e.g., tissue damage [6] and bleeding, that prevent its broad clinical use. One fundamental problem in intensive care is that we can measure tissue PO_2 only in muscles and subcutaneous tissues, and, except in wound healing [25], the role of these tissues in this setting is not yet fully understood. None of these newer techniques will become applicable in the daily bedside routine at any time in the near future.

The more we realize that the cellular O_2 supply may be insufficient despite normal O_2 transport [8, 11, 20, 39] and that the adequacy of tissue oxygenation plays an important role in determining the outcome of critically ill patients [47, 48], the greater the efforts that we must make in searching for more appropriate monitoring devices. Unfortunately, the development of techniques that provide us with better and more direct information as to what is going on at the tissue level does not keep pace with our understanding of the factors that determine tissue oxygenation.

Optimizing O_2 transport and tissue oxygenation is an important task in intensive care, but it should always be kept in mind that sepsis or multiple organ failure cannot thus be prevented as long as the causes of these syndromes are not eliminated. This kind of therapy will always remain symptomatic; it can only help to maintain the body's own defense and repair mechanisms. Nevertheless, treatment and prevention of tissue hypoxia is an ultimate goal in intensive care, since tissue hypoxia stimulates and promotes the same mediator systems as the pathogens or their byproducts [39].

References

1. Adachi H, Stauss W, Ochi H, Wagner HN (1976) The effect of hypoxia on the regional distribution of cardiac output in the dog. Circ Res 39:314
2. Afifi AA, Chang PC, Liu VY, da Luz PL, Weil MH, Shubin H (1974) Prognostic indices in acute myocardial infarction complicated by shock. Am J Cardiol 33:826
3. Barker SJ, Tremper KK (1987) The effect of carbon monoxide inhalation on pulse oximetry and transcutaneous PO_2. Anesthesiology 66:677
4. Barker SJ, Tremper KK, Hyatt J, Zaccari J (1987) Effects of methemoglobinemia on pulse oximetry and mixed venous oximetry. Anesthesiology 67:A171
5. Baue AE (1975) Multiple, progressive or sequential systems failure: a syndrome of the 1970s. Arch Surg 110:779
6. Baumgärtl H (1984) Systematische Untersuchungen der Meßeigenschaften von Nadelelektroden bei polarografischer Messung des lokalen pO_2 im Gewebe. In: Ehrly AM, Heuss J, Huch R (Hrsg) Klinische Sauerstoffdruckmessung. Münchener Wissenschaftliche Publikationen, 1985, S 15
7. Beale PL, McMichan JC, March MB, Sill JC, Southern PA (1982) Continuous monitoring of mixed venous O_2 saturation in critically ill patients. Anesth Analg 61:513
8. Bihari D, Smithies M, Gimson A, Tinker J (1987) The effects of vasodilatation with prostacyclin on oxygen delivery and uptake in critically ill patients. New Engl J Med 317:397
9. Broder G, Weil MH (1964) Excess lactate: an index of reversibility of shock in human patients. Science 143:1457
10. Browning IA, Lindberg SE, Turney SF (1982) The effect of fluctuating FiO_2 on metabolic measurements in mechanically ventilated patients. Crit Care Med 10:82
11. Cain SM (1989) Mechanisms of limited oxygen delivery in sepsis and adult respiratory distress syndrome. In: Reinhart K, Eyrich K (eds) Sepsis – an interdisciplinary challenge. Springer, Berlin Heidelberg New York, p 144
12. Dahn MS, Lange MP, Jacobs LA (1988) Central mixed and splanchnic venous oxygen saturation monitoring. Intensive Care Med 14:373
13. Damsk MC, Forse RA, Kinney JM (1983) Clinical application of gas exchange measurements. Clin Anaesth 1:599

14. Deply DT, Gordon RE, Hope PI et al. (1982) Noninvasive investigation of cerebral ischemia by phosphorus nuclear magnetic resonance. Pediatrics 70:310
15. Fick A (1870) Über die Messung des Blutquantums in den Herzventrikeln. Sitzungsber. Phys Med Ges, Würzburg. BD II:XVI
16. Fleckenstein W, Kersting Th, Schäffer A, Reinhart K, Weiss Ch (1984) Veränderungen des pO_2 im Skelettmuskel von Hunden bei Hämorrhagie und bei Infusion von kolloidosmotisch hypertoner Hydroxyäthylstärkelösung. In: Ehrly AM, Heuss J, Huch R (Hrsg) Klinische Sauerstoffdruckmessung. Münchener Wissenschaftliche Publikationen, 1985
17. Fisher DC, Sahn DI, Friedman MJ, Larson D, Valdes-Cruz LM, Horowitz S, Goldberg SJ, Allen HD (1983) The mitral valve orifice method for noninvasive two-dimensional echo determinations of cardiac output. Circulation 67:872
18. Forsyth RP, Hoffbrand BM, Melmon KL (1970) Redistribution of cardiac output during hemorrhage in the unanesthetized monkey. Circ Res 27:311
19. Gutierrez G, Pohil RJ (1987) Assessment of hypoxia by magnetic resonance spectroscopy and positron emission tomography. In: Bryan Brown CW, Ayres SM (eds) Oxygen transport and utilization. New Horizon. SCCM, Fullerton, Calif., USA
20. Haupt MT, Gilbert EM, Carlson RW (1985) Fluid loading increases oxygen consumption in septic patients with lactic acidosis. Am Rev Respir Dis 131:912
21. Huckabee WE (1961) Relationship of pyruvate and lactate during anaerobic metabolism. V. Coronary adequacy. Am J Physiol 200:1169
22. Jamieson WRE, Turnbull KW, Larrieu AJ, Dodds WA, Allison JC, Tyers GFO (1982) Continuous monitoring of mixed venous oxygen saturation in cardiac surgery. Can J Surg 25:538
23. Jöbsis FF (1977) Noninvasive infrared monitoring of cerebral and myocardial oxygen sufficiency and circulatory parameters. Science 198:1264
24. Jösbis-Vandervliet F, Fos E, Sugioka K (1987) Monitoring of cerebral oxygenation and cytochrome aa_3 redox state. Int Anesth Clinics 25:209
25. Johnsson K, Jensen JA, Goodson WH, West IM, Hunt TK (1987) Assessment of perfusion in post operative patients using tissue oxygen measurements. Br J Surg 74:263
26. Kersting Th, Reinhart K, Dennhardt R, Fleckenstein W, Eyrich K (1985) Effect of low dose dopamine on muscle pO_2 in healthy volunteers and intensive care patients. Eur J Anaesth 2:143
27. Krauss XH, Verdouw PD, Hugenholtz PG, Nauta J (1975) On-line monitoring of mixed venous oxygen saturation after cardiothoracic surgery. Thorax 30:636
28. Lang CH, Bagby GI, Ferguson JL, Spitzer II (1984) Cardiac output and redistribution of oxygen blood flow in hypermetabolic sepsis. Am J Physiol 246:R331
29. Miller MJ (1982) Tissue oxygenation in clinical medicine: a historical review. Anesth Analg 61:527
30. Muir AL, Kirby BJ, King AJ, Miller HC (1971) Mixed venous oxygen saturation in relation to cardiac output in myocardial infarction. Br Med J 4:276
31. Pflüger E (1872) Über die Diffusion des Sauerstoffs, den Ort und die Grenze der Oxydationsprozesse im thierischen Organismus. Pflügers Arch Gesamte Physiol Menschen Thiere 6:43
32. Pinilla JC, Ross DF, Martin T, Crump H (1983) Study of intravascular catheter infection and associated septicemia in critically ill patients. Crit Care Med 11:21
33. Reinhart K, Gramm HJ, Specht M, Föhring U, Mayr O, Schäfer M, Dennhardt R (1986) Physiologische Grundlagen und klinische Erfahrungen mit der kontinuierlichen In vivo-Registrierung der gemischtvenösen Sauerstoffsättigung bei Risikopatienten. Intensivmed 23:346
34. Reinhart K, Kersting K, Föhring U, Schäfer M (1986) Can central-venous replace mixed-venous oxygen saturation measurements during anesthesia? Adv Exper Med Biol 200:67
35. Reinhart K (1988) Zum Monitoring des Sauerstofftransportsystems. Anaesthesist 37:1

36. Reinhart K, Rudolph T, Bredle DL, Hannemann L, Cain SM (1989) Comparison of central venous to mixed venous oxygen saturation during changes in oxygen supply/demand. Chest 95:1216
37. Reinhart K, Föhring U, Kersting Th, Schäfer M, Bredle D, Hirner A, Eyrich K (1989) Effects of thoracic epidural anesthesia on systemic hemodynamic function and systemic oxygen supply-demand relationship. Anesth Analag (in press)
38. Reinhart K, Schäfer M, Rudolph T, Specht M (1989) Mixed venous oxygen saturation. Applied Cardiopulmonary Pathophysiology 2:315
39. Reinhart K (1989) Oxygen transport and tissue oxygenation in sepsis and septic shock. In: Reinhart K, Eyrich K (eds) Sepsis – an interdisciplinary challenge. Springer, Berlin Heidelberg New York, p 125
40. Reinhart K, Specht M, Rudolph T (1989) Aktuelle Aspekte der Oxymetrie. In: Lawin P, Peter K (Hrsg) Intensivmedizin 1989. Intensivmedizin, Notfallmedizin, Anaesthesiologie. Thieme, Stuttgart 71:81
41. Robin ED (1987) Death by pulmonary artery flow-directed catheter (editorial). Chest 92:727
42. Rocha de AG, Edmonds JF, Williams WG, Parier C, Trusler GA (1978) Importance of mixed venous oxygen saturation in the care of critically ill patients. Can J Surg 21:227
43. Rower N, Bednarz F, Kochs E, Schulte am Esch J (1988) Intraoperative Bestimmung des Herzzeitvolumens mit der transösophagealen gepulsten Doppler Echokardiographie. Anaesthesist 37:345
44. Schulte am Esch J, Kochs E, Steinberg B, Bause H (1988) Monitoring of tissue oxygen tension in the skeletal muscle of intensive care patients – effects of crystalloids and colloids. Anesthesiology 69:A292
45. Sendak MJ, Harris AP, Donham RT (1988) Accuracy of pulse oximetry during arterial oxyhemoglobin desaturation in dogs. Anesthesiology 68:111
46. Severinghaus JW, Naifeh KH (1987) Accuracy of response of six pulse oximeters to profound hypoxia. Anesthesiology 76:551
47. Sibbald WJ, Raper F, Bersten D (1989) Circulatory abnormalities in the sepsis syndrome. In: Reinhart K, Eyrich K (eds) Sepsis – an interdisciplinary challenge. Springer, Berlin Heidelberg New York, p 97
48. Sibbald WJ, Bersten A, Rutledge FS (1989) The role of tissue hypoxia in multiple organ failure. In: Reinhart K, Eyrich K (eds) Clinical aspects of oxygen transport and tissue oxygenation. Springer, Berlin Heidelberg New York
49. Smith DS, Chance B (1987) New techniques, new opportunities, old problems (editorial). Anesthesiology 67:157
50. Sottile FD, Durbin CG, Hoyt JW, Swain RF, McLachlan HD (1982) Evaluation of pulmonary artery oximetry as a predictor of cardiac output. Anesthesiology 57:A127
51. Spinale F, Reines HD, Crawford FA (1987) Electrical bioimpedance as a method for continuous noninvasive estimation of cardiac output. Crit Care Med 15:273
52. Waller JL, Kaplan JA, Baumann DI, Craver JM (1982) Clinical evaluation of a new fiberoptic catheter during surgery. Anesth Analg 61:676
53. Weil MH, Afifi AA (1970) Experimental and clinical studies on lactate and pyruvate as indicators of the severity of acute circulatory failure (shock). Circulation 41:989
54. Yelderman N, New W (1983) Evaluation of pulse oximetry. Anesthesiology 59:349

Advantages and Limitations of Pulse Oximetry

H. W. Striebel and F. J. Kretz

Acute hypoxemia is the most serious threat to human life. The pulmonary and cardiovascular system are at the center of oxygen uptake and transport. Every major disease of these organ systems may result in hypoxemia and hypoxia. Many diagnostic and therapeutic measures may also affect the continuous and adequate oxygen supply to the organs. Artificial respiration during anesthesia and in intensive care medicine represents a special danger. Monitoring of oxygenation is therefore at the center of the physician's thoughts and actions.

Physiological Remarks

Oxygen absorbed via the lungs is transported to the cells by the erythrocytes. The oxygen capacity of the arterial blood is calculated from the product of the oxygen content of the blood and the cardiac output. The oxygen content of the blood represents the sum of the oxygen chemically attached to hemoglobin and the low fraction of oxygen physically dissolved in plasma. The oxygen chemically attached to hemoglobin of arterial blood is calculated from the product of hemoglobin content (Hb), arterial oxygen saturation (SaO_2) and Hüfner's number which states that 1 g of hemoglobin fully saturated with oxygen can carry 1.34 ml of oxygen.

Oxygen attached to hemoglobin $= Hb \times SaO_2 \times 1.34$
Example: $15\ g\% \times 0.97 \times 1.34 = 19.5$ vol%

The quantity of oxygen physically dissolved in plasma can be obtained from the solubility coefficient for oxygen in plasma. For each 100 ml blood 0.003 ml oxygen can be dissolved for each mmHg of oxygen tension.

Oxygen dissolved physically in plasma $= PaO_2 \times 0.003$
Example: (at a PaO_2 of 100 mmHg) $= 0.003 \times 100 = 0.3$ vol%

The oxygen fraction chemically attached to hemoglobin is thus approximately 60 times greater than the physically dissolved fraction. The oxygen content is therefore decisively influenced by oxygen chemically attached to hemoglobin, i.e., by hemoglobin and saturation. If the Hb value remains constant, the oxygen content is largely influenced by saturation.

Monitoring of Oxygenation

Monitoring of oxygenation has so far been based on the following.

Clinical Assessment

It is widely assumed that an oxygen deficiency can always be recognized by a cyanosis. But this is not at all true. Saturation is already less than 80% when cyanosis occurs [13]. However, an 80% saturation signifies an arterial PO_2 of about 6.5 kPa. Arterial PO_2 is even lower in unfavorable cases where the oxygen binding curve has shifted to the left. A shift to the left is, for example, seen in newborn infants. Clinical assessment of oxygenation is also difficult in dark-skinned patients and with poor lighting conditions (darkened operating room). Recognition of a cyanosis is apparently not dependent on clinical experience [16].

Laboratory Findings

This may be done with the help of arterial and capillary blood gas analysis. However, it is an invasive technique and requires repeated punctures, and the information provided is intermittent and only available after a delay of at least several minutes. Capillary blood analysis, which is mainly performed in newborn infants because arterial punction is technically often difficult in these patients, also presents a number of interpretation uncertainties concerning PaO_2 [33, 35].

Continuous Transcutaneous PO_2 Measurement

This method is used to measure the PO_2 of the skin. Because of the structure of the skin, transcutaneous PO_2 correlates well with arterial PO_2 only in premature and newborn infants. However, the accuracy of the measurement is largely dependent on the blood supply to the skin. Hypothermia, hypovolemia, edemas, and decreased cardiac output greatly reduce the accuracy of this method [20, 21, 40, 73]. In addition, transcutaneous PO_2 measurement requires a large amount of time and work (calibration, change of sensor position after approximately 2 h) and may present complications (burns).

Clinical assessment, laboratory findings and transcutaneous PO_2 monitoring only permit an insufficient assessment of the patient's oxygenation.

Pulse Oximetric Monitoring

The relatively new method of pulse oximetry has experienced a kind of boom in the past few years. It allows the registration of oxygen saturation of the pulsating and thus the arterial blood. Monitoring of oxygen supply is therefore done via the oxygen saturation of arterial blood. Pulse oximeters are quite easy to handle. A sensor is attached at the finger (see Fig. 1), the ear lobe or the nose. A few seconds after it has been switched on the apparatus shows the ac-

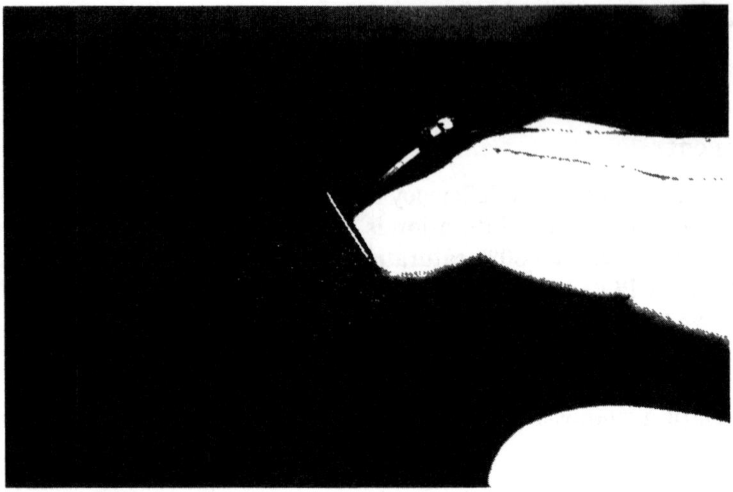

Fig. 1. Finger sensor

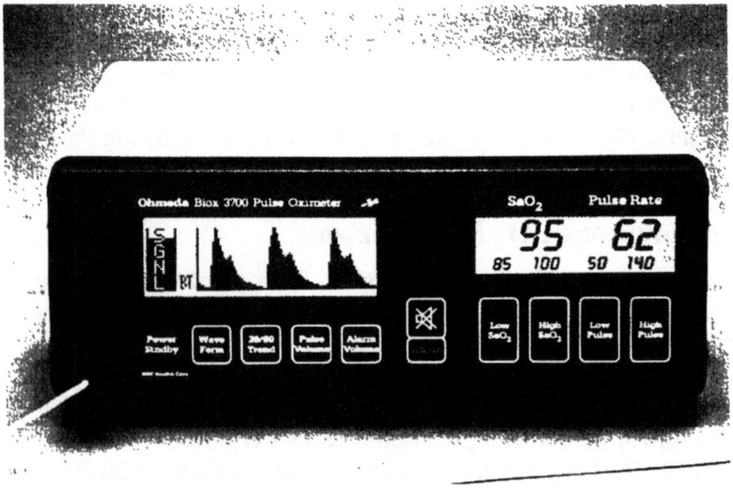

Fig. 2. Pulse oximeter. Biox 3700 (Ohmeda)

tual degree of arterial oxygen saturation as well as the peripheral pulse frequency (see Fig. 2).

The Development of Pulse Oximetry

Already in 1935, Kramer [37] and Matthes [43] published their idea to measure the oxygen saturation in flowing blood on exposed vessels and in the tissue. This idea was based on the finding that oxygenated blood is more easily penetrated by red light than is nonoxygenated blood. The research work done in this area was rapidly pushed ahead in the United States and Great Britain during World War II because of its possible military advantages.

In 1942, Millikan introduced the term "oximetry" for this type of optical method for measuring oxygen. Millikan [46] had already developed a sensor that was easy to use for measuring the saturation of arterial blood in the lobe of the ear. The venous blood was still a problem at that point. It was necessary to arterialize the venous blood by hyperemization in order to eliminate the undesired effects of the venous blood fraction. Calibration of the instruments was also a problem. In later examinations the lobe of the ear was initially compressed to squeeze out the blood to register the absorption by the skin, the pigmentation, and the tissue. This resulted in a zero value [77], which was subsequently subtracted from the measurement value of the resupplied hyperemized lobe of the ear. The light absorbed only by the arterial blood could now be calculated. The conditions for measuring the saturation of arterial blood were now established. However the available light sources and photo cells were not of a sufficiently reproducible and consistent quality.

The idea of combining oximetry and photoplethysmography to obtain pulse oximetry for the selective measurement of arterial oxygen saturation was first published in 1975 by Aoyagi [61] in Japan and by other authors and tested by Asari and Kenmotsu [2] and Yoshiya et al. [80]. Photoplethysmography allows the selective registration of pulsating blood. Since only arterial blood pulsates, but not other components like venous blood, skin, and pigments, oximetry can selectively record saturation of the pulsating, i.e., arterial, blood. Only the development of microprocessors and light-emitting diodes (LEDs) with a very consistent quality of light made it possible to develop of this non-invasive technique. Nowadays, a large number of pulse oximeters are commercially available.

For a historical review of the development of pulse oximetry, see [63].

Pulse Oximetry – How Does It Work?

The light absorbance of oxygenated hemoglobin is normally different from that of reduced hemoglobin. Pulse oximeters measure the different light absorbance of oxygenated and reduced hemoglobin at two distinct wavelengths in the visible red (660 nm) and the invisible infrared range (940 nm) and can calculate the arterial oxygen saturation of the hemoglobin from this difference in absorbance.

The absorption of oxygenated hemoglobin (HbO_2) is markedly less pronounced in the red wavelength range (660) than that of the reduced Hb (see. Fig. 3). Thus, red light penetrates oxygenated hemoglobin better than reduced hemoglobin.

At 660 nm the millimolar extinction coefficient of hemoglobin (Hb) is 0.8 and 0.08 for oxygenated hemoglobin (HbO_2). The absorption rate is reversed

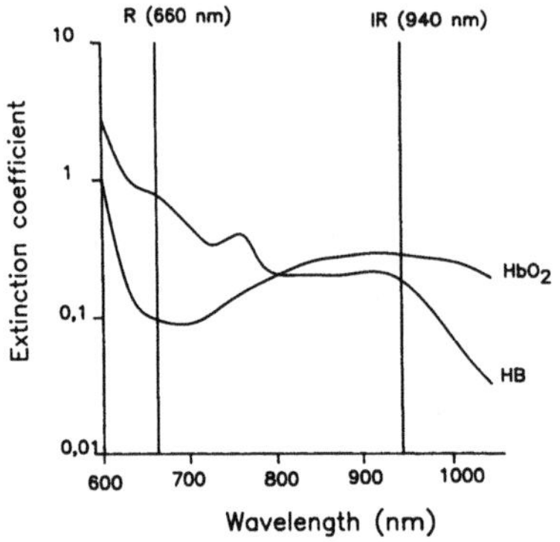

Fig. 3. Extinction curves of oxyhemoglobin (HbO_2) and reduced hemoglobin (Hb)

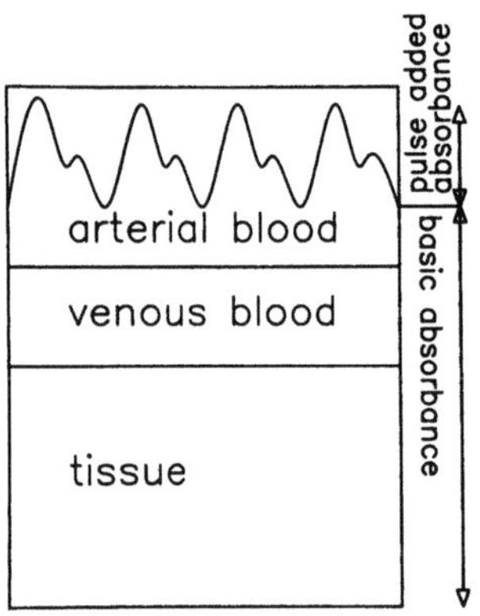

Fig. 4. Light absorption of tissue, venous blood, and arterial blood

at 940 nm. At that wavelength the extinction coefficient of reduced hemoglobin (Hb) is 0.2 and that of HbO_2 0.3 (see Fig. 3).

When tissue is penetrated by light, skin, pigmentation, tissue, bones, and venous blood absorb a constant part of that light. This is called basic absorbance (see Fig. 4). Arterial blood flow causes a pulse-dependent change in blood volume in the transilluminated tissue and thus a pulse-dependent change in the light absorbance. This so-called pulse-added absorbance represents selectively the arterial blood and amounts to a mean of about 3%, and in the most favorable cases to 10%–11% of the basic absorbance [78]. If this value is below 0.2% the Ohmeda Biox 3700 pulse oximeter shows "low quality signal" in the display.

The pulse-added absorbance represents only the arterial blood. It is affected by the intensity of the light source used, the amount of the blood volume change per pulse, and by the arterial O_2 saturation.

The amplitude of the pulse-added absorbance is affected by the intensity of the light source. In order to ensure that the amplitudes of the pulse-added absorbance at the red and infrared wavelength are independent of the light source used and may be compared with each other, the pulse-added absor-

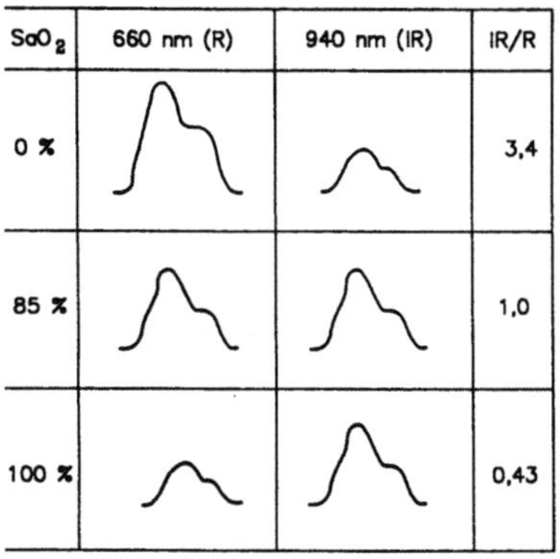

Fig. 5. The ratio between the corrected pulse-added amplitude of the red and infrared light is used to calculate the saturation

bance of each wave length is divided by the basic absorbance, i.e., the pulse-added absorbance is expressed as a fraction of the basic absorbance. Thus, this corrected pulse-added absorbance is independent of the intensity of the light source applied.

Pulse oximeters continually compare the light absorbance at 660 nm and at 940 nm, i.e., in the red (R) and infrared (IR) range. The ratio between the corrected pulse-added amplitude of the red (660 nm, R) and the infrared light (940 nm, IR) is used to calculate saturation (Fig. 5). Saturation is directly dependent on the amplitude ratio of these two corrected plethysmographic curves (R/IR). The pulse oximeter calculates saturation from the corrected amplitude ratio of the pulse-added absorbance with the help of an algorithm. A substantial component of this algorithm is the quotient of these amplitudes in the red (R) and infrared (IR) wave range. Correction factors and constants are also considered. Saturation is 0% at a quotient R/IR of 3.4, 85% at a quotient I/IR of 1.0, and 100% at a quotient of 0.43 (see Figs. 5 and 6). The saturation values associated with a specific R/IR ratio are stored in the pulse oximeter (see Fig. 6).

These are empiricial values obtained in healthy adult subjects with low levels of the dyshemoglobins methemoglobin (MetHb) and carboxyhemoglobin (HbCO; below 2%). When a pulse oximeter thus calibrated is used in a patient with a pathologically high dyshemoglobin fraction, the saturation level stored for a given R/IR value will no longer correspond to the true value. This is so because these dyshemoglobins affect the absorption behavior of red and infrared light. The pulse oximetric measurement is also affected by certain dyes.

The pulse oximetry sensor is equipped with two light-emitting diodes (LEDs). The LED operating in the infrared range is switched off while the LED operating in the red range is emitting light. The photodetector positioned on the opposite side of the tissue receives the unabsorbed residual red light. Then the red LED is switched off while the infrared LED is switched on; the photodetector receives the residual infrared light. Both LEDs are then switched off for the same period of time, during which the photodetector may

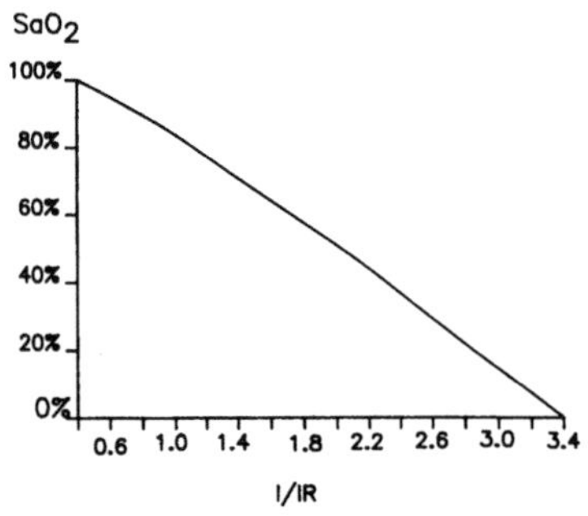

Fig. 6. The empirical relationship between R/IR and the arterial oxygen saturation

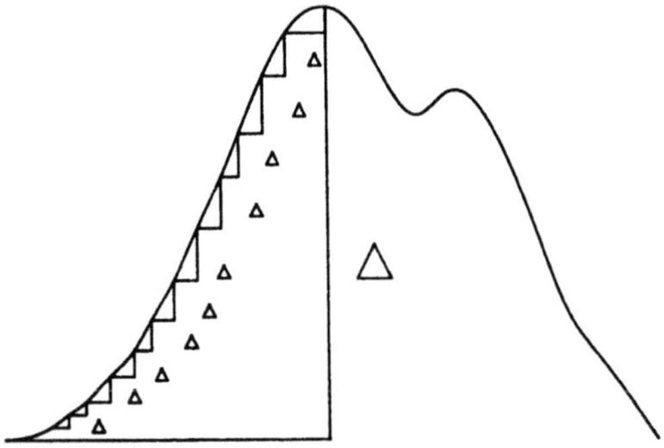

Fig. 7. For achieving an acceptable response time for changes in arterial saturation, the pulse wave changes are calculated in a stepwise procedure

receive ambient light. It is important that the device should also register this ambient light because it may change in the course of pulse oximetric monitoring. The ambient light is then subtracted during each subsequent measurement in the red and infrared range. The Biox 3700, for instance, repeats this cycle – measurement of red, infrared, and ambient light – 480 times per second. For calculation of the saturation, i.e., comparison of the amplitudes of the pulse-added absorbance in the red and infrared range, it would in principle be sufficient to determine the amplitude difference only once per pulse wave and to use this difference for the measurement of saturation. Averaging of several measurements, however, is required to minimize artifacts. If only few measurements are obtained, it is not possible to achieve an acceptable response time for changes in saturation. Pulse wave changes are therefore calculated in a stepwise procedure in order to ensure extremely short response times (see Fig. 7). The Biox 3700 pulse oximeter, for instance, calculates the saturation from this difference 30 times/s. The mean saturation value is computed either for 90 calculations/3 s or 180 calculations/6 s [78]. The newly calculated saturation values are displayed every 3.6 s in the fast response mode and every 7.2 s in the slow response mode.

Interpretation of the Plethysmographic Pulse Curve

The plethysmographic pulse curve is displayed by the Biox 3700 (Ohmeda) and the Satlite 0S-103 (Datex) pulse oximeters. Unfortunately, the signal of the Biox 3700 pulse oximeter is always raised to an optimal screen filling amplitude. Quantitative information about the arterial pulse curve can therefore hardly be obtained. Pulse oximeters like the Datex Satlite 0S-103 and the Hewlett Packard 78352A now permit suppression of this automatic amplitude gain of the plethysmographic curve. Hence it is possible to recognize perfusion reduction by the amplitude decrease of the plethysmographic pulse curve. This makes it possible to gain quantitative as well as qualitative information about the signal quality via the plethysmographic curve. Thus, in addition to cardiac frequency, arterial blood pressure, urine production, and recapillarization time, there now exists another noninvasive parameter for assessing circulatory function.

The displayed plethysmographic pulse curve yields still further information. The arterial pressure curve of hypovolemic patients on controlled ventilation shows a typical undulating course (due to the ventilation-synchronic alteration of the intrathoracic pressure and the concomitant reduction of the venous reflux) [17, 47, 52]; in a similar way, the plethysmographic curve of the pulse oximeter shows a ventilation-synchronic alteration in these patients.

Advantages and Reliability of Pulse Oximetry

The advantages of pulse oximetry are:

1. It is a noninvasive procedure.
2. Values are measured and displayed continuously.
3. No calibration is required prior to use; after switching on, the device runs through a system check and is calibrating automatically.
4. No pretreatment of the site of measurement is required.
5. The accuracy of measurement is high.
6. The per patient costs costs of monitoring are low [12, 55].
7. The number of invasive arterial blood gas analyses can be reduced [50].

The reliability of pulse oximetry in the clinically relevant ranges has been confirmed in numerous studies, both for adults and children [19, 25, 32, 44, 45]. In most studies, the correlation coefficient between the saturation determined in an arterial blood sample by a cooximeter and that obtained by pulse oximetry ranges between 0.9 and 0.98. An even better correlation exists between the heart rate measured by pulse oximetry and that determined by ECG.

The data used for the calibration of pulse oximeters were obtained in healthy subjects breathing in hypoxic air. In most cases, values down to a saturation of 70% were used, and the range below was completed by extrapolation. Errors may, however, occur in that low range, since the relation between light absorption and saturation does not follow strict mathematical laws. Because of this fact some authors question the reliability of pulse oximetry. Fanconi, for instance, concluded from his study in newborns with extremely low saturation values below 65% that pulse oximetry was unreliable [24]. This opinion was also supported by other authors [66]. Fanconi [24] and Kagle et al. [32], however, concluded from their data that this linear error may be corrected by changing the algorithm used by pulse oximeters. Sarnguist reported that the first pulse oximeter models overestimated arterial saturation in the range below 90% [58]. Since the deviation from the correct value was linear ($r=0.973$, $y=0.53x+43$), he also suggested that pulse oximeters should be reprogrammed. This suggestion was supported by Shimada et al. [64], who thought that the linear deviation of the pulse oximetry readings from true arterial saturation values was caused by light scattering occurring at the interface between blood cells and plasma. He changed the algorithm, which considerably improved the reliability of pulse oximetric readings at saturation values between 70% and 100% ($r=0.98$, $y=0.96x+3.97$). Severinghaus and Naifeh [62] investigated the saturation range between 40% and 70%. He could demonstrate a highly improved correlation for two pulse oximetry models after changing the algorithm.

Sendak et al. [60] has recently demonstrated in dogs studied under steady-state conditions that the Nellcor N-100 showed a good correlation at a saturation range between 22% and 100% ($y=0.93x+9.8$, $r^2=0.97$). Only saturation values below 22% showed no correlation. Boxer et al. [8] were also able to demonstrate an excellent correlation for the Nellcor N-100 at values between 35% and 95% in children with cyanotic congenital heart disease ($r=0.95$, $y=1.01x+0.15$). Similar results were reported by Lazzell and Jopling [39] for children with congenital heart disease at a saturation range of 30% to 85%.

Nearly all investigations suggest that pulse oximetry yields accurate readings for the clinically important saturation range of 80% to 100%. Concerning values below that range, the clinician is often interested in the trend only rather than the absolute value. Nevertheless, some of the newer devices with improved calibration and algorithm also give reliable readings at the lower range. But this holds true only if no pathologically high concentrations of dyshemoglobins or dyes are present in the blood (see below).

Factors Influencing the Accuracy of Pulse Oximetry

Point of Measurement

Severinghaus found that ear sensors yield more accurate readings in most cases than finger sensors. This finding was confirmed by Kagle [6, 31, 32], though he mentioned that calibration may likewise solve this problem. Ear sensors furthermore detect changes in arterial saturation slightly earlier [32, 70].

Peripheral Tissue Perfusion

Pulse oximetry can register arterial saturation only in the presence of a sufficiently strong pulsatile signal. Yelderman and New [79] and Mihm and Halperin [45] cautioned that reduced arterial pulsation may affect the accuracy of pulse oximetry readings. Reduced arterial pulsation may be caused by hypothermia, high peripheral resistance (sympatheticotonia, catecholamines), or reduced cardiac output. Lawson and coworkers [38], however, demonstrated that pulse oximeters detect a signal even if the blood flow is reduced to between 4% and 8.6% of the normal. But differences may result from the kind of device used. Vasoconstriction in the presence of moderate hypothermia with a core temperature of 32.3° to 35 °C (mean, 34.2 °C) and a digital skin temperature of 24.4° to 30.6 °C (mean, 26.6 °C) does not impair the accuracy of pulse oximetry [27].

Pulsations in the Venous System

Strong coughing, for example, may lead to extreme volume fluctuations in the venous vascular bed, which may be several orders of magnitude stronger than those in the arterial bed. Such venous pulse waves are registered by the pulse oximeter and measured as arterial pulsations, which may result in a falsely low saturation value.

Movements of the Patient

Movements produce artifacts because of sensor displacement relative to the site of measurement. Motion artifacts are usually more pronounced at a finger sensor than at an ear sensor. Heavy sensors are extremely unfavorable; adhesive sensors are preferable because of their low inert mass and good fixability.

ECG synchronization presents an advance in pulse oximetry (realized, for instance, in the Nellcor N-200). Pulse oximetry readings are obtained only at certain time intervals in relation to the ECG-determined R-peak. This ECG synchronization leads to a considerable reduction of motion artifacts. This method presents an advantage in pediatric anesthesia/intensive care, where motion artifacts are a serious problem. In the presence of prolonged motion artifacts (e.g., when the patient is shivering in the postoperative period), pulse oximeters frequently yield saturation values of approximately 85%. Since motion artifacts produce very strong signals with nearly identical amplitudes in the red and infrared range, the quotient R/IR calculated by the pulse oximeter approximates 1, which corresponds to a saturation value of 85%, as can be seen in Fig. 5 [53].

Dyshemoglobins and Dyes

Any substance in the blood which absorbs light of the wave lengths 660 or 940 nm, at which the pulse oximeter operates, may impair pulse oximetry readings. Of clinical importance are interferences from carboxyhemoglobin

(HbCO) and methemoglobin (MetHb). Problems may also arise from the administration of dyes, such as methylene blue.

HbCO

The carboxyhemoglobin level of the blood is normally below 2% in nonsmokers. In heavy smokers, there may be a concentration of 5% to 10% at the beginning of a day or even 10% to 20% at the end of a day of heavy smoking [81]. The extinction coefficient of HbCO at 660 nm is similar to that of HbO_2. At 940 nm, HbCO does not absorb light and thus does not impair measurement at this wave range. High HbCO concentration therefore leads to falsely high pulse oximetry readings of arterial saturation [3, 4] (see Fig. 8).

MetHb

The fraction of MetHb is normally below 1% but may increase after the administration of certain drugs (e.g., Prilocain for regional anesthesia [36, 74]. MetHb affects absorption at 660 and 940 nm. The pulse oximetry readings exceed the true arterial saturation [4].

HbF

Fetal hemoglobin does not influence the accuracy of pulse oximetry [19].

Skin Color

Skin pigmentation does not influence the accuracy of pulse oximetry [27]. Pulse oximetry can therefore also be used in dark-skinned patients, in whom the clinical monitoring of oxygenation has always been extremely difficult.

Methylene Blue

This substance, which is excreted via the kidneys, is rarely applied intravenously. It is used for the detection of leaks in the urinary tract. The absorption behavior of methylene blue at 660 nm leads to falsely low saturation readings [28, 34, 59, 65, 67].

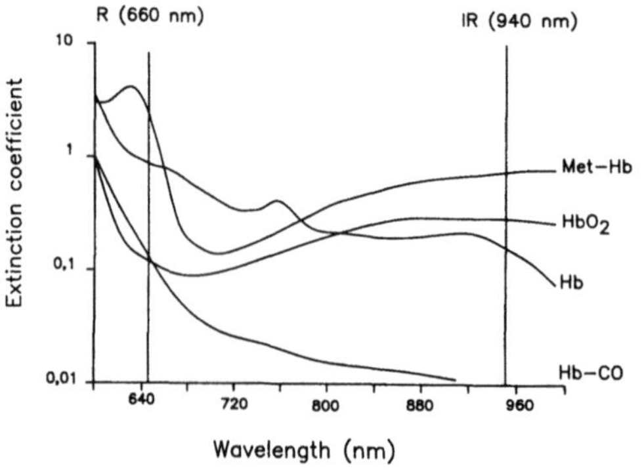

Fig. 8. Absorption spectra of methemoglobin (MetHb), oxyhemoglobin (HbO_2), reduced hemoglobin (Hb), and carboxyhemoglobin (COHb)

Nail Polish

Rubin [57] investigated 31 nail polish colors and found that only a blue nail polish (with a light absorption maximum of 688 nm) affected the pulse oximetry readings (falsely low value).

Intensive Ambient Light

Intensive ambient light, from phototherapy lamps or infrared heat lamps, for instance, can impair pulse oximetry readings [7, 10, 30] and requires shielding of the sensor.

The fact that dyshemoglobins and dyes affect the accuracy is a disadvantage of pulse oximetry. But the latter is nevertheless useful under such conditions, since the anesthesiologist, intensive care and emergency physician are more interested in the trend than in the exact saturation value. And changes in the trend are correctly registered by the pulse oximeter even in these situations.

Indications for Pulse Oximetry

Anesthesiology

The risk of hypoxia is rather high during the perioperative phase. Hypoxemia is by far the most frequent cause of fatal anesthetic mishaps [14, 15, 69]. It therefore seems justified to advocate pulse oximetry as a standard monitoring procedure for all anesthetized patients.

Another argument in favor of pulse oximetric monitoring during anesthesia is the fact that clinical assessment of oxygenation is insufficient, as it was already demonstrated by Comroe and Botelho in a much-quoted paper published in 1947 [13]. It therefore appears to be risky to rely on clinical monitoring alone [29]. Cyanosis is not recognized by the anesthesiologist until saturation falls below 80%, which corresponds to a PO_2 of less than 50 mmHg [13]. The latter has recently been confirmed by Cote et al. [16]. In nine of 24 cases, the anesthesiologist did not recognise a cyanosis even when saturation fell below 72% (P_aO_2 of approximately 40 mmHg). Even in pediatric anesthesia, heart rate changes have to be regarded as late signs of hypoxemia. In Coté's study, bradycardia was observed in only two of 35 patients in whom saturation fell below 85%. Changes in pulse oximetric saturation always occur before clinically apparent changes are noticed. Coté was also able to demonstrate that patients monitored by pulse oximetry had significantly fewer (14%) hypoxemias (saturation below 85%) than those without pulse oximetry monitoring (32%) [16].

The goal should be to use pulse oximetry for continuous monitoring of all patients at risk for hypoxemia. Unfortunately, there are economic limits to this. We do, however, recommend pulse oximetric monitoring to the anesthetist in the following cases:

1. Anesthesia in children. Newborns and infants are predisposed to hypoxemia for the following reasons: (a) The oxygen consumption in babies for

example is about twice as high as in adults. (b) The relation of alveolar ventilation and functional residual capacity (FRC) is about 1.5 : 1 in adults and about 5 : 1 in newborn babies. The buffer function of the FRC therefore is considerably reduced in relation to the alveolar ventilation, and the amount of oxygen stored is therefore much lower than in adults. (c) In addition, responses to anesthesiological and surgical stimuli in infants are more pronounced than in adults, which leads to a higher incidence of laryngo- and bronchospasms. All these factors can lead to fulminant hypoxemias, the dramatic course of which is known to and feared by all anesthetists. Casuistic examples of patients monitored by pulse oximetry are given in Fig. 9.

2. Anesthesia in hip replacement with bone cement. The cardiopulmonary complications associated with cemented hip replacement are well known [1, 54, 56]. Pulse oximetry helps to recognize the often dramatic decrease in saturation and to immediately initiate countermeasures [11] (see Fig. 10).
3. Anesthesia in thoracic surgery [9, 71, 76].

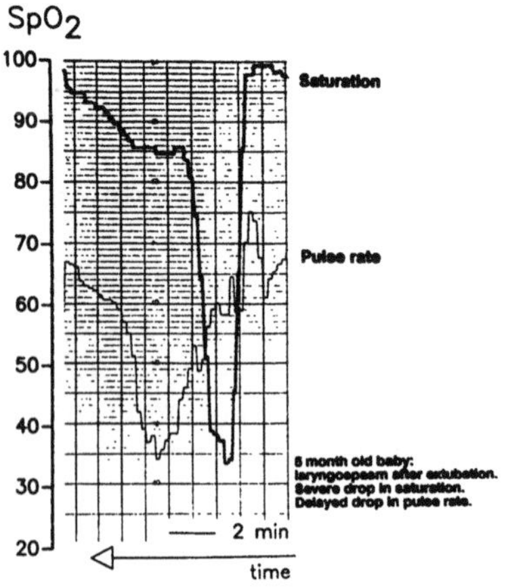

Fig. 9. Case report

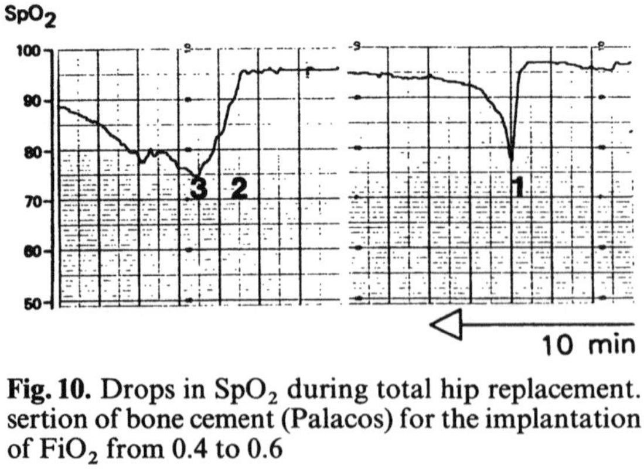

Fig. 10. Drops in SpO_2 during total hip replacement. *1*, endotracheal suctioning; *2*, insertion of bone cement (Palacos) for the implantation of the prosthetic shaft; *3*, increase of FiO_2 from 0.4 to 0.6

4. Monitoring of patients during fiberoptic intubation [41].
5. Anesthesia in darkened rooms and in procedures which require protection of the doctor's eyes by colored classes (e.g.; laser surgery).
6. It would be desirable to use pulse oximetry monitoring in all patients during the immediate postoperative phase [18, 23, 26, 42, 48, 49, 51, 72, 75].

Intensive Care Medicine and Emergency Medicine

Pulse oximetry has been successfully used in these areas. Important indications are:

1. Monitoring of spontaneously breathing patients with borderline respiratory function
2. Monitoring of patients with progressive ARDS
3. Monitoring of patients during weaning following long-term artificial ventilation [45, 50]
4. Transportation of critically ill patients for diagnostic measures [23] (most pulse oximetry devices are also battery-equipped)

Limitations of Pulse Oximetry

Because of the "S"-shaped oxygen dissociation curve, pulse oximeters cannot detect hyperoxemia. It is not possible to distinguish whether, in the presence of a 98%–100% saturation, PaO_2 is 100 or 500 mmHg. The risk of retrolental fibroplasia in premature or newborn babies can be eliminated to a certain extent, if saturation is maintained at 90%–95%.

Complications associated with pulse oximetry are rare. Pressure necroses have been reported to occur after leaving the sensor at the finger for a very long time [5]. One case of burning has been reported in association with a defective finger sensor [68].

Possible Improvements

The reliability and interpretation of pulse oximetric readings may be improved by the following factors:

1. The introduction of new measurement sites (e.g., forehead, tongue) might make it possible to use pulse oximetry in strongly centralized patients.
2. The simultaneous registration of histological parameters at the site of measurement and their inclusion in the calculation of saturation values may improve the accuracy of pulse oximetry.
3. Calibration at extremely low saturation levels may improve the accuracy at these levels.
4. Pulse oximeters measuring with the aid of more than two wave lengths, which are now in the process of being developed, might eliminate false measurements caused by high dyshemoglobin concentrations (especially HbCO).

Summary

Pulse oximetry is an easy-to-handle method for the continuous and reliable monitoring of arterial oxygen saturation at the clinically relevant saturation range. The immediate recognition of hypoxemias makes it possible to initiate therapeutic measures without delay.

References

1. Alexander JP, Barron DW (1979) Biochemical disturbances associated with total hip replacement. J Bone Joint Surg [Br] 61:101–106
2. Asari M, Kenmotsu O (1977) Application of a pulse-type earpiece oximeter in the field of anesthesiology. Jpn J Anesthesiol 26:205–207
3. Barker SJ, Tremper KK (1987) The effect of carbon monoxide inhalation on pulse oximetry and transcutaneous PO_2. Anesthesiology 66:677–679
4. Barker SJ, Tremper KK, Hyatt J, Zaccari J (1987) Effects of methemoglobinemia on pulse oximetry and mixed venous oximetry. Anesthesiology 67:A171
5. Berge KH, Lanier WL, Scanlon PD (1988) Ischemic digital skin necrosis: a complication of the reusable Nelcor pulse oximeter probe (letter). Anesth Analg 67:712–713
6. Berko RS, Kagle DM, Alexander CM, Giuffre M, Gross JB (1988) Evaluation of the Ohmeda 3700 pulse oximeter during rapid changes in arterial oxygen saturation. Anesthesiology 65:A130
7. Block FE (1987) Interference in a pulse oximeter from a fiberoptic light source. J Clin Monit 3:210–211
8. Boxer RA, Gottesfeld I, Sigh S, LaCorte MA, Parnell VA, Walker P (1987) Noninvasive pulse oximetry in children with cyanotic congenital heart disease. Crit Care Med 15:1062–1064
9. Brodsky JB, Shulman MS, Swan M, Mark JBD (1985) Pulse oximetry during one-lung ventilation. Anesthesiology 63:212–214
10. Brooks TD, Paulus DA, Winkle WE (1984) Infrared heat lamps interfere with pulse oximeters. Anesthesiology 61:630
11. Byrick RJ, Forbes D, Waddell JP (1986) A monitored cardiovascular collapse during cemented total knee replacement. Anesthesiology 65:213–216
12. Calaminus JM (1988) Pulsoximetrie. In: Boenick U, Schaldach M (ed) Biomedical Engeneering. Tutorial Polsoximetrie. Schiele and Schön, Berlin, pp 32–33 (Biomedizinische Technik, vol 33, suppl 3)
13. Comroe JH, Botelho S (1947) The unreliability of cyanosis in the recognition of arterial anoxemia. Am J Med Sci 214:1–6
14. Cooper JB, Newbower RS, Long CD, McPeek B (1978) Preventable anesthesia mishaps: a study of human factors. Anesthesiology 49:399–406
15. Cooper JB, Newbower RS, Kitz RJ (1984) An analysis of major errors and equipment failures in anesthesia management: considerations for prevention and detection. Anesthesiology 60:34–42
16. Coté CJ, Goldstein EA, Coté MA, Hoaglin DC, Ryan JF (1988) A single-blind study of pulse oximetry in children. Anesthesiology 68:184–188
17. Coyle JP, Teplick RS, Long MC, Davison JK (1983) Respiratory variations in systemic arterial pressure as an indicator of volume status. Anesthesiology 59:A53
18. Craig DB (1981) Postoperative recovery of pulmonary function. Anesth Analg 60:46–52
19. Durand M, Ramanathan R (1986) Pulse oximetry for continuous oxygen monitoring in sick newborn infants. J Pediatr 109:1052–1056
20. Eberhard P, Mindt W (1977) Skin sensors for continuous oxygen monitoring of newborns. Biotelemetry 4:48–76

21. Eberhard P, Mindt W, Schäfer R (1981) Cutaneous blood gas monitoring in the adult. Crit Care Med 9:702–705
22. Eisenkraft JB (1988) Pulse oximeter desaturation due to methemoglobinemia. Anesthesiology 68:279–282
23. Elling A, Hanning CD (1986) Oxygenation during postoperative transportation. In: Payne JP, Severinghaus JW (eds) Pulse oximetry. Springer, Heidelberg New York, pp 161–164
24. Fanconi S (1988) Reliability of pulse oximetry in hypoxic infants. J Pediatr 3:424–427
25. Fanconi S, Doherty P, Edmonds JF, Barker GA, Bohn DJ (1985) Pulse oximetry in pediatric intensive care: comparison with measured saturations and transcutaneous oxygen tension. J Pediatr 107:362–366
26. Fibuch EE, Rehder K, Sessler AD (1975) Preoperative CC/FRC ratio and postoperative hypoxemia. Anesthesiology 45:481–485
27. Gabrielczyk MR, Buist RJ (1988) Pulse oximetry and postoperative hypothermia. Anesthesia 43:402–404
28. Gormann ES, Shnider MR (1988) Effect of methylene blue on the absorbance of solutions of haemoglobin. Br J Anaesth 60:439–444
29. Hanning CD (1985) "He looks a little blue down this end." Monitoring oxygenation during anaesthesia. Br J Anaesth 57:359–360
30. Hanowell L, Eisele JH, Downs D (1987) Ambient light affects pulse oximeters (correspondence). Anesthesiology 67:864–865
31. Kagle DM, Berko RS, Alexander CM, Giuffre M, Gross JB (1986) Ohmeda biox 3700 pulse oximeters may give falsely low readings when used with finger probes. Anesthesiology 65:A129
32. Kagle DM, Alexander CM, Berko RS, Giuffre M, Gross JB (1987) Evaluation of the Ohmeda 3700 pulse oximeter: steady-state and transient response characteristics. Anesthesiology 66:376–380
33. Karna P, Poland RL (1978) Monitoring critically ill newborn infants with digital capillary blood samples: an alternative. J Pediatr 92:270–273
34. Kessler MR, Eide T, Humayun B, Poppers PJ (1986) Spurious pulse oximeter desaturation with methylene blue pulse injection. Anesthesiology 65:435–436
35. Koch G, Wendel H (1967) Comparison of ph, carbon dioxide tension, standard bicarbonate and oxygen tension in capillary blood and in arterial blood during the neonatal period. Acta Paediatr Scand 56:10–16
36. Konietzke D, Leyser K-H, Lanz E (1985) Vergleichende Untersuchung mit Prilocain 2% bzw. Lidocain 2% jeweils mit Adrenalin zur Periduralanaesthesie. Regional-Anästhesie 8:67–72
37. Kramer K (1935) Ein Verfahren zur fortlaufenden Messung des Sauerstoffgehaltes im strömenden Blute an uneröffneten Gefäßen. Z Biol (Munich) 96:61–75
38. Lawson D, Norley I, Korbon G, Loeb R, Ellis J (1987) Bloodflow limits and pulse oximeter signal detection. Anesthesiology 67:599–603
39. Lazell VA, Jopling MW (1987) Accuracy of pulse oximetry in cyanotic congenital heart disease. Anesthesiology 67:A169
40. Lemke R, Klaus D (1986) Die Bedeutung der nicht-invasiven kontinuierlichen T_cPO_2- und T_cPCO_2-Messung bei kreislaufstabilen Patienten und bei Patienten im Schock. Intensivmed 23:22–26
41. Marian F, Spiss CK, Hiesmayr M, Draxler V (1985) Überwachung der fiberoptischen Intubation mittels nicht invasiver Pulsoximetrie. Anaesthesist 34:630–635
42. Marshall BE, Wyche MQ (1972) Hypoxemia during and after anesthesia. Anesthesiology 37:178–209
43. Matthes K (1935) Untersuchungen über die Sauerstoffsättigung des menschlichen Arterienblutes. Arch Exp Pathol Pharmakol 179:698–711
44. Mendelson Y, Kent JC, Shahnarian A, Welch GW, Giasi RM (1988) Evaluation of datascope accusate pulse oximeter in healthy adults. J Clin Monit 4:59–63

45. Mihm FG, Halperin BD (1985) Noninvasive detection of profound arterial desaturations using a pulse oximetry device. Anesthesiology 62:85–87
46. Millikan GA (1942) The oximeter: an instrument for measuring continuously oxygen saturation of arterial blood in man. Rev Sci Instrum 13:434–444
47. Morgan BC, Crawford EW, Guntheroth WG (1969) The hemodynamic effects of changes in blood volume during intermittent positive-pressure ventilation. Anesthesiology 30:297–305
48. Morris RW, Buschman A, Warren DL, Philip JH, Raemer DB (1988) The prevalence of hypoxemia detected by pulse oximetry during recovery from anesthesia. J Clin Monit 4:16–20
49. Motoyama EK, Glazener CH (1986) Hypoxemia after general anesthesia in children. Anesth Analg 65:267–272
50. Niehoff J, DelGuercio C, LaMorte W, Hughes-Grasberger SL, Heard S, Dennis R, Yeston N (1988) Efficacy of pulse oximetry and capnometry in postoperative ventilatory weaning. Crit Care Med 16:701–705
51. Nunn JF, Payne JP (1962) Hypoxaemia after general anaesthesia. Lancet II:631–632
52. Perel A, Pizov R, Gross D, Cotev S (1986) The systemic blood pressure variation is a sensitive indicator of hypovolemia in ventilated dogs subjected to graded hemorrage. Crit Care Med 14:382
53. Pologe JA (1987) Pulse oximetry: technical aspects of machine design. Int Anesthesiol Clin 25(3):137–153
54. Powell JN, McGrath PJ, Lahiri SK, Hill P (1970) Cardiac arrest associated with bone cement. Br Med J 3:326
55. Raemer DB, Warren DL, Morris R, Philip BK, Philip JH (1987) Hypoxemia during ambulatory gynecologic surgery as evaluated by the pulse oximeter. J Clin Monit 3:244–248
56. Rinecker H (1980) New clinico-pathophysiological studies on the bone cement implantation syndrome. Arch Orthop Trauma Surg 97:263–274
57. Rubin AS (1988) Nail polish color can affect pulse oximeter saturation. Anesthesiology 68:825
58. Sarnquist FH, Todd C, Whitcher C (1980) Accuracy of a new noninvasive oxygen saturation monitor. Anesthesiology 33:S163
59. Scheller MS, Unger RJ, Kelner MJ (1986) Effects of intravenously administered dyes on pulse oximetry readings. Anesthesiology 65:550–552
60. Sendak MJ, Harris AP, Donham RT (1988) Accuracy of pulse oximetry during arterial oxyhemoglobin desaturation in dogs. Anesthesiology 68:111–114
61. Severinghaus JW, Honda Y (1987) History of blood gas analysis. VII. Pulse oximetry. J Clin Monit 3:135–138
62. Severinghaus JW, Naifeh KH (1987) Accuracy of response of six pulse oximeters to profound hypoxia. Anesthesiology 67:551–558
63. Severinghaus JW, Astrup PB (1986) History of blood gas analysis. VI. Oximetry J Clin Monit 2:270–288
64. Shimada Y, Yoshiya I, Oka N, Hamaguri K (1984) Effects of multiple scattering and peripheral circulation on arterial oxygen saturation measured with a pulse-type oximeter. Med Biol Eng Comput 22:475–478
65. Sidi A, Paulus DA, Rush W, Gravenstein N, Davis RF (1987) Methylene blue and indocyanine green artifactually lower pulse oximetry readings of oxygen saturation. Studies in dogs. J Clin Monit 3:249–256
66. Sidi A, Rush W, Gravenstein N, Ruiz B, Paulus DA, Davis RF (1987) Pulse oximetry fails to accurately detect low levels of arterial hemoglobin oxygen saturation in dogs. J Clin Monit 3:257–262
67. Sidi A, Rush WR, Paulus DA, Gravenstein N, Davis RF (1986) Effect of fluorescein, indocyanine green, and methylene blue on the measurement of oxygen saturation by pulse oximetry. Anesthesiology 65:A132

68. Sloan TB (1988) Finger injury by an oxygen saturation monitor probe. Anesthesiology 68:936–938
69. Taylor G, Larson CP, Prestwich R (1976) Unexpected cardiac arrest during anesthesia and surgery. JAMA 236:2758–2760
70. Taylor MB, Whitwam JG (1988) The accuracy of pulse oximeters. Anaesthesia 43:229–232
71. Thys DM, Cohen E, Girard D, Kirschner PA, Kaplan JA (1986) The pulse oximeter: a non-invasive monitor of oxygenation during thoracic surgery. Thorac Cardiovasc Surg 34:380–383
72. Tomkins DP, Gaukroger PB, Bentley MW (1988) Hypoxia in children following general anaesthesia. Anaesth Intensive Care 16:177–181
73. Tremper KK, Shoemaker WC, Shippy CR, Nolan LS (1981) Transcutaneous PCO_2 monitoring on adult patients in the ICU and the operation room. Crit Care Med 9:752–755
74. Tryba M, Kurth H, Lenz M (1987) Klinische und toxikologische Untersuchungen zur axillären Plexusblockade mit Prilocain oder Mepivacain. Regional-Anästhesie 10:31–36
75. Tyler IL, Tantisira B, Winter PM, Motoyama EK (1985) Continuous monitoring of arterial oxygen saturation with pulse oximetry during transfer to the recovery room. Anesth Analg 64:1108–1112
76. Viitanen A, Salmenperä M, Heinonen J (1987) Noninvasive monitoring of oxygenation during one-lung ventilation: a comparison of transcutaneous oxygen tension measurement and pulse oximetry. J Clin Monit 3:90–95
77. Wood E, Geraci JE (1949) Photoelectric determination of arterial oxygen saturation in man. J Lab Clin Med 34:387–401
78. Wukitsch MW, Petterson MT, Tobler DR, Pologe JA (1988) Pulse oximetry: analysis of theory, technology, and practice. J CLin Monit 4:290–301
79. Yelderman M, New W (1983) Evaluation of pulse oximetry. Anesthesiology 59:349–352
80. Yoshiya I, Shimada Y, Tanaka K (1980) Spectrophotometric monitoring of arterial oxygen saturation in the fingertip. Med Biol Eng Comput 18:27–32
81. Zander R, Mertzlufft F (1986) The oxygen status in arterial human blood: terminology, diagnosis and determination of parameters. In: Payne JP, Severinghaus JW (eds) Pulse oximetry. Springer, Berlin Heidelberg New York, pp 31–36

Role of Dual Oximetry in the Assessment of Pulmonary Function

J. Räsänen

Introduction

With the development of critical care medicine, requirements and techniques of patient monitoring have become increasingly complex. Repeated assessment and rapid adjustment of ongoing therapy requires that variables relevant to the patient's disease process be monitored continuously in an on-line fashion. Until recently, monitoring of pulmonary function in critically ill patients has depended upon intermittent sampling of arterial and mixed venous blood, with laborious and time-consuming calculation of derived variables. When monitoring involves significant commitments of time, labor, and cost, its use is likely to be restricted to the most difficult patients and the most critical periods of the patient's disease process. It is possible, then, that some patients at some times would receive suboptimal therapy because of inefficient monitoring. A recently published study assessed the accuracy of such intermittent monitoring with regard to the proper administration of continuous positive airway pressure therapy in a surgical intensive care unit [9]. The results revealed that 8 of 11 patients were receiving unnecessarily high levels of airway pressure, likely because sporadic monitoring did not allow sufficiently rapid detection of the recovery of the patient's pulmonary function. The authors concluded that the ability to continuously monitor pulmonary function would probably result in a significant improvement in the quality of respiratory care.

In an adult intensive care unit, adequacy of alveolar ventilation is a much less often encountered diagnostic and therapeutic problem than is inadequacy of oxygenation. With the exception of sudden airway obstruction, changes in ventilatory status usually occur far more slowly than alterations in arterial blood oxyhemoglobin saturation. Excretion of carbon dioxide also is less readily affected by acute parenchymal lung disease than oxygenation. Therefore, the most crucial event in pulmonary gas exchange to be monitored is oxygen transfer from alveolar air into pulmonary capillary blood. The efficiency of oxygenation in the lungs is commonly assessed by calculating the venous admixture.

Venous Admixture

The calculation of venous admixture or physiologic intrapulmonary shunting of blood (Q_{sp}/Q_t) has been the gold standard for assessment of pulmonary gas exchange for a long time. The determination of venous admixture requires sampling of arterial and mixed venous blood, and measurement of blood oxygen tensions and oxyhemoglobin saturations from these samples. The amount of venous admixture proportional to total blood flow is derived from pulmonary end-capillary ($Cc'O_2$), systemic arterial (CaO_2), and mixed venous ($C\bar{v}O_2$) oxygen contents using the following formula:

$$Q_{sp}/Q_t = (Cc'O_2\text{-}CaO_2)/(Cc'O_2\text{-}C\bar{v}O_2)$$

Pulmonary end-capillary oxygen content is calculated from alveolar oxygen tension by assuming complete equilibration of oxygen tensions between alveolar air and capillary blood. If the calculated venous admixture is to reflect intrapulmonary physiologic shunting, it must be assumed that no extrapulmonary shunts are present.

Although venous admixture is widely used, it is not an unfailing indicator of alterations in pulmonary function. The calculation of venous admixture is based on a two-compartment model of the lung. The calculated "shunt" value represents the amount of right-to-left shunting of blood that would be present if the lung only consisted of two kinds of alveolar units: those that are ventilated ideally and those that are not ventilated at all. The model does not differentiate between the hypoxemia-producing effect of true venoarterial shunting of blood and that of ventilation-perfusion mismatching. This makes the calculated venous admixture sensitive to alterations in the oxygen concentration of the inspired gas (FiO_2). The effect of an alveolar unit with low ventilation-to-perfusion ratio on arterial blood oxygen tension varies with the alveolar oxygen tension and, consequently, with the FiO_2. Alteration of FiO_2 will change the calculated venous admixture even when the gas exchange properties of the lung parenchyma remain stable. Thus, calculated venous admixture often decreases when low to moderate concentrations of oxygen are added to inspired air [5]. Since hypoxemia caused by true left-to-right shunting of blood does not depend on FiO_2, the effect of FiO_2 on venous admixture depends on the relative amount of ventilation-perfusion mismatching. A high level of oxygen supplementation may effect an increase in venous admixture because of absorption atelectasis and release of hypoxic vasoconstriction.

Changes in systemic blood flow are another source of confusion in the interpretation of calculated values of venous admixture. An elevation in cardiac output and pulmonary blood flow may cause a relative improvement in the perfusion of poorly ventilated lung units compared with those with a normal ventilation-perfusion ratio [4]. Such alteration in the distribution of pulmonary blood flow results in an increase in calculated venous admixture. Conversely, diminution of systemic and pulmonary blood flow may decrease venous admixture by allowing disproportionate improvement in the perfusion of well-ventilated areas of the lung. Changes in venous admixture secondary to alterations in systemic blood flow may not bring about fluctuations in arterial blood oxygenation, because of concurrent alterations in mixed venous blood oxygen saturation. As cardiac output and systemic oxygen delivery improve, mixed venous oxygen saturation increases if oxygen consumption remains unchanged. Even though a relatively greater amount of blood flows through areas with a low ventilation-perfusion ratio, the oxygen saturation of the shunting blood is higher and the net effect of venous admixture on arterial blood oxygenation may change little if at all.

Despite its shortcomings, venous admixture still is the most accurate method of evaluating pulmonary gas exchange available for routine clinical use. The tedious calculation and the necessity to draw and analyze both arterial and mixed venous blood samples make it necessary to maintain the search for variables that would accurately reflect venous admixture and be easily and rapidly available at the bedside.

Oxygen Tension-Based Gas Exchange Indices

The simplest of the estimates of venous admixture are based on the measurement of arterial blood oxygen tension (PaO_2). To reduce variability produced by different levels of oxygen therapy, provision usually is made for alterations in FiO_2 or alveolar oxygen tension (PAO_2). Three most commonly used oxygen tension-based gas exchange indices are the alveolar-arterial oxygen tension gradient (PAO_2-PaO_2), the arterial-to-alveolar oxygen tension ratio (PaO_2/PAO_2), and the arterial oxygen tension inspired oxygen concentration ratio (PaO_2/FiO_2) [3]. The most accurate of these, and the easiest to calculate, is the PaO_2/FiO_2. The correlation between venous admixture and the common oxygen tension-based gas exchange indexes are shown in Table 1 [3, 7, 11, 13].

The clinical use of oxygen tension-based gas exchange indexes as estimates of venous admixture is severely limited by several factors. The calculation of venous admixture is based on blood oxygen content which is primarily dependent on oxyhemoglobin saturation. Blood oxygen content is linearly related to oxyhemoglobin saturation, but it has an alinear relationship with oxygen tension. Therefore, the relationship between venous admixture and any oxygen tension-based index will be curvilinear (Fig. 1) [3, 11]. The curvilinearity largely results from the shape of the oxyhemoglobin dissociation curve. Figure 1 shows that as venous admixture increases, the curve relating venous admixture and PaO_2/FiO_2 begins to bend upward at a point that corresponds to a PaO_2 of approximately 115 mmHg. Since the value of PaO_2/FiO_2 at this point decreases when FiO_2 is elevated, the position of the curve becomes a

Table 1. Absolute values of correlation coefficients (*r*) between venous admixture and oxygen tension-based gas exchange indexes in four separate studies

PaO_2/FiO_2	PaO_2/PAO_2	PAO_2–PaO_2	Author
0.69	–	–	Martyn et al. (1979) [7]
0.90	0.88	0.68	Covelli et al. (1983) [3]
0.68	0.67	0.46	Räsänen et al. (1987) [11]
0.51	0.47	0.23	Räsänen et al. (1988) [13]

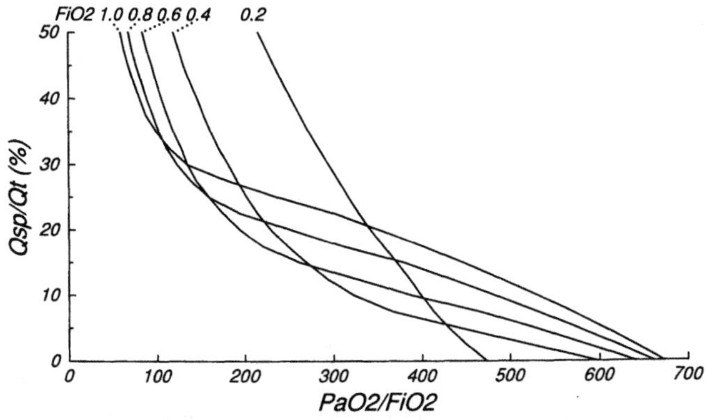

Fig. 1. Mathematical relationships between venous admixture (Q_{sp}/Q_t) and PaO_2/FiO_2 plotted with FiO_2 levels ranging from 0.20 to 1.0. Average normal values were set for Hgb (15.0 g/l), $PaCO_2$ (40 mmHg), and RQ (0.8). The arteriovenous oxygen content difference was assumed to be 4.0 ml/dl

function of the FiO_2. This results in considerable inaccuracy in estimating venous admixture from PaO_2/FiO_2, particularly when accuracy is clinically most needed, i.e., when PaO_2 is low and venous admixture is high [7, 11]. The same phenomenon occurs with the PAO_2-PaO_2 and the PaO_2/PAO_2. The accuracy of the oxygen tension-based gas exchange indices also is affected by factors that alter the position of the oxyhemoglobin dissociation curve.

Further inaccuracy of the oxygen tension-based indexes results from the fact that they include no representation of changes in mixed venous blood oxygenation and therefore are subject to variability induced by variations in systemic blood flow. Alterations in peripheral blood flow bring about changes in mixed venous blood oxygen saturation. Changes in the oxygenation of blood entering the lung and flowing through any existing right-to-left shunts, may effect wide variation in PaO_2 even though the level of venous admixture remains unchanged. Assessment based on arterial and alveolar oxygen tensions does not allow differentiation of such circulatory effects from changes in pulmonary function. This could lead to inappropriate, even harmful therapeutic decisions. Finally, although the oxygen tension-based gas exchange indices are easy to calculate, they still depend on sampling of arterial blood and do not permit continuous monitoring of pulmonary function.

Pulse Oximetry

The introduction of pulse oximetry has improved monitoring of critically ill anesthetized patients considerably by allowing continuous measurement of arterial blood oxyhemoglobin saturation (SaO_2) [16]. By using SaO_2 in place of the oxygen tension-based indices to estimate venous admixture, a nearly linear relationship between the two variables is achieved (Fig. 2). The noninvasive

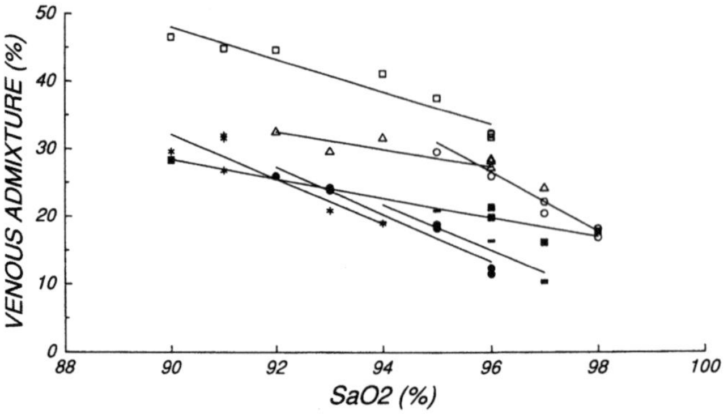

Fig. 2. Response of arterial blood oxyhemoglobin saturation (SaO_2) to alterations in venous admixture induced by changes in continuous positive airway pressure in seven patients with acute respiratory failure. Linear regression lines are drawn for each patient

continuous real-time nature of pulse oximetry constitutes a significant advantage in routine clinical use. When tissue oxygen supply-demand balance is stable, changes in arterial blood oxygenation are effected for the most part by alterations in the FiO_2 and by the efficiency of pulmonary gas exchange. In a large number of patients with mild to moderate acute lung injury, cardiovascular function can be assumed to vary within relatively narrow limits despite the pulmonary disease process and its treatment. During periods of unchanged FiO_2 in such patients, pulse oximetry alone provides a practical guide to the adjustment of respiratory therapy, without invasive monitoring.

Frequently, however, circulatory function and peripheral tissue oxygenation cannot be assumed to remain unchanged in a critically ill patient [6, 8]. The primary disease and therapeutic interventions may bring about rapid and unexpected changes in both pulmonary and cardiovascular functions. In these patients, pulse oximetry alone does not provide an accurate general estimate of venous admixture, because the relationship between venous admixture and SaO_2 is heavily influenced by the FiO_2 and by events that alter the oxygenation of mixed venous blood. Furthermore, currently available pulse oximeter technology allows SaO_2 to be measured to the full percent only, which makes small trends difficult to detect.

Appropriate management of patients with cardiovascular and pulmonary instability requires pulmonary artery catheterization to allow specific separate assessments of circulatory and respiratory functions. The use of continuous mixed venous oximetry provides a means by which venous oxyhemoglobin saturation ($S\bar{v}O_2$) can relatively accurately be estimated continuously in patients who have a pulmonary artery catheter in place. Simultaneous integrated monitoring of both arterial and mixed venous blood oxyhemoglobin saturations, dual oximetry, opens new possibilities for continuous on-line assessment of changes in venous admixture without blood sampling.

Shunt Index

The first report describing use of dual oximetry to estimate venous admixture was published by Carroll in 1987 [2]. This paper introduced a "shunt index" which was calculated from a simplified intrapulmonary shunt equation:

$$\text{Shunt Index} = (1\text{-}SaO_2)/(1\text{-}S\bar{v}O_2)$$

Use of this equation involves the assumption that the amount of oxygen dissolved in pulmonary end-capillary, arterial, and mixed venous blood is negligible and, therefore, can be discounted. Pulmonary end-capillary blood is further assumed to be fully saturated with oxygen.

Computer analysis of the relationship between the shunt index and venous admixture reveals a linear relationship between the two variables (Fig. 3). Since $S\bar{v}O_2$ is included in the formula, alterations in peripheral tissue blood flow and arteriovenous oxygen content differences have little effect on the accuracy with which venous admixture is reflected by the shunt index [11]. The shunt index can be used only when SaO_2 has a value lower than 100%. In the event that arterial blood is fully saturated with oxygen, the shunt index will no longer accurately reflect venous admixture. This limitation has little clinical significance, however, because in clinical practice, an SaO_2 of 100% would call for reduction of oxygen supplementation. The accuracy of the index would be restored as soon as SaO_2 is lowered below 100%. A more serious limitation of the shunt index is its dependence on FiO_2. At high levels of oxygen supplementation, dissolved oxygen contributes significantly to the oxygen content in pulmonary end-capillary blood. Therefore, its omission results in an underestimation of venous admixture by the shunt index when FiO_2 is high. If FiO_2 is changed during monitoring of the shunt index, a new baseline must be established for correct detection of trends. When FiO_2 is kept unchanged at any particular level, linearity of the relationship is maintained and changes in the shunt index should predictably reflect those of venous admixture.

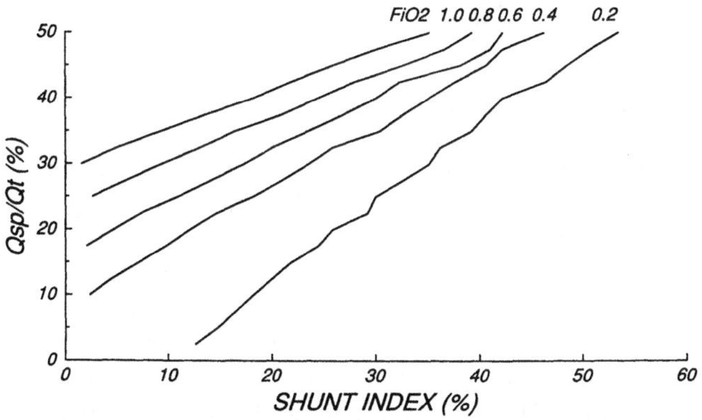

Fig. 3. Mathematical relationships between venous admixture (Q_{sp}/Q_t) and the shunt index plotted with FiO_2 levels ranging from 0.20 to 1.0. Average normal values were set for Hgb (15.0 g/l), $PaCO_2$ (40 mmHg), and RQ (0.8). The arteriovenous oxygen content difference was assumed to be 4.0 ml/dl

The original report that introduced the shunt index described one patient in whom several values of shunt index and venous admixture were plotted over a period of recovery from adult respiratory distress syndrome [2]. A close correlation between the two variables was apparent, with the absolute shunt index values consistently 10% lower than corresponding venous admixture while the patient received 60% oxygen. In a subsequent study, the shunt index was shown to be superior to the oxygen tension-based gas exchange indices in the estimation of venous admixture during heart failure [11]. A later prospective report showed that the shunt index used concomitantly with a saturation-based estimate of oxygen utilization coefficient provided sufficient information for accurate titration of continuous positive airway pressure therapy in 14 of 17 patients with respiratory failure, without blood sampling and analysis [10]. The published reports used shunt index values calculated off-line from data collected from digital readouts of the pulse oximeter and the pulmonary artery oximeter. However, the two monitors can easily be interfaced to perform the calculation automatically, in an on-line fashion.

Manual calculation of the shunt index is a very practical way of determining the approximate level of venous admixture at the bedside in patients with stable oxygen therapy. However, the dependence of the shunt index on FiO_2 makes it cumbersome in long-term clinical usage. To overcome the problem of variable FiO_2, more complex forms of continuous oximetric estimation of venous admixture have been developed recently.

Ventilation-Perfusion Index

When dual oximetry data is collected and displayed using a computer-based automatic interface between the pulse oximeter and the pulmonary artery oximeter, more accurate estimates of venous admixture can be calculated. The ventilation-perfusion index (VQI) also is based on a modified intrapulmonary shunt equation. It resembles the shunt index equation, but includes an estimate of oxygen dissolved in pulmonary end-capillary blood:

$$VQI = \frac{1.32 \cdot Hgb \cdot (1 - SaO_2) + 0.0031 \cdot PAO_2}{1.32 \cdot Hgb \cdot (1 - S\bar{v}O_2) + 0.0031 \cdot PAO_2},$$

where Hgb = blood hemoglobin concentration and PAO_2 = alveolar oxygen tension. Like the shunt index, this calculation discounts the amount of oxygen dissolved in arterial and mixed venous blood and assumes that pulmonary end-capillary blood is fully saturated with oxygen. The VQI formula is applicable whenever SaO_2 is less than 100%. In calculating alveolar oxygen tension, alveolar carbon dioxide tension and the respiratory exchange ratio are assumed to be normal and unchanged. Compared with the shunt index, the calculation of VQI requires two additional variables, hemoglobin concentration and FiO_2, which must be manually entered into the interface device. Since oxygen dissolved in pulmonary end-capillary blood is accounted for, the VQI remains an accurate linear estimate of venous admixture, even with variable

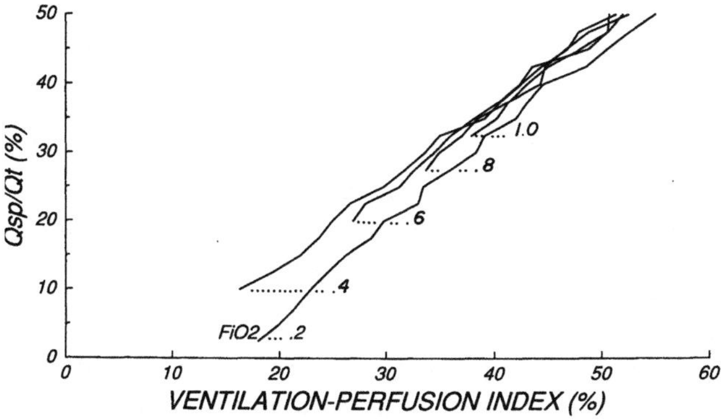

Fig. 4. Mathematical relationships between venous admixture (Q_{sp}/Q_t) and the ventilation-perfusion index plotted with FiO_2 levels ranging from 0.20 to 1.0. Average normal values were set for Hgb (15.0 g/l), $PaCO_2$ (40 mmHg), and RQ (0.8). The arteriovenous oxygen content difference was assumed to be 4.0 ml/dl

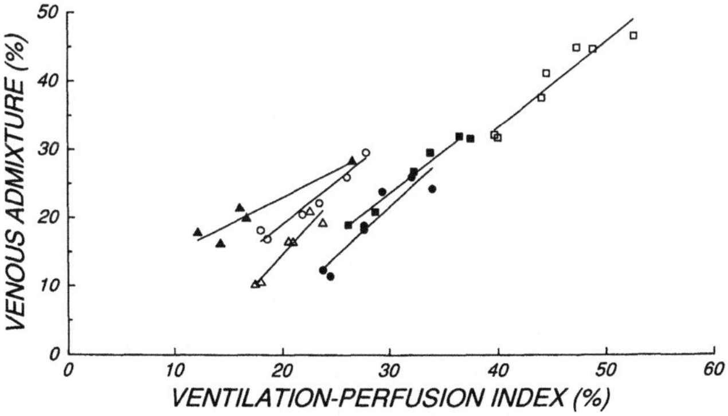

Fig. 5. Response of the ventilation-perfusion index to alterations in venous admixture induced by changes in continuous positive airway pressure in six patients with acute respiratory failure. Linear regression lines are drawn for each patient

FiO_2, and it is little affected by changes in tissue oxygen supply-demand balance (Fig. 4).

The accuracy of the VQI as an estimate of venous admixture has been evaluated in two prospective clinical investigations [13, 14]. In general surgical intensive care unit patients, a correlation coefficient of 0.78 has been calculated for venous admixture and VQI between individual patients. Within patients, change in venous admixture, induced by alteration in continuous positive airway pressure, was reflected by VQI with an average correlation coefficient of 0.94 ± 0.05 (Fig. 5) [13], an accuracy certainly sufficient for clinical use. Maintenance of accuracy during longer periods of monitoring by dual oximetry depends primarily on the drift of the mixed venous oxygen saturation monitor, because the pulse oximeter cannot be calibrated. An absolute drift of $1\% \pm 3\%$ in VQI during 6 h of continuous monitoring has been reported [14].

Technical differences between the pulse oximeter and the pulmonary artery oximeter may effect inaccuracy of continuous estimation of venous admixture by dual oximetry. The pulse oximeter reads dysfunctional hemoglobins, such as carboxy- and methemoglobin, mainly as oxyhemoglobin, while the mixed venous oxygen saturation monitor primarily reads them as deoxyhemoglobin. Since the assumption of 100% oxyhemoglobin saturation of pulmonary end-capillary blood ignores dyshemoglobins, the numerator of the VQI equation remains accurate even in the presence of dysfunctional hemoglobins. The error in the denominator results in slight, systematic underestimation of the absolute level of venous admixture. Since the magnitude of this error is small and remains unchanged in most critically ill patients, it has little clinical significance. In special situations, such as in a patient who is being treated for carboxy- or methemoglobinemia, changing levels of these dysfunctional hemoglobins will impair the accuracy of dual oximetry.

When pulse and pulmonary oximetry are used to calculate the VQI, factors such as the rounding errors of the monitors and spontaneous fluctuations of arterial and mixed venous oxyhemoglobin saturations cause random variability in the measured variables. This random variability must be differentiated from clinically significant trends. It has been estimated that 95% of this random variability of VQI falls within an absolute range of ±5% [14]. This range also is suggested as a guideline for clinical interpretation of changes in VQI.

The feasibility of the combined use of pulse and pulmonary artery oximetry in a surgical intensive care unit has been assessed in a prospective study [14]. The monitoring system remained functional approximately 85% of the time, when no undue attention was focused on the equipment or on the training of the staff. One-half of the 15% failure time (8%) was due to 100% saturation of arterial blood oxyhemoglobin, which renders the VQI formula inaccurate. Other types of equipment failure included malfunctioning of the pulmonary artery catheter (5%), malpositioning of the pulse oximeter probe (3%), and inadvertent disconnect (2%). Most causes of interruption of monitoring would be correctable immediately. Therefore, with proper attention directed to the equipment, training, and appropriate oxygen supplementation, the equipment failure time likely can be reduced to less than 5%.

Absolute values of VQI generally are slightly lower than corresponding values of venous admixture. This is a result of discounting dissolved oxygen in arterial and mixed venous blood. It is suggested that VQI not be taken as an accurate substitute for venous admixture but rather as a separate variable that closely reflects alterations in physiological intrapulmonary shunting of blood.

Real-Time Venous Admixture

To obtain a true real-time equivalent of venous admixture, Scuderi et al. have calculated arterial and mixed venous oxygen tensions from oxyhemoglobin saturations obtained by dual oximetry and included them in their calculated estimate of venous admixture [15]. Off-line values of arterial blood carbon dioxide tension and percentage of dysfunctional hemoglobins were entered into the calculation. Pulmonary end-capillary oxyhemoglobin saturation was calculated. These modifications allowed the authors to continuously record oximeter-based venous admixture values nearly identical to those calculated from blood samples. In a data base consisting of 130 measurements from ten patients, the correlation coefficient was 0.95, the slope of the linear fit was 1.22, and the intercept 0.0. Inclusion of calculated oxygen tensions does not add any independently measured variables into the continuous estimation of venous admixture. Therefore, correlation between the shunt and the estimate would not be expected to improve from that between venous admixture and VQI measured under similar conditions. Whether it is safe under all circumstances to assume an identity between venous admixture and any of its estimates, is not known.

Clinical Considerations

Granted that venous admixture is the gold standard for estimating pulmonary gas exchange, it is evident that pulmonary artery catheterization is necessary if accurate information concerning efficiency of gas exchange is required. Future research may validate the use of central venous blood oximetry as a substitute for pulmonary artery catheterization. The theoretical, experimental, and clinical data available indicate that continuous estimation of venous admixture using dual oximetry is clinically feasible. Oximetric estimation of venous admixture has been shown to permit rapid accurate and effective titration of continuous positive airway pressure therapy in patients with acute lung injury. A significant added advantage of dual oximetry is the simultaneous estimation of the peripheral tissue oxygen utilization coefficient by calculating the oxygen extraction index ($O_2EI = [SaO_2\text{-}S\bar{v}O_2]/SaO_2$) [1, 10]. VQI and O_2EI together allow simultaneous assessment of both circulatory and respiratory functions with no further intervention continuously in an on-line fashion [13, 14]. The obvious advantage of continuous estimation of venous admixture and oxygen utilization is the nearly instantaneous feedback which allows optimization of circulatory and respiratory therapy, without the time lag associated with conventional assessment of patient response.

Monitoring with pulse and pulmonary artery oximetry does not involve an added risk to patients who require a pulmonary artery catheter for routine monitoring. Blood loss for calibration of the equipment is minimal, and repeated patient assessments within one calibration period do not increase blood loss, cost, or risk of bacterial infection. The parent variables estimated by VQI and O_2EI have well-defined physiological significance and are therefore interpreted easily and rapidly. Thus, the information can be applied immediately in therapeutic decision-making without further processing by the observer. It is possible that such continuous cardiopulmonary monitoring makes cardiopulmonary interventions more timely, more clearly focused, and more effective. It is the clinicians responsible for the administration of critical care, however, who ultimately will determine whether the potential advantages of this type of monitoring justify the necessary investment in equipment and training.

References

1. Beach T, Millen E, Grenvik A (1973) Hemodynamic response to discontinuance of mechanical ventilation. Crit Care Med 1:85–90
2. Carroll GC (1987) A continuous monitoring technique for management of acute pulmonary failure. Chest 92:467–469
3. Covelli HD, Nessan VJ, Tuttle WK (1983) Oxygen derived variables in acute respiratory failure. Crit Care Med 11:646–649
4. Dantzker DR, Brook CJ, Dehart P, Lynch JP, Weg JG (1979) Ventilation-perfusion distributions in the adult respiratory distress syndrome. Am Rev Respir Dis 120:1039–1052
5. Douglas ME, Downs JB, Dannemiller FJ, Hodges MR, Munson ES (1976) Change in pulmonary venous admixture with varying inspired oxygen. Anesth Analg 55:688–695
6. Giovannini I, Boldrini G, Sganga G, Castiglioni G, Castagneto M (1983) Quantification of the determinants of arterial hypoxemia in critically ill patients. Crit Care Med 11:644–645
7. Martyn JAJ, Aikawa N, Wilson RS, Szyfelbein SK, Burke JF (1979) Extrapulmonary factors influencing the ratio of arterial oxygen tension to inspired oxygen concentration in burn patients. Crit Care Med 7:492–496
8. Mitchell LA, Downs JB, Dannemiller FJ (1975) Extrapulmonary influences on A-$aDO_2^{1.0}$ following cardiopulmonary bypass. Anesthesiology 43:583–586
9. Räsänen J, Downs JB (1988) Optimum versus clinically established continuous positive airway pressure in respiratory therapy. J Clin Monit 4:235–239
10. Räsänen J, Downs JB, Malec DJ, Seidman P (1987) Estimation of oxygen utilization by dual oximetry. Ann Surg 207:621–623
11. Räsänen J, Downs JB, Malec DJ, Oates K (1987) Oxygen tension and oxyhemoglobin saturation in the assessment of pulmonary gas exchange. Crit Care Med 15:1058–1061
12. Räsänen J, Downs JB, DeHaven B (1987) Titration of continuous positive airway pressure therapy by real-time dual oximetry. Chest 92:853–856
13. Räsänen J, Downs JB, Malec DJ, DeHaven B, Garner W (1988) Real-time continuous estimation of gas exchange by dual oximetry. Int Care Med 14:118–122
14. Räsänen J, Downs JB, Hodges MR (1988) Continuous monitoring of gas exchange and oxygen use with dual oximetry. J Clin Anesth 1:3–8
15. Scuderi PE, Speight KL, Prough DS (1988) Real-time pulmonary shunt fraction in humans. In: Hogt SW (ed) American society of critical care anesthesiologists. San Francisco, CA, USA, p 7
16. Yelderman M, New W (1983) Evaluation of pulse oximetry. Anesthesiology 39: 349–352

Therapy

Nonventilatory Management of ARDS

P. M. Suter, J. Pugin, J.-A. Romand, M. C. Laverriére

The adult respiratory distress syndrome (ARDS) is characterized by a rapid clinical onset of dyspnea, cyanosis, restlessness and usually a hyperdynamic circulatory condition. Associated are diffuse bilateral opacities on chest X-ray, pulmonary arterial hypertension with normal capillary wedge pressure, decreased pulmonary compliance, arterial hypoxemia, and respiratory alkalosis. Respiratory acidosis is a near terminal event and rarely seen in early ARDS.

The cornerstones of efficient therapy include oxygen administration, ventilatory support using positive airway pressure, appropriate intravascular volume and hemodynamic management, prevention of infectious complications, avoidance of pulmonary damage by ventilatory support and early treatment of other organ failures. As most patients with ARDS die today from sepsis and for other organ failure [25], special attention has to be directed to these problems.

Volume Therapy and Hemodynamic Management

Restoration of good cardiocirculatory function is essential to ensure sufficient oxygen transport and normal function of vital organs. Initial intravascular volume loading is necessary in many severe diseases causing ARDS. Subsequently it is however of vital importance to keep fluid balance and cardiac filling pressures as low as possible in order to improve lymph drainage from the edematous lung [2] and increase the chances for survival [33]. The type of solution used for volume therapy seems not to be of great importance, as long as plasma oncotic pressure does not fall below 50% of the normal value. Below this, edema formation increases massively in most tissues. Extravasation of fluid depends primarily on venous pressure and the permeability characteristics of the capillary wall. For instance, the vessels of the gastrointestinal tract have a lower reflection coefficient and are thus more permeable to water and proteins than those in the lung, myocardium, and central nervous system. In the clinical setting, these pathophysiological bases must result in a controlled fluid balance, maintenance of low central venous and pulmonary capillary wedge pressure, and reasonable but not normal serum albumin and total protein levels.

The hemodynamic state in ARDS is frequently characterized by tachycardia, high cardiac output, increased pulmonary artery pressure, and pulmonary vascular resistance. When management of intravascular volume is adequate according to the considerations cited above, tachycardia can persist over several days or even weeks, with no adverse effects in young patients without coronary artery disease. Pulmonary artery hypertension, a hallmark of severe ARDS, can lead to right ventricular distension or failure in some patients. Treatment with vasodilators such as nitroglycerin, nitroprusside, or prostaglandin E_1 can improve pulmonary vascular resistance, cardiac output, and systemic oxygen transport, but does so at the expense of impaired pulmonary gas exchange due to an increased true shunt [30].

Cardiocirculatory depression by mechanical ventilation can be prevented by careful tailoring of ventilatory support to the pulmonary and hemodynamic response of each individual patient. Continuous monitoring of heart rate, blood pressure, central venous pressure, and urine output together with blood gas measurements are essential in the early phase of treatment. In certain situations, measuring cardiac output, mixed venous oxygen saturation, and total respiratory compliance is useful to adjust the level of PEEP or CPAP appropriately. Newer monitors such as pulse oximetry and expiratory CO_2 measurement are valuable for continuous and noninvasive monitoring.

The therapeutic possibilities for reversing cardiocirculatory depression by positive pressure ventilation include intravascular volume expansion or infusion of vasoactive and inotropic agents. Volume expansion is frequently required to increase cardiac output and compensate for decreased venous return and cardiac filling, but has the potential disadvantage of contributing to pulmonary edema [27]. Dopamine infusion can increase venous return, cardiac output, oxygen transport, and urine output [19].

Dobutamine has a marked positive inotropic effect and can be useful in selected situations. Vasoconstrictors such as norepinephrine or phenylephrine are helpful to increase systemic resistance and blood pressure to increase coronary perfusion.

Prevention, Early Recognition and Treatment of Bronchopulmonary Superinfection

Sepsis of respiratory or nonrespiratory origin is the leading cause of death after the first few days following the onset of ARDS [25]. The incidence of secondary respiratory tract infection during mechanical ventilation ranges between 20% and 70% [11], depending on the duration of intubation, the patient's health status, and host defenses as well as concomitant pulmonary disease. Efficient prevention and early appropriate therapy can decrease the mortality from pneumonia.

Pathophysiology of Nosocomial Infection

In critically ill patients gram-negative organisms colonize the oropharynx rapidly. Most of them are "translocated" from the lower part of the gastrointestinal tract by dysfunctional esophageal and intestinal motion, bacterial growth in the stomach being facilitated by drug-induced suppression or neutralization of gastric acid. The presence of a nasogastric tube can increase reflux and contamination of the oropharynx by this flora. Aspiration despite the presence of a high-volume, low-pressure cuff is frequent, and a fraction of a milliliter of highly contamined oropharyngeal secretions contains a sufficient bacterial challenge to cause airway colonization and superinfection.

Contamination of mechanical ventilators, tubing, and humidification devices represents an important risk for the development of respiratory superinfection [8, 9]. However, the quantitatively greater reservoir of microbes is clearly the gastrointestinal tract.

The presence of an open airway, an endotracheal tube made of foreign material, impaired or absent reflexes for coughing and swallowing, decreased ciliary movement, and a severe underlying disease make the elimination of airway infection difficult.

The adherence of bacteria to mucosal cells and foreign surfaces is a central element in the development of nosocomial bronchitis and pneumonia [39]. Microorganisms such as *Staphylococcus aureus* and *Pseudomonas aeruginosa* can excrete a polysaccharide substance, called glycocalyx, which allow these organisms to adhere to cells and foreign material and proliferate.

Sites of Respiratory Infection

A frequent site is the upper airways in a ventilated patient with *tracheobronchitis,* associated with fever, high white cell count with increased band forms in the circulating blood, and increased tracheobronchial aspirate containing numerous white cells and bacteria. Pure colonization of the airways with pathogens is common, but is by definition not associated with systemic signs of infection.

Lower respiratory tract infection or *pneumonia* is characterized by fever, leukocytosis, with numerous band forms, significant impairment of pulmonary gas exchange, new opacities on the chest radiograph, and secretions of the lower respiratory tract containing leukocytes and pathogenic microorganisms. *Sinusitis* is typically associated with fever of "unknown" origin and other systemic signs of infection, sometimes with purulent secretions from the nose and/or the nasopharynx. This diagnosis is confirmed by radiographic techniques including tomography to visualize all sinuses, with direct puncture, lavage and microbiological examination. The incidence is estimated between 25% and 100% in the critically ill, being highest in patients intubated after head injury [5, 17].

Prevention

Routine use of prohylactic antibiotic treatment in ARDS is not justified, but adequate hygienic measures such as sterile endotracheal suction techniques and regular changes of respiratory tubing and humidification devices [7] must be undertaken. In victims of multiple trauma, a new method of selective decontamination of the oropharynx and the digestive tract has been shown in two studies to decrease the incidence of nosocomial pneumonia and mortality [24,

36]. These promising results need to be confirmed in larger patient studies, paying special attention to the emergence of resistant bacteria.

The methods used for stress ulcer prophylaxis seem important: newer agents such as sucralfate appear to protect gastric mucosal cells and maintain low gastric pH values, preventing bacterial overgrowth. Consequently nosocomial pneumonia is less frequent with this regimen than after treatment with histamine-2 blocking agents [15, 37].

Early Diagnosis of Pneumonia

The important differential diagnosis of upper airway colonization and tracheobronchitis versus pneumonia is often difficult to make. Appropriate techniques to confirm lower respiratory tract infection and pneumonia include bronchoalveolar lavage, protected specimen brush, and qualitative *and* quantitative bacteriological analysis [6, 20].

The direct coloration and search for leukocytes and microorganisms in samples collected by bronchial aspiration is an inexpensive and efficient means for recognizing a significant infection realy. This type of daily surveillance, combined with good clinical judgement, allows a hopeful outlook for the patient with ARDS.

Treatment

Antibiotics should only be used if clear clinical and bacteriological evidence of an important infection is present. The gram stain will allow specific treatment to be given, avoiding the use of large-spectrum drugs and multiple combinations. This restrictive approach delays or prevents the emergence of resistant stains.

Other therapeutic measures for sepsis or severe infection include adequate nutrition, changes of intravenous lines and other devices when indicated.

Avoidance of Pulmonary Damage by Ventilatory Support

Positive pressure ventilation interferes with the normal function of mucociliary movement and alveolar surfactant. The pathophysiologic mechanisms involved are not well understood in man, and the data derived from short term animal studies may not necessarily apply to the patient in the intensive care unit. It is evident that impairment of mucociliary clearance contributes to the development and persistence of nosocomial superinfection (see above). Changes of surfactant turnover may influence alveolar distensibility and collapse as well as the formation of alveolar edema.

The mechanical complications of increased intrapulmonary pressure are airway enlargement and barotrauma. Permanent distension of small airways with morphologic changes of the mucosa has been reported at postmortem examination [34]. The incidence of permanent airway damage in patients surviving prolonged periods of positive pressure ventilation is not known.

Table 1. Risk factors for barotrauma

Trauma	Pulmonary contusion or penetrating lung trauma Rib fractures
Mechanical ventilation	Elevated peak inflation pressure "Fighting" the respirator, coughing
Pulmonary disease	Lung abscess Aspiration pneumonia Parenchymal consolidation (ARDS) – infarction necrosis Emphysema Asthma Necrotizing pneumonia

Barotrauma is defined as a leak of alveolar gas into the interstitial space, mediastinum, subcutaneous tissue, peritoneum, retroperitoneum, or pleural space. The reported incidence varies from 0.5% to 25% [11, 28]. The risk factors (Table 1) include certain underlying traumatic, infectious, or degenerative lung diseases, alveolar overinflation, and a large pressure gradient between alveoli and interstitial or pleural spaces [16]. Early signs of alveolar rupture can be detected on the chest X-ray [3]. The mechanism of progression of alveolar air to extrapulmonary tissues is schematically represented in Fig. 1 [23]. Regular and careful clinical observation, including auscultation, palpation, and daily chest radiographs, can help to detect early signs of barotrauma. Tension pneumothorax is a potentially life-threatening complication for which pleural drainage must be instituted as early as possible.

High peak inspiratory pressures must be avoided by proper adjustment of mechanical ventilation and the alarm/pressure relief settings on the ventilator; these are efficient preventive measures to decrease the incidence of barotrauma. A large bronchopleural fistula is a severe form of barotrauma that is often difficult to treat. Whenever possible, partial or total spontaneous breathing should be maintained. When mechanical ventilatory support is necessary, the lowest possible peak inspiratory, mean and end-expiratory pressures should be applied. The lowest effective level of chest-tube suction should be used. Nursing in the lateral position should be tried, with the leaking lung dependent. Only if these strategies do not reduce the air-leak, more aggressive therapy such as high frequency jet ventilation, independent ventilation of left and right lungs using a double lumen endotracheal tube, or surgical repair should be considered.

Additional ventilation-induced lungs damage includes oxygen toxicity, high inflation pressure pulmonary edema, and formation of hyaline membranes. Evidence for the toxic effect of high inspired oxygen concentrations in adults is mainly derived from post-mortem studies or investigations in animals [12, 31, 32]. These data together with reports suggesting the formation of resorption atelectasis during ventilation with 100% oxygen suggest caution, but oxygen toxicity in adults remains controversial [13]. Recent animal experiments [14] confirm the possibility of diffuse alveolar damage and permeability

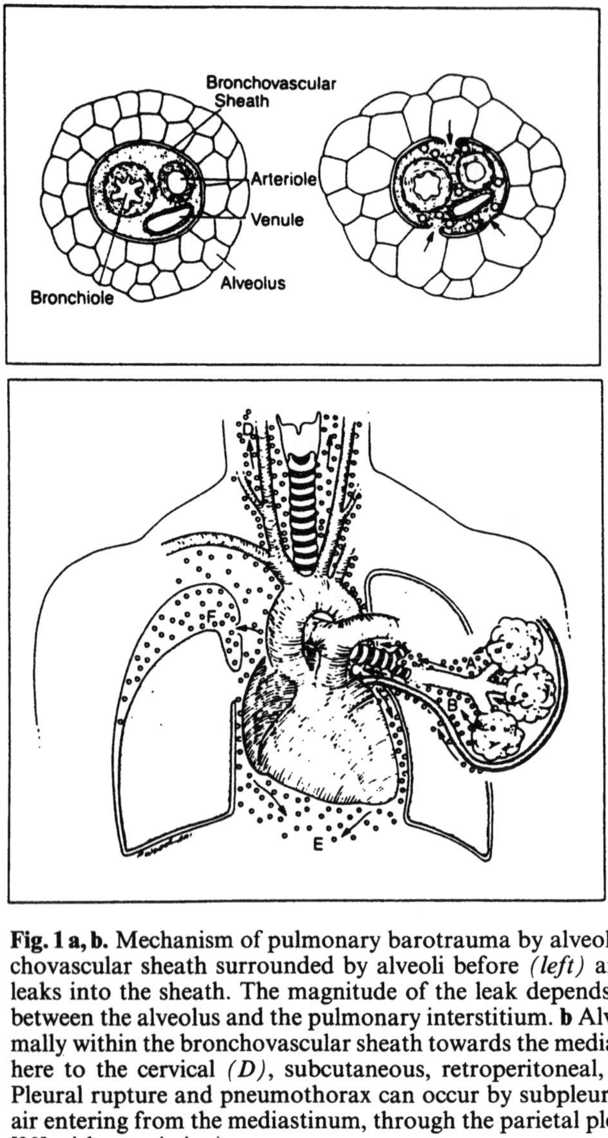

Fig. 1 a, b. Mechanism of pulmonary barotrauma by alveolar disruption. **a** Small bronchovascular sheath surrounded by alveoli before *(left)* and after *(right)* alveolar air leaks into the sheath. The magnitude of the leak depends upon the pressure gradient between the alveolus and the pulmonary interstitium. **b** Alveolar air *(A)* dissects proximally within the bronchovascular sheath towards the mediastinal area *(B, C)*, and from here to the cervical *(D)*, subcutaneous, retroperitoneal, and peritoneal *(E)* spaces. Pleural rupture and pneumothorax can occur by subpleural alveolar dysruption or by air entering from the mediastinum, through the parietal pleura *(F)*. (Reproduced from [23] with permission)

edema caused by high tidal volume ventilation. These lesions require large tidal volumes, because employing positive end-expiratory pressure and lower tidal volumes, resulting in similar peak airway pressure, does not produce alveolar damage. Although no similar studies have been reported in man, it seems advisable to employ moderate tidal volumes, i.e., 10–15 ml/kg ideal body weight, adding positive end-expiratory pressure to improve pulmonary gas exchange and thereby possibly avoiding lung tissue damage.

References

1. Abramson MS, Wald KS, Grenvik ANA, Robinson D, Snyder JV (1980) Adverse occurrences in intensive care units. JAMA 244:1582–1584
2. Allen SJ, Drake RE, Katz J, Gabel JC, Laine GA (1987) Elevation of superior vena cava pressure increases extravascular lung water after endotoxemia. J Appl Physiol 62:1006–1009
3. Altmann AR, Johnson TH (1979) Roentgenographic findings in PEEP therapy – indicators of pulmonary complications. JAMA 242:727–730
4. Andrivet P, Adnot S, Brun-Buisson C, Chabrier PE, Darmon JY, Braquet P, Lemaire F (1988) Involvement of ANF in the acute antidiuresis during PEEP ventilation. J Appl Physiol 65:1967–1974
5. Caplan ES, Hoyt NJ (1982) Nosocomial sinusitis. JAMA 247:639–641
6. Chastre J, Fagon JY, Soler P, Bornet M, Domart Y, Trouillet JL, Gibert C, Hance AJ (1988) Diagnosis of nosocomial bacterial pneumonia in intubated patients undergoing ventilation: comparison of the usefulness of bronchoalveolar lavage and the protected specimen brush. Am J Med 85:499–506
7. Craven DE, Connolly MG, Lichtenberg DA, Primeau PJ, McCabe WR (1982) Contamination of mechanical ventilators with tubing changes every 24 or 48 hours. N Engl J Med 306:1505–1509
8. Craven DE, Goularte TA, Make BJ (1984) Contaminate condensate in mechanical ventilator circuits. A risk factor for nosocomial pneumonia? Am Rev Respir Dis 129:625–628
9. Craven DE, Kunches LM, Kilinsky V, Lichtenberg DA, Make BJ, McCabe WR (1986) Risk factors for pneumonia and fatality in patients receiving continuous mechanical ventilation. Am Rev Respir Dis 133:792–796
10. Cross AS, Roup B (1981) Role of respiratory assistance devices in endemic nosocomial pneumonia. Am J Med 70:681–685
11. Cullen DJ, Caldera DL (1979) The incidence of ventilator-induced pulmonary barotrauma in critically ill patients. Anesthesiology 50:185–190
12. De Los Santos R, Seidenfeld JJ, Anzueto A, Collins JF, Coalson JJ, Johanson WG Jr, Peter JI (1987) One hundred percent oxygen lung injury in adult baboons. Am Rev Respir Dis 136:657–661
13. Deneke SM, Fanburg BL (1980) Normobaric oxygen toxicity of the lung. N Engl J Med 303:76–86
14. Dreyfuss D, Soler P, Basset G, Saumon G (1988) High inflation pressure pulmonary edema. Respective effects of high airway pressure, high tidal volume, and positive end-expiratory pressure. Am Rev Respir Dis 137:1159–1164
15. Driks MR, Craven DE, Celli BR, Manning M, Burke RA, Garvin GM, Kunches LM, Farber HW, Wedel SA, McCabe WR (1987) Nosocomial pneumonia in intubated patients given sucralfate as compared with antacids or histamine type 2 blockers. N Engl J Med 317:1376–1382
16. Haake R, Schlichtig R, Ulstad DR, Henschen RR (1987) Barotrauma. Pathophysiology, risk factors, and prevention. Chest 91:608–613
17. Hansen M, Poulsen MR, Bendixen DK, Hartmann-Andersen F (1988) Incidence of sinusitis in patients with nasotracheal intubation. Br J Anaesth 61:231–232
18. Hemmer M, Suter PM (1979) Treatment of cardiac and renal effects of PEEP with dopamine in patients with acute respiratory failure. Anesthesiology 50:399–403
19. Hemmer M, Viquerat CE, Suter PM, Vallotton MB (1980) Urinary antidiuretic hormone excretion during mechanical ventilation and weaning in man. Anesthesiology 52:395–400
20. Johanson WG JR, Seidenfeld JJ, Gomez P, De Los Santos R, Coalson JJ (1988) Bacteriologic diagnosis of nosocomial pneumonia following prolonged mechanical ventilation. Am Rev Respir Dis 137:259–264
21. Leithner C, Frass M, Pacher R, Hartter E, Pesl H, Woloszczuk W (1987) Mechanical ventilation with positive end-expiratory pressure decreases release of alpha-atrial natriuretic peptide. Crit Care Med 15:484–488

22. Matuschak GM, Pinsky MR, Rogers RM (1987) Effects of positive end-expiratory pressure on hepatic blood flow and performance. J Appl Physiol 62:1377–1383
23. Maunder RJ, Pierson DJ, Hudson LD (1984) Subcutaneous and mediastinal emphysema: pathophysiology, diagnosis, and management. Arch Intern Med 144:1447–1453
24. McA Ledingham I, Alcock SR, Eastaway AT, McDonald JC, McKay IC, Ramsay G (1988) Triple regimen of selective decontamination of the digestive tract, systemic cefotaxime, and microbiological surveillance for prevention of acquired infection in intensive care. Lancet I:785–790
25. Montgomery AB, Stager MA, Carrico CJ, Hudson LD (1985) Causes of mortality in patients with the adult respiratory distress syndrome. Am Rev Respir Dis 132:485–489
26. Natanson CH, Fink MP, Ballantyne HK, MacVittie TJ, Conklin JE, Parrillo JE (1986) Gram-negative bacteremia produces both severe systolic and diastolic cardiac dysfunction in a canine model that stimulates human septic shock. J Clin Invest 78:259–270
27. Noble WN, Colin KJ (1986) The effects of dobutamine, nitroprusside, or volume expansion on cardiac output and lung water after CPPV. Can Anaesth Soc J 33:48–56
28. Petersen GW, Baier H (1983) Incidence of pulmonary barotrauma in a medical ICU. Crit Care Med 11:67–69
29. Priebe HJ, Heimann JC, Hedley-Whyte J (1981) Mechanisms of renal dysfunction during positive end-expiratory pressure ventilation. J Appl Physiol 50:643–649
30. Radermacher P, Santak B, Becker H, Falke KJ (1989) Prostaglandin E_1 and nitroglycerin reduce pulmonary capillary pressure by worsen ventilation-perfusion distributions in patients with adult respiratory distress syndrome. Anesthesiology 70:601–606
31. Repine JE, Cheronis JC, Rodell TC, Linas SL, Patt A (1987) Pulmonary oxygen toxicity and ischemia-reperfusion injury. Am Rev Respir Dis 136:483–485
32. Royer F, Martin DJ, Benchetrit G, Grimbert FA (1988) Increase in pulmonary capillary permeability in dogs exposed to 100% O_2. J Appl Physiol 65:1140–1146
33. Simmons RS, Berdine GG, Seidenfeld JJ, Prihoda TJ, Harris GD, Smith JD, Gilbert J, Mota E, Johanson WG Fr (1987) Fluid balance and the adult respiratory distress syndrome. Am Rev Respir Dis 135:924–929
34. Slavin G, Nunn JF, Crow J, Doré CJ (1982) Bronchiolectasis – a complication of artificial ventilation. Br Med J 285:931–934
35. Stauffer JL, Olson DE, Petty TL (1981) Complications and consequences of endotracheal intubation and tracheotomy. A prospective study of 150 critically ill adult patients. Am J Med 70:65–76
36. Stoutenbeek CP, Van Seane HKF, Miranda DR, Zanstra DF, Langrehr D (1987) The effect of oropharyngeal decontamination using topical nonabsorbable antibiotics on the incidence of nosocomial respiratory tract infections in multiple trauma patients. J Trauma 27:357–364
37. Tryba M (1987) Risk of acute stress bleeding and nosocomial pneumonia in ventilated intensive care patients: sucralfate versus antacids. Am J Med 83 [Suppl 3B]:117–124
38. Vincent JL, Suter PM (1987) Cardiopulmonary interactions in acute respiratory failure. Springer, Berlin Heidelberg New York
39. Woods DE, Straus DC, Johanson WG, Bass JA (1981) Role of salivary protease activity in adherence of gram-negative bacilli to mammalian buccal epithelial cells in vivo. J Clin Invest 68:1435–1440

Current Concepts and Future Perspectives in the Treatment of the Acute Respiratory Distress Syndrome in Neonate

H. Schachinger

Chronic respiratory disorders in the early days of the life of a newborn, i.e., during the first 4 weeks after birth, often become apparent as the result of aggressive treatment of acute respiratory disorder, such as bronchopulmonary dysplasia. Other respiratory disorders, often not related to pulmonary disorders, develop slowly, symptomless, and remain unnoticed for a long period of time, like hemangioma of the larynx or of the trachea. Acute respiratory disorders also very often are so symptomatic just after birth that they have to be treated immediately within the first hours of life.

Before the various types of therapy for acute respiratory disorders are dealt with the definitions for such disorders should be differentiated. In general, the term "respiratory distress syndrome" is used – according to its symptoms – for all pulmonary ventilation disorders in newborns; but specifically, it is understood to mean surfactant deficiency and its effects, atelectasis as well as hyaline membrane disease (HMD). In such instances and because of immaturity, surfactant deficiency refers specifically to the premature infant. The surfactant deficiency is also possible after intensified loss or deficient reproduction of the lipoprotein; for example, if the production center of the surfactant, namely, the type II alveolar pneumocytes, are damaged by severe acidosis, hypoxia, or shock in premature or maturely born neonates. However, this phenomenon can also be observed in adults.

Symptoms

The symptoms of respiratory insufficiency in neonates are usually the same, in spite of the different causes for such disorders. Among the symptoms are tachypnea, dyspnea, tachycardia, thoracic retraction on inspiration, expiratory grunting, nasal flaring, and often very severe cyanosis, as well as muscular hypotension and an increased inclination for apneas.

Causes

A variety of acute ventilation disorders are hidden behind the aforementioned symptoms. These include:

1. *Obstructions* of the respiratory tract, such as choanalatresia, macroglossia, subglottic stenosis, hemangioma, vocal chords paralysis, tracheal malacia, tracheoesophageal fistulas, or stenosis in the tracheal or bronchial area

2. *Deformities* such as hypoplasia or aplasia of the lungs, diaphragmatic hernia, intrathoracic cysts or tumors, congenital lobar emphysema, or chylothorax
3. *Nonpulmonary related causes* such as heart defects, respiratory disorders caused by the central nervous system or by metabolism, respiratory disorders after severe acidosis, hypothermia and hypoglycemia or caused by a persistent fetal circulation (PFC) [= persistent pulmonary hypertension of the neonate (PPHN)]. In considering these, the interaction between circulation and respiration becomes apparent.
4. *Pulmonary illnesses* such as the aspiration syndrome (meconium aspiration), the so-called hyaline-membrane disease (HMD), air-leak syndromes and the transient tachypnea of neonates (TTN), or serious pneumonias.

Assisted Ventilation of the Neonate

The basic treatment of the aforementioned respiratory disorders is initially the same because, more often than not, they occur most intensively immediately after birth. This uniform treatment especially occurs in instances where intensive clinical symptoms are accompanied by the appropriate laboratory results: an arterial PO_2 below 50 mmHg at a FiO_2 of 0.6, a PCO_2 above 60 mmHg (already above 50 mmHg in the case of very low birth weight neonates) and with a pH below 7.20, and also when repeated and/or persistent apnea are found. In these cases, an effort has to be made to control the clinical symptoms and to normalize the blood gases, through the use of oxygen treatment or possibly through artificial ventilation.

Oxygen

The simplest form to support ventilation is the administering of oxygen through a funnel, an oxygen mask, or oxygen hood. However, with a hood the oxygen or respiratory gas has to be warmed; the oxygen concentration has to be regulated according to the principle "as much as necessary and as little as possible."

Increasing the Mean Airway Pressure (Continuous Distending Pressure)

The next step in the treatment is to increase the mean airway pressure while continuously maintaining spontaneous breathing. This continuous distending pressure (CDP) can be achieved through two methods (see Table 1): (1) by achieving continuous positive airway pressure (CPAP) through the use of short double-sided or single-sided nasal tubes or a tracheal tube, although a closed hyperbaric oxygen hood provides similar results according to the CPAP principle [11, 31]; (2) through application of continuous suction on the entire thorax area, in keeping with the principle of continuous negative pressure (CNP) [15], in this case the body of the neonate is placed in a small hypobaric chamber. As previously mentioned, both methods require the prerequisite of

Table 1. Continuous distending pressure (CDP) with spontaneous breathing of the neonate

CPAP	CNP
Practice	*Practice*
Heat chamber	Pulmarca
Face chamber	Isolette respirator
Nasal tube	
Endotracheal tube	
Oxygen blender	
Flow meter	
Heated humidifier	
Pressure gauge	
Water seal	

CPAP, continuous positive airway pressure; CNP, continuous negative pressure

good spontaneous breathing. The clinical protocol, as well as frequent and repeated evaluation of the blood gases, should determine whether or not this form of therapy is adequate and if the breathing process is too difficult for the patient. It is of paramount importance that the next higher form of therapy be initiated before the patient becomes exhausted, i.e., the use of continuous controlled artificial ventilation.

All forms of postpartum maladaptions indicate the need for CPAP treatment, especially with children weighing 1200 to 1500 g, or in instances of a mild respiratory distress syndrome. The prompt initiation of CDP therapy usually prevents the need for extended respiratory therapy [16]. CPAP therapy has been proven beneficial in the weaning stage after extended respiration therapy for children of varying weights and diagnosis. Recurring apnea are also favorably treated in this way [14, 28].

Indications for CPAP therapy include maladaptation, mild respiratory distress, weaning after long mechanical ventilation, and recurrent apnea. The therapy can be implemented through the use of one or two short nasal or tracheal tubes, with a diameter of 2.5 or 3.5 mm, inserted into one or both nostrils, depending on the size of the child. If a singel nasal tube is used it is better to take a tube of 3 or more mm. During a laryngoscopic examination, the short nasal tubes should not be visible in the epipharynx. A flow meter should be used to set the gas flow at 3–5 (–6) l/min; the gas flow depends on the size of the child and the prescribed regulation of the end-expiratory pressure. If possible, the distending pressure should be held steady. Constant bubbling in a water seal is both protection against extreme distending pressure and an indicator for constant gas flow. In cases of extreme respiratory distress syndromes, where the oxygen supply is inadequate, end-expiratory pressure of 7–8 cm H_2O can be employed. A CPAP system consists of: an oxygen mixer, a flowmeter, a heated humidifier, a pressure gauge, and a water seal (see Table 1). The prompt use of the CPAP system is usually adequate to provide the child with temporary breathing assistance and prevent the worsening of the pulmonary condition, for example, during transport from the delivery room to the intensive care unit [24].

Mechanical Ventilation

If the clinical condition of the patient requires respiratory therapy and has not yet been diagnosed, the respirator can be regulated as indicated (see Table 2). Initially, a constant respiratory frequency of 50–60 bpm (i.e., beats per minute) should be used and, depending on the clinical condition, an oxygen concentration (FiO_2) of 0.8–1. With mature neonates, an inspiration/expiration ratio (I/E) of 1:1.5, and a positive end-expiratory pressure (PEEP) of 3 cm H_2O should be used. Initially, an inspiratory pressure ($P_{insp.}$) of 25 cm H_2O is called for. With premature neonates weighing between 1500 and 2500 g, a $P_{insp.}$ of 20 cm H_20, a PEEP of 3 cm, and an I/E ratio of 1:1 should be used. With particulary small neonates (i.e., those under 1 500 g) a $P_{insp.}$ of 18 cm H_2O should initially be used, a PEEP of 2 cm H_2O, and an I/E ratio of 1:1. At this stage, it is imperative that a blood-gas analysis be performed, within 10–15 min and following a brief clinical observation, to determine the clinical reaction of the patient to the respirator, whether the respiration is being resisted, and to determine how the blood gases have developed. Should the respirator frequency prove unaccommodating (fighting against the respirator), the patient should be disconnected. At this point, a respiratory bag can employed to manually immitate the patient's spontaneous frequency and afterwards to adjust the respirator, accordingly. This method is definitely preferred to sedation.

Since the beginning of the 1970s, supportive ventilation or artificial respiration of neonates with end-expiratory pressure (spontaneous breathing, CPAP, as well as artificial ventilation and PEEP) has unquestionably established itself, as opposed to treatment with positive-negative pressure ventilation or negative pressure respirators. The described plan (see Table 3) can provide reference points for end-expiratory pressure respiration. In the various neonate intensive care units, however, it is especially the respiratory frequency and/or the I/E ratio which is frequently varied.

Table 2. Initial respirator adjustment (before diagnosis)

	Newborn	Preterm	VLBW
Rate (bpm)	(50–)60	60	60
FiO_2	0.8–1	0.8–1	0.8–1
I/E ratio	1:1.5	1:1	1:1
$P_{insp.}$ (cm H_2O)	25	20	18
PEEP (cm H_2O)	3	3	2

VLBW, very low birth weight (under 1500 g); FiO_2, forced inspiratory oxygen; I/E, inspiratory/ expiratory; $P_{insp.}$, inspiratory pressure; PEEP, positive end-expiratory pressure; bpm, beats per minute

Table 3. Initial respirator adjustment (following the diagnosis)

	RDS	Meconium aspiration	PFC	Pneumo-thorax
Rate (bpm)	60	60	60–80	60
FiO_2	0.8–1	0.8–1	1	0.4–1
$P_{insp.}$ (cm H_2O)	25	Up to 30–35	25–35	25–30
PEEP (cm H_2O)	4 (−6)	2	3	1
MAP (cm H_2O)	12–14	14–16	12–14	8–12
I/E	1:1–1.5	1:2	1:1	1:2–3
Insp. time (s)	0.5–0.4	0.3	0.5	0.3–0.25

MAP, mean arterial pressure; Insp., inspiratory; RDS, respiratory distress syndrome; PFC, persistent fetal circulation

In addition to these "standardized" controlled methods of artificial ventilation, there are various and sundry others which, however, have hardly succeeded beyond the experimental stage; nonetheless, these should be employed as a final option in cases of emergency.

Ventilation with Sedation and/or Relaxation

In general, neonates do not require sedation or relaxation when the oxygen supply is adequate; finding the optimal respiratory frequency is the ideal solution to circumvent the need for sedation. Sedation or relaxation should be employed to prevent the child from fighting against the respirator, in light of the danger of a pneumothorax, other respiratory damage, or a cerebral hemorrhage [3, 9]. The practicality of sedation and relaxation should be considered with the following disorders: the artificial respiration of large newborns (respiratory distress syndrome in neonates of diabetic mothers, for example), severe meconium aspiration, hyperexcitability and convulsive newborns (which is often the case with meconium aspiration), and with interstitial emphysema. Phenobarbital sedation is often adequate in order to synchronize the neonate's respiratory frequency to that of the respirator.

Phenobarbital dosage:

Saturation dosage V:15 mg/kg body weight/24 h

Sustenance dosage: 5 ml/kg body weight/24 h

Depending on their age and weight, the phenobarbital half-life period in neonates is particularly long and can exceed 100 h [22]. Consequently, additional doses should be determined by drug monitoring.

Pancuronium dosage:

0.05–0.1 mg/kg body weight (single dosage)

The preconditions for relaxation involve regularly turning the patient over, regularly voiding the bladder, and exclusively parenteral feeding. The advantages of sedation/relaxation are fewer cerebral hemorrhages and a lesser occurrence of respiratory damage. The disadvantages are that the neurological diagnosis of the child is impossible, the circulation is very often influenced, and there is a danger of hypotension.

Intermittent Mandatory Ventilation (IMV)

With this particular type of artificial ventilation, the respiratory frequency is fractionally lower than the child's respiratory frequency. The respirator frequency is usually set at <20/bpm or less, in accordance with the appropriate PEEP. The patient can and should breathe spontaneously between each slow respirator cycle. The patient adjusts to this breathing assistance after a short habituation period. This type of breathing assistance readily accommodates a slow and agreeable weaning period from the respirator, by gradually reducing the respiratory frequency, subsequently increasing the neonate's involvement in spontaneous breathing. The respirator frequency can eventually be diminished to just a few breathing cycles per minute, to 1–5 bpm, for example, allowing an effortless transition to CPAP therapy. Reiterating, the IMV procedure particularly accommodates the weaning process, even in cases of mild to moderately acute respiratory disorders [4].

Assisted Mechanical Ventilation

In principle, the respiratory frequency should be synchronized to the neonate's breathing in such a manner that it suffers no resistance. In the simplest instance this is achieved by precisely counting the neonate's personal breathing frequency and then setting the respirator accordingly. This is also achieveable by disconnecting the respirator and briefly respirating the neonate manually with an air bag (see above).

In respirators which allow assisted mechanical ventilation, the neonate's inspiration trigger impulse is used to initiate the breathing cycle of the respirator. Whereas many neonates, especially small premature neonates, have particularly low inspiration volumes, the trigger impulse often does not respond and the respirator is therefore not initiated. The impedance-controlled respiration monitor (the respiration rate of apnea monitors) is an alternative possibility for the so-called assisted mechanical ventilation. With this instrument the impedance signal from the monitor is retransmitted to the respirator. During inspiration, the thorax movement instantaneously initiates the respirator cycle. This method of assisted mechanical ventilation also readily accommodates weaning [26]. Careful breathing frequency synchronization often alleviates respiratory damage (interstitial emphysema, pneumothorax) [10].

Hyperventilation

A frequency of (80–) 100–150 bpm is strived for with this particular respiratory technique. The intensity of the patient's disorder often makes it commonplace to use inspiration pressure of up to 40 cm H_2O. This technique can be employed in instances of persistent pulmonary hypertension in neonates (PPHN, or persistent fetal circulation, i.e., PFC syndrome) [5], and as well in instances of severe infections and meconium aspiration. This respiration technique is used to try to diminish the pulmonary vascular resistance by reducing the PCO_2 and by improving oxidation. In addition to the damage done by mechanical ventilation, which occassionally may occur, with this type of respiration there is the added danger of cerebral circulation deficiency (resulting from drastic PCO_2 reduction). It is therefore of utmost necessity that the patient remain under continuous scrutinizing observation (by monitoring the transcutaneous PO_2 and the PCO_2).

High Frequency Ventilation (HFPPV)

A respirator frequency from 60–150 (–180) bpm should be chosen, if the patient exhibits low mean airway pressure [6, 7], when HFPPV is employed. Usually, a frequency of over 75–100 bpm should be strived for; subsequently, the child's spontaneous breathing is often interrupted by reflex. This method can be attempted in cases of PFC syndrome and also in instances of respiratory distress syndrome in small premature neonates weighing less than 1000 g, especially if they are fighting against the respirator. Improved oxidation should be achievable through improved molecular gas diffusion [30]. The choice of a lower mean airway pressure also provides a lower risk of respiratory damage.

High frequency jet ventilation (HFJV) is a special type of high frequency ventilation [2]. With this type of ventilation breathing gas is injected into the lungs in short inspiration intervals and at a high frequency (150–900 bpm) through an extra-thin catheter in the tracheal tube. This type of respiration has, however, not been categorically employed because its use is often accompanied by severe tracheal tissue transformation [12].

High Frequency Oscillation Ventilation (HFOV)

Breathing gas at the entrance of the tracheal tube is made to vibrate by the use of an oscillating piston pump or a membrane pump (at a rate of between 7–40 Hz, 400–2400 bpm) [27]. This method is only employable in instances where the lungs are expanded and in combination with the CPAP system. Analogous to high frequency respiration, the use of HFOV results in the patient experiencing a reflex-incited apnea. To date, there is no detailed explanation for the gas exchange which occurs when HFOV is used. Since 1915 theoretical hypotheses and associated research have been available, formulated and presented by Henderson et al. (in [13], quoted from [30]). The gas exchange appears to take place as the result of an increased diffusibility, which results from the oscillating stream of gas. This, in turn, supposedly results from the interaction between the central gas flow in the airway passages and its very high molecular velocity and the gas flow at the edge of the breathing gas column, where an increased molecular diffusion is possible. This is referred to as the "Taylor dispersion" (in [29], quoted from [30]). High frequency oscillation has not been widely accepted for the treatment of respiratory disorders in neonates.

Extracorporeal Membrane Oxygenation (ECMO)

If the patient's oxygenation, that is, the entire gas exchange rate, can not be regulated by mechanical ventilation, then some other technique should be used. Instead of gas, the neonate is given oxygen-enriched blood and CO_2 is filtered from the blood. This method, called "artificial lung" or extracorporeal membrane oxygenation (ECMO), will be addressed in detail at a later point. To date, oxygenation assistance to the neonate is only available through the use of an enormous battery of instruments.

Avoidance of High Technology – Improved Prophylaxis

Prevention of Prematurity

The sometimes overly aggressive therapeutic methods used in the treatment of severe respiratory distress syndrome should not discourage future efforts to assist suffering neonates in every possible manner and efforts to completely avoid this clinical disorder, i.e., to principally address the very cause of the disorder.

The first concern should be to prevent early interruption of pregnancy, i.e., premature delivery, considering the fact that the most commonly found sufferers of breathing disorders are premature neonates. Prenatal medicine should be commended for the excellent possibilities which are available today to prolong pregnancy, through the use of medicine (with fenoterol, for example) and also operatively (cerclage, for example), if premature delivery threatens. In the event that this necessity arises, efforts should be made to accelerate the maturing process of the fetal lungs by administering ambroxol, or the mother should be given glucocorticosteroids [1, 18, 32]. Through this treatment respiratory distress syndrome can often be avoided, or at least its severity diminished.

Initial Care

If the neonate is premature, in spite of preventive measures having been taken or the unavailability of such, the only remaining option is the basic rule of initial care: the prevention of hypothermia should be given priority. The morbidity rate rises markedly if hypothermia is not sufficiently controlled (increased cerebral hemorrhage and respiratory disorders, for example). Accordingly, the mortality rate is also higher. It has been repeatedly reported that about 50% of the neonates who die after being hospitalized are diagnosed as hypothermic upon arrival. Today, although not categorically adhered to, professional initial care includes the following procedure: correct suctioning (endotracheal, for example, in a meconium aspiration and lavage), the prevention of both asphyxia and brief instances of oxygen deficiency (i.e., properly administering oxygen), and circulatory stabilization treatment (the administration of plasma protein after measuring the blood pressure). A future goal should be to ensure that the neonatalogist supervises all high-risk deliveries and that these neonates are born in specialized facilities. Clinical reality repeatedly shows definite

Table 4. Clinical results of surfactant replacement

Improvements	Uncertain effects
PaO_2	BPD
FiO_2	PDA
MAP	IVH
$P_{insp.}$	Air leak syndrome

advantages in the use of these techniques for the prevention of respiratory disorder in newborn neonates, especially in small premature neonates.

Surfactant Replacement

In instances where premature neonates suffer from respiratory distress syndrome with a surfactant deficiency, endotracheal surfactant can be administered. As the result of over a decade of research this substance has almost become a general standard for treatment of this disorder. The surfactant is injected endotracheally into the lungs, through a tracheal tube. Different surfactants are utilized by the extensive number of research centers and pharmaceutical companies who work with this substance. Simply stated, there are principally three groups: surfactant extracted from human amnion fluid [18]; synthesized surfactant, principally created from the chemical building blocks [19]; and, animal surfactants, extracted from the lungs of calves [17], bovines [8], or pigs [23]. A synopsis of the results of numerous medical studies concludes that through the use of surfactants, oxidation can be substancially improved, and the forced inspiratory oxygen (FiO_2) and ventilation pressure could be reduced (see Table 4). The treatment remains effective for only 20–24 h and its effectiveness varies greatly from neonate to neonate.

Using surfactants prophylactically, immediately after birth, poses a number of problems. Many preterms as well as neonates with very low birth weight experience no respiratory distress syndrome whatsoever and patients who have not shown an immediate positive reaction to surfactants have been treated unnecessarily. In addition, the side-effects of the otherwise unavoidable use of mechanical ventilation, like respiratory damage to the lungs (bronchopulmonary dysplasia, air-leak syndrome), or an open ductus Botalli and cerebral hemorrhage, could not completely be avoided by the use of surfactants.

Within the current framework of clinical research, it is imperative that the different surfactants be evaluated, as a single group, to ascertain why they are sometimes completely ineffective and why the reactions and responses vary so drastically.

Conclusion

Clinical research, within the past 20 years, has provided enormous benefits for neonates with respiratory disorders, particularly for small premature neonates. This progress is particularly documented by the reduced mortality rate, especially among these severely afflicted patients [25]. To facilitate gas exchange, conventional ventilation methods have been improved, often in combination with spectacular new technical discoveries. The ECMO oxygenation principle, i.e., extracorporeal gas exchange or membrane oxygenation, which ensures the protection of damaged lungs, is successful and quite promising, at present depicting only the mere beginning of its future potential. The problems as yet unsolved with ECMO include the use of nonthreatening catheter techniques as well as heparin-coated catheters, the threat of coagulation, the development techniques which would allow reduced blood flow, and the monitoring of circulation in individual organs – especially the cerebrum and the kidney, and the problems of long-term follow-up of the children. The use of surfactants, as a substitute for alveolar stabilizing substances, provides indisputable advantages, in spite of the fact that there are still unanswered compatibility questions. The all-encompassing future goals of further research in this field should be to create and develop gentler therapeutic methods and to prevent the side-effects of therapy, thereby giving neonates the opportunity to live more rewardingly. At this point, it is indisputable that, as an initial step, the best and most practical means to acheive this goal lie in the use these simple methods of initial care and in the establishment of a regional care center.

References

1. Ballard P, Benson B, Brehier A (1977) Glucocorticoid effects in the fetal lung. Am Rev Respir Dis 115:29–36
2. Boros SR, Mammel MC, Coleman JM, Lewallen PK, Gordon MJ, Bing DR, Ophoven JP (1985) Neonatal high-frequency jet ventilation: 4 years experience. Pediatrics 75:95–100
3. Donn SM, Roloff DW, Goldstein GW (1981) Prevention of intraventricular haemorrhage in preterm infants by phenobarbitone: a controlled trial. Lancet II:211–215
4. Downs JB, Klein EF Jr, Desantels D et al. (1973) Intermittent mandatory ventilation: a new approach to weaning patients from mechanical ventilators. Chest 64:331
5. Duara S, Gewitz MH, Forx WW (1984) Use of mechanical ventilation for clinical management of persistent pulmonary hypertension of the newborn. Clin Perinatol 11:641–652
6. Eyal FJ, Arad ID, Goddes K, Robinson MJ (1984) High frequency positive-pressure ventilation in neonates. Crit Care Med 12:793–797
7. Frantz ID, Werthammer J, Stork AR (1983) High frequency ventilation in premature infants with lung disease: adequate gas exchange at low tracheal pressure. Pediatrics 71:482–488
8. Fujiwara T, Maeta H, Chida S, Morita T, Watabe Y, Tadaahi A (1980) An artificial surfactant therapy in hyaline membrane disease. Lancet I:55–59
9. Greenough A, Wood S, Morley CJ, Davis JA (1984) Pancuronium prevents pneumothoraces in ventilated premature babies who actively expire against pressure ventilation. Lancet I:1–4
10. Greenough A, Greenall F, Gamsu H (1987) Synchronous respiration: which ventilator rate is best? Acta Paediatr Scand 76:713–718
11. Gregory GA, Kittermann JA, Phibbs RH, Tooley WH, Hamilton WK (1971) Treatment of the idiopathic respiratory distress syndrome with continuous positive airway pressure. N Engl J Med 284:1333

12. Harris T, Gouch W, Wilson JF (1984) Necrotizing tracheobronchitis associated with high frequency jet ventilation in neonates. Clin Res 32:132
13. Henderson Y, Chillingworth FP, Whitney JL (1915) The respiratory dead space. Am J Physiol 38:1
14. Kattwinkel J, Nearman HS, Fanaroff AA et al. (1976) Apnea of prematurity: comparative therapeutic effects of cutaneous stimulation and nasal CPAP. J Pediatr 86:588
15. Kisling JA, Schreiner RL, Liechty EA (1982) Mechanical ventilation in the newborn. In: Schreiner RL, Kisling JA (eds) Practical neonatal respiratory care. Raven, New York, pp 329–350
16. Kronskop RW, Brown EG, Sweet AY (1975) The early use of continuous positive airway pressure in the treatment of idiopathic respiratory distress syndrome. J Pediatr 87:263
17. Kwong MS, Egan EA, Notter RH, Shapiro DL (1985) Double-blind clinical trial of calf lung surfactant extract for the prevention of hyaline membrane disease in extremely premature infants. Pediatrics 76:585–592
18. Liggins GC, Howie RN (1972) A controlled trial of antepartum glucocorticoid treatment for prevention of the respiratory distress syndrome in premature infants. Pediatrics 50:515
19. Merritt TA, Hallman M, Bloom BT et al. (1986) Prophylactic treatment of very premature infants with human surfactant. N Engl J Med 315:785–750
20. Morley CJ, Bangham AD, Miller N et al. (1981) Dry artificial surfactant and its effects on very premature babies. Lancet I:64–68
21. Ortiz RM, Cilley RE, Bartlett RH (1987) Extracorporal membrane oxygenation in pediatric respiratory failure. Pediatr Clin North Am 34:39–46
22. Pitlick W, Painter M, Pippenger C (1978) Phenobarbital pharmacokinetics in neonates. Clin Pharmacol Ther 23:346
23. Robertson B et al. (1988) Surfactant replacement therapy for severe neonatal respiratory distress syndrome. An international randomized clinical trial. Pediatrics 82:683–691
24. Schachinger H, Frank HD, Ruhe B (1976) Further improvements in the transport of high-risk neonates. J Perinat Med 4:131–133
25. Schachinger H, Hanefeld F, Frank HD, Schneider H (1982) Entwicklung langzeitbeatmeter kleiner Frühgeborener. In: Huch A, Huch R, Duc G, Rooth G (eds) Klinisches Management des „kleinen“ Frühgeborenen. Thieme, Stuttgart, pp 23–26
26. Schmid HJ, Frank HD, Schachinger H (1984) Impedanzgesteuerte assistierte Beatmung des Neugeborenen. In: Dudenhausen JW, Saling E (eds) Perinatale Medizin, vol 10. Thieme, Stuttgart: 338–339
27. Smith R (1982) Ventilation at high respiratory frequencies. Anaesthenia 37:1011
28. Speidel BD, Dunn PM (1977) Use of nasal CPAP to treat severe recurrent apnea in very preterm infants. Lancet II:658
29. Taylor GI (1953) Dispersion of soluble matter in solvent flowing slowly through a tube. Proc R Soc London 219:186–203
30. Wetzel RC, Gisia FR (1987) High frequency ventilation. Ped Clin North Am 34:15–38
31. Williams TJ (1975) Continuous positive airway pressure. In: Lough MD, Williams TJ, Rawson JE (eds) Newborn respiratory care. Chicago, Year Book Medical Publisher
32. Wolff F, Ponnath H, Wiest W (1987) Induktion der fetalen Lungenreifung durch Ambroxol und Betamethason. Geburtshilfe Frauenheilkd 47:19–25

New Trends in Ventilatory Therapy

R. Rossaint, K. Slama, and K. J. Falke

With the various new possibilities of supporting spontaneous breathing mechanically – also called augmented spontaneous breathing – changes have occurred in the nomenclature and the systematics of ventilatory techniques. We can therefore distinguish between partial and total ventilatory support. Partial ventilatory support (PVS) comprises all methods used in connection with spontaneous breathing; complete or total ventilatory support (TVS) includes all forms of controlled ventilation.

Partial Ventilatory Support

Intermittent Mechanical or Mandatory Ventilation

Downs et al. were the first, in 1973, to report on intermittent mandatory mechanical ventilation (IMV) as a new method of weaning adults from mechanical ventilation [1]. IMV was developed out of the combination of spontaneous breathing with continuous positive airway pressure (CPAP) and mechanical ventilation. This was done by connecting a CPAP system to an Emerson respirator's valve for spontaneous inhalation. In this way it was possible to let patients breathe spontaneously in between or simultaneously with mechanical/mandatory breaths. In the beginning breaths delivered by the machine could only be applied nonsynchronized but later they could also be synchronized to spontaneous inspiration (synchronized IMV = SIMV; Fig. 1). Although IMV and SIMV are now widely used, especially in weaning, this technique is still controversial [2].

Some of the main advantages and disadvantages that have been postulated and, to some extent, proved are listed in Table 1.

IMV and SIMV today do not only, as Downs et al. initially described, serve as a method of weaning, but are often used as the basic setting of the ventilator, so that the patient can breathe spontaneously whenever he or she feels the need.

IMV/SIMV with CPAP can be implemented technically in two ways: with a continuous flow system or with a demand-valve system. When a continuous flow system is used, a continuous high gas flow (25–60 l/min) is delivered, independent of mechanical ventilation, into the inspiratory part of the ventilatory circuit. With the help of an elastic reservoir (20–25 l) the pressure throughout spontaneous inspiration is kept constant as far as possible. Under

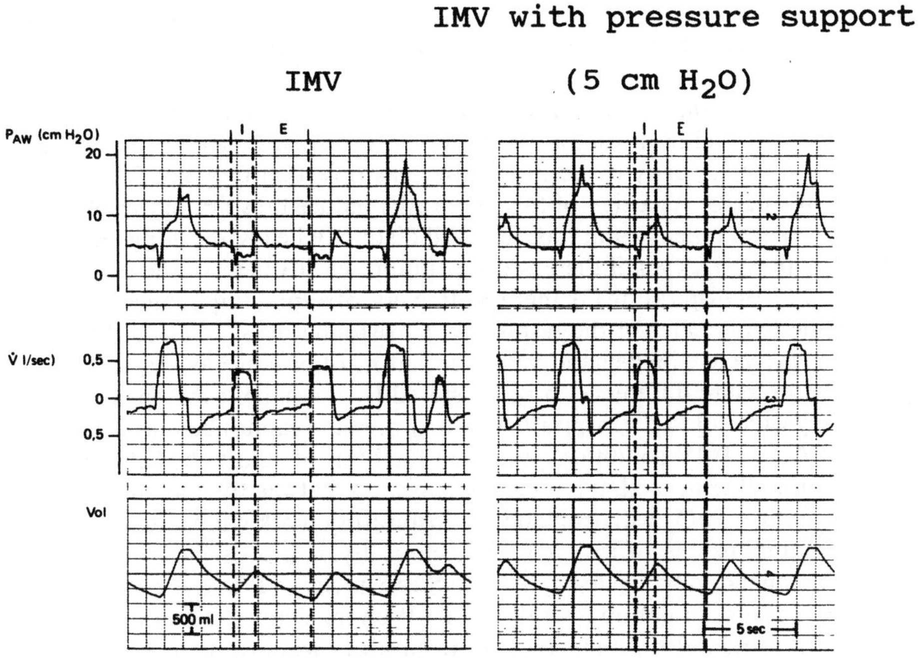

Fig. 1. Simultaneous respiratory pressure, respiratory flow, and volume recording (pneumotachograph) in a patient during IMV with and without pressure support. Puritan Bennett 7200. IMV frequency 5/min. Trigger sensitiveness 1 cm H_2O, PEEP 5 cm H_2O. The recording was made between tube and Y-piece. Without IPS the airway pressure decreases slightly over the whole inspiratory phase; in expiration it increases slightly for a short period. With IPS without any change in the apparatus adjustment there is only a very short decrease in pressure with a subsequent increase in pressure over the PEEP level. At the same time the inspiratory flow and the tidal volume increase

Table 1. Advantages and disadvantages of IMV and SIMV

Advantages	Disadvantages
SV in connection with MV is possible without deterioration of bloodgases [3]	Risk of ineffective ventilation
SV does not always has to be suppressed pharmacologically to maintain optimal bloodgases	Risk of inspiratory muscle fatigue
Risk of disconnection incidents is reduced through preservation of spontaneous breathing	Permanent "weaning" condition, therefore high level of monitoring required
Gradual weaning from high ventilatory pressure is possible	Spontaneous breathing activity can increase LV dysfunction [5]
Impairment of circulation and kidney function less than with CMV [4]	

SV, spontaneous ventilation; MV, mandatory ventilation; LV, left ventricular; CMV, controlled mechanical ventilation these conditions the patient can breathe without having to overcome external resistance – with the exception of the resistance caused by the endotracheal tube.

In contrast to this, demand-flow systems always require the patient to perform apparatus-induced respiratory work. This is caused partly by the "trigger" function and partly by an inspiratory gas flow that may not fully meet the patient's needs. As a sign of this apparatus-induced respiratory work, the airway pressure, taken at the tube, can fall distinctly below the adjusted end-expiratory pressure, even if there was maximum sensitiveness of the trigger at the beginning of inspiration [3]; there is often no corresponding change of pressure on the manometer of the respirator. Christopher et al. showed that the internal manometers on demand-valve ventilators often considerably underestimate the pressure difference to be mustered by the patient for opening the inspiratory valve [6]. If the inspiratory airway pressure cannot be kept constant under CPAP or IMV conditions, then, on the basis of studies by Schlobohm et al. [7] and Gherini et al. [8], it can be expected that the functional residual capacity and the PaO_2 will drop and the inspiratory work will increase.

This requirement is difficult to fulfill technically, so that on the first respirators with demand-valve systems, like the Siemens Servo B and the Engström Erica, in contrast to continuous flow CPAP under defined conditions (V= 0.5 l/sec, sinusoidal flow) an increase of inspiratory work of up to 22% could be noticed, even though the trigger was adjusted to maximum sensitiveness [9].

Modern respirators like the Servo C, the Eva, and the Puritan Bennett 7200, however, guarantee an almost as effective inspiratory pressure constancy as continuous flow CPAP systems during spontaneous breathing, if the inspiratory peak flow of the patient lies below 60 l/min. Yet it is necessary to adjust the inspiratory flow of the mandatory ventilatory pressure to the patient's needs with regard to peak flow and flow pattern.

The necessity to keep up spontaneous breathing with demand-flow-respirators without additional inspiratory work, even in critical phases of weaning, has led to the development of new methods for the support of spontaneous breathing.

Inspiratory Pressure Support

Another form of augmented spontaneous breathing, inspiratory pressure support (IPS), was introduced in 1982. With IPS, each inspiration of the patient is supported after triggering with an additional inspiratory flow until a preselected pressure difference is reached. Expiration remains passive and starts either after the IPS level has been exceeded by 1–3 cm H_2O (e.g. Servo C, Puritant Bennett 7200) or after the inspiratory flow has fallen below a certain level (Fig. 2). In some respirators this switch-over occurs when the inspiratory flow has sunk to 25% of the peak flow (Servo C, Intermed Bear 5, Hamilton Veolar, Bird 6400 ST, Dräger Evita), in others an absolute flow level between 2 and 6 l/min has been established as the end of inspiration (Puritan Bennett

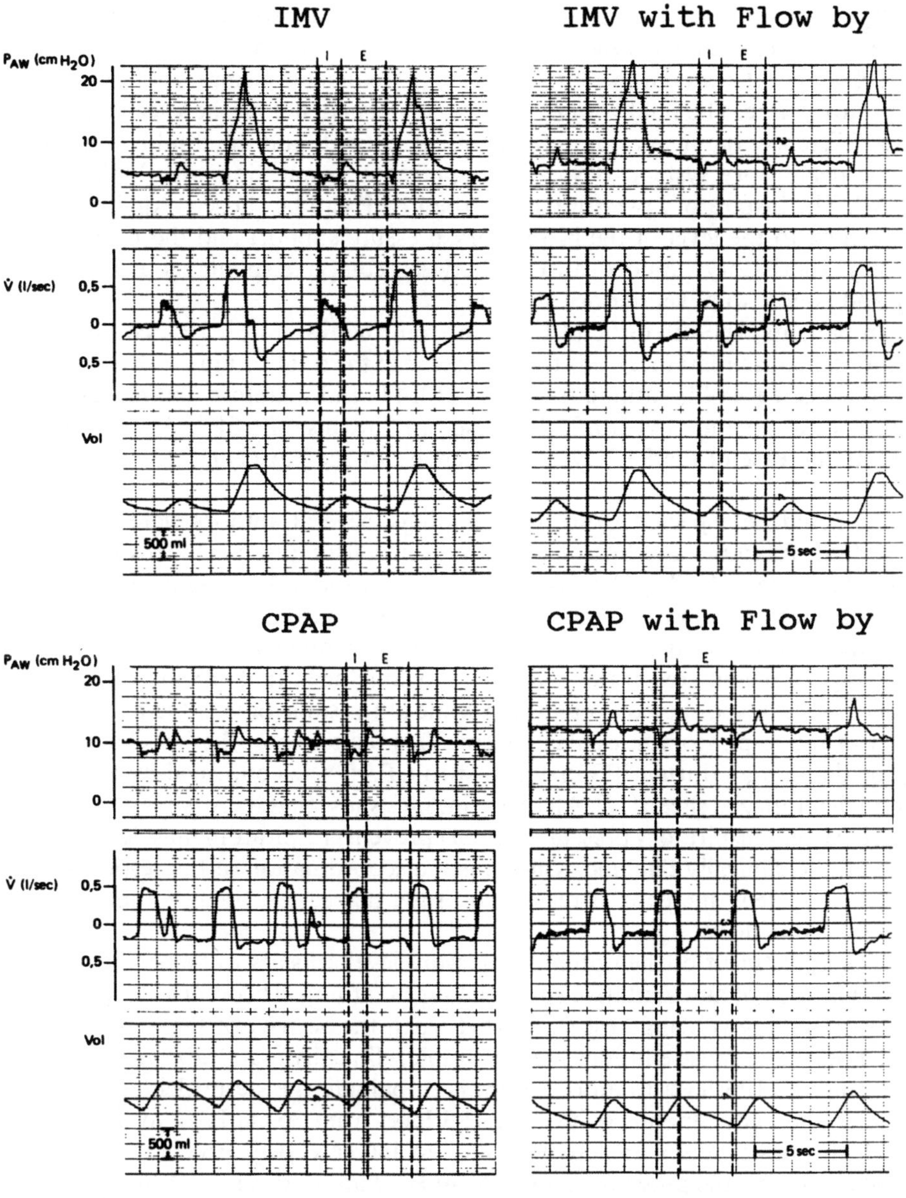

Fig. 2. Simultaneous respiratory pressure, respiratory flow, and volume recording (pneumotachograph) in a patient during IMV *(upper panel)* and CPAP *(lower panel)* with demand flow and with flow by. Puritan Bennett 7200. IMV frequency 5/min. PEEP 5 cm H_2O. Demand-flow: trigger sensitiveness 1 cm H_2O; flow by: basic flow 20 l/min, sensitiveness 1 l/sec. The recording was made between tube and Y-piece. While spontaneous breathing in the demand-flow mode *(left)* causes a decrease in pressure over the whole inspiratory phase with PEEP as well as during IMV and CPAP, the combination of IMV or CPAP with flow by *(right)* causes an initially almost similar but very brief decrease in airway pressure. In both cases an increase of pressure over PEEP can be noticed with the beginning of expiration

7200, Engström Erica, Ohmeda, Dräger Evita). This allows the patient to continue to inspire even when the preselected pressure level has been reached.

IPS allows the patient to control breathing frequency, inspiratory flow, and inspiratory time. The tidal volume changes in dependence on the selected pressure difference, the inspiratory efforts of the patient, and the total resistance of the respiratory system. IPS can be applied in connection with IMV and CPAP. The inspiratory pressure above the PEEP can be chosen individually. According to the level of the inspiratory pressure support and the IMV frequency, ventilatory support can vary between complete spontaneous breathing and almost total ventilatory support.

In patients who are difficult to wean from the respirator, IPS, compared to spontaneous breathing, leads to an increase of the tidal volume with a simultaneous decrease of breathing frequency [10, 11] and therefore diminishes the danger of a dynamic hyperinflation resp. an "intrinsic PEEP." At the same time an increase of the $PaCO_2$ and a decrease of the $PaCO_2$ [11,12] could be noticed.

As could be expected from these findings, several authors were able to show that IPS causes a reduction of the oxygen consumption in the respiratory muscular system [13–16]. Brochard et al. [11] proved a decrease of the transdiaphragmatic pressure and the diaphragmatic pressure–time index parallel to a decrease of the electric diaphragmatic activity among patients who were recovering from acute respiratory failure, and concluded that IPS increases the effectiveness of spontaneous breathing while at the same time reducing the activity of the respiratory muscular system. This reduction of the EMG activity of the diaphragm during IPS in contrast to CPAP was confirmed by a study on tracheotomized sheep [12]. All these findings show that there is every reason to believe that inspiratory pressure support prevents respiratory muscle fatigue with all the clinically tangible symptoms – discoordination of the respiratory muscular system, increase of respiration rate, decrease of tidal volume, and respiratory acidosis.

The adjustment of the optimum pressure level appears to be problematic with this form of augmentative spontaneous breathing. Theoretically, spontaneous breathing is being best supported when the activity of the diaphragm does not lead to muscle fatigue [17]. A simple, clinically practicable method of adjusting the IPS level to an optimum is to palpate the sternocleidomastoid muscles and simultaneous reduce the IPS level from 30 cm H_2O to the level at which phasic muscular activity seems to increase [18]. Brochard recommends adjusting the pressure support 5 cm H_2O above this level. With the occurrence of diaphragmatic fatigue there is an increase in the activity of the sternocleidomastoid muscles that can be recorded on the EMG, while during optimum pressure support only minimal activity is registered [19]. However, further studies on the optimum adjustment of pressure support remain to be seen.

Since IPS cuts down the apparatus-induced inspiratory work of breathing to that share that is determined by the trigger of the inspiratory valve (Fig. 3), and can furthermore eliminate the breathing work caused by the tube, the gen-

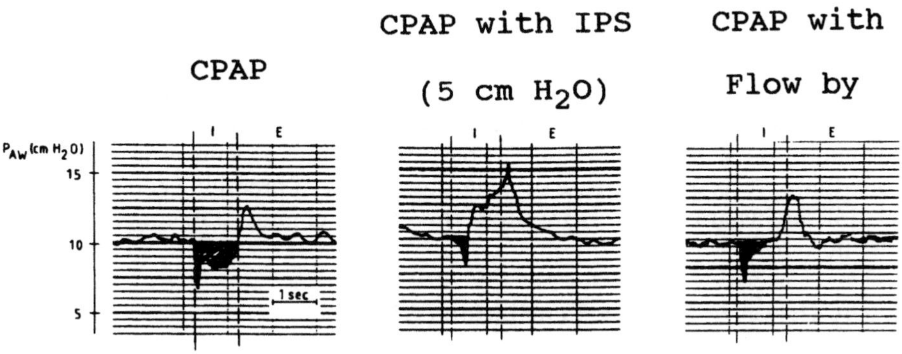

Fig. 3. Respiratory pressure recording in a patient during CPAP with demand-flow, with IPS (5 cm H_2O), and with flow by. Puritan Bennett. Trigger sensitiveness with demand-flow and IPS: 1 cm H_2O; flow by: basic flow 20 l/min, sensitiveness 1 l/sec. The recording was made between tube and Y-piece. While spontaneous breathing in the demand-flow mode causes a decrease in pressure with PEEP over the whole inspiratory phase, there is only a brief decrease in respiratory pressure caused by the trigger during IPS *(middle)*. CPAP in combination with flow by, in contrast to demand-flow CPAP, causes an initially similar but only brief inspiratory pressure decrease. The decrease in inspiratory pressure *(hatched area)* leads to a decrease in the functional residual capacity and the PaO_2 and to an increase in inspiratory work. CPAP in combination with IPS requires the least respiratory work

eral employment of an inspiratory pressure support of at least 3–5 cm H_2O during IMV as well as CPAP conditions seems to be sensible [20, 21].

"Flow By"

A further technical innovation, also with the aim of reducing inspiratory breathing work during spontaneous breathing, was introduced in 1986 – the "flow by" option of the Puritan Bennett 7200. "Flow by" allows a continuous, variably adjustable basic fresh gas flow between 5 and 20 l/min. The trigger mechanism here is not released through a decrease of pressure in the ventilatory system but through a gas flow inhaled by the patient; the sensitiveness of the trigger – the flow-sensitiveness – can be chosen between 1 and 10 l/min. When it is triggered, the apparatus should within 20 msec supply the gas flow that is immediately needed – which can amount to 180 l/min. With the beginning of the expiratory phase the basic flow is reduced to 5 l/min for 0.5 sec or for half the average time of the three previous expiratory phases. The "flow by" mode is possible during IMV as well as with CPAP, the combination of IPS and "flow by", however, is excluded for technical reasons.

Contrasting spontaneous breathing with demand-flow to spontaneous breathing with "flow by", the airway pressure decrease measured at the tube and caused by inspiration turns out to be less in the "flow by" mode (Fig. 2). While under the CPAP-conditions with "demand-valve" of the Bennett 7200 a pressure decrease under the PEEP-level can be stated over the whole inspiratory phase, the decrease of airway pressure in CPAP in combination with "flow by" is only short (Fig. 3).

Unanimously, Cox et al. found only a minimal temporal delay until the release of the gas flow required by spontaneously breathing patients under "flow by" conditions [19]; an initial decrease of airway pressure, however, was not proved. These observations allow the expectation that "flow by", in contrast to demand-flow without IPS, causes a reduction of the early inspiratory work of breathing. A further decrease of inspiratory work of breathing could be expected if the inspiratory pressure support could be employed in combination with "flow-by".

Airway Pressure Release Ventilation (APRV)

This form of ventilatory support is actually CPAP with intermittent pressure decrease. APRV was first described by Downs and Stock in 1987 [23, 24]. This method serves to support spontaneous breathing during CPAP for a better elimination of CO_2. The setup of an APRV-system resembles – but for an additional expiratory valve equipped with a timer – the continuous CPAP-system. When the timer opens this additional valve for about 1,5 sec, the airway pressure drops from the initial PEEP-level to a lower PEEP that can be adjusted through another valve (Fig. 4). The pressure decrease causes an addi-

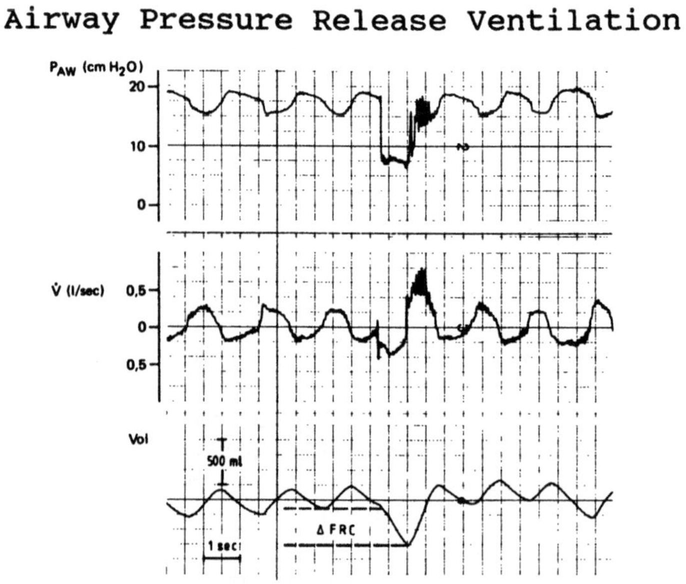

Fig. 4. Simultaneous respiratory pressure, respiratory flow, and volume recording (pneumotachograph) in a volunteer with a modified continuous flow CPAP system during airway pressure release ventilation. Flow 1.5 l/sec, elastic reservoir 2 l, PEEP 17.5 cm H_2O. The pressure decrease in the CPAP system from a higher to a lower PEEP level for about 1.5 s causes an increase in the expiratory flow as well as in the expiratory volume. In connection with this there follows a decrease in the functional residual capacity *(FRC)*. Due to the high continuous gas flow and the characteristics of the expiratory valve, the airway pressure increases distinctly during expiration

tional expiration and therefore CO_2 is expirated. As soon as the additional expiratory valve closes, the airway pressure, due to the high system gas flow (approx. 100 l/min), quickly increases to the former PEEP-level, comparable to a mechanical breath. The extent of the additional CO_2 elimination is dependent on the duration as well as on the frequency of the pressure decrease.

In this method of augmentative ventilation the average airway pressures are equivalent to those in mechanical ventilation but with the advantage that the peak pressures exceed the average airway pressure only little and the danger of a barotrauma is probably reduced [25]. As the airway pressure never exceeds the PEEP-level this method can also be used on patients who are not intubated by using a mask [26].

However, so far there are only few reports on APRV, a clinical multi-center study on the use of this method for patients with a moderate acute respiratory failure is being conducted at the moment. It remains to be seen which rank APRV will occupy in a future strategy of ventilation.

Total Ventilatory Support

Differential Lung Ventilation

Through the introduction of double-lumen tracheotomy tubes at the beginning of 1986 differential ventilation was reevaluated. This method is used either pronounced unilateral or bilateral lung disease to improve the ventilation–perfusion ratio.

While standard ventilation through a normal endobronchial tube can, in unilateral lung disease with different lung compliances, lead to hyperdistension of the side not afflicted and to alveolar collapse of the afflicted side, selective intubation of the main bronchi allows ventilation of both lungs according to their compliance with different tidal volumes and "selective" PEEP. Differential ventilation can be applied synchronously or asynchronously. Most clinicians favor two synchronously working respirators. The distribution of the tidal volume between the two lungs and a selective PEEP seem to be more important in relation to the success of this ventilation technique than the manner of the technical realization. Usually both lungs are ventilated with an identical tidal volume because it has been shown in animal tests that identical tidal volumes – compared to differential tidal volumes, which led to identical end-expiratory CO_2 and airway pressure – produce the best oxygenation [27–29]. The effectiveness and the therapeutic success of this method can be calculated by means of the end-expiratory CO_2 and CO_2 elimination measured separately.

If the indication for differential lung ventilation is given on the strength of asymmetrical bilateral lung disease, the PEEP is increased on the basal side and at the same time contralaterally reduced in the lateral position. In this way the ventilation–perfusion ratio and the PaO_2 are improved through increased ventilation of the lower well-perfused lung and increased vascularity in the better ventilated upper lung with cardiac output constant [28].

In addition to unilateral injury of the lung through contusion, aspiration, edema, embolism, therapy-refractory atelectasis, pneumonia, and bilateral asymmetric lung diseases, the treatment of bronchopleural fistulas counts among the indications for differential lung ventilation [31]. Here it is possible not to ventilate the lung with the bronchopleural fistula but to keep it inflated with CPAP. The PEEP should be adjusted just under the critical opening point of the fistula while the contralateral lung is ventilated conventionally.

Prone Position

In the therapy of the adult respiratory distress syndrome (ARDS), moving the patient from the supine to the prone position can be tried as an additional possibility to improve the PaO_2 [33]. Although this has been performed in two small retrospective studies [34, 35] with 11 patients altogether on 10 of whom it was successful so far little use has been made of this possibility in the therapy of ARDS.

Recent CT studies on ARDS patients show that compression atelectasis is often seen in the form of distinct condensations in posterobasal lung sections [36, 37]. In these cases a change of position from supine to prone can sometimes lead to an improvement in the ventilation–perfusion ratio and an equivalent increase of the PaO_2. In a prospective study by Langer et al. the gas exchange and the hemodynamics of 13 patients with moderate to severe ARDS were analyzed before, during, and after a 2-h period in the prone position [38]. Eight of the patients responded with a significant increase in the PaO_2, while in five the PaO_2 did not change. On two patients computer tomography of the lung was conducted before and after the prone position. Both patients showed dissolution of the posterobasal densities in the prone position, while at the same time new densities appeared in the anterior region. In animal studies it could be proved that the increase in PaO_2 in the prone position cannot be attributed to a change in cardiac output, pulmonary arterial pressures, or the functional residual capacity [39].

As a result of these studies it can be recommended that patients suffering from ARDS with impaired arterial oxygenation ($FIO_2 > 0.5$, PEEP > 5 cm H_2O) and possible posterobasal compression atelectasis should be brought into the prone position at least for a test period. If PaO_2 increases this could have a positive influence on outcome, if the PaO_2 does not improve or deteriorates, conventional therapy should be continued.

References

1. Downs JB, Klein EF et al. (1973) Intermittent mandatory ventilation: a new approach to weaning patients from mechanical ventilators. Chest 64:331–335
2. Weisman IM, Rinaldo JE, Rogers RM, Saunders MH (1983) State of the art: Intermittent mandatory ventilation. Am Rev Resp Dis 127:641–647
3. Steinhoff H, Falke K, Schwarzhoff W (1982) Enhanced renal function associated with intermittent mandatory ventilation in acute respiratory failure. Intensive Care Med 8:69–74

4. Steinhoff H, Kohlhoff RJ, Falke K (1984) Facilitation of excretory function and hemodynamics of the kidneys by intermittent mandatory ventilation. Intensive Care Med 10:59–64
5. Lemaire F, Teboul JL et al. (1988) Acute left ventricular dysfunction during unsuccessful weaning from mechanical ventilation. Anesthesiology 69:171–179
6. Christopher KL, Neff TA et al. (1985) Demand and continous flow intermittent mandatory ventilation systems. Chest 87:625–630
7. Schlobohm RM, Falltrick RT et al. (1981) Lung volumes, mechanics, and oxygenation during spontaneous positive pressure ventilation: the advantage of CPAP over EPAP. Anesthesiology 55:416–422
8. Gherini S, Peters R, Virgilio R (1979) Mechanical work on the lungs and work of breathing with positive end-expiratory pressure and continuous positive airway pressure. Chest 76:251–256
9. Samodelov LF, Falke K (1988) Total inspiratory work with modern demand valve devices compared to continous flow CPAP. Intensive Care Med 14:632–639
10. MacIntyre NR (1986) Respiratory function during pressure support ventilation. Chest 89:677–683
11. Brochard L, Pluskwa F, Lemaire F (1987) Improved efficacy of spontaneous breathing with inspiratory pressure support. Am Rev Respir Dis 136:411–415
12. Kacmarek RM, Torres A et al. (1988) Diaphragmatic function during pressure support ventilation and CPAP in the adult sheep. Int. symposium: Inspiratory muscle function during partial ventilatory support. Abstract Tutzing
13. Kanak R, Fahey P, Vanderwarf C (1985) Oxygen cost of breathing: changes dependent upon mode of mechanical ventilation. Chest 87:126–127
14. Brochard L, Harf A, Lorino H, Lemaire F (1987) Pressure support decreases work of breathing and oxygen consumption during weaning from mechanical ventilation. Am Rev Respir Dis 135:A51
15. Viale JP, Annat GJ et al. (1988) Pressure support ventilation vs continuous positive airway pressure. Chest 93:506–509
16. Viale JP, Annat GJ et al. (1988) Oxygen cost of breathing during inspiratory pressure support ventilation. Int. symposium: Inspiratory muscle function during partial ventilatory support. Abstract Tutzing
17. Brochard L, Harf A, Lorino H, Lemaire F (1987) Optimum level of pressure support in patients with unsuccessful weaning from mechanical ventilation. Am Rev Resp Dis 135:A51
18. Brochard L, Lemaire F (1988) Inspiratory pressure support. Update in intensive care and emergency medicine, 767–771 Bd 5. Springer, edited by JC Vincent
19. Brochard L, Harf A et al. (1988) Prevention of diaphragmatic fatigue with inspiratory pressure support during weaning from mechanical ventilation. Int. symposium: Inspiratory muscle function during partial ventilatory support. Abstract Tutzing
20. Kacmarek RM (1988) The role of pressure support ventilation in reducing work of breathing. Respir Care 33:99–120
21. Falke K (1988) Intermittent mandatory ventilation: revisited. Update in intensive care and emergency medicine, 759–766 Bd 5. Springer, edited by JC Vincent
22. Cox D, Tinloi SF, Farrimond JG (1988) Investigation of the spontaneous modes of breathing of different ventilators. Intensive Care Med 14:532–537
23. Down JB, Stock C (1987) Airway pressure release ventilation: a new concept in ventilatory support. Editorial. Crit Care Med 15:459–461
24. Stock C, Downs JB, Frolicher D (1987) Airway pressure release ventilation. Crit Care Med 15:462–466
25. Garner W, Downs JB, Stock MC, Räsänen J (1988) Airway pressure release ventilation. Chest 94:779–781
26. Jousela IT, Nikki P, Tahvanainen J (1988) Airway pressure release ventilation by mask. Crit Care Med 16:1250–1251

27. East TD, Pace L et al. (1983) Differential lung ventilation with unilateral PEEP following unilateral hydrochloric acid aspiration in the dog. Acta Anaesthesiol Scand 27:356–360
28. Baehrendtz S, Hedenstierna G (1984) Differential ventilation and selective positive endexpiratory pressure: effects on patients with acute bilateral lung disease. Anesthesiology 61:511–517
29. Hedenstierna G, Baehrendtz S et al. (1984) Differential ventilation in acute respiratory failure. Indications and outcome. Bull Eur Physiopathol Respir 21:281–285
30. Zandstra DF, Stoutenbeek ChP (1988) Monitoring differential CO_2 excretion during differential lung ventilation in asymmetric pulmonary contusion. Clinical implications. Intensive Care Med 14:106–109
31. Rafferty TD, Palma J et al. (1980) Management of a bronchopleural fistula with differential lung ventilation and PEEP. Respir Care 25:654–657
32. Dantzker DR, Wagner PD, West JB (1975) Instability of lung units with low VA/Q ratios during O2 breathing. J Appl Physiol 38:886
33. Bryan AC (1974) Comments of a devil's advocate. Am Rev Respir Dis 110 [Suppl]:143–144
34. Phiel MA, Brown RS (1976) Use of extreme position changes in acute respiratory failure. Crit Care Med 4:13–14
35. Douglas WW, Rehder K et al. (1977) Improved oxygenation in patients with acute respiratory failure: the prone position. Am Rev Respir Dis 115:559–566
36. Gattinoni L, Mascheroni D et al. (1986) Morphological and functional changes induced by PEEP in ARF. Intensive Care Med 12:136–142
37. Maunder RJ, Shuman WP et al. (1986) Preservation of normal lung region in the adult respiratory distress syndrome: analysis by computed tomography. JAMA 255:2463–2466
38. Langer M, Mascheroni D, Marcolin R, Gattinoni L (1988) The prone position in ARDS patients. Chest 94:103–107
39. Albert RK, Leasa D et al. (1987) The prone position improves arterial oxygenation and reduces shunt in oleic-acid-induced acute lung injury. Am Rev Respir Dis 136:628–633

Principles and Present Role of Extracorporal Elimination of CO_2 in the Therapy of Respiratory Failure

H. Lennartz

Introduction

Adult respiratory distress syndrome (ARDS), defined by Ashbaugh et al. [1] as an acute arterial hypoxia, has a high mortality. In the NIH study [8] in the early 1970s mortality was 80%–90%, and in the most recent European study by Artigas [3], for patients in Morel's stages III–IV [7], the percentage is 70%. In this study we discuss ARDS patients in stages III and IV. Death, however, is not only caused by ARDS but also by the basic disease. The lungs of patients with severe progressive ARDS, i.e., with ARDS developing continuously for days or even weeks, show disturbances of ventilation and perfusion that are not only regionally distributed. They range from ventilated nonperfused to perfused nonventilated alveolar regions without fixed boundaries.

Disturbances of the ventilatory process reach the same degree as in the ventilatory-perfusory process. Finally, they even cannot be suppressed by changing the method of ventilation. In these patients, continued aggressive ventilation with continuously growing pressure and necessarily increasing forced inspiratory oxygen (FiO_2) causes barotrauma, right heart failure, and hepatonephritic failure.

Numerous therapeutic devices such as interventions into the prostaglandin metabolism and administration of antioxidants have failed to influence mortality among these patients. Earlier efforts to improve their prognosis by extracorporeal membrane oxygenation (ECMO) must also be regarded as failures after the ECMO study by Zapol [9]. In the same way, expectations concerning high-frequency ventilation and jet ventilation have been disappointed.

Patients and Method

Extracorporeal elimination of CO_2 by a partial venovenous bypass corresponding to the method introduced by Kolobow et al. [6] was applied by us in 50 patients aged 5–51 years. All patients had ARDS stage IV (Morel's classification [7]; Table 1) which had developed continuously for 6–14 days on average under progressive ventilation therapy. In all patients, X-rays and thoracic CT scans revealed infiltrations relating to an infection and pneumothoraces to different degrees, interstitial accumulations of air, and so-called lung hernias as signs of severe barotrauma (Fig. 1).

Table 1. Degrees of severity of ARDS in 50 patients (classification according to Morel [7]

Stage	X-ray findings	$AaDO_2F_1O_2$ [a] (mmHg)	C_T (ml/cmH_2O)	MPAP (mmHg)
1	Low-grade symptoms of interstitial edema	300–375	70–80	20–25
2	Clear symptoms of interstitial edema	375–450	50–70	25–30
3	Patchy infiltrations	450–525	30–50	30–35
4	Extensive infiltrations	>525	<30	>35

[a] PEEP >5 cm H_2O

Own patients	In all cases extensive infiltrations	559	27	36

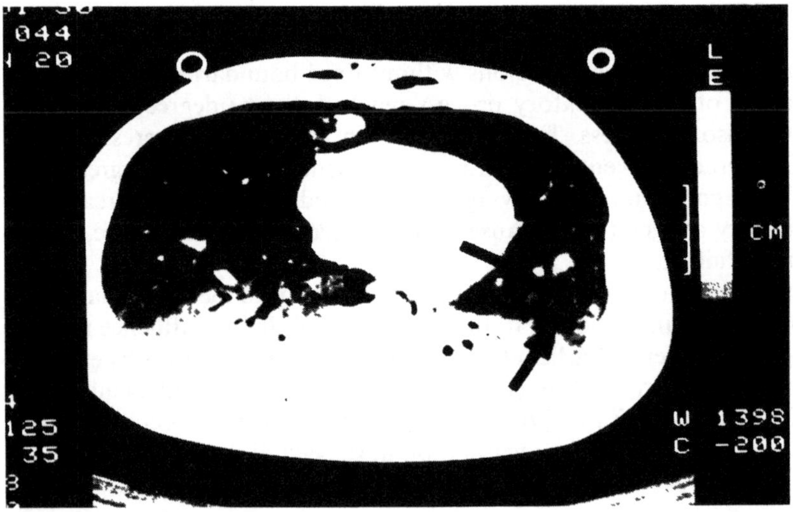

Fig. 1. Thoracic CT of a patient suffering from ARDS. Note interstitial accumulation of air *(arrows)*

All patients were treated for 12–24 h by conventional ventilation with all assisting measures. In spite of all means of therapeutic assistances, i.e., inverse ratio ventilation (IVR), inversed-ratio ventilation, higher positive end-expiratory pressure (PEEP), hemodynamic stabilization, and excessive cleaning of the respiratory tract, together with dehydrating measures, there was no significant improvement in the status of any patient.

The indications (Table 2) used in the patients treated upto now were established strictly according to the quick or slow entry criteria of the ECMO study

Table 2. Indication for $ECCO_2$-R and LFPPV

$PaO_2 < 70$ mmHg bei FiO_2 1.0 and/or positive pressure respiration > 50 cm H_2O	
at	
PEEP	10 cm H_2O
I:E	1:1
AF>	15
AMV>	15 ml/kg
If after 24 h no improvement under differentiated respiration with: PEEP-increase change of I:E 2:1 or simultaneously positive pressure respiration > 50 cm H_2O or simultaneously $S_VO_2 < 60\%$	

LFPPV,
PEEP = Positive endexpiratory pressure

[9]. Arterial hypoxia takes first place in the list of indications. Contraindications for extracorporeal elimination of CO_2 include:

1. Craniocerebral trauma with fresh intracerebral bleeding
2. Acute bleeding
3. Hypoxic cerebral damage
4. Long-term obstructive disease of the respiratory tract in its final stage
5. Large parenchymatous fistula
6. Progressive fibrosis
7. Cardiac lung edema
8. Infaust carcinoma disease
9. Immunosuppression including AIDS
10. Age over 65 years

Results

Of 50 patients treated with extracorporeal elimination of CO_2 27 survived. Thirty-three of the 50 have so far been evaluated with regard to duration of previous respiration, $AaDO_2$ (alveolar-arterial O_2 tension difference), extravascular lung water, PIF (aggressiveness of respirator treatment by PIF-Index from Benzer), shunt, respiratory mean pressure, and pulmonary arterial pressure (Fig. 2). We found 24 responders and 9 nonresponders among the 33 patients. There were no statistical differences between the responders and nonresponders with regard to the measured values. We therefore employed a step-by-step multiple discrimination analysis with about 15 variables in gas exchange and hemodynamics.

By summing all factors we succeeded in developing a system of equations that divides patients into responders and nonresponders. The accuracy of the Jackknife classification in dividing the patients was stable at 93.1% (Fig. 3). This result demonstrates that before beginning extracorporeal elimination of

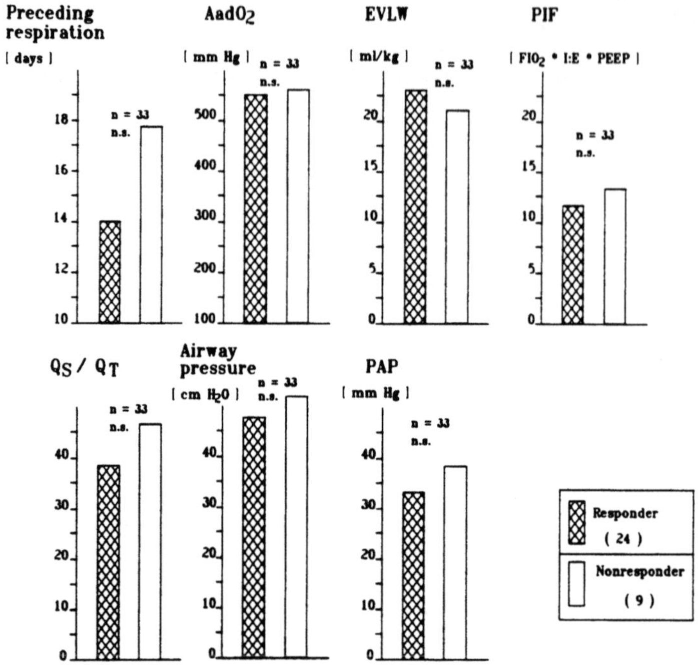

Fig. 2. Respiratory variables (extravascular lung water, oxygenation, and hemodynamics) of responders and nonresponders before treatment with extracorporeal elimination of CO_2

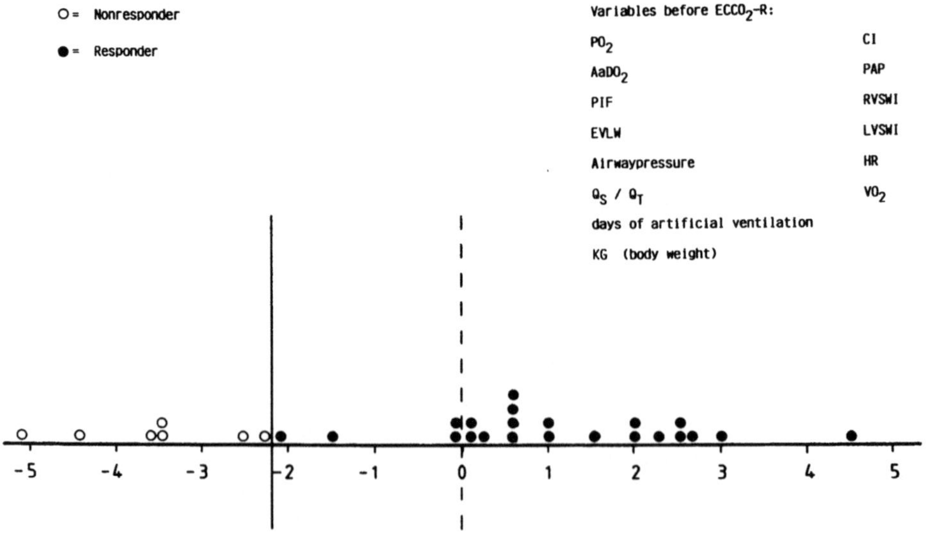

Fig. 3. Jackknife classification (93.1% accurate)

'able 3. Procollagen III peptide in the serum of patients suffering rom ARDS

Name	Before $ECCO_2$-R (ng/µl)	After $ECCO_2$-R (ng/µl)
Responders		
M. K. ♀	194	37
J. S. ♂	204	28
S. D. ♀	180	20
H. M. ♂	166	21
M. F. ♀	8	21
I. R. ♀	180	38
Nonresponders		
S. K. ♀	204	204
A. d. P. ♀	94	130

$ECCO_2$-R, extracorporeal elimination (removal) of CO_2

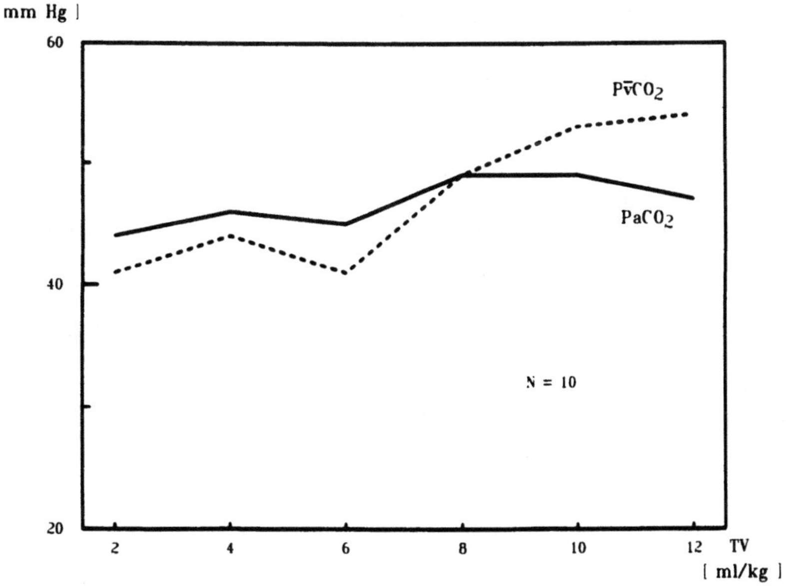

'ig. 4. Inverse reaction of $P\bar{v}CO_2$ and $PaCO_2$ relative to dependence on tidal volume

O_2 we are able, by means of this equation, to separate responders from non-sponders almost perfectly.

The data we had collected before the treatment were evaluated by a com-uter program, and with one exception all patients were separated into re-ponders or nonresponders. This proves that it is not gas exchange alone that etermines a patient's prognosis, but the combination of gas exchange and he-odynamics.

During the treatment the responders showed a clear reduction of $AaDO_2$, ulmonary arterial mean pressure, and shunt, and an increase of compliance as well as a normalization of the previously increased extravascular lung water. In eight patients we examined the procollagen III peptide as an indicator of "progressive fibrosis of the lung" in the responders we found a clear reduction of this peptide, which had previously been pathologically increased (Table 3).

When we started the extracorporeal venovenous bypass, the pulmonary arterial values of PCO_2 were lower in all patients than the arterial values of PCO_2 in relation to the inspiratory volume. This inverse proportion of $P\bar{v}CO_2$ and $PaCO_2$ during extracorporeal elimination of CO_2 and low frequency positive pressure ventilation was evaluated in ten patients (Fig. 4).We found progressive reduction of PEEP during the treatment and augmentation of inspiratory volume together with an obvious normalization of $P\bar{v}CO_2$ and $PaCO_2$, i.e., $P\bar{v}CO_2$ again surpasses $PaCO_2$.

Discussion

Kolobow et al. [6] having experimentally demonstrated the dissociation of the respiratory function in animals, formulated the concept of apneic oxygenation in extracorporeal elimination of CO_2 and low frequency positive pressure ventilation. He demonstrated that ventilation is not necessary to maintain a normal oxygen partial pressure, if only a quantity of oxygen corresponding to the oxygen required is delivered by a bronchoalveolar oxygen supply and pulmonary blood flow is normal. The ventilation, that is, the removal of the CO_2 proceeding from the metabolism, can then be performed by a venovenous bypass and a membrane lung that may be hyperventilated if necessary. There is no restriction of pulmonary blood flow. The reaction of $P\bar{v}CO_2$ and $PaCO_2$ during extracorporeal elimination of CO_2 and the ventilation diagram (Fig. 5) prove that the method we applied is in fact an apneic oxygenation.

The effect observed is the Christiansen-Douglas-Haldane (CDH) effect which was recently outlined experimentally under clinical conditions by

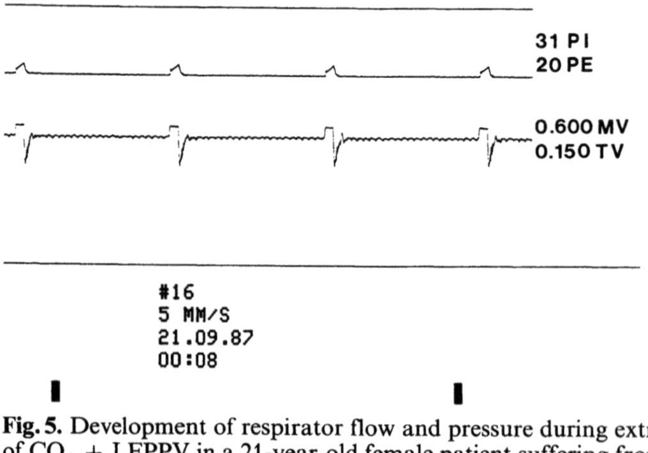

Fig. 5. Development of respirator flow and pressure during extracorporeal elimination of CO_2 + LFPPV in a 21-year-old female patient suffering from ARDS

Table 4. Comparison of ECMO [9] and $ECCO_2$-R [4]

ECMO	$ECCO_2$-R
Purpose of treatment	
Short-term overcoming of oxygenation and reduction of FiO_2	Long-term lung rest and reduction of positive respiration pressure and FiO_2 but apneic oxygenation by the affected lung
Extracorporeal circulation	
Venoarterial for oxygenation of the arterial blood. Substitution of the oxygenation	Venovenous to eliminate CO_2 Substitution of ventilation
Respiration	
Conventional CPPV Frequency: 8–15, maximum pressure 50 cm H_2O, PEEP: 5–10 cm H_2O	LFPPV, Frequency: 2–4 Maximum pressure: 35–40 cm H_2O PEEP: 20–30 cm H_2O
Bypass flow	
3–6 l/min	30% of cardiac output 1.5–2.5 l/min
Haemodynamics	
Influenced by the venoarterial bypass	Not influenced
Lung blood flow	
1/10–1/5 of cardiac output	100% of cardiac output, increase of mixed-venous O_2 saturation
Duration	
2–10 days	Up to 25 days
Success	
Ca. 10% under comparable indications	Ca. 50% under comparable indications

CPPV, continuous positive pressure ventilation

Brandt [2] and his team. In the unphysiological situation of a closed system, resembling the situation of hyperoxic apnea, i.e., reception of O_2 and lack of elimination of CO_2, the arterial partial pressure can not only reach the mixed-venous value but can even surpass it. The graph of CO_2 absorption shifts to the right. This is the CDH effect. The resulting increase of PCO_2 causes a difference between the arterial and the mixed-venous PCO_2 of 2–3 mmHg.

The method of extracorporeal elimination of CO_2 with low frequency positive pressure ventilation, which was developed by Kolobow et al. [6], differs from the ECMO principle in a number of respects (Table 4). The aim of ECMO is to overcome the breakdown of arterial oxygenation and with it the reduction of FiO_2 at the respirator. Extracorporeal elimination of CO_2, however, rests the lung and reverses the therapeutic principle from high frequency respirator ventilation and ventilation by high pressure to low frequency ventilation with reduced pressure. In contrast to ECMO, CO_2 elimination is characterized by a venovenous bypass with low blood flow and high gas flow, i.e.,

Table 5. Saturation of mixed venous blood (SvO_2) – before and during treatment with ECMO and $ECCO_2$-R (%)

ECMO (from [5])		
Before	During	*n*
56	55	10
$ECCO_2$-R (own results)		
Before	During	*n*
56.7	79.8	10

high ventilation – perfusion ratio in the membrane lungs. The adjustment of the respirator during the extracorporeal bypass is therefore exactly opposite in the two methods. Applying ECMO means maintaining the respirator therapy, whereas applying extracorporeal elimination of CO_2 with low frequency positive pressure ventilation and apneic oxygenation means only inflating the lung by the respirator at a PEEP level of 20–30 cm H_2O. Unlike the venoarterial bypass, the low-ranging venovenous bypass flow does not interfere with the hemodynamics (Table 5).

It is true that pulmonary arterial pressure is reduced by ECMO, but this is caused not only by the clearly reduced cardiac output but also by the decrease of pulmonary blood circulation to one-fifth or one-tenth of its normal level. In contrast, maintaining blood circulation in the affected organ together with increased mixed-venous oxygen saturation must be regarded as the leading therapeutic principle of extracorporeal elimination of CO_2. ECMO is largely seen as a short-term therapy, whereas we were able to treat a patient for 25 days successfully with extracorporeal elimination of CO_2 + LFPPV (Low Frequency Positive Pressure Ventilation). In our opinion, the reduction of mortality in patients with severe progressive ARDS to below 50% worldwide answers the question of whether this method will influence the survival of patients with progressive ARDS in stage IV [7]. This means that for these patients extracorporeal elimination of CO_2 is superior to any form of respiratory treatment. With regard to future improvements, extracorporeal elimination of CO_2 has to be applied earlier to effect a further reduction of mortality. However, first the question must be answered whether in Morel's stage III extracorporeal elimination of CO_2 is superior to conventional respiration. To answer this question, a controlled randomized study is needed and can be ethically justified. Its projected principles are as follows:

Patients with ARDS, Morel's stage III, are admitted to clinical treatment (Fig. 6). The therapy is composed of inverse-ratio ventilation, invasive monitoring including measurement of compliance and thoracic CT, and 24-h intensive treatment.

Patients who are improving, i.e., patients on conventional treatment progressing from Morel stage III to Morel stage II continue to receive conven-

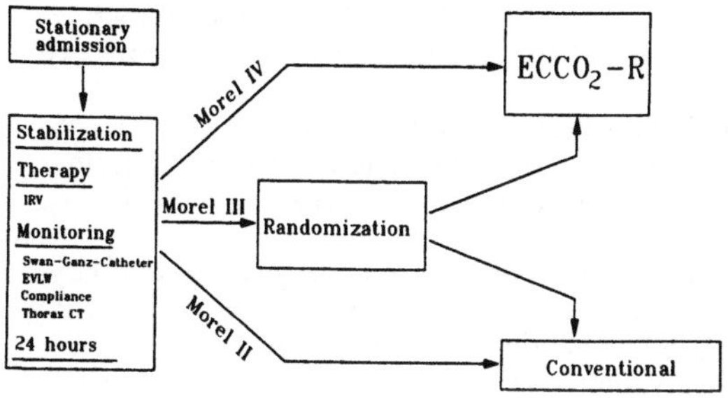

Fig. 6. Diagram of the treatment of patients with progressive ARDS classified according to Morel. *$ECCO_2$-R*, extracorporeal elimination (removal) of CO_2

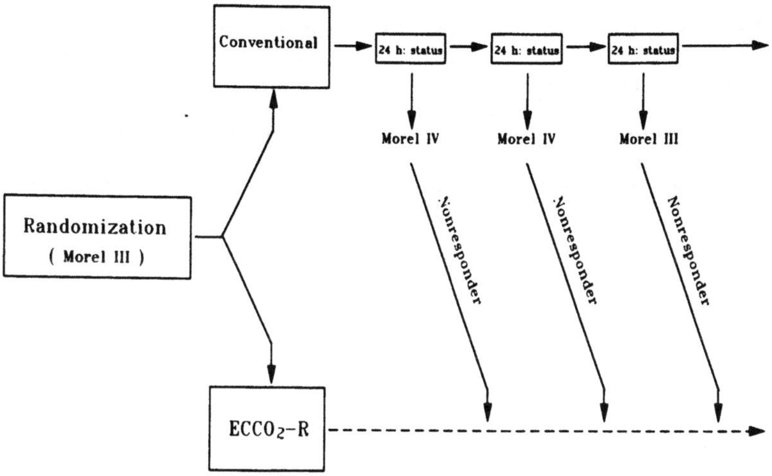

Fig. 7. Diagram of randomization and treatment

tional treatment. Patients whose condition is deteriorating, i.e., developing from Morel stage III to Morel stage IV, at once undergo extracorporeal elimination of CO_2. Patients remaining in Morel stage III are randomized (Fig. 7). The patients treated conventionally are tested every 24 h for 3 days. Those who deteriorate within the first 24–48 h are designated nonresponders to conventional therapy and subjected to extracorporeal elimination of CO_2. Patients still in Morel stage III after 72 h are also classified as nonresponders to conventional therapy and subjected to extracorporeal elimination of CO_2.

Our results to date do not allow us, for ethical reasons, to undertake a controlled randomized study using the above-listed criteria in patients in Morel stage IV.

References

1. Ashbaugh DG, Bigelow DB, Petty TL, Levine BE (1967) Acute respiratory distress in adults. Lancet II:319–333
2. Brandt L, Mertzlufft FO, Rudolf B, Dick W (1988) In-vivo-Nachweis des Christiansen-Douglas-Haldane-Effektes unter klinischen Bedingungen. Anaesthesist 37:529–534

3. European ARDS Collaborative Working Group (1988) Adult respiratory distress syndrome (ARDS). Clinical predictors, pronostic factors and outcome. Intensive Care Med 14 [Suppl 1]:300
4. Gattinoni L, Agostoni A, Pesenti A, Pelizzola A, Rossi G, Langer M, Vesconti S, Uziel L, Fox U, Longoni F, Kolobow T (1980) Treatment of acute respiratory failure with low frequency positive-pressure ventilation and extracorporeal removal of CO_2. Lancet II:29
5. Jardin F (1979) Pulmonary hemodynamics and gas exchange during venoarterial bypass with membrane–lung oxygenation. In: Unger, Regnier B, Gastine H, Lemaire F (eds) Assisted circulation. Springer, Berlin Heidelberg New York
6. Kolobow T, Gattinoni L, Tomlinson TA, Pierce JE (1977) Laboratory report. Control of breathing using an extracorporeal membrane lung. Anaesthesiology 46:138–141
7. Morel DR, Dargent F, Bachmann M, Suter PM, Junod AF (1985) Pulmonary extraction of serotonin and propranolol in patients with adult respiratory distress syndrome. Am Rev Respir Dis 132:479
8. National Heart Lung and Blood Institute. Division of Lung Diseases (1970) Extracorporeal support for respiratory insufficiency: a collaborative study. Nahonal Institute of Health, Bethesda
9. Zapol WM, Snider MT, Hill JD (1979) Extracorporeal membrane oxygenation in severe acute respiratory failure. JAMA 242:2193

Extracorporeal Oxygen Delivery and Life Support in Neonatal Respiratory Failure

R. H. Bartlett

Introduction

Most of the variables which influence oxygen delivery and oxygen consumption are controlled during extracorporeal circulation, hence it is appropriate to include this topic in the Steglitz Symposium. In fact, extracorporeal circulation is an exercise in applied physiology of oxygen kinetics. Whether in the laboratory or at the bedside the physiologist or physician can address problems which can not be solved in any other way. Prolonged extracorporeal circulation has been described by the acronym ECMO (extracorporeal membrane oxygenation), but this represents only one of the variables. Extracorporeal life support (ECLS) is a better term, describing oxygen exchange, CO_2 exchange, perfusion, and temperature control.

The technique of extracorporeal life support has been most successful in newborn infants with severe respiratory failure. During the past 5 years this technique has grown from a clinical research curiosity practiced in a few research institutions to the standard method of treatment for severe newborn respiratory failure, offered in more than 50 centers throughout the world. Experienced centers regularly report 95% survival in a group of patients who are considered moribund when ECLS is begun. Understanding and control of oxygen delivery kinetics is central to the success of this procedure.

Physiology of Extracorporeal Life Support

Most of the experience with neonatal ECLS has used venoarterial cardiopulmonary bypass. That is, venous blood is drained from the right atrium, through the extracorporeal circuit including a membrane lung, and reinfused into the aortic arch. It is possible to collect all the venous return in the drainage catheter, constituting total venoarterial bypass as is practiced during cardiac surgery. However, the technique is usually conducted as partial venoarterial bypass, taking 50% to 80% of the venous return into the drainage catheter. The amount of venous drainage is determined by the amount of support required; the extracorporeal flow rate is regulated to the minimum level which will support gas exchange and perfusion. Extracorporeal flow is balanced against normal flow through the right ventricle and pulmonary artery. If the lung is not functioning at all then 80% or more of the venous return must be diverted through the extracorporeal circuit. As lung function improves the

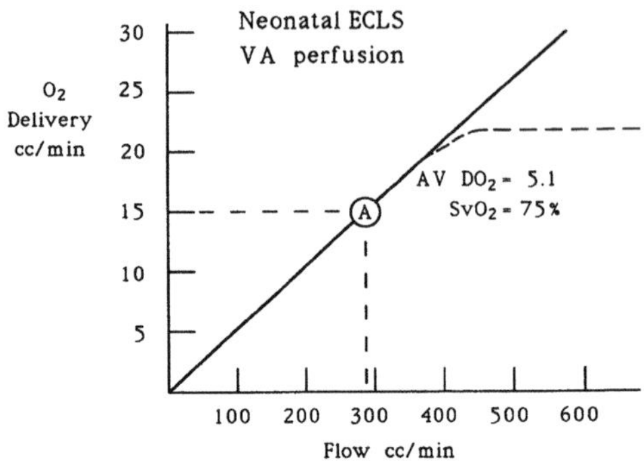

Fig. 1. Oxygen delivery through the extracorporeal circuit is controlled by venous blood characteristics and blood flow. In this example hemoglobin is 15 g per deciliter and the venous blood saturation is 75%. Point *A* identifies a typical newborn with 15 cc/min oxygen requirement. The *dotted line* identifies the rated flow for a membrane lung capable of 22 cc/O_2 transfer per min

amount of extracorporeal flow can be decreased. The amount of oxygen that can be supplied through the extracorporeal circuit is a function of the flow, hemoglobin concentration, and saturation of the venous blood.

Obviously the membrane lung can do no more than fully saturate the flowing blood, hence the amount of oxygen that can be added per minute can be calculated as the difference in oxygen content from the inlet to the outlet of the membrane lung times the blood flow. A typical example is shown in Fig. 1. In this example the hemoglobin concentration is 15 g per deciliter and the venous blood is 75% saturated with oxygen. Therefore, the venous (oxygenator inlet) oxygen content is 15.3 cc/O_2 per deciliter, and the arterial (oxygenator outlet) oxygen content is 20.4 cc/O_2 per deciliter, discounting the small amount of extra oxygen dissolved in plasma. Thus, the amount of oxygen that can be delivered to the patient each minute is a function of blood flow, as shown in Fig. 1. The oxygen requirement for a 3 kg newborn at rest is 15 cc/min, which would require 300 cc/min of blood flow. Oxygen delivery could be increased by increasing blood flow, or by increasing hemoglobin concentration, or by decreasing venous saturation. If, for example, oxygen consumption increased to 20 cc/min because of muscular activity or catecholamine effect, venous saturation would drop to approximately 50%, and the arterial venous oxygen content difference would increase to 10.2 cc/O_2 per deciliter. The ECLS operator could improve oxygen delivery by increasing blood flow, or increasing hemoglobin. Or the operator could decrease oxygen consumption by paralyzing or cooling the patient.

The oxygen transfer characteristics of the membrane lung are limited by the membrane surface area. Suppose that the membrane lung had a maximal oxygen transfer of 16 cc/min. In the example given, increasing flow or hemoglobin could not increase oxygen delivery to 20 cc/min, and a larger membrane lung would be required. In practice membrane lungs are used which are large enough to permit oxygen transfer more than twice the resting metabolic rate

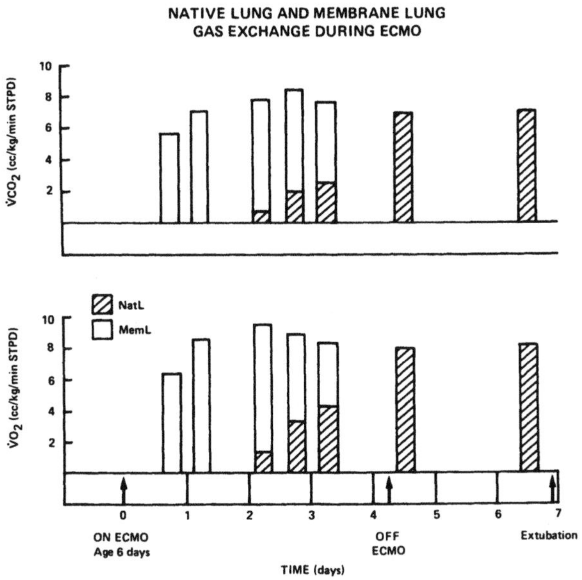

Fig. 2. Oxygen uptake across the native lung compared with the extracorporeal lung during a typical case of VA neonatal ECLS. (From Cilley et al. [28] with permission)

of the patient. This surface area related oxygen transfer limitation is usually described in terms of the amount of venous blood which can be fully saturated by the membrane lung. For example, as shown by the dotted line in Fig. 1, a membrane lung which is limited to 22 cc of oxygen transfer per minute has a rated flow of 440 cc/min of venous blood.

Although oxygen uptake is limited by the amount of unsaturated hemoglobin, CO_2 elimination is limited only by the gradient between the venous blood PCO_2 and the ventilating gas. CO_2 elimination is always more efficient than oxygenation during extracorporeal circulation. Since this gradient is relatively constant at about 45 torr, the amount of CO_2 elimination is essentially a function of the membrane lung surface area. Therefore, if ECLS is conducted with the sole intent of removing carbon dioxide (as advocated by Kolobow et al. [1] and Gattinoni et al. [2]), then extracorporeal circulation can be conducted at relatively low blood flow using a very large membrane lung surface area. This technique has been very successful in adult patients who retain most of the ability to oxygenate blood via the native lung. However, in newborn infants the lung usually goes through a stage of no gas exchange, hence both CO_2 and oxygen requirements must be supplied.

This point is illustrated by the studies of Cilley et al. [3] from our laboratory. Oxygen exchange across the native lung and the extracorporeal membrane lung during a typical ECLS run are shown in Fig. 2. Before ECLS the oxygen consumption across the native lung is 8 cc/kg/min, but this is being accomplished by using 100% O_2 and very high ventilator pressure. Despite these efforts the arterial PO_2 is only 30 torr. During venoarterial ECLS, the venti-

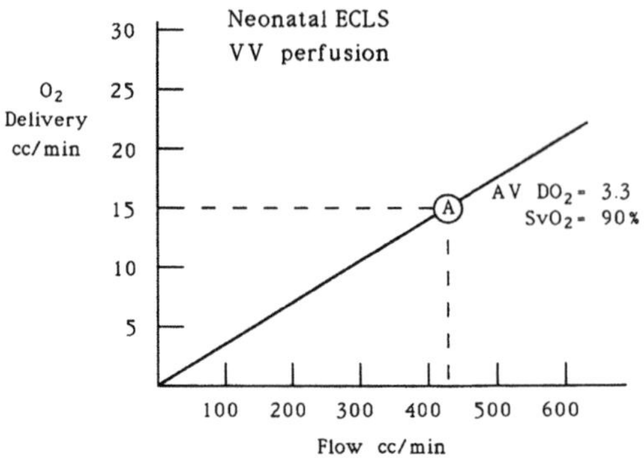

Fig. 3. Oxygen delivery related to blood flow, when the venous saturation is 90%, as occurs during venovenous perfusion or arteriovenous perfusion. Point *A* identifies requirements for a typical newborn infant

lator is turned down to allow lung rest, and oxygen transfer across the native lung ceases. Oxygen requirements are supplied by the extracorporeal circuit. During the next few days gas transfer across the native lung resumes, and when the lung function has returned to normal and oxygenation is adequate at low ventilator settings, extracorporeal support can be discontinued.

With venoarterial bypass systemic perfusion is controlled, in addition to gas exchange. The arterial pulse contour and pulse pressure are minimal, but as long as the flow is adequate this has no major physiologic side effects. Cardiac function in these infants is usually normal, and it is possible to conduct ECLS in the venovenous mode. In this fashion, the arterialized blood is returned to the venous circulation rather than the aorta, achieving pre pulmonary gas exchange and leaving the patient totally dependent on his own cardiovascular system for systemic oxygen delivery. It is relatively simple to achieve total CO_2 elimination during venovenous bypass, for the reasons discussed above. However, the ability to deliver oxygen is limited because the right atrial venous blood oxygen saturation is high, limiting the extracorporeal oxygen uptake capability. Of course the intent of venovenous bypass is to raise the venous oxygenation to 90% or greater. In venovenous ECLS we rely on the native lung to provide a significant portion of the systemic oxygen requirement. However, even if there is no oxygen uptake across the native lung, the total oxygen requirement can be supplied during venovenous ECLS by using higher extracorporeal flow, and accepting the fact that the patient's arterial saturation will be between 80%–90%. In Fig. 3, oxygen delivery related to flow during venovenous ECLS is shown. In this example the venous drainage saturation is 90% (compared with 75% in Fig. 1). Otherwise the characteristics of the circuit and the membrane lung are the same. Comparing Fig. 3 with Fig. 1 identifies the difference in flow required for total oxygen support when using venovenous compared with venoarterial circulation. Venovenous circulation can be achieved by continuous flow through two separate catheters, continuous flow through a single double lumen catheter, or intermittent tidal flow through a single catheter. The disadvantage of venovenous circulation is the requirement for higher extracorporeal blood flow rate, and the advantage is simplicity of vascular access [4, 5].

Current Status of Neonatal ECLS

Between 1980 and December 1988, 2171 cases from 53 centers were collected in the Neonatal ECMO Registry [6]. The survival rate was 83% (Table 1). Approximately one-third of the patients had mechanical complications and two-thirds had physiologic complications. From 1980 through 1988 160 neonates with respiratory failure have been treated with ECLS at the University of Michigan (U of M). The presenting diagnoses in these patients, in order of frequency, are meconium aspiration syndrome (MAS), respiratory distress syndrome (RDS), sepsis, persistent fetal circulation (PFC), and congenital diaphragmatic hernia (CDH). In total, 147 patients survived (92%); 96 of the last 100 patients survived. At U of M, for newborns greater than 34 weeks EGA, the success rate is 145 out of 151 (96%), while in less mature neonates the survival is 2 out of 9 (22%). Most of the deaths in the latter group are associated with intracranial hemorrhage. In the U of M experience, 16 of 17 (94%) neonates with CDH survived. Similar results have been reported in individual series by Weber et al. [7], Short and Pearson [8], and Redmond et al. [9].

The follow-up on the first 72 neonatal survivors ranged from 3 months to 11 years [10]. Ten children (14%) were lost to follow-up. Of those followed, 45 (63%) were normal or near-normal and 12 (17%) had major neurologic dysfunction and/or developmental delay. These results are similar to the findings of Andrews et al. [11], Towne et al. [12], and Krummel et al. [13], who noted normal mental function in 70%–80% of the patients in their individual studies. Additionally, all these results are comparable with the 77% normal mental ability noted in the 3-year follow-up of patients treated with conventional mechanical ventilation therapy [14]. This suggests that the neurologic damage is secondary to events that precede the onset of ECLS, although we have observed some right-brain ischemia in venoarterial patients [15].

Eight of the first 72 neonatal ECLS survivors (10%) had residual lung disease when discharged from the hospital [10]. This bronchopulmonary dys-

Table 1. Neonatal ECMO registry data December 1988

	Total cases	Survival (%)
Meconium aspiration syndrome	861	799 (93)
Respiratory distress syndrome	288	228 (79)
Congenital diaphragmatic hernia	336	218 (65)
Sepsis	224	170 (76)
Persistent pulmonary hypertension	323	281 (87)
Other	139	111 (80)

plasia (BPD) resolved in two patients. This compares with a 0%–35% incidence of BPD in survivors of conventional therapy. We currently are evaluating the effect of late versus early ECLS upon the incidence of BPD in a prospective, randomized fashion.

This increased survival in high-risk neonates with relatively low morbidity is gratifying. However, ECLS also appears to have economic advantages as noted in a study by Pearson and Short [16]. The average daily charge for ECLS was approximately $4000, almost $2000 more than the daily charge for conventional therapy patients. However, the number of hospital days was substantially reduced in the ECLS patients (21 vs 37.4 days). The total hospitalization charge of survivors in the ECLS group was 43% less than that of survivors among the conventional mechanical ventilation therapy patients.

Complications

The complications of ECLS fall into three major categories: a) bleeding associated with heparinization, b) technical failure, and c) sequelae of the hypoxia and hemodynamic instability which occur in the patient's course before onset of bypass.

Because of systemic heparinization, bleeding complications are the most common. Intracranial bleeding is the most feared of all ECLS complications. The overall incidence of ICH in our first 100 newborns was 29% [10]. ICH has occurred in only 4 of the last 100 ECLS patients in our series. These patients were full-term newborns with EGA greater than 34 weeks. Some abnormal bleeding, such as oozing from the cannulation site, occurs in almost all patients on ECLS. However, major bleeding complications other than ICH occur in about 10% of cases. These include pericardial tamponade, postoperative intrathoracic bleeding, gastrointestinal bleeding, and retroperitoneal hemorrhage. Bleeding is managed by lowering the ACT to approximately 200 s and by ensuring that the platelet count is greater than 100,000. If tolerated by the patient, ECLS support may be temporarily discontinued with reinstitution of full ventilator support. The patient's ACT is allowed to normalize for 1–2 h before return to bypass. If the bleeding persists at a significant rate in spite of these manipulations, aggressive surgical intervention or discontinuation of ECLS support is indicated.

Technical complications occurred in one-third of all patients. Oxygenator failure occurred in 20% of our cases [10]. Other technical complications included malfunction of the heat exchanger, electrical or mechanical pump failure, and tubing leak or rupture. Three patients had complications related to cannula placement or removal resulting in two deaths. Otherwise, there was no resulting mortality from any technical complication, although temporary physiologic instability was often observed until the problem could be corrected.

Neonatal venoarterial ECMO is routinely performed via right internal jugular vein and carotid artery access. The common carotid artery is ligated during cannulation and no attempt is made to repair it after decannulation. Collateral flow is established after carotid ligation in neonates and the symptoms of right hemispheric dysfunction have been minimal [10]. However, a predominance of right-sided findings have been demonstrated by auditory evoked potentials, computerized tomography, and EEG [17, 18]. Additionally, Schumacher and associates have noted a predominance of mild left-sided tone abnormalities on physical exam in some of our post-ECMO infants [15]. The incidence of such abnormalities is low, but any steps to improve neurologic outcome are justified. Successful use of venovenous ECLS would make carotid artery ligation unnecessary.

Kolobow has used venovenous ECLS in newborn lambs [19]. Tidal flow is established by intermittently draining and reinfusing through a single large catheter placed in the right atrium. Durandy et al. [20] have reported a similar system, using the Rhone-Poulene self-regulating roller pump. They reported successful venovenous neonatal perfusion in animals and patients. Otsu [21] reported a similar tidal flow system in dogs. Our group has experimented with a double lumen catheter for continuous flow venovenous ECLS [22], and recent clinical trials look very promising. If the adequacy of life support is equivalent, the advantage of avoiding carotid ligation makes venovenous access the method of choice for most newborn patients.

Seizures have been noted during ECLS in 24 of our first 100 neonates [10]. It is sometimes difficult to distinguish between seizure activity and the twitching and involuntary movements that are often seen in newborns on ECLS. EEG documentation of seizures is sometimes necessary. Other less frequent complications include cardiac arrest prior to and while on ECLS support, hypertension requiring vasoactive drug therapy, global myocardial dysfunction, and renal failure. Treatment of the latter is usually approached with the use of extracorporeal hemofiltration [23].

Technique of ECLS

The circuit includes a servoregulated roller pump, membrane lung, heat exchanger, and polyvinylchloride tubing and connectors (Fig. 4). Blood is drained via a cannula in the right internal jugular or femoral vein by a gravity siphon (100 cm) to a small distensible bladder. The bladder and a "bladder box" microswitch act as a servoregulator of the roller pump. The pump is turned off whenever the pump flow exceeds the venous blood return. In addition, this system turns off the pump if a large air bubble is entrained in the venous line, avoiding air embolism. Blood passes through an occlusive roller pump and is perfused through a silicone rubber membrane Kolobow Sci-Med lung. The size of the artificial lung is selected to provide *total* cardiopulmonary support. A given artificial lung has a "rated flow" which specifies the maximum blood flow rate at which normal venous blood perfusate leaves the oxygenator 95% saturated. Therefore, the artificial lung chosen for a given case must have a rated flow equivalent to or greater than the cardiac output of the patient. Routine blood flow rates are 70–90 cc/kg/min in adults, 80–100 cc/kg/min in children, and 120–170 cc/kg/min in neonates. Routine lung sizes are

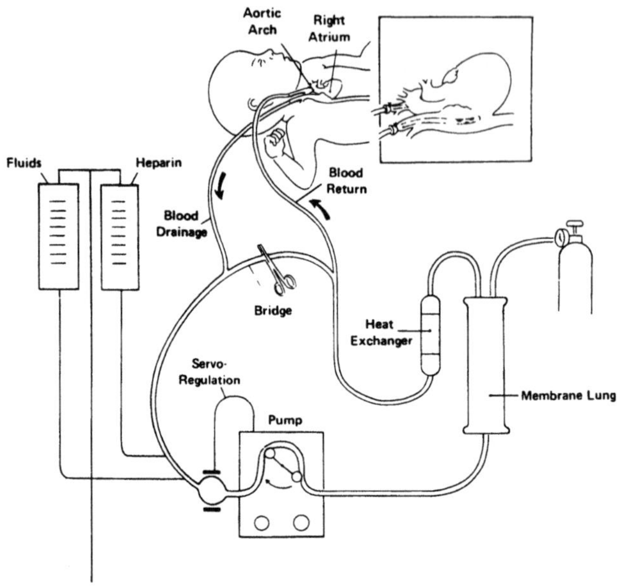

Fig. 4. Diagram of a typical neonatal extracorporeal life support (ECLS) circuit

3.5–4.5 m^2 in adults, 1.5–2.5 m^2 in children, and 0.4–0.8 m^2 in neonates. As the blood is oxygenated, CO_2 and water vapor are removed into the gas phase of the artificial lung. Blood flows through a countercurrent heat exchanger. The arterialized blood is then perfused at body temperature through a carotid, femoral, or axillary artery cannula into the aortic arch. A bridge exists between the arterial perfusion and venous drainage tubing in order to permit recirculation when the patient is off bypass. While operative placement of the cannulae is taking place, the circuit is primed sequentially with CO_2, electrolyte solution, albumin, and, finally, fresh blood. In neonates, the final prime is approximately 400 cc in volume. This is approximately double the newborn's blood volume and the prime must therefore be carefully adjusted for pH, temperature, and hematocrit. Circulation of the prime takes place through the circuit via the bridge until cannulation is complete.

Cannulation is performed at the bedside in the intensive care unit with an operating room team present. In neonates, the right common carotid artery and internal jugular vein are exposed via a right transverse cervical incision. Heparin, 100 units/kg, is administered intravenously after exposure of the vessels is complete. Through transverse arteriotomy and venotomy incisions, the largest cannulae which may be easily advanced are placed with the tips respectively in the aortic arch and the right atrium. The internal diameter of the venous catheter is the limiting factor which determines maximal flow. The venous catheter must be large enough to allow total cardiopulmonary bypass. Rarely, a second venous access site is necessary to achieve adequate flow. The cannulae are carefully secured in place and connected to the circuit. Cardiopulmonary bypass is initiated and flow is increased over the ensuing 10–15 min until levels of near total bypass are achieved. Venovenous access can be used, as discussed previously.

The complexity of ECLS support limits application to medical centers willing to dedicate themselves to formation of an established program. Maintaining a patient on extracorporeal support for days or weeks depends upon a prepared, organized, well-trained, and highly skilled team of physicians, respiratory therapists, nurses, perfusionists, and ECLS technicians. It is not a technique to be undertaken in a haphazard fashion on the spur of the moment without prior preparation and organization. With an established team available, ECLS routinely can be initiated within 2 h after a decision to use ECLS is made. Simplification of the circuit along with improved automated systems will someday allow application of ECLS on a wider clinical basis.

Once on ECLS support, the transformation of the patient's cardiopulmonary status is remarkable. All paralyzing agents, vasoactive drugs, and other infusions are discontinued. Ventilator settings are adjusted to minimal levels to allow "lung rest" (Fig. 2). Typical neonatal settings are a pressure limit (PIP) of 20, a positive end-expiratory pressure (PEEP) of 4, a rate of 10/min, and an FiO_2 (forced inspiratory oxygen) of 30%. The patient is allowed to awaken and is often alert. Pulmonary physiotherapy is started an extensive percussion and pulmonary lavage, especially in the newborn with meconium aspiration syndrome or pneumonia, is accomplished. As ventilator pressures are minimized, air leaks begin to seal.

Blood flow is maintained at a level sufficient to keep the venous saturation above 60%. Venous saturation is conveniently monitored by a fiberoptic Oximetrix catheter in the venous circuit. A normal venous saturation insures that the combined oxygen delivery from the patient's cardiopulmonary system and the circuit is adequate for oxygen consumption requirements. A continuous noninvasive arterial oxygen saturation monitor is placed on the patient in an area of postductal blood flow distribution. With this monitoring available, arterial blood gases need only be drawn every 8 h once the patient is stable. The PaO_2 is maintained between 50 and 70 and is manipulated by adjusting the extracorporeal blood flow rate. The PCO_2 is maintained between 35 and 50 and is inversely proportional to the flow rate of gas ventilating the membrane lung. The ventilating gas used is routinely 100% oxygen. Frequently a mixture of 5% CO_2 and 95% O_2 is used to ventilate the membrane lung since CO_2 removal from the artificial lung is very efficient and may potentially induce a respiratory alkalosis.

A continuous heparin infusion is mandatory throughout the ECLS course. Maintenance infusion is 30–60 units/kg/h [8]. The level of anticoagulation is monitored hourly by the whole blood activated clotting time (ACT). The heparin dose is adjusted to maintain the ACT between 220 and 260 s (normal is approximately 100 s). There is a fall in platelet count at onset of bypass secondary to dilution, blood-surface interactions, and complement activation [24]. Platelet consumption continues during and for up to 4 days after termination of the ECLS course [25]. In infants, platelet transfusions are required to maintain a level greater than 50000–70000. The hematocrit is maintained between 45% to 50% and occasional red blood cell transfusion is required. In general, hemolysis is minimal and free serum hemoglobin levels are usually <20 mg%/dl during an ECLS course (normal <5 mg%/dl).

The extracorporeal flow is gradually decreased, as the native lung function increases. When the flow is approximately 20 cc/kg/min a trial-off bypass is attempted. If tolerated for a 1- to 3-h period, the cannulae are removed and the vessels are ligated.

Future of Neonatal ECLS

In 1989, ECLS is the treatment of choice for infants with severe respiratory failure who fail to respond to conventional management. In the next decade, conventional management will undoubtedly improve, resulting in less lung injury and less mortality, decreasing the need for radical approaches such as extracorporeal life support. At the same time, however, ECLS will become safer and simpler, so that management of the critically ill newborn infant will probably include both mechanical ventilation and extracorporeal support. ECLS will be simplified by the use of single catheter venovenous access and perhaps arterial venous access via the umbilical vessels in some infants. A major complication of ECLS is bleeding which is in part related to heparinization. The use of heparin-coated circuits has been demonstrated to be effective in the laboratory [26], and in clinical trials in Europe [27]. We anticipate that neonatal ECLS with minimal systemic heparinization will decrease the risk of bleeding and expand the indications for use of ECLS. Single catheter low heparin ECLS will permit a return to clinical trials in premature infants, where the risk of intracranial bleeding is prohibitive with current techniques.

Summary and Conclusions

Extracorporeal life support has become standard treatment for term and near-term newborn infants with severe respiratory failure which is unresponsive to conventional ventilator and pharmacologic management. Pulmonary hypertension with right to left shunting is the underlying pathophysiology in these infants, regardless of the primary diagnosis. With the lung rest provided by extracorporeal support, pulmonary hypertension resolves in 3 or 4 days and lung recovery occurs in almost all of these infants. The survival rate for 2171 cases in the Neonatal ECMO Registry was 83%. The survival in our last 100 cases was 96%. The lesson learned from neonatal experience is similar to the lesson learned from the adult experience with extracorporeal life support: avoiding high pressure, high oxygen, mechanical ventilation by means of extracorporeal life support will result in recovery of the lung and patient survival.

References

1. Kolobow T, Gattinoni L, Tomlinson T et al. (1978) An alternative to breathing. J Thorac Cardiovasc Surg 75(2):261–266
2. Gattinoni L, Pesenti A, Pelizzola A et al. (1981) Reversal of terminal acute respiratory failure by low frequency positive pressure ventilation with extracorporeal removal of CO_2 (LFPPV-$ECCO_2R$). ASAIO Trans 27:289–293
3. Cilley RE, Polley TZ, Zwischenberger JB, Toomasian JM, Bartlett RH (1989) Independent measurement of oxygen consumption and oxygen delivery. J Surg Res (in press)
4. Klein MD, Andrews AF, Wesley JR, Toomasian J, Nixon C, Roloff D, Bartlett RH (1985) Venovenous perfusion in ECMO for newborn respiratory insufficiency: a clinical comparison with venoarterial perfusion. Ann Surg 201:520–526
5. Ladowski JS, Borovetz HS, Brant AM, Griffith BP, Hardesty RL (1984) Flow characteristics of Kolobow system for extracorporeal CO_2 removal ($ECCO_2$-R). ASAIO Trans 30:635
6. Neonatal ECMO Registry (1989) Ann Arbor, Michigan, January 1989
7. Weber TR, Pennington DG, Connors R et al. (1986) Extracorporeal membrane oxygenation for newborn respiratory failure. Ann Thorac Surg 42:529
8. Short BL, Pearson GD (1986) Neonatal extracorporeal membrane oxygenation: a review. J Intensive Care Med 1:47
9. Redmond CR, Graves ED, Falterman KW et al. (1987) Extracorporeal membrane oxygenation for respiratory and cardiac failure in infants and children. J Thorac Cardiovasc Surg 93:199
10. Bartlett RH, Gazzaniga A, Toomasian J, Roloff D, Rucker R (1986) Extracorporeal membrane oxygenation (ECMO) in neonatal respiratory failure: 100 cases. Ann Surg 204:236–245
11. Andrews AF, Nixon CA, Roloff DW (1986) One-to-three year outcome of fourteen neonatal ECMO survivors. Pediatrics 78(4):692–698
12. Towne BH, Lott IT, Hicks DA et al. (1985) Long-term follow-up of infants and children treated with extracorporeal membrane oxygenation (ECMO). A preliminary report. J Pediatr Surg 20:410–414
13. Krummel TM, Greenfield LJ, Kirkpatrick BV et al. (1984) The early evaluation of survivors after extracorporeal membrane oxygenation for neonatal pulmonary failure. J Pediatr Surg 19(5):585–590
14. Cohen RS, Stevenson DK, Malackowski N et al. (1980) Late morbidity among survivors of respiratory failure treated with tolazoline. J Pediatr 97:644–647
15. Schumacher RE, Barks JDE, Johnston MV et al. (1988) Right-sided brain lesions following ECMO. Pediatr 82(2):155–161
16. Pearson GD, Short BL (1989) An economic analysis of extracorporeal membrane oxygenation. (in press)
17. Voorhies TM, Tardo CI, Starrett AL et al. (1985) Evaluation of the cerebral circulation in neonates following extracorporeal membrane oxygenation. Ann Neurol 18:380
18. Cilley RE, Zwischenberger JB, Andrews AF (1986) Intracranial hemorrhage during extracorporeal membrane oxygenation in neonates. Pediatrics 78:699–704
19. Kolobow T, Moretti MP, Mascheroni D et al. (1983) Experimental meconium aspiration syndrome in the preterm fetal lamb: successful treatment using the extracorporeal artificial lung. ASAIO Trans 29:221–226
20. Durandy Y, Batisse A, Chevalier JY (1988) A new extracorporeal respiratory assist device: initial clinical experience in paediatric patients. Intensive Care Med [Suppl]:268
21. Saito Y, Terasaki H, Otsu T, Ezaki K, Nogami T, Morioka T (1985) Extracorporeal lung assist with a single catheter in puppies. Crit Care Medicine 13:501–503

22. Zwischenberger JB, Toomasian JM, Drake K, Andrews AF, Kolobow T, Bartlett RH (1985) Total respiratory support with single cannula venovenous ECMO: double lumen continuous flow vs single lumen tidal flow. ASAIO Trans 31:610–615
23. Heiss KH, Pettit BJ, Hirschl RB et al. (1987) Renal insufficiency and volume overload managed in neonatal ECMO by continuous ultrafiltration. ASAIO Trans 33:557–560
24. Bartlett RH, Fong SW, Bruns NE et al. (1974) Prolonged partial venoarterial bypass: physiologic, biochemical, and hematologic responses. Ann Surg 180(6):918–932
25. Anderson HL III, Cilley RE, Zwischenberger JB et al. (1986) Thrombocytopenia in neonates after extracorporeal membrane oxygenation. ASAIO Trans 32:534–537
26. Toomasian JM, Hsu L-C, Hirschl RB, Heiss KF, Hultquist KA, Bartlett RH (1988) Evaluation of Duraflo II heparin coating in prolonged extracorporeal membrane oxygenation. ASAIO Trans 34:410–414
27. Bindslav L (1988) Adult ECMO performed with surface-heparinized equipment. ASAIO Trans 34:1009–1013
28. Cilley RE, Wesley JR, Zwischenberger JB, Toomasian JM, Bartlett RH (1986) Method of pulmonary and membrane lung gas exchange during extracorporeal membrane oxygenation. ASAIO Trans 32:525–529

Effects of Vasoactive Substances on Oxygen Transport and Tissue Oxygenation

L. Hannemann and K. Reinhart

There is one important unifying principle relevant to all aerobic organisms: a constant oxygen supply is required for cellular oxidative phosphorylation. There is some variation in the specific mechanisms of O_2 transport among the different animals, but all transport systems employ the same basic principles. These basic principles of gas transport are convection, diffusion, and gas exchange.

Convection is mass transfer of gaseous molecules by an external force. An example of convection is the pumping of blood by the heart. In this case, the flow of gas is equivalent to the product of the volume flow rate and the carrying capacity of the carrier (the blood). In the specific case of oxygen transport in humans and higher animals, systemic O_2 transport (QO_2) is the product of the cardiac output (Qt) and the arterial oxygen content (CaO_2):

$$QO_2 = Qt \times CaO_2 \times 10$$

Transport of oxygen from air to mitochondria in all large animals involves a series of transfer steps utilizing two separate serial gas exchangers joined by the convective flow of blood [74]. The oxygen transport system is made up of the following steps: the convection of O_2 from the external environment into the external gas exchange apparatus, i.e., the lungs; the diffusion of O_2 from the gas within the lungs into the blood; the respiratory gas exchange; the convection of blood to the tissues; the diffusion of oxygen from capillary blood to the mitochondria; the peripheral gas exchange; and, in the last step, utilization of O_2 by the respiratory enzymes of the mitochondria.

Recent clinical studies have led to a new approach to the physiology and therapy of shock states [61]. Traditionally, shock syndromes are assessed according to their etiologic categories, which include hemorrhagic, cardiogenic, traumatic, and septic shock. It is now well accepted that, from the viewpoint of circulatory physiology, the reduced or inadequate oxygen consumption (VO_2), which limits body metabolism, is the common fundamental alteration of all these shock syndromes. Retrospective and prospective clinical trials have shown that monitoring of the oxygen transport system – especially volume, flow, oxygen delivery (DO_2), and VO_2 – and maintaining the measured variables at empirically determined "optimal values" [cardiac index (CI) $>50\%$ above normal, $DO_2 > 600$ ml/min/m^2, VO_2 about 30% above normal (170 ml/min/m^2) and blood volume 500 ml above normal leads to markedly lower morbidity and mortality than in control groups with conventional therapy

[62–64]. These findings suggest that it is of utmost importance to restore defective physiological parameters not just to their normal values but to optimal values empirically defined by groups of survivors of life-threatening illnesses [61].

To reach these therapeutic goals, especially an above normal oxygen delivery and oxygen consumption, it is necessary to optimize the convective oxygen transport of the body. After initial adequate volume replacement, it may be necessary to administer catecholamines, if sufficient perfusion pressures cannot be obtained. The endogenous catecholamines are key regulators of many physiological events in human beings. Norepinephrine primarily acts as a neurotransmitter which is released from sympathetic nerve terminals, and epinephrine functions as a circulating hormone released from the adrenal medulla. Catecholamines initiate target-cell responses by binding to specific recognition sites, the adrenergic receptors. These receptors are the initial decoders of extracellular messages. This concept has guided extensive research on hormone and neurotransmitter action [51].

The effects of the catecholamines commonly used in critically ill patients – i.e., dopamine, dobutamine, and norepinephrine – are dose-related. While much knowledge has been acquired concerning the effects of these substances on the macrocirculation and the heart, the influence of catecholamines on the microvasculature is poorly investigated. Dopamine, the third naturally occurring catecholamine, is an intermediate compound in the synthesis of epinephrine and norepinephrine. At infusion rates of 0.5–1.5 µg/kg/min, the compound acts predominantly on DA1- and DA2-receptors to produce vasodilation in the renal, mesenteric, cerebral, and coronary vascular beds [24, 40]. Sodium and urine excretion usually increases; the natriuresis may be due to renal vascular effects which possibly also involve DA1-receptors located on renal tubules [18].

At infusion rates of 2–4 µg/kg/min, an activation of β1-adrenoceptors results in increasing cardiac contractile force and heart rate. Dopamine also causes release of norepinephrine from cardiac sympathetic nerves [3]. At higher dose ranges, the action of dopamine on alpha1- and alpha2-adrenoceptors dominates with evidence of increasing blood pressure. Due to the diverse effects it produces by activation of DA1-, DA2-receptors and postsynaptic alpha1- and alpha2-adrenoceptors, dopamine exhibits marked individual variations in the infusion rate necessary to elevate diastolic blood pressure. An increase in blood pressure has been observed with infusion rates as low as 2 µg/kg/min to greater than 10 µg/kg/min in normal subjects. In critically ill patients, infusion rates of 50 µg/kg/min or more have sometimes been used to increase blood pressure [33].

Fleckenstein et al. [20] and Kersting et al. [35] have demonstrated a dopamine-induced increase of mean muscle PO_2 in nine healthy volunteers and seven critically ill patients with on-line registration of tissue PO_2 histograms of the skeletal muscle (m. quadriceps femoris). The initially maldistributed histograms became progressively more symmetrical. The dosage of dopamine ranged from 2–10 µg/kg/min in the critically ill patients to 3 µg/kg/min in the volunteers. The authors also revealed that mean muscular PO_2 rose significantly not only under increased or unchanged total body oxygen supply, but also at decreased oxygen delivery. They interpreted these findings as an indication for redistribution of microflow. Because of the striking increase they observed in mean tissue PO_2, it was assumed that, under the conditions of the study, dopamine not only induced a redistribution of microflow but also increased muscular blood flow, though there is no evidence that dopamine enhances muscular blood flow in humans [53].

Dobutamine is the synthetic catecholamine which comes closest to being a pure positive inotropic drug. The drug is a powerful $\beta 1$-adrenergic agonist which augments ventricular contractility, stroke volume, and cardiac output. At higher dosages, it increases sinus node automaticity and enhances AV nodal and intraventricular conduction, but, at low dosages, the increase in inotropy is much greater than in chronotropy [38]. Though some of the dobutamine-induced positive inotropic effects, e.g., vasoconstriction, may also be mediated through stimulation of myocardial alpha1-adrenergic receptors, they are offset by concomitant $\beta 2$-receptor stimulation which produces vasodilatation. The net effect is a mild vasodilatation, since the $\beta 2$-agonist properties tend to override the peripheral alpha1-adrenergic vasoconstrictive effects [55]. Unlike dopamine, dobutamine does not stimulate dopaminergic receptors in the kidney to produce specific renal vasodilatation and it does not release norepinephrine from presynaptic terminals.

As a naturally occurring catecholamine, norepinephrine mediates sympathetic nervous system activity and stimulates the myocardium directly. The stimulatory effect of alpha-adrenergic receptors is clinically apparent at relatively lower doses than with epinephrine. The drug produces a powerful vasoconstriction in all vascular beds with a striking increase in systemic vascular resistance (SVR). The increased blood pressure results in a reflex bradycardia due to baroreceptor reflexes with possible reduction of cardiac output in normal humans. This reflex bradycardia is normally not seen if norepinephrine is used to treat severe hypotension in cases where cardiac output is maintained [26, 65]. The clinical use of the drug is indicated when peripheral vascular resistance is markedly reduced in connection with severe hypotension secondary to extreme vasodilatation in cases of septic shock or anaphylaxis. Such situations call for the maintenance of an adequate coronary perfusion pressure, and this can often be achieved with the use of norepinephrine. It may be advantageous to add low-dose dopamine to the norepinephrine infusion to reduce renal vascular resistance and augment renal blood flow [56]. Of course it is of utmost importance to provide for adequate volume loading before initiating norepinephrine therapy.

Concerning the influence of the catecholamines on the microvasculature, there is evidence that they are major controllers of vascular smooth muscle, but the extent to which they contribute to the regulation of smooth muscles of the lymphatic vessels remains obscure. In an experimental sheep model, McChale et al. [46] found that intravenous infusion of adrenaline and noradrenaline increased the frequency of lymphatic contraction and the lymph flow in popliteal, prefemoral, and mesenteric efferent lymphatic vessels in conscious sheep. In experimental studies it was shown that the slow intravenous injection of epinephrine or the intraarterial infusion of epinephrine or norepinephrine in large doses causes an increase in flow from the thoracic duct [22].

Dabney et al. [14] investigated the regulation of lymphatics by sympathetic nerves or hormones using an experimental in vivo study with dogs. His findings clearly demonstrate that canine lymphatic vessels in vivo respond to adrenergic drugs and sympathetic nervous activity. This substantiates the existence of intrinsic mechanisms for control of the lymphatic vessels by the sympathoadrenal system. Hayashi et al. [30] showed that hemorrhage in anesthetized sheep increased pulsatile pumping of postnodal mesenteric lymphatics. In the study of Dobney et al. [14], intraarterial catecholamine infusion or hemorrhage produced sustained contraction, but no pulsations, of perfused forelimb lymphatics. An increase in the pumping of lymphatics would be of value during stress. Like compression by skeletal muscle during exercise, it would result in an almost immediate translocation of lymph into the blood and a shortened time for the return of newly formed lymph.

Leier et al. [29] showed that dobutamine was superior to dopamine in patients with cardiomyopathic heart failure by comparing the systemic and regional hemodynamic effects of the two drugs. His crossover study included 13 patients with congestive cardiomyopathy (NYHA III,IV). Dose-response data demonstrated that dobutamine (2.5–10 µg/kg/min) progressively and predictably incrases cardiac output by increasing the stroke volume while simultaneously decreasing the systemic and pulmonary vascular resistance as well as the pulmonary pressure and pulmonary capillary wedge pressure (PcWP). At this dose range, there were no changes in heart rate or premature ventricular contractions (PVCs)/min. Dopamine (2–8 µg/kg/min) increased the stroke volume and cardiac output at 4 µg/kg/min. Dopamine at >4 µg/kg/min had hardly any additional effect on the cardiac output, but increased the pulmonary wedge pressure and the number of PVCs/min. Dopamine at >6 µg/kg/min increased the heart rate. The inability of dopamine to further improve the stroke volume and cardiac output in these patients was probably related to an increase in afterload and the rise in cumulative heart rate (sinus beats plus PVCs/min). The elevation of PcWP with dopamine probably resulted from an increase in afterload; other possible explanations may be the drug-induced decrease of ventricular compliance or the venoconstriction-determined emptying of the venous blood pool [39, 76].

The superiority of dobutamine to dopamine in patients with severe congestive cardiomyopathy or low-output cardiac failure (NYHA III,IV) has been confirmed by other clinical studies [6, 29, 66]. Dopamine was found to have a greater tendency to cause persistent elevation of vascular resistance, to increase left-ventricular filling pressure, and to produce clinical signs of pulmonary congestion and edema. The heart rate and filling pressures, two important determinants of myocardial oxygen consumption, were relevantly elevated during dopamine infusion at dose ranges >4 µg/kg/min; thus dobutamine may be preferable in treating patients with coronary artery disease [66].

During a 24-h maintenance-dose infusion of either dopamine (3.7–4 μg/kg/min) or dobutamine (7.3–7.7 μg/kg/min), only dobutamine maintained a significant increase of stroke volume, cardiac output, urine flow, urine sodium concentration, creatinine clearance, and peripheral flow. Renal and hepatic blood flow were not significantly altered by the maintenance dose of either drug. The mean upper extremity blood flow (forearm and hand blood flow) was measured by the method of venous occlusion using a water-containing plethysmograph. Dobutamine produced a significantly greater increase of blood flow in the upper extremity than dopamine.

Concerning the undesirable side-effects of dopamine, some authors have recommended the combination of dopamine with nitroglycerin (NTG) to compensate the increase in the filling pressures and afterload in patients with coronary heart disease and congestive heart failure [31].

There are striking differences in response to dopamine between hypotensive patients with clinical shock and normotensive patients with chronic low-output cardiac failure and end-stage heart disease. Loeb et al. [42] administered dopamine in 62 patients with shock of various etiologies at dosages above 10 μg/kg/min. Of these patients, 38 in whom left-ventricular end-diastolic pressure (LVEDP) was measured directly, showed only a slight increase of this parameter from 13 to 16 mmHg during dopamine infusion; the drug was remarkably well tolerated and increased the cardiac output by a mean of 37%. In shock patients, especially in septic shock, there is a relevant decrease in vascular resistance due to vasodilatation. Under such circumstances, volume loading alone may be insufficient to elevate perfusion pressure to normal ranges; thus, even large doses of dopamine may lead to satisfactory restoration of arterial pressure by improving coronary and systemic perfusion [24, 42].

Dopexamine, a synthetic catecholamine, is structurally related to dopamine, but differs both in its receptor activity and pharmacodynamic profile. It has a potent effect on $\beta 2$-adrenoceptors as well as on dopaminergic receptors of the DA1 and DA2 subtypes, but does not activate alpha1- and alpha2-adrenoceptors, and the $\beta 1$-adrenoceptor activation seems to be poor. Compared with dopamine, there is considerably less affinity for the DA2-receptor. The DA1 action increases renal blood flow, while the $\beta 2$-adrenoceptor action causes decreased peripheral resistance and a reflex increase in the heart rate [21, 69]. Dopexamine has a rapid onset and short duration of action [10, 11].

The effects of dopexamine have been investigated in a large number of patients with chronic heart failure. The dosage ranged from 1 to 4 and maximally 6 μg/kg/min [13, 15, 67]. At the mentioned dosage ranges, there were corresponding dose-related increments in the cardiac index, stroke volume index, and heart rate, whereas the systemic vascular resistance and pulmonary vascular resistance were reduced. One randomized crossover study compared dopexamine and dobutamine in 12 patients with chronic congestive heart failure [9]. Infusion of 2 μg/kg/min of dopexamine produced increments in the cardiac index comparable with those achieved by infusion of 10 μg/kg/min dobutamine. The systemic vascular resistance was reduced to a greater extent by dopexamine, but the reduction of the pulmonary artery capillary wedge pressure was similar with both drugs.

With regard to the question of whether dopexamine possesses a substantial positive inotropic action, there are marked differences between the results of experimental and clinical studies. In the former, dopexamine exhibits very weak direct positive inotropic action [2, 10, 11]. In contrast, clinical studies by Jaski [34] and Tan [68] have demonstrated clear positive inotropism when dopexamine was infused. One explanation could be that dopexamine increases the cardiac contractile force in the clinical setting by direct action on myocardial β2-adrenoceptors, which may exert a greater influence in patients with congestive heart failure, who have a reduced number of β1-adrenoceptors [34]. Another possible mechanism may be the proven powerful competitive dopexamine-induced inhibition of neuronal norepinephrine reuptake [2]. Patients with congestive heart failure have high levels of circulating norepinephrine; thus, the prevention of uptake may increase norepinephrine levels at the β1-adrenoceptors, which in turn may result in a positive inotropic effect.

Vasodilators

Many studies have confirmed that vasodilator therapy can shift the Starling function curve upwards and to the left, thus reducing the symptoms of both pulmonary congestion and low-cardiac output states. In this way, the improvement in hemodynamics is associated with an increase of the convective oxygen transport and a decrease in myocardial oxygen consumption (MVO_2). The addition of vasodilators to the inotropic therapy of patients with congestive heart failure (CHF) has been one of the cornerstones in the actual management of heart disease [45].

The mechanisms by which vasodilators correct the abnormalities in CHF are:

1. Reduction of afterload or impedance
2. Venodilatation and reduction of intracardiac volume
3. Reduction of myocardial ischemia
4. Increase of the diastolic compliance of the left ventricle

In decreasing impedance to ejection, vasodilators may reduce preload and thus shift the patient too far to the left of the filling-pressure axis of the Starling curve, which leads to a limited improvement of cardiac output. This preload/afterload mismatch should be corrected by adequate volume infusion to restore the normal left-ventricular filling volume. The principle of treatment with vasodilators to augment cardiac output should be minimizing afterload while maximizing preload.

Intravenous nitroprusside (NP) has a uniform effect on arterioles and veins, thus dilating both types of vessels to the same degree. The characteristic hemodynamic effects of NP are a significant increase in the cardiac output and stroke volume combined with a decrease in the pulmonary artery pressure, pulmonary capillary wedge pressure, and central venous pressure, as well as in the systemic and pulmonary vessel resistances [48]. Rebound hemodynamic effects may occur after abrupt withdrawal of NP from patients with CHF. The mechanism of this rebound is the activation of reflex and humoral vasoconstrictive forces during administration of the vasodilator; this partially involves the activation of the renin angiotensin system, which can be blocked by either alpha-adrenergic blockers or angiotensin antagonists [30].

The hemodynamic effects of nitroglycerin have been extensively studied in patients with acute or chronic CHF [1]. At low doses, nitrates predominantly dilate the large veins and do not greatly affect the arteries, while, at high doses, they have a significant arteriolar vasodilating capacity. There is evidence that, at high doses, the hemodynamic profile of nitroglycerin in patients with heart failure is similar to that of nitroprusside [19]. By virtue of these effects, administration of nitroglycerin in patients with CHF results in a constant reduction of the pulmonary artery pressure, the pulmonary capillary wedge pressure, the central venous pressure, and the pulmonary vascular resistance. Variable responses occur in the blood pressure, heart rate, cardiac output, and systemic vascular resistance. Nitroglycerin dilates the pulmonary circulation, thus causing pooling of blood in the lungs, which may also play a role in the therapy of CHF. In contrast to the effect of NP administration, renal blood flow usually falls with nitroglycerin [1].

There is evidence indiciating that the effects of sodium nitroprusside and nitroglycerin on the microvasculature different widely. Hauss et al. [28] studied the effects of both drugs on the microvasculature in 16 mongrel dogs. He recorded the hemodynamic effects with invasive catheterization and simultaneously measured the partial oxygen pressure with Kessler-Lübbers multiwire surface electrodes in the gracilis muscle, the myocardium, and the liver. Sodium nitroprusside (NP) was given at low (4 µg/kg/min) and high (8 µg/kg/min) dosages; nitroglycerin (NTG) was likewise applied (12 µg/h and 24 µg/h respectively). Electron-microscopic investigations of different tissues were carried out at the end of the study.

The essential result of these investigations is that, unlike nitroglycerin, NP lowers the partial oxygen pressure in the myocardium, skeletal muscle, and liver, although the oxygen pressure of the arterial blood shows hardly any change. The initial PO_2 histogram of the skeletal muscle in animals of the NP group had a physiological shape with a mean value of 34.6 mmHg. Under low-dosage NP, the histogram changed and showed a shift to the left. Under high NP dosage, numerous anoxic and hypoxic regions were evident, and the mean value had fallen to 12.3 mmHg. These were clear signs of a pathological disturbance of the local oxygen supply. In contrast, the compiled PO_2 histograms of the NTG group reevidenced only a slight fall in mean values from 39.6 mmHg to 32.9 mmHg under high dosage. On the other hand, all PO_2 histograms showed an unchanged physiological local oxygen supply; thus, there were no hypoxic or anoxic regions in the tissue. Continuous registration demonstrated that local oxygen pressures in the myocardium (left ventricle) and the liver showed a similarly marked decrease dependent on the NP dosage, whereas the local PO_2 remained unaltered during nitroglycerin infusion. Similar results could be obtained during measurements in intensive-care patients [41].

Electron microscopy of various organs demonstrated that alterations of the oxygen supply found after NP administration correlated impressively with changes in ultrastructure. The heart muscle tissue revealed marked lesions in almost all mitochondria. In some cases, myocardial cells showed incipient cristolysis, indicating severe mitochondrial damage, characteristic of a hypoxic lesion. Similar massive changes were not found in dogs of the NTG group.

If the blood pressure decrease following drug administration were accompanied by a decreasing flow, the left shift could easily be explained, but, in an organism with intact regulation, the blood pressure can vary within a certain range without affecting local flow or changing the PO_2 histogram. The study shows that this regulatory mechanism is well maintained after application of NTG, but that massive disturbance impairing the oxygen supply is evident after administration of NP. It is still unclear to what extent these changes are modified by capillary-flow alterations or metabolic factors. Though blood cyanide and thiocyanate concentrations were never at a toxic level in this study, it is nevertheless possible that the doses used might have disturbed the metabolism of some organs. Investigations of Michenfelder [47] have revealed that not all of the free cyanide is quickly converted into thiocyanate by rhodanase, thus there are enough free cyanide molecules left to cause cyanide cell poisoning through cytochrome oxidase inhibition with a subsequent anaerobic status of the total metabolism.

On the other hand, the low partial oxygen pressure in a tissue can also be caused by a changing of blood distribution in the microcirculatory bed. Zweifach [77] explains this redistribution as follows: NP-induced vasoplegia causes maximal dilation of the muscularized "preferential channels," so the bulk of perfusion at the microvasculatory level would then be drained through these "preferential channels," which are less important for the tissue oxygen supply. The peripheral resistance will decrease, and the arterial pressure will no longer be sufficient to perfuse the "nutritive capillary channels" that are without muscles and therefore not distended. As a result of this redistribution, the cell regions situated further away from the "preferential channels" no longer receive an adequate oxygen supply [28, 77].

The different lengths and sizes of the capillaries make the microcirculatory bed nonhomogeneous. It is hypothesized that there are capillaries with "high flow" and others with "a normally adapted flow" [36]. The shift of the PO_2 histogram could also be interpreted as being due to a disproportionately greater perfusion of the "high flow capillaries." Tountas et al. [73] found a 72% rise in coronary blood flow and an increase of PO_2 in the sinus venosus after application of NP. These findings together with the local decrease of PO_2 in the study of Hauss et al. may be explained in terms of a redistribution of this kind. The results demonstrate once more that a quantitative increase in the blood flow does not necessarily improve the oxygen supply to the tissue.

Using the xenon-133 washout technique, Mann et al. [44] studied the effects of NP on regional myocardial blood flow in 25 patients and compared them with those observed in 31 patients treated with NTG. Despite similar hemodynamic effects, the influence exerted on the regional myocardial specific blood flow differed significantly. In patients with coronary artery disease and well-developed collateral vessels, regional myocardial blood flow was significantly decrased after nitroprusside, but substantially increased after nitroglycerin. It was concluded that NP caused a redistribution of blood flow away from ischemic areas and could potentially increase the injury in patients with coronary artery disease. It is thus pointed out that a mere supervision of arterial oxygen pressure is by no means sufficient for assessing the supply to the most important organs.

Endrich et al. [17] has recently investigated the effects of sodium NP and NTG on the microvasculature of striated muscles in the hamster during hypotension induced by these substances. Their methods of examination included intravital microscopy with quantitative video image analysis, platinum multiwire electrodes for local PO_2 measurements, and a micropuncture system for determination of the microvasculatory pressure. Using NP, they found that, during a mean arterial pressure reduction to 70 or 40 mmHg, the precapillaries dilated and precapillary resistance decreased, but there were no significant changes in venular diameter. NP-induced hypotension was associated with a constant increase in intravascular pressure within the venules; thus, the resulting arteriolar-venular pressure gradient was reduced by more than 50%. Moreover, NP-induced hypotension was accompanied by reduced functional capillary density as well as by tissue hypoxia. In contrast, NTG dilated both arterioles and venules within the microvascular network. Despite the lower blood cell velocity in all segments, functional capillary density and local PO_2 remained unchanged, most probably because there was only a 10% reduction of the arteriolar-venular pressure gradient.

The observations of Endrich et al. relating to NP are in accordance with those of other authors [40, 41]. Using intravital microscopy and quantitative analysis of TV images, he was able to reveal that there was a preferential dilation of precapillaries but not of venules during NP infusion; this finding is in agreement with data from Longnecker et al. [43], who investigated the rat cremaster muscle. As a consequence, the lower arteriolar pressure after NP hypotension associated with a constant pressure in drainage vessels reduces the pressure gradient in the microvasculature, thus facilitating the development of microvascular dysfunction.

These results are also important for other organ systems like the liver, whose sinusoids receive the bulk of their blood supply from the portal vein. Because portal venous pressure is only 7–10 mmHg, changes in the pressure and pressure gradient, especially along the sinusoids, are very critical for liver perfusion and oxygenation. Both these findings are in contrast with the assumption that NP produces venodilation, as has been suggested in the literature [37, 48, 70].

Effects on the microvasculature contrary to those of NP were found by Tillmanns et al. [71], who used intravital microscopy to investigate the influence which NTG exerts on the microvasculation of the left myocardium in cats and rats. He found that intravenous administration of this drug resulted in a dilatation of large arterioles (70–240 μm) with a concomitant pressure decrease in small coronary arterioles and venules and a slight decrease in the distances between perfused myocardial capillaries. These data are in good agreement with the results of Endrich et al. and confirm statements favoring the preferential use of NTG to induce hypotension.

Prostaglandins

In recent years, the prostaglandins have been extensively evaluated as therapeutic agents for influencing the oxygen supply/demand ratio in different organ systems during treatment of critically ill patients. Both iloprost, a stable prostacyclin (PGI2) analogue with a nearly identical potency and pharmacological profile [57, 58], and prostacyclin have been shown to increase blood flow to the periphery even at doses below those that elicit a systemic hypotensive response [49]. Because the efficiency of tissue oxygen extraction at a constant metabolic rate and given oxygen diffusion gradient is mainly a function of the ratio of the perfused capillary surface to the blood flow, a mere increase in tissue blood flow does not automatically reflect parallel increases in tissue oxygen delivery. Thus, a vasodilator which increases the blood flow and erythrocyte flow velocity, but has no effect on the perfused capillary density, will not increase and might even decrease tissue PO_2 [27].

Müller et al. [50] studied the microvascular effects which iloprost produced in the hamster cheek pouch. Using intravital videomicroscopy and, for quantification of vascular permeability, venular leakage of fluorescin-labelled dextran, he found that intravenous application of iloprost at a nonhypotensive, platelet-aggregation inhibiting dosage of 0.5 µg/kg/min significantly increased the diameters of arterioles and venules as well as the density of perfused capillaries; it also antagonized vasoconstriction and the decrease of perfused capillary density induced by leukotriene D4. The drug antagonized venular leakage induced by histamine (10/5 *M*), bradykinin (10/6 *M*), and reperfusion after 30 min of ischemia. Topical application of iloprost (10/8 *M*) and intraarterial infusion of prostaglandin E1 (PGE1) also attenuated histamine-induced venular leakage.

Concerning the mechanism by which iloprost attenuates the increased permeability induced by all three above-mentioned inflammatory mediators as well as by reperfusion after ischemia, it is assumed that the drug exerts its antipermeability effects via functional inhibition of a mediated increase in cyclic adenosine-monophosphate (cAMP) [16]. The possible beneficial effects that can be derived from the ability of the prostaglandins PGE1 and PGI2 to increase tissue oxygenation may provide a therapeutic approach in preventing multiple organ failure, which has become the major challenge facing the intensive-care physician [4]. These are as follows:

1. Improvement in microcirculatory blood flow with the prevention of tissue hypoxia; with regard to microcirculatory vasodilatation, inhibition of platelet-activation/aggregate-formation with thromboxane A2 release, fibrinolysis (reported with PGI2 only)

2. Inhibition of polymorphonuclear leukocyte activation (PGE1) and adhesion to vascular endothelium (PGI2)
3. Inhibition of monocyte activation and the release of monokines (PGE2 and PGI2)
4. "Cytoprotection" (reported with PGE1, PGE2, and PGI2)
5. Pulmonary vasodilation with a reduction in pulmonary artery pressure and calculated resistance
6. Increased delivery of antimicrobial agents to septic foci [4]

To examine the influence of PG infusion on survival in critically ill humans, Holcroft et al. [32] studied the effect of a 7-day continuous infusion of PGE1 (30 ng/kg/min) in patients with acute respiratory failure (ARDS) associated with trauma and sepsis. The PGE1 group had a significantly improved 30-day survival: 15 of 21 (71%) treated patients survived as opposed to only 7 of the 20 (35%) controls. Remarkably, none of the PGE-treated patients, with only ARDS (i.e., no other organ dysfunction) developed multiple organ failure, and all survived. Unfortunately, a multicenter study with 150 PGE1-treated patients did not confirm these promising results [75].

Shoemaker et al. [60] and Tokioka et al. [72] have both demonstrated in clinical studies with ARDS patients that PGE1, like PGI2, not only reduces pulmonary vascular resistance, but also increases oxygen delivery (DaO_2) and oxygen consumption.

Bihari et al. [5, 8] studied 27 patients with sepsis and dysfunction of two or more organ systems. He stated that, in both low and high cardiac output states, the development of irreversible multiple organ failure and subsequent death might be predicted early in the course of a patient's illness by the response to an increase in DaO_2 obtained by a 30-min infusion of PGI2. He has found that patients who subsequently die have a significantly greater percentage increase in the oxygen uptake index during the PGI2 infusion than survivors. PGI2 produced an increase in the oxygen extraction ratio in 10 of the 13 patients who died in contrast to the reductions observed in all normal controls and surviving patients.

Gimson et al. [23] and Bihari et al. [6, 7] studied the effect of increasing oxygen flux by the infusion of PGI2 at 5 ng/kg/min for 30 min in 11 patients with acute liver failure and stage III or IV encephalopathy. These patients represent a homogeneous group with a hemodynamic disturbance similar to that in sepsis, but much more profound. The authors observed that increases in DaO_2 were associated with significant increases in oxygen consumption. In another eight patients, given the same dosage of PGI2 over a 1-h period, there was not only an increase in oxygen consumption but also a fall in the mixed venous lactate concentration from a median of 3.8 to 3.2 mmol/l.

In summary, catecholamines and vasodilators both have a profound influence on securing an adequate oxygen transport not only within the macrocirculation, but also in the microcirculation. The principal function of the circulation is to guarantee an oxygen transport that is sufficient to satisfy the needs of the organ systems and the periphery. Presently, great efforts are being made to prevent the multiple organ failure syndrome (MOFS) during intensive care in patients with severe trauma associated with sepsis or ARDS. One relevant reason for developing MOFS is the insufficient supply of the organism with oxygen under these stressful circumstances. Because the organ systems have an increased need for oxygen due to an enhanced metabolic load and a loss of microcirculatory autoregulation, which leads to a greater DO_2 demand, efforts must be made toward increasing oxygen delivery. Physiological experiments [12] and clinical studies [59] suggest that, under the special pathophysiological conditions mentioned above, an oxygen supply dependency exists; this means that oxygen consumption of the organism is largely, if not always, dependent on oxygen delivery.

Depending on the actual hemodynamic profile and naturally also the volume status of the patient, catecholamines and/or vasodilators may be helpful in increasing the oxygen delivery, but it is also of considerable relevance to take into account the effects of these substances within the microvasculature of the tissues of the organ systems with an eye to securing aerobic metabolism at this target. If the increased cardiac output is not distributed where it is needed, pharmacological support of the circulation may lead to further damage.

More comprehensive research seems to be necessary to elucidate the complex interactions and effects of these substances on the microvasculature.

References

1. Armstrong PW et al. (1980) Pharmacokinetic-hemodynamic studies of intravenous nitroglycerin in congestive heart failure. Circulation 62:160–166
2. Bass AS et al. (1987) Mechanisms mediating the positive inotropic and chronotropic changes induced by dopexamine in the anesthetized dog. J Pharmacol Exp Ther 242:940–944
3. Beregovich J et al. (1974) Dose-related hemodynamic and renal effects of dopamine in congestive heart failure. Am Heart J 87:550–557
4. Bihari D (1988) Oxygen delivery and consumption in the critically ill: their relation to the development of multiple organ failure. In: Kox W et al. (eds) Shock and the adult respiratory distress syndrome. Springer, Berlin London, pp 95–121
5. Bihari D et al. (1987) The effects of vasodilation with prostacyclin on oxygen delivery and uptake in critically ill patients. N Engl J Med 317:397–403
6. Bihari D et al. (1986) Disturbances in cardiovascular and pulmonary function in fulminant hepatic failure. In: Williams R (ed) Liver failure. Clinics and Critical Care Medicine. Churchill, Livingstone Edinburgh, pp 47–71
7. Bihari D et al. (1986) Cardiovascular, pulmonary and renal complications of fulminant hepatic failure. Semin Liver Dis 6:119–128
8. Bihari D et al. (1986) Unrecognised tissue hypoxia in the critically ill: its relation to survival. Crit Care Med 14:349
9. Bonnier JJ (1986) Dopexamine hydrochloride, haemodynamic effects in haemochronic cardiac failure, a comparison with dobutamine. Abstracts of X World Congress of Cardiology, Washington DC, September, 188# 1076
10. Brown RA et al. (1985) Dopexamine: a novel agonist at peripheral dopamine receptors and beta2-adrenoceptors. Br J Pharmacol 85:599–608
11. Brown RA et al. (1985) The effect of dopexamine on the cardiovascular system of the dog. Br J Pharmacol 85:609–619
12. Cain S (1977) Oxygen delivery and uptake in dogs during anaemic and hypoxic hypoxia. J Appl Physiol 42:228–234

13. Colardyn F et al. (1986) Acute and long-term haemodynamic effects of dopexamine hydrochloride in patients with chronic cardiac failure. Abstracts of X World Congress of Cardiology, Washington DC, September, 346# 1980
14. Dabney JM et al. (1988) Constriction of lymphatics by catecholamines, carotid occlusion, or hemorrhage. Am J Physiol 255 (Heart Circ Physiol 24):H514–H524
15. Dawson JR et al. (1985) Acute haemodynamic and metabolic effects of dopexamine, a new dopaminergic receptor agonist, in patients with chronic heart failure. Br Heart J 54:313–320
16. Dembinska-Kiec A et al. (1980) Effects of PGI2 and PGI2-analogues on c-AMP levels in cultured endothelial and smooth muscle cells derived from bovine arteries. Naunyn-Schmiedebergs Arch Pharmacol 311:67
17. Endrich J et al. (1987) Induced hypotension: action of sodium nitroprusside and nitroglycerin on the microvasculature. A micropuncture investigation. Anesthesiology 66:605–613
18. Felder RA et al. (1984) Dopamine receptors in the proximal tubule of the rabbit. Am J Physiol 247:F499–F505
19. Flaherty J (1983) Comparison of intravenous nitroglycerin and sodium nitroprusside in acute myocardial infarction. Am J Med 53:60
20. Fleckenstein W et al. (1984) Dopamine effects on the oxygenation of human skeletal muscle. In: Brunley S et al. (eds) Advances in experimental medicine and biology, vol 180: Oxygen transport to tissue. Plenum Press, New York London, pp 609–622
21. Foulds RA et al. (1986) The renovascular effects of dopexamine hydrochloride, a dopaminergic and beta2-adrenergic agonist. Abstracts of X World Congress of Cardiology, Washington DC, September, 201# 1151
22. Gesler RM et al. (1956)Observations on the histoaminolytic activity of dog thoracic duct lymph. J Pharmacol Exp Ther 116:356–365
23. Gimson A et al. (1984) Delivery dependent oxygen consumption in acute liver failure. Clin Sci 66:12P
24. Goldberg LI et al. (1978) A comparison of the vascular dopamine receptor with other dopamine receptors. Ann Rev Pharmacol Toxicol 18:57–79
25. Goldberg LI (1988) Dopamine agonists in intensive care medicine: from receptors to clinical applications. In: Vincent JL (ed) Update in intensive care and emergency medicine, vol 5. Springer, Heidelberg, pp 684–692
26. Gunnar RM et al. (1970) The hemodynamic effects of myocardial infarction and results of therapy. Med Clin North Am 54:235
27. Harper SL et al. (1985) Vasoactive agents and the mesenteric microcirculation. Am J Physiol 249:G309
28. Hauss J et al. (1982) Nitroprusside and nitroglycerin-induced hypotension: effects on hemodynamics and on the microcirculation. World J Surg 6:241–250
29. Hauss J et al. (1978) Die kontrollierte Hypotension mit Natriumnitroprussid. Herz/Kreislauf 8:379
30. Hayashi A et al. (1987) Increased intrinsic pumping of intestinal lymphatics following hemorrhage in anesthetized sheep. Clin Res 60:265–272
31. Hess W et al. (1979) Haemodynamic effects of dopamine and dopamine combined with nitroglycerin in patients subjected to coronary bypass surgery. Br J Anaesth 51:1063–1069
32. Holcroft J et al. (1986) Prostaglandin E1 and survival in patients with adult respiratory distress syndrome. Ann Surg 203:371–378
33. Horwitz D et al. (1962) Effects of dopamine in man. Circ Res 10:237–243
34. Jaski BE et al. (1986) The haemodynamic and myocardial effects of dopexamine: a new beta-2-adrenoceptor and dopaminergic agonist. Br J Clin Pharmacol 21:393–400
35. Kersting T et al. (1985) The effect of dopamine on muscle PO_2 in healthy volunteers and intensive care patients. Eur J Anaesthesiol 2:143–153
36. Kessler M et al. (1973) Oxygen supply. Urban and Schwarzenberg, Munich

37. Kötter W et al. (1977) Comparison of hemodynamic effects of phentolamine, sodium nitroprusside, and glyceryl trinitrate in acute myocardial infarction. Br Heart J 39:1196–1204
38. Leier CV et al. (1983) Dobutamine. Ann Intern Med 99:490
39. Leier CV et al. (1978) Comparative systemic and regional hemodynamic effects of dopamine and dobutamine in patients with cardiomyopathic heart failure. Circulation 58:3 466–475
40. Levinson PD et al. (1985) Endocrine, renal, and hemodynamic responses to graded dopamine infusions in normal men. J Clin Endocrinol Metab 60:821–826
41. Loeb HS et al. (1977) Superiority of dobutamine over dopamine for augmentation of cardiac output in patients with chronic low output cardiac failure. Circulation 55:375–381
42. Loeb HS et al. (1971) Acute hemodynamic effects of dopamine in patients with shock. Circulation 44:163
43. Longnecker DE et al. (1979) A microvascular site of action of sodium nitroprusside in striated muscle of the rat. Anesthesiology 50:111–117
44. Mann T et al. (1978) Effect of nitroprusside on regional myocardial blood flow in coronary artery disease. Results in 25 patients and comparison with nitroglycerin. Circulation 57:732
45. Mason DT et al. (1980) Treatment of acute and chronic congestive heart failure by vasodilator-afterload reduction. Arch Intern Med 140:1577–1581
46. McHale NG et al. (1983) The effect of intravenous adrenaline and noradrenaline infusion on peripheral lymph flow in the sheep. J Physiol 341:517–526
47. Michenfelder JD (1977) Cyanide release from sodium nitroprusside in the dog. Anesthesiology 46:196
48. Miller RR et al. (1976) Pharmacologic mechanism for left ventricular unloading and clinical congestive heart failure: differential effects of nitroprusside, phentolamine, and nitroglycerin on cardiac function in the peripheral circulation. Circ Res 39:127–133
49. Müller B et al. (1986) Effects of prostacyclin and iloprost on regional blood flow in rats. Naunyn-Schmiedebergs Arch Pharmacol [Suppl] 332:R36
50. Müller B et al. (1987) Action of the stable prostacyclin analogue iloprost on microvascular tone and permeability in the hamster cheek pouch. Prostaglandins Leukotrienes Med 29:187–198
51. Motulsky HJ et al. (1982) Adrenergic receptors in man. Direct identification, physiologic regulation, and clinical alterations. N Engl J Med 307:1:18–29
52. Parker M et al. (1979) Rebound hemodynamic events after the abrupt withdrawal of nitroprusside in patients with severe congestive heart failure. N Engl J Med 301:1193–1197
53. Ramdohr B et al. (1972) Vergleichende Untersuchungen über die Wirkung von Dopamin und Orciprenalin am gesunden Menschen: Muskeldurchblutung, Nierendurchblutung, Nierenfunktion. Klin Wochenschr 50:149–157
54. Ross JJR (1976) Afterload mismatch and preload reserve. A conceptual framework for the analysis of ventricular function. Prog Cardiovasc Dis 18:255–264
55. Ruffolo RR (1984) On the mechanism of action of dobutamine. Ann Intern Med 100:313
56. Schaer GL et al. (1985) Norepinephrine alone versus norepinephrine plus low-dose dopamine: enhanced renal blood flow with combination pressor therapy. Crit Care Med 13:492–496
57. Schillinger E et al. (1981) Prostacyclin Drugs of the future. 6:676
58. Schrör K et al. (1981) The antiplatelet and cardiovascular actions of a new carbacyclin derivative (ZK 36.374) equipotent to PGI2 in vitro. Naunyn-Schmiedebergs Arch Pharmacol 316:252
59. Schumacker P et al. (1984) Limitations of aerobic metabolism in critical illness. Chest 85:453–454

60. Shoemaker W et al. (1986) Effects of PGE1 in the adult respiratory distress syndrome. Surgery 99:275–282
61. Shoemaker WC et al. (1987) A new approach to physiology, monitoring, and therapy of shock states. World J Surg 11:133–146
62. Shoemaker WC et al. (1982) Clinical trial of survivors' cardiorespiratory patterns as therapeutic goals in critically ill postoperative patients. Crit Care Med 10:398
63. Shoemaker WC et al. (1983) Use of physiologic monitoring to predict outcome and to assist in clinical decision in critically ill postoperative patients. Am J Surg 146:43
64. Shoemaker WC et al. (1985) Comparison of two monitoring methods (central venous versus pulmonary artery catheter) and two protocols (normal values vs values of survivors) in a prospective randomized clinical trial of critically ill surgical patients. Crit Care Med 13:304
65. Shubin H et al. (1965) The hemodynamic effects of vasopressor agents in shock due to myocardial infarction. Am J Cardiol 15:147
66. Stoner JB et al. (1977) Comparison of dobutamine and dopamine in treatment of severe heart failure. Br Heart J 39:536–539
67. Svensson G et al. (1986) Short-term haemodynamic effects of dopexamine in patients with chronic congestive heart failure. Eur Heart J 7:697–703
68. Tan LB et al. (1987) Beneficial haemodynamic effects of intravenous dopexamine in patients with low-output heart failure. J Cardiovasc Pharmacol 10:280–286
69. Tan LB et al. (1986) Renal response to dopexamine infusion in low output heart failure. Clin Sci 71 [Suppl 15]:56P# 155
70. Tarnow J (1981) Vasodilatatoren. Therapie des Herzversagens und der akuten Myocardischämie. Anaesthesist 30:269–279
71. Tillmanns H et al. (1980) Einfluß von Nitroglycerin auf die Mikrozirkulation des Katzen- und Rattenherzens. In: Rudolf W et al. (eds) Nitrate II. Urban and Schwarzenberg, Munich, pp 119–123
72. Tokioka H et al. (1985) The acute effects of prostaglandin E1 on the pulmonary circulation and oxygen delivery in patients with the adult respiratory distress syndrome. Intensive Care Med 11:61–64
73. Tountas CJR et al. (1965) The effect of sodium nitroprusside on coronary circulation. J Cardiovasc Surg 6:100
74. Weibel ER (1984) The pathway for oxygen. Cambridge: Harvard University Press
75. Weigelt JA (1989) Acute respiratory failure: current concepts. In: Vincent JL (ed) Update in intensive care and emergency medicine, vol 8. Springer, Heidelberg, pp 51–57
76. Wirtzfeld A et al. (1978) Dopamin und Dobutamin in der Behandlung der schweren Herzinsuffizienz. Dsch Med Wochenschr 103:1915–1921
77. Zweifach BW (1961) Functional behavior of the microcirculation. Charles C Thomas, Springfield

Sympathomimetic vs Non-Sympathomimetic Drugs in the Treatment of Heart Failure

G. Baumann and S. B. Felix

Introduction

The syndrome of congestive heart failure is characterized by a reduced stroke volume and peripheral circulatory changes that redistribute blood flow to metabolically active tissues. Conventional inotropic therapy has been limited by the moderate potency and marked toxicity of the glycosides [1] and the obligate i.v. route of administration of the catecholamines. Recent studies suggest that the potent effects of the catecholamines are also subject to tolerance after prolonged administration [2–5]. Thus, it is not surprising that considerable effort has been expended on developing new inotropic therapies that produce their effects by novel mechanisms of action and – in addition – exert considerable vasodilator properties at the same time. Whereas conventional therapeutic strategy attempts to improve ventricular performance by eliciting a "contractile reserve" from the failing heart, it now seems apparent it is the peripheral circulatory changes that predominantly govern functional capacity. An inotropic agent's ability to reverse these peripheral circulatory changes is determined by its inotropic potency, vasodilating capacity, and sustained efficacy. The limitations of conventional therapies have therefore led to the development of new classes of nonglycosidic, nonadrenergic inotropic agents that seem to exert their effects by myocardial phosphodiesterase inhibition, by H_2-receptor mediated adenylate cyclase stimulation and by calcium-sensitizing of myocardial contractile proteins. Although these potent inotropes enhance exercise and aerobic capacity, they are palliative rather than curative agents.

Physiological and Pathophysiological Considerations in Heart Failure

Myocardial failure causes peripheral circulatory derangements mediated by vasoconstriction and a redistribution of blood flow [6]. The peripheral vasoconstriction is probably caused by an enhanced sympathetic tone [3–5, 7], a decrease in arteriolar compliance [8] an increase in interstitial fluid pressure [6], and activation of the renin-aldosterone-angiotensin system [9]. Blood is directed toward the heart and skeletal muscle [10] and as ventricular dysfunction progresses, a deterioration in renal, hepatic, peripheral vascular, and respiratory function ensues. The limited contractile reserve of the failing heart especially limits its ability to provide enough blood flow to metabolizing tissues during exercise. Although blood is directed to exercising skeletal muscle and away from the renal, cutaneous, and mesenteric beds, skeletal muscle blood flow is limited by a fixed vasodilating capacity of the skeletal muscle circulation [11, 12]. The fixed vasodilating capacity probably reflects an increased sodium and water content of the vessel walls and may explain why inotropic agents and vasodilators do not immediately improve exercise capacity despite their beneficial acute hemodynamic effects [13–15]. Even if cardiac output is enhanced, the skeletal muscle circulation cannot effectively lower its impedance and blood is directed to metabolically less active tissues [13, 14].

Chronic therapy with inotropic agents or vasodilators does permit a gradual reversal of the peripheral circulatory changes that compensate for the low output state in heart failure. Presumably, the subsequent hemodynamic and peripheral circulatory improvement permit more effective perfusion of exercising tissues, allowing the patient greater participation in various activities. Physical conditioning improves and functional capacity is enhanced [16].

A combination of inotropy and vasodilation provides the most pronounced improvements in peripheral circulatory hemodynamics [17]. Indeed, inotropes that also have vasodilating properties effect a rapid functional improvement in patients with heart failure [17–19]. Chronic therapy with these agents permits even greater improvements in peripheral circulatory hemodynamics, and the enhanced functional capacity seen initially is sustained and often improved [17].

It is apparent that peripheral circulatory hemodynamics are important determinants of a patient's functional capacity – and in fact, may be more influential on exercise capacity than cardiac output and pulmonary circulatory congestion [20, 21]. The poor correlation between left ventricular performance and exercise capacity is consistent with this conclusion [22].

Inotropic Therapy

Inotropic therapy for heart failure is predicated on the assumption that residual myocardial function, or a "contractile reserve" can be elicited from the failing heart [1]. Residual contractile activity in failing hearts has been demonstrated by post-extrasystolic potentiation of myocardial contractility [22] and paired electrical stimulation [22, 23].

Catecholamines

The sympathetic amines are potent inotropes but their utility in the management of heart failure has been limited by their chronotropic and arrhythmogenic potentials and the obligate i.v. route of administration [24]. They enhance myocardial cyclic AMP by increasing β-receptor mediated adenylate cyclase activity. Protein kinases are subsequently activated, and phosphorylation of sarcolemmal membrane proteins increases the number of active calcium channels. The slow inward current is enhanced, and calcium release from the sarcoplasmatic reticulum is increased [25].

While in the United States the original catecholamines (norepinephrine, epinephrine) are still widely used for therapy of acute heart failure, in Western Europe dobutamine probably is the most clinically important sympathomimetic agent [24, 26]. A derivative of isoproterenol, it has a high affinity for β_1-receptors and a weak affinity for α_1, α_2 and β_2-receptors [27]. Its cardiotonic effects are relatively free of concomitant increases in heart rate leading some investigators to suggest that β_2-receptors are primarily responsible for determinating heart rate. Dobutamine improves the hemodynamic profile of patients with chronic heart failure, but tolerance to its acute effects develops within 2–3 days after initiation of therapy [28, 29]. The mechanism of tolerance development is most likely due to a specific damage of sarcolemmal β_1-receptors ("receptor down-regulation") due to enhanced levels of circulating endogenous catecholamines [3, 4, 7]. The higher the degree of left ventricular dysfunction, the higher catecholamine plasma concentrations are found with the result of a proportionally decreased number and affinity of cardiac β_1-receptors [4, 7, 29, 30]. Exogenous catecholamines may accelerate and intensify this pathophysiologic cycle leading to a catecholamine-insensitive heart failure state [4, 28]. This has been shown for both, i.v. and orally effective catecholamines [2, 5, 28, 30]. Dobutamine does not immediately enhance functional capacity [13], but persistant functional benefits have been reported in patients treated with continuous 72 h infusions [31]. Improved clinical status and functional capacity have also been reported in patients receiving weekly 4-h infusions of dobutamine. The clinical improvement probably was mediated by peripheral circulatory changes, since resting ventricular function was not changed [32].

Several new orally effective catecholamines have been developed and are being studied. These agents, including pirbuterol and prenalterol, are partial β-agonists with different specifities for β_1- and β_2-receptors [33]. The partial β-agonists increase cardiac output and decrease filling pressures and systemic vascular resistance [34, 35]. Their efficacy is limited, however, by side effects (nervousness, tremulousness) and also tolerance development that is mediated by β-adrenoceptor down-regulation after chronic administration [2]. Since partial agonists must stimulate a large portion of available receptors to exert an effect on the target tissue, their maximal action diminishes as β-adrenoceptor density is reduced. If β-receptor density declines enough, the partial β-agonists exert no β-adrenergic effect but continue to occupy the remaining receptors. In this setting these agents competitively inhibit other more potent catecholamines and may effectively act as beta-blocker thus inducing "β-adrenoceptor up-regulation." This concept has been proposed earlier for prenalterol [30, 35] and recently for xamoterol, a novel β_1-selective partial agonist with obvious long-term efficacy [36].

The recent demonstration of decreased β-adrenoceptor density in failing human hearts [2–4, 7] suggests that the overall efficacy of full β-receptor-agonists may be limited from the very onset of therapy [7]. Myocardial contractility may be enhanced in such situations by β-adrenoceptor independent inotropes, such as phosphodiesterase III inhibitors, H_2-receptor agonists, or compounds directly sensitizing myocardial myofibrils for Ca^{2+}-ions (see below). A further reduction in β-receptor density after chronic treatment with sympathomimetic agents may be minimized by alternating β-agonists with these other inotropes, since β-receptor number and affinity return to pretreatment levels when sympathomimetic drugs are withdrawn [2, 37–39].

In this context it seems of interest that cardiac β_2-receptors were found to be present at the sarcolemmal surface mediating a positive inotropic action by also increasing adenylate cyclase activity [40]. Evidence has been produced that there is a large proportion of β_2-receptors (approximately 20% in nonfailing hearts vs 80% β_1-receptors) [40–43].

In contrast, in the failing human ventricular myocardium almost all of the decrease in total β-receptor density is due to "selectivity" for β_1-receptors and not due to a reduction of cardiac β_2-receptor density [44, 45]. Thus, the relatively stable β_2-receptor population may be of value for therapeutic interventions. A recently developed, highly selective β_2-agonist, dopexamine hydrochloride, resembles a relatively new addition for treatment of congestive heart failure and preliminary studies in patients with idiopathic congestive cardiomyopathies are promising in terms of both acute and long-term efficacy [44, 47]. Besides that dopexamine hydrochloride proved to markedly improve diuresis and renal creatinine clearance when given over a period of 48 h, due to a pronounced agonistic action of renal dopaminergic DA_2-receptors [47]. However, further studies are needed to ultimately determine the therapeutic value of this compound especially in acute heart failure, where up to now no systematic investigations have been carried out.

Non-Catecholamine Mediated Inotropic Pathways

The limitations of conventional inotropic therapy (including digitalis) prompted a worldwide stimulus for the search of new inotropic agents and culminated in the development of bipyridine derivatives. Amrinone is the prototype of this group of drugs [48], and the i.v. form has recently been approved for the treatment of congestive heart failure in the USA and the Federal Republic of Germany (FRG).

Phosphodiesterase III Inhibitors

Considerable attention has been given to the role of phosphodiesterase inhibitors in the treatment of congestive heart failure, all compounds being more or less specific inhibitors of myocardial phosphodiesterase (PDE) III fraction. Three classes of pharmacologic agents share this ability to selectively inhibit the enzyme and thereby increase intracellular cyclic AMP levels: bipyridine derivatives (amrinone, milrinone), imidazolone derivates (enoxymone, piroxymone), and benzimidazole derivatives (pimobendane, UDCG 115 BS). The mechanism of action and clinical utility has recently been reviewed [52–54]. Although they increase cyclic AMP accumulation and thereby enhance contractility in normal myocardium, their ability to augment contractility in failing human hearts has been questioned [55]. Nevertheless, amrinone is the first commercially available PDE III inhibitor in the USA and FRG.

Amrinone was first shown to augment myocardial contractility in papillary muscle preparations and in intact dogs [48]. It causes a nonspecific smooth muscle relaxation in vitro [49] and induces substantial vasodilation at high doses in animals and humans [50]. Although the mechanism of amrinone's inotropic and vasodilating action is not fully understood at present, its effects are thought to be caused by PDE III inhibition [51].

In our clinical experience amrinone has produced favorable effects in patients with severe heart failure, although the more recently developed piroximone seems to have a clearly superior profile of action with an apparent redistribution of blood flow in favor of skeletal muscle perfusion, resulting in an increase in exercise capacity and work load in these critically ill patients. Additionally, there may be an important role for the combined use of a PDE inhibitor and an agent that stimulates cardiac adenylate cyclase activity at a more proximal site (β_1-, β_2-, or H_2-receptors) in the receptor-adenylate cyclase complex [56, 57].

Amrinone and piroximone decrease atrial and atrioventricular (AV) nodal refractory periods and improve AV nodal conduction [58, 59]. No significant change in electrocardiographic intervals or AH and HV intervals has been demonstrated. Sinus node refractory time seems unaltered [58]. Amrinone causes a dose-dependent augmentation of dp/dt in animal studies [60]. It improves cardiac output and reduces systemic vascular resistance and filling pressures. The acute and chronic administration enhances functional capacity at submaximal levels of exercise [61–63]. It has salutary effects on peripheral circulatory hemodynamics and potentiates renal blood flow and improves renal function [64]. These effects can even be enhanced by concomitant administration of vasodilators, which also permit the use of lower doses of PDE III inhibitors [17]. Tachyphylaxis and tolerance do not occur with either amrinone (up to 14 days) [61] or piroximone (up to 6 months) [65]. Amrinone, but not piroximone, causes several disturbing side effects including dose-related thrombocytopenia, sometimes gastrointestinal disturbance, and in a few patients hepatotoxicity and fever [64, 66, 67]. None of these side effects have been observed for piroximone during short- and long-term administration [65]. Also milrinone, another bipyridine derivative, which is 10 to 30 times more potent than amrinone, seems to have none of amrinone's side effects as well.

The H_2-Histamine Receptor Pathway, Possible Role of Cardiac H_2-Receptor Agonists in Patients with Chronic and Acute Heart Failure

The H_2-histamine receptor pathway in nonfailing and failing ventricular myocardium was assessed by measuring inotropic responses in isolated perfused hearts [2, 4, 7] and adenylate cyclase stimulation rates in particulate membrane preparations. Baumann et al. directly measured H_2-receptors by ^{3}H-tiotidine binding [4]. In human ventricular myocardium histamine activates adenylate cyclase activity through H_2-receptors to a degree comparable with isoproterenol [4]. No differences have been found between failing and nonfailing hearts for either adenylate cyclase activation, muscle contraction, or radioligand binding [4], thus indicating, that the myocardial H_2-receptor adenylate cyclase system is not involved in the pathophysiologic process of receptor down-regulation as described for the β_1-adrenoceptor system in the development of congestive heart failure [3–5, 7, 38, 45, 74–78].

Since cardiac H_2-receptors appear to be relatively undisturbed in the failing human heart, they could be used for inotropic support and in fact there are reports of favorable hemodynamic effects from administration of the high-affinity H_2-agonist impromidine in patients with severe NYHA IV congestive heart failure [68]. It seems remarkable that H_2-receptor stimulation still induced a marked positive inotropic effect in patients who did not respond to catecholamine treatment as a consequence of a specific β_1-receptor damage occurring during the development of heart failure [68]. Dobutamine was without any significant effect in these studies, while the H_2-receptor agonist impromidine elicited potent hemodynamic actions. The increase in cardiac output and decrease in right atrial, pulmonary capillary wedge pressures, as well the decline in pulmonary and systemic vascular resistance were not only due to a pure vasodilator action of impromidine, since sodium-nitroprusside elicited only 40% of the overall hemodynamic properties in the same patients. This implies that the overall effect of H_2-receptor stimulation is due to vasodilation by approximately 40%, and, on the other hand, is based upon a direct positive inotropic effect on the heart, which may account for about 60%.

Agents that Sensitize the Contractile Proteins to Calcium

As the interaction of calcium with subunits of the contractile proteins is the final step in excitation-contraction coupling, it may be the most important. Therefore, a change in the sensitivity of the contractile proteins to Ca^{2+} ions would substantially alter contractility. Several new inotropics appear to exert their inotropic effects at least in part via increasing the activation potency of Ca^{2+} ions at the myofibrils: DPI 201-106 [69] and UDCG 115 BS (pimobendane) [70]. Both compounds have undergone phase I and II studies. Although sulmazole (ARL 115) has been withdrawn from clinical studies, pimobendane, a compound with structural similarities and an ability to enhance Ca^{2+} affinity of the contractile proteins [70], is in phase II clinical trials with obviously favorable results [39]. Meanwhile, these agents, which have already shown their potent inotropic effects in vitro, have proved their safety and efficacy in patients with congestive cardiomyopathy. The acute hemodynamic effects are very impressive and the overall profile of pimobendane was superior compared with dobutamine in patients with severe end stage heart failure [39]. Furthermore, it could be shown that pimobendane is capable of potentiating the hemodynamic effects of β_1- and β_2-receptor mediated adenylate cyclase stimulation under clinical conditions [37, 38] in a very impressive way. The most interesting finding is reflected in a recent clinical study, in which 5 days treatment with pimobendane resulted in a marked improvement of the β_1-receptor mediated inotropic response to dobutamine in eight patients with initial catecholamine-insensitive heart failure [57]. During this 5-day treatment period with pimobendane endogenous catecholamines declined to nearly normal values with the results of a regeneration of the β-receptor population. This – in turn – improved functional capacity in these patients so that it was concluded that the transient inotropic stimulation with pimobendane restored the physiological ability of the heart to adapt to stress situations and physical requirements of the body. Similar results were also obtained with the H_2-receptor agonist impromidine [57, 58]. Hence, it seems important to stimulate the heart independently of the β_1-receptor-adenylate cyclase mechanism, if inotropic support is needed.

Inotropic Agents and Disease Progression

It has been suggested that inotropic agents may accelerate the progressive myocardial deterioration in heart failure by exhausting limited myocardial energy supplies and increasing oxygen demands in the setting of ischemia [71]. Only controlled, randomized, double-blind studies will fully address this issue. Theoretically, cardiotonic agents may actually be beneficial to the failing heart. Subendocardial perfusion is decreased in a dilated heart with elevated filling pressure because of wall tension and a narrow coronary artery perfusion pressure gradient. Cardiotonic agents decrease systemic vascular resistance, left ventricular filling pressure, and chamber size, and thereby decrease wall tension. The net result is a decrease in myocardial oxygen demands and an increase in the coronary perfusion pressure gradient, with increased oxygen delivery to ischemic tissues [72].

The arrhythmogenic potential of the inotropes is also of particular concern and is well documented for the digitalis glycosides and sympathomimetic amines. Few studies have examined the arrhythmogenic properties of the bipyridine derivatives [58] and further work is necessary to define whatever role these potent inotropes may have in contributing to sudden death in patients with heart failure [73].

Most of the patients we have treated with new inotropes like impromidine and pimobendane have had advanced pump dysfunction. One can only speculate as to what effect earlier intervention would have had on the progression of the disease. Perhaps inotropic stimulation will delay or even reverse ventricular dilatatioin in heart failure states. In dilated hearts inotropic agents shorten the length of sarcomeres at end systole and end diastole, thus leading to a reduction in ventricular chamber size and functional improvement of the sliding filaments of the contractile apparatus. Alternatively, patients with mild or moderate failure without ventricular dilatation and elevated filling pressure may be the least likely to benefit from these agents. Indeed, the increased myocardial energy expenditure required to support an increase in inotropy would not be compensated for by a fall in wall tension and enhanced subendocardial perfusion. Thus, potent inotropic agents should be used cautiously in patients with mild heart failure at present. Future efforts must be directed at the preservation of myocardium during early stages of ventricular dysfunction. Once ventricular dilatation and fibrosis is established, only transplantation offers a reasonable expectation of cure. Thus, inotropic therapy provides palliation for an inexorably progressive disease.

References

1. Selzer A (1981) Digitalis in cardiac failure: do benefits justify risks? Arch Intern Med 141:18
2. Colucci WS, Alexander W, Williams GH et al. (1981) Decreased lymphocyte beta-adrenergic receptor density in patients with heart failure and tolerance to the beta-adrenergic agonist pirbuterol. N Engl J Med 305:185
3. Baumann G, Rieß G, Erhardt WD, Felix STB, Ludwig L, Blümel G, Blömer H (1981) Impaired beta-adrenergic stimulation in the uninvolved ventricle post-acute myocardial infarction: reversible defect due to decline in number and affinity of beta-receptors. Am Heart J 101:569
4. Baumann G, Mercader D, Busch U et al. (1983) Effects of H_2-receptor agonist impromidine in human myocardium and patients with heart failure due to mitral and aortic valve disease. J Cardiovasc Pharmacol 5:618–625
5. Baumann G, Felix STB (1983) Zur pharmakologischen Stellung von Prenalterol. II. Versuch einer kritischen Wertung aus experimenteller und klinischer Sicht. Herz/Kreislauf 2:65
6. Zelis R, Lee G, Mason DT (1974) The influence of experimental edema on metabolically determined blood flow. Circ Res 34:482
7. Bristow MR, Ginsburg R, Minobe W et al. (1982) Decreased catecholamine sensitivity and beta-adrenergic receptor density in failing human hearts. N Engl J Med 307:205
8. Zelis R, Delea CS, Coleman H et al. (1970) Arterial sodium content in experimental congestive heart failure. Circulation 41:213
9. Watkins L, Burkin LA, Haven E et al. (1976) The renin-angiotensin system in congestive heart failure in conscious dogs. J Clin Invest 57:1606
10. Mason DT, Zelis R, Longhurst J et al. (1977) Cardiocirculatory responses to muscular exercise in congestive heart failure. In: Sonnenblick EH, Lesch M (eds) Exercise and heart disease. Grune and Stratton, New York, p 229
11. LeJemtel TH, Maskin CS, Sinoway L et al. (1983) Fixed vasodilating capacity in exercising leg muscles: a limitation of aerobic capacity in heart failure. Clin Res 31:2 (abstr)
12. Zelis R, Longhurst J, Capone RJ et al. (1974) A comparison of regional blood flow and oxygen utilization during dynamic forearm exercise in normal subjects and patients with congestive heart failure. Circulation 50:137
13. Maskin CS, Forman R, Sonnenblick EH et al. (1983) Failure of dobutamine to increase exercise capacity. Am J Cardiol 51:177
14. Kugler J, Maskin C, Frishman WH et al. (1982) Regional and systemic metabolic effects of angiotensin converting enzyme inhibition during exercise in patients with severe heart failure. Circulation 66:1258
15. LeJemtel TH, Kugler J, Maskin CS et al. (1982) Captoril therapy in severe heart failure: delayed improvement in maximal oxygen uptake despite immediate hemodynamic effects. Acta Cardiol [Suppl] (Brux) 28:61
16. Lee AP, Ioe R, Blusey R et al. (1979) Long-term effects of physical training on coronary patients with impaired ventricular function. Circulation 60:1519
17. Siegel LA, Keung E, Siskind SJ et al. (1981) Beneficial effects of amrinone-hydralazine combination on resting hemodynamics and exercise capacity in patients with severe congestive heart failure. Circ Res 63:838

18. Siskind SJ, Sonnenblick EH, Forman R et al. (1981) Acute substantial benefits of inotropic therapy with amrinone on exercise hemodynamics and metabolism in severe congestive heart failure. Circulation 64:966
19. Maskin CS, Sinoway L, Chadwick B et al. (1983) Sustained hemodynamic and clinical effects of a new cardiotonic agent WIN 47203 in patients with severe congestive heart failure. Circulation 67:1065
20. Wilson JR, Ferraro N (1983) Exercise intolerance in patients with chronic left heart failure: relation to oxygen transport and ventilatory abnormalities. Am J Cardiol 51:1358
21. Franciosa JA, Park M, Levine TB (1981) Lack of correlation between exercise capacity and indexes of resting left ventricular performance in heart failure. Am J Cardiol 47:33
22. Dyke SH, Urschel CW, Sonnenblick EH et al. (1975) Detection of latent function in acutely ischemic myocardium in the dog. Circ Res 36:490
23. Braunwald E, Ross J, Frommer PL et al. (1964) Clinical observations on paired electrical stimulation of the heart. Am J Med 37:700
24. Sonnenblick EH, Frishman WH, LeJemtel TH (1979) Dobutamine: a new synthetic cardioactive sympathetic amine. N Engl J Med 300:17
25. Scholz H (1984) Inotropic drugs and their mechanism of action. J Am Coll Cardiol 4:389
26. Klein G, Wirtzfeld A, Schnelle K, Holzmüller W, Schinz A (1980) Hämodynamische und metabolische Wirkungen von Dobutamin und Prenalterol bei gesunden Probanden. In: Bleifeld W, Gattinge R, Schaper W, Brade W (eds) Internationales Dobutamin Symposium. Urban and Schwarzenberg, Munich
27. Williams RJ, Bishop Z (1981) Selectivity of dobutamine for adrenergic receptor subtypes: in vitro analysis by radioligand binding. J Clin Invest 67:1703
28. Unverferth DV, Blauford M, Kates RE et al. (1980) Tolerance to dobutamine after a 72-hour continuous infusion. Am J Med 69:262
29. Baumann G, Pfafferott C, Klein G (1988) Acute hemodynamic effects of dopexamine, dobutamine and sodium-nitroprusside in chronic heart failure. Eur Heart J 9:503
30. Baumann G, Felix STB, Rieß G, Loher U, Ludwig L, Blömer H (1984) Apparent superiority of H_2-receptor stimulation and simultaneous β-blockade over conventional treatment with β-sympathomimetic drugs post-acute myocardial infarction. Agents Actions 15:216–228
31. Unverferth DV, Magorien RD, Altschuld R et al. (1983) The hemodynamic and metabolic advantages gained by a 3-day infusion of dobutamine in patients with congestive cardiomyopathy. Am Heart J 106:29
32. Leier CV, Huss P, Lewis RP et al. (1982) Drug-induced conditioning in congestive heart failure. Circulation 65:1382
33. Kenakin TP, Ferris RM (1983) Effects of in vivo beta-adrenoceptor down regulation on cardiac responses to prenalterol and pirbuterol. J Cardiovasc Pharmacol 5:90
34. Awan NA, Evensen MK, Needham KE et al. (1981) Hemodynamic effects of oral pirbuterol in chronic severe congestive heart failure. Circulation 63:96
35. Erbel R, Meyer J, Lambertz H et al. (1982) Hemodynamic effects of prenalterol in patients with ischemic heart disease and congestive cardiomyopathy. Circulation 66:361
36. Pouleur H, van Eyll CH, Hanet C et al. (1988) Long-term effects of xamoterol on left ventricular function and late remodeling: a study in patients with anterior myocardial infarction and single-vessel disease. Circulation 77:1081
37. Baumann G, Busch U, Permanetter B et al. (1986) Occurrence and function of histamine receptors – possible significance of H_2-receptor stimulation in catecholamine-insensitive myocardial insufficiency. In: Schölmerich P, Holtmeier HJ, Kroneberg HG (eds) Cardiovascular receptors – new pharmacologic and clinical aspects. Thieme, Stuttgart, p 169
38. Baumann G, Busch U, Permanetter B et al. (1987) Mögliche Bedeutung einer kardialen H_2-Rezeptorstimulation bei Katecholamin-refraktärem Myokardversagen

unterschiedlichster Ätiologie. In: Brisse B, Bender F (eds) Autonome Inervation des Herzens. Steinkopff, Darmstadt, p 183
39. Baumann G, Ningel K, Permanetter B (1989) Cardiovascular profile of UDCG 115 BS – pimobendane and reversibility of catecholamine subsensitivity in severe congestive heart failure secondary to idiopathic dilated cardiomyopathy. J Cardiovasc Pharmacol 13:730
40. Brodde OE, Schuler S, Kretsch R et al. (1986) Regional distribution of β-adrenoceptors in the human heart: coexistence of functional β_1- and β_2-adrenoceptors in both atria and ventricles in severe congestive cardiomyopathy. J Cardiovasc Pharmacol 8:1235
41. Stiles GL, Taylor S, Lefkowitz RJ (1983) Human cardiac β-adrenergic receptors: subtype heterogeneity delineated by direct radioligand binding. Life Sci 33:467
42. Heitz A, Schwartz J, Velly J (1983) β-Adrenoceptors of the human myocardium: determination of β_1 and β_2 subtypes by radioligand. Br J Pharmacol 80:711
43. Golf S, Lovstad R, Hnsson V (1985) β-Adrenoceptor density and relative number of β-adrenoceptor subtypes in biopsies from human right atrial, left ventricular and right ventricular myocardium. Cardiovasc Res 19:636
44. Bristow MR, Ginsburg R, Fowler M et al. (1986) β_1- And β_2-adrenergic receptor subpopulations in normal and failing human ventricular myocardium: coupling of both receptor subtypes to muscle contraction and selective β_1 receptor down-regulation in heart failure. Circ Res 59:297
45. Bristow MR, Ginsburg R (1986) β Receptors are present on myocardial cells in human ventricular myocardium. Am J Cardiol 57:3F
46. Baumann G, Felix STB, Sackmann I, Klein G (1989) An open study to assess the effects of dopexamine on urinary output and haemodynamics in patients with chronic cardiac failure and to compare these effects with those produced by dobutamine. Eur Heart J (in press)
47. Baumann G, Gutting M, Pfafferott C et al. (1988) Comparison of acute haemodynamic effects of dopexamine hydrochloride, dobutamine and sodium nitroprusside in chronic heart failure. Eur Heart J 9:503
48. Alousi AA, Farah AE, Lesher GY et al. (1979) Cardiotonic activity of amrinone – WIN 40680 (5-amino-3,4′-bipyridine-6(1H)-one). Circ Res 45:666
49. Ross G, Dobestani AI, Patel AL (1981) Effect of amrinone on vascular smooth muscle. Fed Proc 40:659 (abstr)
50. Sonnenblick EH, Mancini DM, LeJemtel TH (1989) New inotropic drugs for the treatment of heart failure: promises and limitations. Am J Cardiol (in press)
51. Levine SD, Jacoby M, Satriano JA et al. (1981) The effects of amrinone on transport and cAMP metabolism in toad urinary bladder. J Pharmacol Exp Ther 216:220
52. Scholz H, Meyer W (1986) Phosphodiesterase inhibiting properties of newer inotropic agents. Circulation [Suppl III] 73:III–108
53. Rapundalo St, Grupp I, Grupp G et al. (1986) Myocardial actions of milrinone: characterization of its mechanism of action. Circulation 73 [Suppl III]:III–134
54. Colucci WS, Wright RF, Braunwald E (1986) New positive inotropic agents in the treatment of congestive heart failure (pt 2). N Engl J Med 314:349
55. Feldman MD, Copelas L, Gwathmey JK et al. (1987) Pharmacologic evidence of an important cause of contractile dysfunction in patients with end-stage heart failure. Circulation 75:331
56. Baumann G, Mercader D, Permanetter B, Busch U, Ningel K, Wirtzfeld A, Blömer H (1985) A new therapeutic approach on congestive heart failure: combined phosphodiesterase inhibition with simultaneous H_2-receptor stimulation. In: Ganellin CR, Schwartz JC (eds) Frontiers in histamine research. Pergamon, New York, p 325 (Advances in the biosciences, vol 54)
57. Baumann G, Buschauer A, Permanetter B et al. (1988) New aspects for the treatment of congestive heart failure. Innere Medizin 15:30
58. Naccarelli GV, Gray EL, Dougherty AH et al. (1984) Amrinone: acute electrophysiologic and hemodynamic effects in patients with congestive heart failure. Am J Cardiol 54:600

59. Nasrat A, Tepper D, Hertzberg J et al. (1983) Effects of amrinone on atrioventricular conduction in the intact canine heart. J Clin Pharmacol 23:257
60. Alousi AA, Farah AE, Lesher GY et al. (1979) Cardiotonic activity of amrinone – WIN 40680. Circ Res 45:666
61. Maskin CS, Forman R, Klein NA et al. (1982) Long-term amrinone therapy in patients with severe heart failure. Am J Med 72:113
62. Weber KT, Andrews V, Janicki JS et al. (1981) Amrinone and exercise performance in patients with chronic heart failure. Am J Cardiol 48:164
63. Siskind SY, Sonnenblick EH, Forman R et al. (1981) Acute substantial benefits of inotropic therapy with amrinone on exercise hemodynamics and metabolism in severe congestive heart failure. Circulation 64:966
64. LeJemtel TH, Keung E, Ribner HS et al. (1980) Sustained beneficial effects of oral amrinone on cardiac and renal function in patients with severe congestive heart failure. Am J Cardiol 45:123
65. Baumann G, Felix STB, Ningel K, Klein G (1989) Piroximone. Vasodilatation versus inotropy: a group comparative study of hemodynamic responses in chronic congestive heart failure with sodium nitroprusside, piroximone (MDL 19205) and dobutamine. Eur Heart J (in press)
66. Wynne J, Malacoff RF, Benotti JR et al. (1980) Oral amrinone in refractory congestive heart failure. Am J Cardiol 45:1245
67. Sterling Winthrop Research Institute (1982) Clinical experience with amrinone: overall summary for NDA amendment. Sterling Winthrop Research Institute, Rensselaer NY
68. Baumann G, Permanetter B, Wirtzfeld A (1984) Possible value of H_2-receptor agonists for treatment of catecholamine-insensitive congestive heart failure. Pharmacol Ther 24:177
69. Scholtysik G, Salzmann R, Berthold R et al. (1985) DPI 20106, a novel cardioactive agent. Combination of cAMP-independent positive inotropic, negative chronotropic action potential prolonging and coronary dilatory properties. Naunyn-Schmiedeberg's Arch Pharmacol 329:316
70. Rüegg JC (1986) Effects of new inotropic agents on Ca^{2+} sensitivity of contractile proteins. Circulation 73 [Suppl III]:III–78
71. Katz AM (1978) A new inotropic drug: its promise and a caution. N Engl J Med 29:1409
72. Kirk ES, LeJemtel TH, Nelson GR et al. (1976) Mechanisms of beneficial effects of vasodilators and inotropic stimulation in the experimental failing ischemic heart. Am J Med 65:189
73. LeJemtel TH, Sonnenblick EH (1984) Should the failing heart be stimulated? N Engl J Med 310:1384
74. Baumann G, Rieß G, Felix STB et al. (1981) Catecholamines and β-adrenergic receptors in the non-ischemic myocardium after coronary occlusion. In: Delius W, Gerlach E, Grobecker X, Kübler W (eds) Catecholamines and the heart, vol 72. Springer, Berlin Heidelberg New York, p 91
75. Baumann G, Felix STB, Schrader J et al. (1981) Cardiac contractile and metabolic effects mediated via the myocardial H_2-receptor adenylate cyclase system: characterization of two new specific H_2-receptor-agonists, impromidine and dimaprit, in the guinea pig and human myocardium. Res Exp Med (Berl) 179:81–98
76. Baumann G, Felix STB, Rieß G, Loher U, Ludwig L, Blömer H (1982) Effective stimulation of cardiac contractility and myocardial metabolism by impromidine and dimaprit – two new H_2-agonistic compounds – in the surviving, catecholamine-insensitive myocardium after coronary occlusion. J Cardiovasc Pharmacol 4:542–553
77. Baumann G, Rieß G, Erhardt WD, Felix STB, Blömer H (1980) Reduzierte β-adrenerge Ansprechbarkeit im nicht ischämischen Myokard nach experimentellem Herzinfarkt. Z Kardiol 69:209
78. Baumann G, Schrader J, Gerlach E (1981) Inhibitory action of adenosine on histamine- and dopamine-stimulated cardiac contractility and adenylate cyclase in guinea pigs. Circ Res 48:259–266

Proven Therapeutic Uses for Hyperbaric Oxygen

C. D. Wan Lu and E. M. Camporesi

Definition

Hyperbaric oxygen therapy consists of the inhalation of oxygen at partial pressures greater than that which can be achieved at sea level. These pressures are expressed as atmospheres absolute (ATA) such that 1 ATA represents 760 mmHg or normal barometric pressure at sea level. Hyperbaric oxygen therapy can be accomplished in monoplace and multiplace chambers. Monoplace chambers accommodate one patient at a time, with the entire chamber pressurized with 100% oxygen. Multiplace chambers are larger and can expose two or more people simultaneously, including support personnel. In this situation, the chamber is usually pressurized with air while patients breathe 100% oxygen via a face mask, head tent, or through an endotracheal tube.

Brief History

Hyperbaric conditions were first used clinically in the midnineteenth century. Decompression sickness was first described as a complication of bridge construction using compressed air in France (caissons disease). Some of the earliest and most astute observations on the effects of changes in barometric pressure were made by Paul Bert (1843, first published in 1878). He demonstrated that pure oxygen could cause seizures and death in animals if inhaled at pressures greater than approximately 4 ATA and thus felt that the use of hyperbaric oxygen was only justified in carbon monoxide poisoning. He felt, however, that hyperbaric pressure could be used therapeutically in the treatment of decompression sickness. Another complication, pulmonary damage, due to inhalation of pure oxygen at 1 ATA was described in the early 1900s (the Lorrain Smith effect; Smith 1899). Cunningham (1927) had insight enough to propose the use of compressed air in the therapy of hypoxic states, however due to incorrect selection of patients and poor results, enthusiasm diminished. The use of hyperbaric oxygen fell into disrepute when it was claimed to be a panacea for many ailments. In the 1930s the British first used oxygen inhalation during decompression. Simultaneously the US Navy investigated hyperbaric oxygen therapy for treating decompression sickness. Since then, there have been extensive studies on safe depth-time parameters for decompression as well as tolerated limits for oxygen toxicity. A revival in the use of hyperbaric oxygen therapy for nondiving disorders occurred in the 1960s following scientific studies by Boerema et al. (1956, 1960). He and others investigated hyperbaric oxygen as therapy for gas gangrene and cardiac surgery. In the hopes of overcoming difficulties with hypothermic arrest during cardiac surgery, he demonstrated that pigs with insufficient hemoglobin levels to sustain life, could survive due to dissolved oxygen in plasma at 3 ATA.

Today the field encompasses about one dozen diverse indications for which there are excellent rationale and clinical experience. Despite this, hyperbaric oxygen therapy has not been without criticism (Gabbs and Robin 1987).

Physical and Physiologic Principles of Hyperbaric Oxygen Therapy

Pressure

Pressurization of the body above atmospheric pressure causes a variety of physiologic alterations. Most importantly, it must be remembered that for an enclosed volume, gas volume is inversely proportional to absolute pressure (Boyle's Law). Gas-containing cavities in the body therefore undergo volume changes with compression and decompression. This principle is used therapeutically for the treatment of air embolism and decompression sickness since the volume of intravascular and tissue gas bubbles are decreased by increased ambient pressures. During decompression, disastrous consequences of Boyle's Law may occur; if there is inadvertent obstruction of airways or air trapping and overdistension, such pulmonary overinflation on decompression may lead to pneumothorax or air embolism. Middle ear and paranasal sinus problems, often aggravated by upper respiratory tract infection, may cause discomfort during compression and decompression. These problems are helped by training, practice, and judicious use of intranasal vasoconstrictor agents. Acutely ill or unconscious patients, or those chronically unable to equalize pressures in the ear, may require myringotomy to avoid trauma to or rupture of tympanic membranes during pressurization.

Oxygen

The total pressure of a gas mixture can be expressed as the sum of the partial pressures of each gas present in the mixture (Dalton's Law). In practical terms, atmospheric air contains just two gases: oxygen (20.9%) and nitrogen (78.1%). The most frequent pressures and partial pressures used during therapeutic regimes are shown in Table 1.

Transport of oxygen in blood occurs by chemical binding to hemoglobin and by physical solution in plasma. As per Henry's Law, the volume of gas in physical solution in body fluids is directly proportional to the partial pressure of the gas to which the fluid is exposed. Whole blood with a hemoglobin concentration of 15 g/dl has an oxygen capacity of about 20 vol%. Oxygen solubility at 37 °C in plasma is equal to 0.0031 vol% O_2/mmHg. Therefore additional dissolved oxygen amounts to about 0.3 vol% at a PO_2 of 100 mm/Hg.

Table 1. Range of ideal partial pressures of oxygen in hyperbaric oxygen therapy

ATA	P_{tot} (mmHg)	Gas species	Alveolar PO_2[a] (mmHg)	Arterial PO_2[a, b] (mmHg)	Dissolved O_2 content[d] (vol %)	Total O_2 content[b] (vol %)
1	760	Air	110	110	0.32	20.4
1	760	100% O_2	673	673	2.09	22.2
2	1520	100% O_2	1433	1433	4.40	24.3
3	2280	100% O_2	2193	2193	6.80	26.9
4	3040	Air or Nitrox[c]	582		1.80	
5	3800	Air or Nitrox[c]	742		2.30	
6	4560	Air or Nitrox[c]	902		2.40	

[a] Modified from Moon et al. (1987) with the assumption that $PA_{CO_2} = Pa_{CO_2}$ and $R = 0.8$ and where PA_{O_2} is calculated using the formula:

$$PA_{O_2} = PI_{O_2} - PA_{CO_2}\left[FI_{O_2} + \frac{1 - FI_{O_2}}{R}\right]$$

PA_{O_2}, PA_{CO_2} = alveolar gas tensions; PI_{O_2} = inspired oxygen tension; Pa_{CO_2} = arterial P_{CO_2}; FI_{O_2} = fractional inspired oxygen concentration; R = respiratory quotient = $\dot{V}_{CO_2}/\dot{V}_{O_2}$

[b] Modified from Saltzman et al. (1965)

[c] No supplemental oxygen is used at pressures greater than 3 ATA due to risk of oxygen toxicity. Nitrox, a mixture of oxygen and nitrogen is used instead

[d] Modified from Bakker (1984)

The total oxygen content in the blood can be expressed by the following equation:

$$SaO_2 \times 1.39 \times Hb + PaO_2 \times 0.0031 \text{ (vol\%)}$$

where

SaO_2 = oxygen saturation

PaO_2 = arterial partial pressure of oxygen

Thus, hemoglobin-bound oxygen normally accounts for more than 98% of the oxygen carrying capacity in the blood. However, it can be seen from Table 1 that the total oxygen requirement of the body (approximately 6.0 vol% O_2 with normal cardiac output) can be satisfied by just dissolved oxygen in plasma at 3 ATA (2280 mmHg). This has been substantiated by animal studies (Boerema et al. 1960). This method of oxygen transfer, rather than an increase in saturation of hemoglobin, is primarily responsible for the improvement in tissue oxygenation during hyperbaric oxygen therapy.

Carbon Dioxide

Carbon dioxide produced in the body by metabolism is transported in blood predominantly in the form of carbonic acid/bicarbonate ion (70%) or combined with hemoglobin as carbaminohemoglobin (25%). A small amount is dissolved in plasma (5%). Under hyperbaric conditions, a small rise in $PaCO_2$ (2–4 mmHg) and a decrease in pH has been measured (Saltzman et al. 1965) due to increased oxygen saturation of venous hemoglobin which becomes unavailable to carry carbon dioxide. This phenomenon is usually not significant as only 20% of the carbon dioxide carried is affected. The displaced carbon dioxide is instead transported in the dissolved form in plasma; however, in conditions of carbon dioxide retention (e.g., large right-to-left shunting or inadequate alveolar ventilation), the effect may become clinically relevant.

Nitrogen

Nitrogen is highly soluble in plasma (0.067 ml N_2/ml/per atmosphere) and lipids. Because of high lipid solubility, nitrogen has an anesthetic affect (nitrogen narcosis) when present at sufficiently high partial pressures. The degree to which this effect becomes significant varies among individuals; however, it usually does not occur until pressures exceed 4 ATA (Behnke et al. 1935). Clinical practice usually involves treatment at pressures between 2 to 3 ATA, therefore nitrogen narcosis is rarely a problem in clinical practice. Since nitrogen is readily taken up by the body during compression, the additional nitrogen absorbed during the treatment time may be released as bubbles on decompression. Thus rapid ascent can cause decompression sickness in multiple chambers, where clinical personnel are breathing air at pressure. Commonly, US Navy or other safe diving tables are followed in order to minimize the possibility.

Cardiovascular Effects

Increased tissue oxygen tensions cause generalized vasoconstriction, however arterial blood pressure remains stable or slithly increased. Autoregulatory changes such as reduction in cardiac output by 10% to 20% (Saltzman et al. 1965), and a concomitant 7% reduction of heart rate and stroke volume (Plewes and Farhi 1983), are responsible for this stability. Savitt et al. (1989) showed that in a dog preparation with normal coronary anatomy, decreases in coronary blood flow and cardiac output during hyperbaric oxygenation are not due to primary changes in myocardial energetic function. Despite vasoconstriction, an increased amount of oxygen is available to the tissues at higher ambient pressures due to the large increase in dissolved oxygen.

Complications of Hyperbaric Therapy

Oxygen Toxicity

Oxygen toxicity is recognized as a potential hazard of hyperbaric oxygen therapy and must be guarded against. It can affect any tissue in the body, however pulmonary tissue is exposed to the highest oxygen concentrations. Hyperbaric exposures at 1.5 to 3.0 ATA are limited by pulmonary oxygen toxicity (Clark and Lambertsen 1971 a). Acute central nervous system toxicity occurs at pressures of 2.0 ATA or more; however the length of exposure at any particular depth is also a factor in the development of toxicity.

Smith (1899) was the first to describe the inflammatory changes of pulmonary oxygen toxicity; since that time, pulmonary effects have been studied extensively (Clark and Lambertsen 1971 a, b; Crapo 1986). Pathologic manifestations include acute changes with accumulation of edema in the perivascular, interstitial, and alveolar spaces, and progression to alveolar hemorrhage and pulmonary endothelial and type I epithelial cell necrosis. Chronically (in hours and days) there is proliferation of the type II cells and interstitial cells and increased elastin and collagen production. Ultimately oxygen induces irreversible pulmonary fibrosis. Symptoms begin (approximately 4 h after breathing pure oxygen at 2 ATA) as a mild tickling cough from tracheal irritation and worsen to a burning sensation, persistent cough, and dyspnea. Following exposure, symptoms subside over a few hours and resolve in 1–3 days. Pulmonary function studies show progressive decreases in vital capacity and thoracic compliance. Gas exchange abnormalities are late and are characterized by widening of the alveolar-arterial oxygen gradient. Guidelines have been developed (Bardin and Lambertson 1970) to compare the pulmonary effects of different hyperbaric oxygen treatment tables using a scale to quantitate oxygen exposure, the Unit Pulmonary Toxic Dose (UPTD).

The central nervous system effects of oxygen toxicity were studied extensively by Donald (1947). He described a large variation in oxygen tolerance in humans and a wide range of symptoms including: anxiety, behavioral changes, sweating, nausea, twitching of the lips and face, visual field and auditory changes, vertigo, syncope, and tonic-clonic seizures which also may occur without any prodrome.

During hyperbaric therapy, premonitory symptoms of central nervous system toxicity are treated by switching the breathing gas from pure oxygen to chamber air. Insertion of "air breaks" or reduction of pressure is often used to avoid these symptoms. If seizures occur in the chamber at pressure, decompression must be delayed until tonic-clonic movements have ceased (as the patient may be breath-holding), to prevent lung rupture and air embolism.

Ocular changes include a relatively frequent (20%–40%) occurrence of reversible myopia of lenticular origin in elderly patients receiving weeks of daily exposure to oxygen at 2 ATA (Anderson and Shelton 1987). Retrolental fibroplasia has been demonstrated in 25% of 28 infants receiving 60% oxygen for 4–6 weeks (Patz et al. 1952). Despite meticulous restriction and even absence of oxygen administration to these infants, retrolental fibroplasia continues to occur, suggesting that other factors must also be important in the etiology of this syndrome (Patz 1976). Retinal separation, destruction of visual cells, visual field contraction, and blindness have also been documented after hyperbaric oxygenation (Behnke et al. 1936; Beehler 1964).

Susceptibility to oxygen toxicity is related to the level of inspired oxygen and the duration of exposure; it also varies between individuals or in the same individual from day to day (Donald 1947). The cause of this variability is not known. Animal studies have also shown that adrenocortical hormones, carbon dioxide inhalation, catecholamines, insulin, hyperthermia, hyperthyroidism, and vitamin E deficiency hasten the onset or increase the severity of oxygen toxicity. On the other hand, acclimatization to hypoxia, adrenergic and ganglionic blocking drugs, antioxidants, glutathione, hypothyroidism, hypothermia, intermittant exposure to oxygen, disulfiram, and vitamin E may delay or lessen the severity of oxygen toxicity. In general, toxic effects can be reversed with cessation of oxygen therapy; however, with continued exposure, permanent deficits may occur (Clark 1982).

The precise mechanisms of oxygen toxicity are still under investigation but may be related to the production of oxygen-free radicals (e.g., superoxide and hydroxyl radicals). Reactive oxygen species may overwhelm the normal antioxidant defenses of the cell (Gilbert 1963) causing enzyme inactivation, DNA damage, and lipid membrane destruction. Protective enzymes such as glutathione peroxidase, superoxide dismutase (McCord and Fridovich 1978), catalase, and cytoplasmic antioxidants may also be inactivated (Frank and Massero 1980).

Other Complications

Psychological complications consist mainly of claustrophobia which can be minimized by empathetic staff, patient education, and orientation. Tranquilizers may be used if supportive therapy is not sufficient.

The risk of fire in the chamber is increased due to high oxygen concentrations. This requires careful monitoring of the chamber oxygen tension as well as use of fire-retardant materials, conductive flooring, and removal of electrical equipment from the chamber. A fire in a closed environment, in the presence of high oxygen concentrations is almost always disastrous.

Contraindications to Hyperbaric Therapy

Absolute contraindications to hyperbaric oxygen therapy are rare. Each patient must be considered individually in terms of the potential decrease in morbidity and mortality offered by hyperbaric therapy, as opposed to the possible risks. Oxygen toxicity, pneumothorax, air embolism, and fire in the chamber though serious, occur very rarely. Seizure-prone patients should receive prophylactic anticonvulsant therapy prior to hyperbaric oxygen therapy. Common side effects such as middle ear and paranasal sinus problems and claustrophobia may be bothersome; however, these symptoms are usually easily managed. Myopic visual changes in the elderly occur quite frequently; however, these are completely reversible after cessation of hyperbaric therapy. The most common situation which warrants consideration is the evaluation of the patient with chronic pulmonary disease, at times at an advanced stage, for an indication which is not life-threatening. In this case, individual risk assessment must be applied. In life-threatening diseases such as decompression sickness, air embolism, carbon monoxide poisoning, and clostridial myonecrosis, the benefit gained from hyperbaric oxygen therapy usually outweighs the risks.

Table 2. Accepted conditions for hyperbaric therapy

Bubble-mediated diseases	Air or gas embolism (acute)[a] Decompression sickness[a] Altitude decompression sickness
Toxicosis	Carbon monoxide poisoning[a] Cyanide poisoning Hydrogen sulfide poisoning
Acute infections	Clostridial myonecrosis (gas gangrene) Necrotizing infections
Chronic infections	Osteomyelitis[a]
Acute ischemic processes	Crush injury Compartment syndrome
Chronic ischemic processes	Selected nonhealing wounds[a] Radiation necrosis Skin graft preparation
Exceptional blood-loss anemia	
Special considerations	Burns

[a] Diseases most frequently seen in clinical practice

Accepted Conditions for Hyperbaric Therapy

In this section, we will review the rationale and clinical basis for the therapeutic use of hyperbaric oxygen. Table 2 outlines the indications currently accepted by the Hyperbaric Oxygen Therapy Committee Report of the Undersea and Hyperbaric Medical Society (Myers 1986). This report is reviewed every 2–3 years on the basis of scientific evidence, and constitutes the most complete document in the field.

Air and Gas Embolism

The entry of air or gas into the intravascular space probably occurs more often than it is recognized. It can occur as an iatrogenic process (Peirce 1980), or may evolve in accidental rapid decompression (J.C. Davis and Elliott 1982). Almost any procedure may lead to iatrogenic embolism such as complication of head, neck, or thoracic surgery, cardiopulmonary bypass (Stoney et al. 1980), penetrating chest injury (Halpern et al. 1983), needle or catheter placement for monitoring or diagnostic purposes, renal dialysis, obstetric or gynecologic manipulation, and urologic procedures (Vourc'h et al. 1982). The pathologic mechanism of intravascular air bubbles involves not only mechanical obstruction of blood flow but also secondary platelet aggregation and activation of hemostatic mechanisms (Hallenbeck et al. 1973).

Manifestations of gas embolism are varied depending on the size of the bubbles, volume of gas entrained, rapidity of the event, position of the patient at the time of the event, and whether gas is located intraarterially or intravenously (Peirce 1980). Intraarterial gas emboli usually present with symptoms involving the central nervous system or the myocardium. Common presentations include: dizziness, nausea, sensory or motor deficits, visual disturbances, coma, and seizures (Gillen 1968). Myocardial manifestations of ischemia such as chest pain and changes on electrocardiogram may occur. Venous air emboli may present with pulmonary symptoms such as chest pain, cough, dyspnea, and hemodynamic instability. Mortality and morbidity is significant. The confirmation of air embolism may be difficult unless air entry is actually witnessed, a characteristic "millwheel murmur" is present on cardiac auscultation, or air is found on aspiration from a central line. New Doppler and neuroimaging modalities add to the diagnostic armamentarium. A recent study by Warren et al. (1988) found that magnetic resonance imaging is more sensitive in detecting focal cerebral ischemia due to air embolism than conventional computerized tomography scanning.

The rationale for the use of hyperbaric oxygen therapy in gas embolism is based upon rapidly increasing ambient pressure to decrease bubble size and improve blood flow to the affected area. Ventilation with 100% oxygen induces the largest possible gradient for the inert gas (usually nitrogen) in the bubble to be reabsorbed. Vasoconstriction due to high tissue oxygen tension may contribute to the decrease in the amount of cerebral edema, while increased tissue oxygen tension will improve survival of marginally viable and ischemic areas (Sukoff et al. 1968; Sukoff and Ragatz 1982). Numerous cases of successful hyperbaric oxygen therapy of air embolism have been reported (Gillen 1968; Peirce 1980; Bove et al. 1982; Takahashi et al. 1987).

The treatment of choice for air or gas embolism is compression in a hyperbaric chamber, instituted as close to the time of insult as possible. However, improvement has been documented after delay in treatment of 7 h (Bove et al. 1982), and up to 42 h by Massey et al. (1989) who have recommended that delay in referral does not preclude successful hyperbaric treatment. Treatment varies from administering oxygen at 2.8 ATA to using compressed air or Nitrox at 6.0 ATA, utilizing US Navy Table VI or VIA with repeated treatments until there is no further improvement.

Decompression Sickness

Decompression sickness (DCS) is a diverse clinical syndrome produced when inert gas in bodily tissues (usually nitrogen) is released from physical solution, forming bubbles during decompression. The details of bubble formation and growth remain unknown, but they may affect virtually any part of the body.

Decompression sickness presents in a great variety of ways, therefore a high index of suspicion and a history of recent decompression play an important role in diagnosis. Correct diagnosis is vital; without proper treatment, permanent neurologic deficits can ensue in previously healthy individuals. The commonest symptom (in 91.8% of cases) is deep, dull pain occurring in any joint ("bends" or type I DCS). The central nervous system is affected in approximately 25% of cases of decompression sickness with a predominance of spinal cord involvement (type II DCS). Dizziness, nausea, behavioral changes, visual disturbances, seizures, and coma are among the most common presentations. Presence of motor and sensory deficits, paraplegia, bowel or bladder incontinence, and loss of sexual function usually indicate spinal cord involvement. Symptoms attributable to the peripheral nervous system occur in approximately 22% of sport divers presenting with decompression sickness. These manifest as low back pain, paresthesia, weakness, or proprioceptive deficits (Rivera 1964). Rarely, labyrinthine effects occur, presenting with nystagmus, vertigo, nausea, and vomiting. This syndrome must be treated within 45 min of onset to avoid permanent damage. "Chokes" or pulmonary involvement are rare and present with chest pain, dyspnea, nonproductive cough, and cyanosis. Decompression sickness shock is a serious complication characterized by plasma leakage through capillaries causing hypovolemia, shock, and pulmonary edema. Other manifestations of decompression sickness include drowsiness, extreme fatigue, transient skin itch, and, more serious, skin mottling.

Various factors predispose to decompression sickness: cramped position during or after decompression, recent strain or sprain of muscle or joint, hard exercise during or after decompression, hyperthermia, post-alcoholic state, age over 40, and hypercarbia. In addition, Moon et al. (1989) have shown that out of 23 divers with serious decompression sickness there was an increased incidence (39%) of patent foramen ovale, compared with an incidence of 5% in 176 normal volunteers. They hypothesize that a patent foramen ovale may allow otherwise innocuous venous gas bubbles to enter the arterial circulation and become symptomatic.

The definitive treatment for decompressive disease is recompression in a hyperbaric chamber. Often the patient must be transported some distance to the nearest hyperbaric facility and should be kept as close to sea level as possible by using pressurized or low-flying aircraft (maximum altitude 1000 feet). To hasten the elimination of nitrogen from the tissues, 100% oxygen via tight-fitting face mask or endotracheal tube should be used in the interim time period prior to hyperbaric treatment. Resuscitation with intravenous crystalloids or colloid is used to maintain tissue perfusion. This also may aid in the elimination of nitrogen gas. Steroids may be used whenever central nervous system or spinal cord edema is presumed, although they may take several hours to have an effect. Steroids have been shown to increase the risk of oxygen toxicity in animals, but this has not proven to be clinically significant in humans.

Hyperbaric treatments vary according to clinical picture but US Navy Table 6 is used most commonly. Multiple treatments may be given until there is no further clinical improvement. The faster the patient can be recompressed, the better the results, particularly in labyrinthine decompression sickness; however, treatment may still be effective after a delay of several days (Myers and Bray 1985).

Altitude decompression sickness is similar to diving decompression sickness in its mechanism and clinical manifestation. Return to sea level and oxygen breathing are usually sufficient to treat mild cases. Compression to hyperbaric pressures may be needed in more serious cases. J.C. Davis et al.

(1977) reported complete resolution of symptoms in 143 out of 145 cases of altitude decompression sickness when treated with recompression at 2.8 ATA.

Toxicosis: Carbon Monoxide Poisoning

Carbon monoxide poisoning is common, often accidental, and may present with nonspecific, generalized symptoms. It occurs predominantly during could weather. Sources of carbon monoxide include motor vehicle exhaust, space-heaters, industrial furnaces, and smoke inhalation. Neurologic and cardiovascular involvement is common; patients may present acutely with nausea, vomiting, hypotension, headache, syncope, vasomotor collapse, behavioral abnormalities, seizures, and coma. The classic description of a cherry-red facies is rarely seen. Acutely, carboxyhemoglobin (HbCO) levels may range from 10%–20% in asymptomatic patients to 50%–60% in comatose patients. However, HbCO measurements performed hours after exposure do not correlate well with clinical findings as blood levels do not reflect intracellularly bound carbon monoxide. Norkool and Kirkpatrick (1985) showed that the mean carboxyhemoglobin level in patients who survived (29.3%) was not significantly different from those who died (30.8%). In addition, Myers et al. (1985) found that psychometric testing may be necessary to demonstrate subtle neuropsychiatric abnormalities. The duration of exosure, activity during that period, and interval between exposure and assessment are also factors in judging the severity of intoxication (Sokal 1975).

Subacute neurologic sequelae have been described by Myers et al. (1985). They reported that out of 213 patients treated for carbon monoxide poisoning, none of the patients treated with hyperbaric oxygenation suffered clinically significant sequelae; however, 12.1% of those not treated with hyperbaric oxygenation developed subacute neurologic deficits. Symptoms such as headache, memory loss, abnormal psychometric testing, and personality change have developed up to 21 days after initial exposure, and have been treated successfully with hyperbaric oxygen therapy.

Haldane (1895) demonstrated that the poisonous action of carbon monoxide was due to its combination with hemoglobin and that this effect could be reversed with oxygen administration at increased tensions. Carbon monoxide binds to hemoglobin in competition with oxygen, forming carboxyhemoglobin. The affinity of carbon monoxide for hemoglobin is over 200 times greater than the affinity of oxygen for hemoglobin (Sendroy et al. 1929). Once carbon monoxide is bound, less hemoglobin is then available for oxygen transport and the oxygen dissociation curve of the remaining oxyhemoglobin is shifted to the left, resulting in functional tissue hypoxia. It has been discovered more recently that intracellular binding of carbon monoxide to cytochrome oxidase a,a_3 in mitochondria may occur in vivo. In some cases intracellular binding may contribute to the pathophysiology of carbon monoxide poisoning, due to persistent disruption of intracellular respiration (Piantadosi 1987).

Hyperbaric oxygen therapy speeds the dissociation of carboxyhemoglobin as the rate of carbon monoxide elimination is inversely related to the inspired oxygen partial pressure. Pace et al. (1950) found that in healthy males, initial carboxyhemoglobin levels of 20%–30% could be halved in 249 min breathing room air at 1 ATA, in 47 min breathing 100% oxygen at 1 ATA, or in 22 min breathing 100% oxygen at 2.5 ATA. Hyperbaric oxygen therapy also improves tissue oxygenation by increasing the amount of physically dissolved oxygen and by hastening the liberation of carbon monoxide from cytochromes (Piantadosi 1987). Goulon et al. (1969) demonstrated a decrease in mortality from 30% to 13.5% if hyperbaric oxygen therapy was administered within 6 h of discovery as compared with patients who received 100% oxygen at the surface and later hyperbaric oxygen more than 6 h after discovery. They also found that the group treated within 6 h had a reduced incidence of long-term sequelae. These findings have been confirmed by Myers et al. (1985) and Norkool and Kirkpatrick (1985).

Administration of hyperbaric oxygen for carbon monoxide intoxication during pregnancy has recently been reported by Van Hoesen et al. (1989). They concluded that short hyperoxic exposures attained during hyperbaric therapy for carbon monoxide poisoning should be tolerable by the fetus in all stages of pregnancy and may reduce the risk of death to the mother and deformity or death to the fetus.

Hyperbaric oxygen therapy is the treatment of choice in patients with carbon monoxide poisoning. Generally, patients with heavy exposure, as suggested by carboxyhemoglobin levels greater than 25%, any neurologic symptoms, circulatory or respiratory collapse, and ischemic changes on electrocardiogram, should receive treatment regardless of their carboxyhemoglobin levels. The patient should be given 100% oxygen via a tight-fitting face mask during transport and evaluation prior to hyperbaric therapy. Therapy is recommended at 2.5 to 3.0 ATA for up to 90 min depending on the clinical picture. Follow-up treatments may be administered 12 to 24 h after initial therapy in patients presenting with severe manifestations of carbon monoxide poisoning or residual symptoms.

Cyanide Intoxication

The mechanism of cyanide intoxication is thought to be through the inhibition of cytochrome oxidase, impairing intracellular respiration. The mainstays of treatment are sea level oxygen and chemical antidotes. The use of sodium nitrite enhances cyanmethemoglobin formation and sodium thiosulfate treatment provides sulfur to hasten thiocyanate formation, which is less toxic than cyanide. Some animal studies have shown improvement with hyperbaric therapy, when used as an adjunct to chemical antidotes. Although case reports in humans have shown conflicting results (Litovitz et al. 1983), good outcomes have been reported in humans by Trapp (1970) and F. M. Davis and Ewer (1988).

Hydrogen Sulfide Poisoning

Hydrogen sulfide has also been shown to have a toxic effect on cytochrome oxidase. For this reason, hyperbaric oxygenation has been suggested as adjunctive therapy when conventional treatment fails. Isolated case reports have documented improved outcome (Smilkstein et al. 1985; Hsu et al. 1987).

Acute Infection: Gas Gangrene

Clostridial myonecrosis is a dramatic form of necrotizing infection involving rapidly spreading muscle necrosis. Traumatic, contaminated, or ischemic wounds in diabetic or debilitated patients are particularly at risk for clostridial infection. The presence of foreign bodies or compound fractures also increase the risk of this type of infection. Clostridial myonecrosis is caused by a variety of organisms; principally *Clostridium perfringens* in the majority of cases. This organism is an anaerobic, spore-forming, gram-prositive rod present abundantly in soil and in normal flora of the gastrointestinal tract. Despite preferring anaerobic conditions, *Clostridium perfringens* can also grow freely in oxygen tensions of approximately 30 mmHg (similar to body tissue oxygen tensions) and in a restricted fashion even in the presence of 70 mmHg oxygen (McLeod 1930). *Clostridium novii, C. Septicum, C. histolyticum, C. fallax,* and *C. bifermentans* have also been cultured from these wounds (Bakker 1988). The pathophysiologic picture is mainly attributed to the production of numerous exotoxins; *C. perfringens* can produce nine types. The most important is alpha-toxin, an oxygen-stable lecithinase-C, which causes rapidly progressive hemolysis, tissue liquefaction, and necrosis. In the tissue surrounding the wound, there is extreme pain, swelling, brownish discoloration, gas production, and a brownish sweet-smelling drainage. Systemic effects of the infection include septic shock, hemolysis leading to anemia, renal failure, disseminated intravascular coagulation, cardiotoxicity, and neurologic abnormalities, leading to a fulminant clinical course in the absence of early treatment.

The rationale for hyperbaric oxygen therapy in this group of anaerobic infections is varied but centers on the fact that anaerobic organisms lack antioxidant enzymes (superoxide-degrading enzyme, dismutase; and hydrogen peroxide-degrading enzyme, catalase). This enables oxygen exposure to be lethal for anaerobic organisms (McCord et al. 1971). Demello et al. (1970) demonstrated that hyperbaric oxygen at 2 and 3 ATA stopped spore germination and inhibited bacterial growth in a bacteriostatic fashion. More importantly, Van Unnik (1965) found that elevated oxygen tensions at 3 ATA for 1.5 h can totally inhibit the production of alpha-toxin in vitro (although alpha-toxin already present in stable at 3 ATA). Another mechanism of hyperbaric oxygen in this disease process involves hyperoxia-induced vasoconstriction which decreases edema and improves oxygenation of ischemic tissue, particularly in enclosed compartments.

Hyperbaric oxygen is recommended as an adjunct to surgical debridement and broad spectrum antibiotic therapy. Other organisms are often found with clostridia in these wounds. Prior to the use of hyperbaric oxygen, mortality rates in gas gangrene ranged from 30% to 50% (MacLennan 1962). The 20-year experience of Boerema and Brummelkamp in the treatment of this disease was summarized in 1984 by Bakker. He reported a 20% overall mortality rate; however, death attributed directly to gas gangrene is 10.6%. Treatment commenced within the first 24 h of diagnosis achieved the best results. There was a decrease in amputation rate from 50% with primary surgical therapy to 24% with surgery after completion of a series of hyperbaric oxygen treatments. These findings have been substantiated by many investigators. Hart et al. (1983) compiled 15 years of experience of combined therapy consisting of surgery, antibiotics, and hyperbaric oxygen for clostridial infections. Out of 139 consecutive patients, 81% survived. Patients who were treated early and did not have shock or other debilitating medical disease fared better. This study also demonstrated a reduction in the amputation rate to 17% with combined treatment. Hitchcock et al. (1975) showed that 44 patients treated with surgery and antibiotics had a survival rate of 55% compared with a 78.2% survival rate in 89 patients who received hyperbaric oxygen therapy. The closer the patients were to a hyperbaric facility, the quicker the therapy was instituted and the greater was the survival rate.

In suspected gas gangrene, hyperbaric oxygenation should be initiated as quickly as possible. This may be done before the diagnosis is confirmed microbiologically, and before definitive surgical treatment. Surgical intervention is better performed after hyperbaric therapy has helped to delineate nonviable tissue, in the hopes of saving tissue and limb. A protocol which has been found to be useful consists of three treatments within the first 24 h at 3 ATA for 90 min each, followed by treatments twice per day for 4 to 5 days.

Other Necrotizing Infections

Although clostridial myonecrosis is the most prominent and lethal of the necrotizing infections, other gas-forming organisms (anaerobic and aerobic) cause distinguishable clinical syndromes. Like clostridial myonecrosis, these infections occur in debilitated patients with traumatic or surgical wounds which typically have conditions of local tissue hypoxia encouraging bacterial growth. Prognosis appears to be related to the underlying diseases often present.

Crepitant anaerobic cellulitis is a localized soft tissue infection with abundant gas production and absence of muscle involvement. Onset is gradual occurring usually after trauma to the lower extremities. Systemic involvement and mortality rate is lower (10%–15%) than other disease entities in this group. Species of Bacteroides, Peptostreptococcus, Enterobacteriaceae, and Clostridium and are frequently isolated from the wounds (Mader 1988).

Progressive bacterial gangrene commences about 2 weeks after injury or surgery, as an indurated site slowly progressing to a painful, ulcerating lesion of the skin and subcutaneous tissue of the abdominal or thoracic wall. Meleney (1931), who first described the condition, found it to be due to the synergistic infection of anaerobic streptococci with *Staphylococcus aureus* or Enterobacteriaceae. Mortality ranges between 10%–25% (Mader 1988).

Necrotizing fasciitis is a disease involving extensive necrosis of the superficial and deep fascia, spreading between tissue planes, but without muscle involvement.

Fournier's disease is a necrotizing fasciitis involving the perineal or scrotal areas. Systemic toxicity is marked and a mortality rate of 30% has been reported (Rea and Wyrick 1970). Anaerobic (species of Bacteroides, Peptostreptococcus, and Fusobacterium), as well as aerobic (*Staphylococcus aureus, Streptococcus pyogenes,* and Enterobacteriaceae) organisms have been isolated.

Nonclostridial myonecrosis is similar to clostridial myonecrosis in terms of muscle and systemic involvement, aggressive spread, and high mortality rate (75%, Stone and Martin 1970). Clinically, these are painful lesions exuding foul-smelling "dish-water pus," occurring particularly in association with perirectal abcesses and peripheral vascular disease. Mixed gram-positive and gram-negative, aerobic and anaerobic organisms have been implicated.

Hyperbaric oxygen has been recommended for most necrotizing infections as adjuvant therapy together with surgical debridement and antibiotic therapy. The rationale for the use of hyperbaric oxygenation is based on the direct lethal effect of oxygen on anaerobic and microphilic aerobic organisms which is related to antioxidant enzyme activity (Rolfe et al. 1978). Furthermore, it has been shown that the number and size of experimentally induced intra-abdominal abscesses caused by *Fusobacterium necrophorum* with either *Bacteroides fragilis* or *Fusobacterium nucleatum* are reduced by hyperbaric oxygen therapy (Hill 1976). Hypoxic environments diminish the oxygen-dependent intracellular killing of organisms such as *Staphylococcus aureus, Escherichia coli, Klebsiella pneumoniae,* and *Proteus vulgaris* by polymorphonuclear leukocytes (Mandell 1974). Another oxygen-dependent mechanism is the neutrophil myeloperoxidase-hydrogen peroxide-halide system which is postulated to aid in bacterial cell wall destruction (Zgliczynski and Stelmaszyńska 1975). Knighton et al. (1986) demonstrated that prophylactic antibiotics in conjunction with administration of increased inspired oxygen produced an additive effect in the reduction of infectious necrosis. Good clinical results with adjunctive hyperbaric oxygen therapy have been reported by workers such as Gozal et al. (1986) and Riegels-Nielsen et al. (1984).

The contribution of oxygen administration at increased pressures in these syndromes is varied. Hyperbaric therapy may be useful in all necrotizing infections; however, it is most cost-effective in situations where the patient is compromised, not responding to conventional therapy, or in those diseases carrying high morbidity and mortality rates such as progressive bacterial gangrene, necrotizing fasciitis, and nonclostridial myonecrosis. Twice daily treatments at 2.0 to 2.5 ATA for 90 to 120 min are recommended until the patient's condition stabilizes, after which daily treatments are used.

Chronic Infection: Chronic Refractory Osteomyelitis

Osteomyelitis usually involves mixed infection of bone and surrounding soft tissue by organisms such as *Staphylococcus aureus, Escherichia coli,* and species of Klebsiella, of *Pseudomonas,* Proteus, and *Enterobacter.* Patients with local bone ischemia, foreign bodies, and compromising diseases such as diabetes mellitus, peripheral vascular disease, and immunosuppression are particularly at risk of developing a refractory, chronic form of osteomyelitis. This is defined as continuing infection, after 6 months of combined antibiotic and surgical therapy. In cases of refractory chronic osteomyelitis hyperbaric oxygen therapy may be beneficial in conjunction with aggressive surgical debridement and antibiotic therapy.

In osteomyelitis oxygen penetrates necrotic tissue, edema, fibrous tissue, pus, and avascular bone poorly. Hypoxia can also interfere with the activities of leukocytes, antibodies, and antibiotics. Infection develops and persists in such hypoxic areas (Strauss 1987). Several studies have shown multiple modes of action by which hyperbaric oxygen therapy acts in the treatment of chronic osteomyelitis. Controlled animal studies have demonstrated hypoxia in infected bone and that oxygen therapy is successful in increasing bone oxygen tension (Niinikoski and Hunt 1972). Hyperbaric oxygen may increase tissue oxygen tensions by tenfold (Wells et al. 1977). Aminoglycoside transport across the bacterial cell wall is also oxygen dependent. Verklin and Mandell (1977) demonstrated that in anaerobic tissue, up to 20 times the amount of aminoglycosides is required to inhibit bacterial growth of *Escherichia coli, Proteus mirabilis,* and *Klebsiella pneumoniae.* Mader et al. (1978) demonstrated that hyperbaric oxygen is at least as effective as cephalothin in the treatment of chronic osteomyelitis due to *Staphylococcus aureus.* Later, this group determined that phagocytic killing of *Staphylococcus aureus* was decreased in hypoxic bone and could be corrected when bone oxygen tensions were increased by hyperbaric oxygen (Mader et al. 1980). Oxygen-dependent osteoclast activity to remove necrotic tissue, osteoneogenesis (Steed et al. 1982), and wound healing are also stimulated by hyperbaric oxygenation. Hamblen (1968) administered hyperbaric oxygen therapy to rats with staphylococcal osteomyelitis and demonstrated increased numbers of healed wounds using radiologic, microbiologic, and histologic criteria. The response appears related mainly to improvement of host factors rather than direct bactericidal or bacteriostatic effects.

Clinical studies have supported the improvement of chronic refractory osteomyelitis with hyperbaric oxygen therapy. Morrey et al. (1979) followed 40 patients with chronic refractory osteomyelitis, treated with debridement, antibiotics, and hyperbaric oxygen therapy (mean of 40 treatments). Eighty-five percent of patients were clinically free of disease after a mean period of 23 months, and 75% were free of disease after a mean of 8.4 years (J. C. Davis 1986). In a different study, J. C. Davis et al. (1986) reported 38 consecutive patients treated with a similar regimen including an average of 48 daily treatments of hyperbaric oxygen. They found that 89.5% remained disease-free after an average of 34 months while only four patients in this group had been free of clinical signs of osteomyelitis for as long as 3 months during the 2 years prior to treatment. Gates et al. (1989) recently reported 28 patients treated with local wound debridements, prolonged parenteral antibiotics, and an average of 36 daily hyperbaric oxygen treatments with 100% oxygen at 2 ATA for 2 h. They found that 70% of cases were free of clinical signs of osteomyelitis after hyperbaric oxygen therapy for an average of 41 months, while the pretreatment drainage period averaged 15 years. Not all studies have shown improved patient outcomes, however, partly because of differences in patient populations. Esterhai et al. (1987) studied 28 cases of chronic refractory osteomyelitis where there wer no complications of persistent fracture, nonunion, septic arthritis, total joint arthroplasty or major systemic disease. They classified the patients according to a staging system, assigned them to control and treatment groups, and found no difference in outcome between those treated with hyperbaric oxygen and controls.

Treatment with hyperbaric oxygen at 2.0 to 2.5 ATA for 90 to 120 min is recommended twice daily in the acute stage and once daily after chronic presentation. A therapeutic trial of 30 treatments is recommended with repeated wound debridement, wicking, and daily dressing changes to determine if the wound will granulate and close over healthy tissue.

Acute Ischemic Processes

Crush injury is defined as severe diffuse trauma to two or more tissues producing varying degrees of tissue and microvascular damage, leading to ischemia. Compartment syndrome likewise involves ischemia due to swelling and edema in areas confined by fascia. Commonly the anterior compartment of the leg and volar aspect of the forearm are involved. Local hypoxia causes vasodilatation, leading to further swelling and compromised perfusion. Muscle necrosis ultimately leads to deposition of fibrous tissue and contractures. The rationale for the use of hyperbaric therapy hinges on the demonstrated reduction of edema and improvement of tissue oxygenation. Restoring adequate tissue oxygen tension increases the survival of marginally viable tissue and aids in the demarcation of nonviable tissue at the time of debridement.

Animal models of compartment syndrome have shown significant improvement of muscle necrosis and edema and an increase in tissue viability with hyperbaric oxygen therapy (Strauss et al. 1983). Nylander et al. (1985) demonstrated reduction of postischemic edema in rats by as much as 50%, an effect which persisted for 40 h after the last hyperbaric treatment. Clinical studies summarized by Strauss (1981) show that up to 60% of patients with acute ischemic and crush injuries benefit from hyperbaric therapy. In addition, the best results have been seen with prompt and more frequent treatments.

Hyperbaric oxygen therapy is recommended particularly in the interim period before surgery, while waiting for operating room availability or, after surgical decompression, in patients where there is neural deficit or necrotic tissue. Therapy should be commenced as soon as possible after injury to maximize limb-saving potential and benefit to tissues. Twice daily treatments at 2.0 to 2.5 ATA for 90 to 120 min are recommended for 5 to 7 days with frequent observation of the extremity.

Chronic Ischemic Processes: Selected Non-Healing Wounds

Slow healing of wounds is attributable to poor perfusion and hypoxic tissue beds which are more likely to occur in compromised hosts prone to infection. Multiple factors such as peripheral vascular disease, diabetes mellitus, irradiation, infection, trauma, immunosuppression, anemia, malnutrition, and presence of foreign bodies contribute to poor healing. The rationale for hyperbaric oxygen is to provide intermittently increased tissue oxygen tension to hypoxic wounds and prevent infection by improving the bactericidal activity of leukocytes.

Animal studies have demonstrated improved wound healing after treatment with hyperbaric oxygen. Kivisaari and Niinikoski (1975) determined that rats with compromised circulation and full thickness wounds, in contrast to animals with intact vasculature, showed delay in wound healing. After treatment with hyperbaric oxygenation healing approached normal rates. In addition, they documented that local and systemic hypoxia retarded healing in wounds. Tissue oxygen can be measured by several methods including implanted miniature electrodes or by transcutaneous measurements in skin adjacent to the wound. Using these techniques, Sheffield and Dunn (1977) and Sheffield (1985) demonstrated oxygen tensions of 10 to 20 mmHg in human nonhealing wounds. These wounds responded to hyperbaric oxygen with tissue oxygen tensions increasing to greater than 30 mmHg but showed no response to 100% oxygen at 1 ATA.

Anaerobic metabolism, however, is also a necessary element in some stages of wound healing. Hypoxia has been shown to stimulate angiogenesis (Manson et al. 1980); however, hyperoxia is the stimulus for the growth of support tissues for these vessels. It appears that alternating periods of both conditions may be necessary to aid blood vessel and granulation tissue growth.

Due to the multifactorial nature of wound healing and problems in objectively measuring wound progress, it is difficult to conduct randomized controlled clinical studies. Baroni et al. (1987) have shown in a small prospective study that diabetic foot wounds significantly improved with hyperbaric therapy. Sixteen out of 18 patients in the hyperbaric treatment group healed as opposed to 1 out of 10 patients in the control group who did not receive hyperbaric oxygen. Several cases have been described by others, such as J. C. Davis et al. (1988), also demonstrating benefit in diabetic wounds. Cianci et al. (1988 b) recently reported on 39 patients with lower limb wounds treated with an aggressive multidisciplinary approach including hyperbaric oxygen therapy. They demonstrated a 92% salvage rate of the limb using this protocol which was more cost effective when compared with the cost of primary amputation and rehabilitation. Diabetic patients with additional large vessel disease tend not to improve with hyperbaric oxygen administration until reconstructive vascular surgery has been performed. Adjunctive therapy includes aggressive daily debridement of wounds with appropriate analgesic cover, antibiotics if necessary, timely surgical debridement or split skin grafting, nutritional support, and strict metabolic control.

Radiation Necrosis

Radiation therapy can damage microvasculature resulting in altered perfusion and tissue or bone necrosis. Osteonecrosis is thought to occur in about 10% to 15% of cases of therapeutic irradiation with a resolution rate of only 15% (Epstein et al. 1987). Two processes in particular which appear to be helped by hyperbaric oxygen therapy are reconstructive surgery in irradiated tissues and osteoradionecrosis.

Hyperbaric oxygen has been recommended as adjunctive therapy to reconstructive surgery, particularly in cases involving the mandible or jaw, where radical surgery is disfiguring, psychologically disabling, and physiologically nonfunctional. This is because reconstructive surgery in irradiated tissues is traditionally associated with a complication rate of 68.8% and a graft failure rate of 25% (Adamo and Szal 1979). Complications involve poor host granulation tissue formation and infection of graft sites due to microvascular destruction and an ischemic environment. These conditions manifest as wound dehiscence, graft exposure, and complete graft loss, graft infection, bone resorption, and pathologic fracture, and functionally inadequate results. Hyperbaric oxygen therapy is thought to increase collagen synthesis (Hunt and Pai 1972), neovascular formation (Manson et al. 1980), and osteoneogenesis (Mainous et al. 1973), which may help to prepare the area for debridement and reconstruction. Clinical studies have shown that using hyperbaric therapy prior to reconstructive surgery of irradiated tissue, 92% of 276 patients undergoing elective facial reconstruction had successful procedures with a complication rate of only 9% (Marx and Johnson 1988).

Osteonecrosis of the mandible may also benefit from hyperbaric oxygen. Farmer et al. (1978) established that in patients who showed no improvement despite adequate nonhyperbaric oxygen therapy for 3 months, 54% of cases resolved and 23% improved once treated with hyperbaric oxygen in conjunction with surgery. Marx (1984) demonstrated that all 70 cases of osteonecrosis (65 of whom were refractory) showed resolution with a combined protocol of wound debridement, hyperbaric oxygen, and reconstructive surgery. In a different study, Marx and Johnson (1988) showed 100% success in 268 patients treated with a similar combined approach. They documented remarkable cost-effectiveness and lack of recurrence after treatment, unlike those treated without hyperbaric oxygen therapy. Prevention of osteoradionecrosis development after surgery has also been demonstrated. A randomized prospective trial conducted by Marx et al. (1985) showed that in patients previously treated with radiation to the mandible, there was a reduction in the development of osteoradionecrosis after tooth extraction from 29% in those treated with penicillin alone to 5.4% in those treated with hyperbaric oxygen alone.

The recommended hyperbaric oxygen protocol for the therapy consists of 2.0 to 2.4 ATA treatments for 60–120 min daily for approximately 40 treatments after which reevaluation is indicated.

Radiation-induced cystitis has also been reported to be responsive to hyperbaric oxygen therapy (Weiss et al. 1985; Schoenrock and Cianci 1986). The condition manifests as hemorrhagic cystitis and cystoscopic changes and is otherwise often refractory to other forms of therapy, requiring urinary diversion.

Skin Graft Preparation

Hyperbaric oxygenation may be useful in selected patients with poor wound healing where skin grafts are being planned. The rationale of use in this situation is to prepare a healthy bed of granulation tissue on which the graft can be placed as well as to promote faster, more complete healing postoperatively. Studies have shown that animals exposed to hyperbaric oxygenation have better flap survival than those breathing room air (Champion et al. 1967; Manson et al. 1980). Perrins (1967) conducted a controlled clinical trial on 48 patients undergoing split thickness skin grafting by the same surgeon. Ninety-five percent of the graft area survived in 64% of patients treated with hyperbaric oxygen at 2 ATA, 2 h twice daily after operation for 3 days, as opposed to 17% of untreated patients. There was an overall mean improvement of 91.7% in the hyperbaric treatment group compared with 62.7% in controls. Hyperbaric therapy has been recommended for approximately 20 treatments in preparation for skin grafting and for ten treatments postgrafting.

Exceptional Blood-Loss Anemia

Hyperbaric oxygenation should be used in exceptional anemia only when blood transfusion is not yet available (usually due to major blood typing incompatibilities) or has been rejected due to religious reasons in a hemodynamically unstable patient. Boerema et al. (1960) documented that life can be supported at 3 ATA solely by physically dissolved oxygen in plasma. The rationale behind hyperbaric therapy in this rare circumstance is that the patient can be sustained temporarily until blood is available or until there is sufficient time for erythropoiesis. It is also of concern, however, that hypoxia is the primary stimulus for erythropoiesis. Hart et al. (1987) have summarized their experience over the past 17 years in the treatment of 26 patients with hyperbaric oxygen for exceptional blood-loss anemia. There were 8 deaths; of these, 7 patients were decerebrate on arrival, 1 had no neurologic response, and 1 died of anaphylactic reaction (presumed due to iron dextran). The remainder were treated with hyperbaric oxygen intermittently for several days and survived.

Thermal Burns

Treatment of burn victims with hyperbaric oxygen is somewhat controversial. The rationale for treatment is related to the fact that burn wounds are characterized by edema, increased vascular permeability, stasis of circulation, and intravascular coagulation. They are thus prone to hypoxia, spread of ischemic areas, poor wound healing, infection, and scar formation (Arturson 1980). In addition to soft tissue damage, smoke inhalation injuries occur in combination with carbon monoxide and cyanide poisoning. The treatment of these intoxications has been discussed above. Carbon monoxide and cyanide poisoning should be suspected in all cases where unconscious patients have been rescued from fires.

Animal studies (Wells and Hinton 1977) show reduction in plasma extravasation in dogs with third-degree flame burns over 40% of their bodies from 37% in controls to 20% after treatment with oxygen at 2 ATA. Similar results are seen using hyperbaric oxygen at 3 ATA. Korn et al. (1977) demonstrate benefit from hyperbaric oxygen therapy with faster epithelialization, earlier reversal of capillary stasis, reduced conversion of partial to full-thickness injury, and reduction of edema and inflammation.

Hart et al. (1974) showed similar gains in a small randomized, controlled, double-blinded study in humans. Grossman et al. (1977) compared 181 patients treated at the Sherman Oaks Burn Center (which includes hyperbaric therapy as a treatment modality) with results from the National Burn Information Exchange. They found a decrease in the length of hospital stay as well as an increase in the number of patients surviving 40% total body surface area burns and third-degree burns. Cianci et al. (1988 a) recently reported on 12 patients with total body surface area burns of 40% to 80%. A decrease in the number of surgeries was shown in patients given adjunctive hyperbaric oxygen therapy. Duration and cost of hospital stay were also reduced in those who underwent hyperbaric oxygen therapy.

Duke University Hyperbaric Center

The Duke University Hyperbaric Center is a system of multiplace chambers affiliated with a 1000-bed tertiary level institution utilizing a multidisciplinary approach involving anesthesia and medical and surgical expertise in the treatment of patients with selected disorders. The center receives referrals from all over the country as well as being headquarters for the Divers Alert Network (DAN), a service providing 24-h telephone consultation service with a hyperbaric physician. The center is also one of the leading research groups in hyperbaric and diving medicine. Table 3 summarizes the number of patients undergoing treatment and the changing patient population over the past 3 years.

Conclusion

With the growing body of evidence documenting the mechanism and effectiveness of hyperbaric oxygen therapy, indications have become more precise and

Table 3. Compilation of patient diagnosis by year at Duke University Hyperbaric Center

Diseases	1986	1987	1988
Air embolism	1	4	4
Decompression sickness	13	23	17
Carbon monoxide intoxication	19	26	37
Osteomyelitis	12	17	22
Osteo/soft tissue radionecrosis	23	23	22
Skin graft preparation	19	30	45
Necrotizing infection	15	26	24
Miscellaneous (lung lavage, multiple sclerosis)	10	7	13
Total	112	156	184
Total number of treatment hours	4342	6426	7462

limited. The development of accurate determination of localized tissue oxygen tension will provide more objective evidence of treatment efficacy, which so far must be limited to repeated patient observation over several days. When such instruments (for example, interstitial PO_2 detectors and optical monitoring of tissue oxygenation) become more accurate and available, hyperbaric oxygen therapy will be delivered more effectively and titrated more easily to therapeutic effects. The establishment of safe and experienced hyperbaric therapy centers with formally trained technical and medical staff will allow those patients in whom this mode of therapy is beneficial and cost-effective to receive appropriate therapy without significant complication.

References

Adamo AK, Szal RL (1979) Timing, results and complications of mandibular reconstructive surgery: report of 32 cases. J Oral Surg 37:755–763

Anderson BJ, Shelton DL (1987) Axial length in hyperoxic myopia. In: 9th International symposium on underwater and hyperbaric physiology. Undersea and Hyperbaric Medical Society, Bethesda MD, pp 607–611

Arturson G (1980) Pathophysiology of the burn wound. Ann Chir Gynaecol 69:178–190

Bakker DJ (1984) The use of hyperbaric oxygen in the treatment of certain infectious diseases especially gas gangrene and acute dermal gangrene. Veenman, Wageningen

Bakker DJ (1988) Clostridial myonecrosis. In: Davis JC, Hunt TK (eds) Problem wounds. Elsevier, New York, pp 153–172

Bardin H, Lambertson CJ (1970) A quantitative method for calculating cumulative pulmonary oxygen toxicity – use of the unit pulmonary toxicity dose (UPTD). University of Pennsylvania, Philadelphia. (Institute for Environmental Medicine report)

Baroni G, Porro T, Faglia E et al. (1987) Hyperbaric oxygen in diabetic gangrene treatment. Diabetes Care 10(1):81–86

Beehler CC (1964) Oxygen and the eye. Surv Ophthalmol 9:549–560

Behnke AR, Thompson RM, Motley EP (1935) The psychologic effects from breathing air at 4 atmospheres pressure. Am J Physiol 112:554–558

Behnke AR, Forbes HS, Motley EP (1936) Circulatory and visual effects of oxygen at 3 atmospheres pressure. Am J Physiol 114:436–442
Bert P (1943) Barometric pressure. Researches in experimental physiology. College Book, Columbus. Translation of: la pression barométrique. Masson, Paris, 1878
Boerema I, Kroll JA, Meijne NG et al. (1956) High atmospheric pressure as an aid to cardiac surgery. Arch Chir Neerl 8:193–211
Boerema I, Meijne NG, Brummelkamp WK et al. (1960) Life without blood: a study of the influence of high atmospheric pressure and hypothermia on dilution of the blood. J Cardiovasc Surg 13:133–146
Bove AA, Clark JM, Simon AJ, Lambertsen CJ (1982) Successful therapy of cerebral air embolism with hyperbaric oxygen at 2.8 ATA. Undersea Biomed Res 9(1):75–80
Champion WM, McSherry CK, Goulian D Jr (1967) Effect of hyperbaric oxygen on the survival of pedicled skin flaps. J Surg Res 7(12):583–586
Cianci P, Lueders H, Lee H et al. (1988 a) Adjunctive hyperbaric oxygen reduces the need for surgery in 40%–80% burns. J Hyperbaric Med 3(2):97–101
Cianci P, Petrone G, Drager S et al. (1988 b) Salvage of the problem wound and potential amputation with wound care and adjunctive hyperbaric oxygen therapy: an economic analysis. J Hyperbaric Med 3(3):127–141
Clark JM (1982) Oxygen toxicity. In: Bennett PB, Elliott DH (eds) The physiology and medicine of diving, 3rd edn. Bailliere-Tindall, London, pp 200–238
Clark JM, Lambertsen CJ (1971 a) Pulmonary oxygen toxicity: a review. Pharmacol Rev 23(2):37–133
Clark JM, Lambertsen CJ (1971 b) Rate of development of pulmonary oxygen toxicity in man during oxygen breathing at 2.0 ATA. J Appl Physiol 30(5):739–752
Crapo JD (1986) Morphologic changes in pulmonary oxygen toxicity. Annu Rev Physiol 48:721–731
Cunningham OJ (1927) Oxygen therapy by means of compressed air. Anesth Analg 6:64
Davis FM, Ewer T (1988) Acute cyanide poisoning: case report of the use of hyperbaric oxygen. J Hyperbaric Med 3(2):103–106
Davis JC (1986) Adjunctive hyperbaric oxygen in chronic refractory osteomyelitis: long-term follow-up results (letter). Clin Orthop 205:310
Davis JC, Elliott DH (1982) Treatment of decompression disorders. In: Bennett PB, Elliott DH (eds) The physiology and medicine of diving, 3rd edn. Bailliere-Tindall, London, pp 473–486
Davis JC, Sheffield PJ, Schuknecht L et al. (1977) Altitude decompression sickness: hyperbaric therapy results in 145 cases. Aviat Space Environ Med 48(8):722–730
Davis JC, Heckman JD, DeLee JC, Buckwold FJ (1986) Chronic non-hematogenous osteomyelitis treated with adjuvant hyperbaric oxygen. J Bone Joint Surg [Am] 68(8):1210–1217
Davis JC, Buckley CJ, Barr P (1988) Compromised soft tissue wounds: correction of wound hypoxia. In: Davis JC, Hunt TK (eds) Problem wounds. Elsevier, New York, pp 143–152
Demello FJ, Hashimoto T, Hitchcock CR, Haglin JJ (1970) The effect of hyperbaric oxygen on the germination and toxin production of *Clostridium perfringens* spores. In: Wada J, Iwa T (eds) Proceedings of the Fourth International Congress on Hyperbaric Medicine. Williams and Wilkins, Baltimore, pp 276–281
Donald KW (1947) Oxygen poisoning in man, pt 1 and pt 2. Br Med J 1:667–672; 712–717
Epstein JB, Wong FL, Stevenson-Moore P (1987) Osteoradionecrosis: clinical experience and a proposal for classification. J Oral Maxillofac Surg 45:104–110
Esterhai JL Jr, Pisarello J, Brighton CT et al. (1987) Adjunctive hyperbaric oxygen therapy in the treatment of chronic refractory osteomyelitis. J Trauma 27(7):763–767
Farmer JC, Shelton DL, Angelillo JD, Bennett PB, Hudson WR (1978) Treatment of radiation-induced injury by hyperbaric oxygen. Ann Otol 87:707–715
Frank L, Massero D (1980) Oxygen toxicity. Am J Med 69:117–126

Gabbs G, Robin ED (1987) Hyperbaric oxygen: a therapy in search of diseases. Chest 92(6):1074–1082
Gates HS, Levin LS, Harrelson JM, Moon RE, Camporesi EM (1989) Adjunct hyperbaric oxygen therapy in the treatment of chronic osteomyelitis in the lower extremities. Orthopedics (submitted for publication)
Gilbert DL (1963) The role of pro-oxidants and antioxidants in oxygen toxicity. Radiat Res [Suppl] 3:44–53
Gillen HW (1968) Symptomatology of cerebral gas embolism. Neurology 18:507–512
Goulon M, Barois A, Rapin M et al. (1969) Carbon monoxide poisoning and acute anoxia due to breathing coal gas and hydrocarbons. Republished in (1986) J Hyperbaric Med 1(1):23–41
Gozal D, Ziser A, Shupak A, Ariel A, Melamed Y (1986) Necrotizing fasciitis. Arch Surg 121:233–235
Grossman AR, Hart GB, Yanda RL (1977) Thermal burns. In: Davis JC, Hunt TK (eds) Hyperbaric oxygen therapy. Undersea Medical Society, Bethesda MD, pp 267–279
Haldane J (1895) The relation of the action of carbonic oxide to oxygen tension. J Physiol 18:201–207
Hallenbeck JM, Bove AA, Moquin RB, Elliott DH (1973) Accelerated coagulation of whole blood and cell-free plasma by bubbling in vitro. Aerosp Med 44:712–714
Halpern P, Greenstein A, Melamed Y et al. (1983) Arterial air embolism after penetrating chest injury. Crit Care Med 11(5):392–393
Hamblen DL (1968) Hyperbaric oxygenation: its effect on experimental staphylococcal osteomyelitis in rats. J Bone Joint Surg [Am] 50(6):1129–1141
Hart GB, O'Reilly RR, Broussard ND et al. (1974) Treatment of burns with hyperbaric oxygen. Surg Gynecol Obstet 139:693–696
Hart GB, Lamb RC, Strauss MB (1983) Gas gangrene. J Trauma 23(11):991–1000
Hart GB, Lennon PA, Strauss MB (1987) Hyperbaric oxygen in exceptional acute blood-loss anemia. J Hyperb Med 2(4):205–210
Hill GB (1976) Hyperbaric oxygen exposures for intrahepatic abscesses produced in mice by nonsporeforming anaerobic bacteria. Antimicrob Agents Chemother 9(2):312–317
Hitchcock CR, Demello FJ, Haglin JJ (1975) Gangrene infection: new approaches to an old disease. Surg Clin North Am 55(6):1403–1410
Hsu P, Li H-W, Lin Y-T (1987) Acute hydrogen sulfide poisoning treated with hyperbaric oxygen. J Hyperb Med 2(4):215–221
Hunt TK, Pai MP (1972) The effect of varying ambient oxygen tensions on wound metabolism and collagen synthesis. Surg Gynecol Obstet 135:561–567
Kivisaari J, Niinikoski J (1975) Effects of hyperbaric oxygenation and prolonged hypoxia on the healing of open wounds. Acta Chir Scand 141:14–19
Knighton DR, Halliday B, Hunt TK (1986) Oxygen as an antibiotic: a comparison of the effects of inspired oxygen concentration and antibiotic administration on in vivo bacterial clearance. Arch Surg 121:191–195
Korn HN, Wheeler ES, Miller TA (1977) Effect of hyperbaric oxygen on second-degree burn wound healing. Arch Surg 112:732–737
Litovitz TL, Larkin RF, Myers RAM (1983) Cyanide poisoning treated with hyperbaric oxygen. Am J Emerg Med 1:94–101
MacLennan JD (1962) The histotoxic clostridial infections of man. Bacteriol Rev 26:177–276
Mader JT (1988) Mixed anaerobic and aerobic soft tissue infections. In: Davis JC, Hunt TK (eds) Problem wounds. Elsevier, New York, pp 173–186
Mader JT, Guckian JC, Glass DL, Reinarz JA (1978) Therapy with hyperbaric oxygen for experimental osteomyelitis due to *Staphylococcus aureus* in rabbits. J Infect Dis 138(3):312–318
Mader JT, Brown GL, Guckian JC, Wells CH, Reinarz JA (1980) A mechanism for the amelioration by hyperbaric oxygen of experimental staphylococcal osteomyelitis in rabbits. J Infect Dis 142(6):915–922

Mainous EG, Boyne PS, Hart GB, Terry BC (1973) Restoration of resected mandible by grafting with combination of mandible homograft and autogenous iliac marrow and postoperative treatment with hyperbaric oxygen. Oral Surg Oral Med Oral Pathol 35(1):13–20

Mandell GL (1974) Bactericidal activity of aerobic and anaerobic polymorphonuclear neutrophils. Infect Immun 9(2):337–341

Manson PN, Im MJ, Myers RAM, Hoopes JE (1980) Improved capillaries by hyperbaric oxygen in skin flaps. Surg Forum 31:564–566

Marx RE (1984) Osteoradionecrosis of the jaws: review and update. HBO Rev 5(2):78–126

Marx RE, Johnson RP (1988) Problem wounds in oral and maxillofacial surgery: the role of hyperbaric oxygen. In: Davis JC, Hunt TK (eds) Problem wounds. Elsevier, New York, pp 65–124

Marx RE, Johnson RP, Kline SN (1985) Prevention of osteoradionecrosis: a randomized prospective clinical trial of hyperbaric oxygen versus penicillin. J Am Dent Assoc 111:49–54

Massey EW, Shelton DL, Moon RE, Camporesi EM (1989) Hyperbaric treatment of iatrogenic air embolism. In: Undersea and Hyperbaric Medical Society Annual Scientific Meeting (abstr). Undersea and Hyperbaric Medical Society, Bethesda MD

McCord JM, Fridovich I (1978) The biology and pathology of oxygen radicals. Ann Intern Med 89:122–127

McCord JM, Keele BB Jr, Fridovich I (1971) An enzyme-based theory of obligate anaerobiosis: the physiologic function of superoxide dismutase. Proc Natl Acad Sci USA 68(5):1024–1027

McLeod JW (1930) Variations in the periods of exposure to air and oxygen necessary to kill anaerobic bacteria. Acta Pathol Microbiol Scand [Suppl] 3:255

Meleney FL (1931) Bacterial synergism in disease processes with a confirmation of the synergistic bacterial etiology of a certain type of progressive gangrene of the abdominal wall. Ann Surg 94(6):961–981

Moon RE, Camporesi EM, Shelton DL (1987) Prediction of arterial PO_2 during hyperbaric treatment. In: 9th Int symp on underwater and hyperbaric physiology. Undersea and Hyperbaric Medical Society, Bethesda MD, pp 1127–1131

Moon RE, Camporesi EM, Kisslo JA (1989) Patent foramen ovale as a risk factor for decompression sickness in compressed air divers. Lancet (accepted for publication)

Morrey BF, Dunn JM, Heimbach RD, Davis JC (1979) Hyperbaric oxygen and chronic osteomyelitis. Clin Orthop 144:121–127

Myers RAM (chairman) (1986) Hyperbaric oxygen therapy: a committee report. Undersea Medical Society, Bethesda MD

Myers RAM, Bray P (1985) Delayed treatment of serious decompression sickness. Ann Emerg Med 14(3):254–257

Myers RAM, Snyder SK, Emhoff TA (1985) Subacute sequelae of carbon monoxide poisoning. Ann Emerg Med 14:1163–1167

Niinkoski JC, Hunt TK (1972) Oxygen tensions in healing bone. Surg Gynecol Obstet 134:746–750

Norkool DM, Kirkpatrick JN (1985) Treatment of acute carbon monoxide poisoning with hyperbaric oxygen: a review of 115 cases. Ann Emerg Med 14:1168–1171

Nylander G, Lewis D, Nördstrom H, Larsson J (1985) Reduction of postischemic edema with hyperbaric oxygen. Plast Reconstr Surg 76(4):596–601

Pace N, Strajman E, Walker EL (1950) Acceleration of carbon monoxide elimination in man by high pressure oxygen. Science 111:652–654

Patz A (1976) Current status of role of oxygen in retrolental fibroplasia. Invest Ophthalmol 15(5):337–339

Patz A, Hoeck LE, De La Cruz E (1952) Studies on the effect of high oxygen administration in retrolental fibroplasia. Am J Ophthalmol 35:1248–1252

Peirce EC (1980) Cerebral gas embolism (arterial) with special reference to iatrogenic accidents. Hyperbaric Oxygen Rev 1(3):161–184

Perrins DJD (1967) Influence of hyperbaric oxygen on the survival of split skin grafts. Lancet I:868–871
Piantadosi CA (1987) Carbon monoxide, oxygen transport, and oxygen metabolism. J Hyperbaric Med 2(1):27–44
Plewes JL, Farhi LE (1983) Peripheral circulatory responses to acute hyperoxia. Undersea Biomed Res 10(2):123–129
Rea WJ, Wyrick WJ Jr (1970) Necrotizing fasciitis. Ann Surg 172:957–964
Riegels-Nielsen P, Hesselfeldt-Nielsen J, Bang-Jensen E, Jacobsen E (1984) Fournier's gangrene: 5 patients treated with hyperbaric oxygen. J Urol 132:918–920
Rivera JC (1964) Decompression sickness among divers: an analysis of 935 cases. Milit Med 129:314–334
Rolfe RD, Hentges DJ, Campbell BJ, Barrett JT (1978) Factors related to the oxygen tolerance of anaerobic bacteria. Appl Environ Microbiol 36(2):306–313
Saltzman HA, Smith WW, Fuson RL et al. (1965) Hyperbaric oxygenation. Monogr Surg 2(1):1–68
Savitt MA, Elbeery JR, Owen CH, Rankin JS, Camporesi EC (1989) Mechanism of decreased coronary and systemic blood flow during hyperbaric oxygenation. In: Undersea and Hyperbaric Medical Society Annual Scientific Meeting (abstr). Undersea and Hyperbaric Medical Society, Bethesda MD
Schoenrock GJ, Cianci P (1986) Treatment of radiation cystitis with hyperbaric oxygen. Urology 27(3):271–272
Sendroy J Jr, Liu SH, Van Slyke DD (1929) The gasometric estimation of the relative affinity constant for carbon monoxide and oxygen in whole blood at 38 °C. Am J Physiol 90:511
Sheffield PJ (1985) Tissue oxygen measurements with respect to soft-tissue wound healing with normobaric and hyperbaric oxygen. HBO Rev 6(1):18–46
Sheffield PJ (1988) Tissue oxygen measurements. In: Davis JC, Hunt TK (eds) Problem wounds. Elsevier, New York, pp 17–51
Sheffield PJ, Dunn JM (1977) Continuous monitoring of tissue oxygen tension during hyperbaric oxygen therapy – a preliminary report. In: Smith G (ed) Proceedings of the 6th Inernational Congress on Hyperbaric Medicine. Aberdeen University Press, Aberdeen, pp 125–129
Smilkstein MJ, Bronstein AC, Pickett HM, Rumack BH (1985) Hyperbaric oxygen therapy for severe hydrogen sulfide poisoning. J Emerg Med 3:27–30
Smith LJ (1899) The pathological effects due to increase of oxygen tension in the air breathed. J Physiol 24:19–35
Sokal JA (1975) Lack of the correlation between biochemical effects on rats and blood carboxyhemoglobin concentrations in various conditions of single acute exposure to carbon monoxide. Arch Toxicol 34:331–336
Steed DS, Kolodny SC, Wilcox JW, Malloy RB (1982) Enhancement of osteogenesis with hyperbaric oxygen. A clinical study. J Dent Res 61A:288
Stone HH, Martin JD Jr (1970) Synergistic necrotizing cellulitis. Ann Surg 175:702–711
Stoney WS, Alford WC Jr, Burrus GR, Glassford DM Jr, Thomas CS Jr (1980) Air embolism and other accidents using pump oxygenators. Ann Thorac Surg 29(4):336–340
Strauss MB (1981) Role of hyperbaric oxygen therapy in acute ischemias and crush injuries – an orthopedic perspective. HBO Rev 2(2):87–106
Strauss MB (1987) Refractory osteomyelitis. J Hyperbaric Med 2(3):147–159
Strauss MB, Hargens AR, Gershuni DH et al. (1983) Reduction of skeletal muscle necrosis using intermittent hyperbaric oxygen in a model compartment syndrome. J Bone Joint Surg 65 [Am] (5):656–662
Sukoff MH, Ragatz RE (1982) Hyperbaric oxygenation for the treatment of acute cerebral edema. Neurosurgery 10(1):29–38
Sukoff MH, Hollin SA, Espinosa OE, Jacobson JH (1968) The protective effect of hyperbaric oxygenation in experimental cerebral edema. J Neurosurg 29:236–241

Takahashi H, Kobayashi S, Hayase H, Sakakibara K (1987) Iatrogenic air embolism: a review of 34 cases. In: 9th International symposium on underwater and hyperbaric physiology. Undersea and Hyperbaric Medical Society, Bethesda MD, pp 931–948

Trapp WG (1970) Massive cyanide poisoning with recovery: a Boxing Day story. Can Med Assoc J 102:517

Van Hoesen KB, Camporesi EM, Moon RE, Hage ML, Piantadosi CA (1989) Should hyperbaric oxygen be used to treat the pregnant patient for acute carbon monoxide poisoning?: A case report and literature review. JAMA 261(7):1039–1043

Van Unnik AJM (1965) Inhibition of toxin productioin in *Clostridium perfringens* in vitro by hyperbaric oxygen. Antonie Van Leeuwenhoek 31:181–186

Verklin RM Jr, Mandell GL (1977) Alteration of effectiveness of antibiotics by anaerobiosis. J Lab Clin Med 89(1):65–71

Vourc'h G, Berreti E, Trichet B, Moncorge C, Camey M (1982) Two unusual cases of gas embolism following urethral surgery under laser. Intensive Care Med 8:239–240

Warren LP, Djang WT, Moon RE et al. (1988) Neuroimaging of scuba diving injuries to the CNS. AJNR 9:933–938

Weiss JP, Boland FP, Mori H et al. (1985) Treatment of radiation-induced cystitis with hyperbaric oxygen. J Urol 134:352–354

Wells CH, Hinton JG (1977) Effects of hyperbaric oxygen on post-burn plasma extravasation. In: Davis JC, Hunt TK (eds) Hyperbaric oxygen therapy. Undersea Medical Society, Bethesda MD, pp 259–265

Wells CH, Goodpasture JE, Horrigan DJ, Hart GB (1977) Tissue gas measurements during hyperbaric oxygen exposure. In: Smith G (ed) Proceedings of the 6th International Congress on Hyperbaric Medicine. Aberdeen University Press, Aberdeen, pp 118–124

Zgliczyński JM, Stelmaszyńska T (1975) Chlorinating ability of human phagocytosing leucocytes. Eur J Biochem 56:157–162

Anesthesia

The Influence of Anesthesia on the Respiratory System

J. F. Nunn

The influences of anesthesia on the respiratory system are complex and varied. Apart from obvious changes, such as the depression of breathing and interference with arterial oxygenation, the effects could not easily be predicted and their precise causation is still unclear in many cases. It is untrue to say that all aspects of the system are simply "depressed" and certain functions are actually enhanced. The plan of this review is to commence with a consideration of the effects of anesthesia on the pattern of contraction of the respiratory and ancilliary muscles because this underlies many of the secondary changes.

Effect on the Pattern of Contraction of the Respiratory Muscles

The Inspiratory Muscles

It has long been known that deepening anaesthesia causes a decrease in thoracic respiratory excursion, usually interpreted as progressive failure of the intercostal muscles, with preservation of the action of the diaphragm. These changes appear to play a major part in the effect of anesthesia on the ventilatory response to PCO_2, since the major part of the ventilatory response to PCO_2 seems to be in the rib cage rather than in the abdominal component of the total respiratory excursion (Tusiewicz et al. 1977).

The other major change is in the diaphragm which, during normal breathing by the conscious subject in the supine (but probably not in the upright) position, retains considerable tone at the end of expiration. Muller and his colleagues (1979) have used diaphragmatic electromyography to demonstrate that this residual end-expiratory tone is lost during anaesthesia with halothane. It seems likely that this phenomenon is the main cause of the important change in functional residual capacity (see below).

The Expiratory Muscles

For no obvious reason, general anesthesia appears to cause phasic activity of the expiratory abdominal muscle, which are normally silent in the conscious supine subject (Freund et al. 1964). This activation of expiratory muscles seems to have no functional significance (except perhaps for a surgeon trying to operate on the abdomen) and it is extremely difficult to abolish without resorting to neuromuscular blockade (Kaul et al. 1973).

Other Muscles

The genioglossus muscle contracts rhythmically in phase with breathing. In the cat, there is interference with its activity during anesthesia (Nishino et al. 1985), and it is reasonable to believe that anaesthesia may interfere with activity of the genioglossus in man. This would provide an explanation for the well-known fact that the tongue falls back against the posterior pharyngeal wall during anesthesia. This together with changes in the position of the soft palate is the cause of the airway obstruction which almost always occurs when anesthesia is induced. The down-folding of the epiglottis reported by Boidin (1985) has not been confirmed by soft tissue radiography by the present author.

Changes in Lung and Trunk Volumes

(see reviews by Rehder 1985; Froese 1985)

Change in Functional Residual Capacity (FRC)

In the supine position, the FRC is about a litre less than in the upright position (Nunn 1987). There is now widespread agreement that FRC is further reduced during anesthesia. This occurs with all anaesthetic drugs which have been investigated, and the mean change is about 16%–20%. FRC decreases immediately after induction and appears to reach its final value within the first few minutes of anesthesia. Inhalation of high concentrations of oxygen does not appear to be a factor in the change. FRC is reduced to the same extent whether the patient is paralysed or not and expiratory muscle activity has no significant effect on the change in FRC. The reduction in FRC has a weak but significant correlation with the age of the patient. Artificial ventilation of the conscious

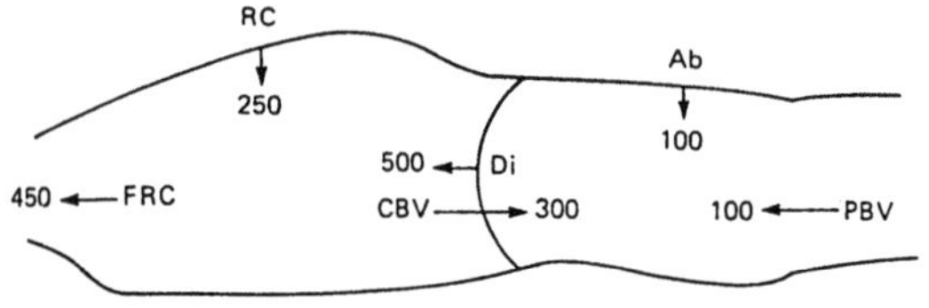

Thoracic volume			
thoracic area	− 250 ml	FRC	− 450 ml
diaphragm shift	− 500 ml	CBV	− 300 ml
	− 750 ml		− 750 ml
Abdominal volume			
abdominal area	− 100 ml	CBV	+ 300 ml
diaphragm shift	+ 500 ml	PBV	+ 100 ml
	+ 400 ml		+ 400 ml

Fig. 1. Mean changes in volume (ml) of rib cage *(RC)* and abdomen *(Ab)*, and movement of central blood volume *(CBV)* and peripheral blood volume *(PBV)*, resulting from anesthesia. *FRC* indicates the measured change in functional residual capacity and *Di* the calculated volume change resulting from movement of the diaphragm. [Redrawn from the data of Hederstierna et al. (1985) with permission, and reproduced from Nunn (1987) with the permission of Butterworths]

subject causes only a small reduction in FRC and anesthesia does not change FRC in the sitting position.

Froese and Bryan (1974) in a classical study of lateral chest radiographs during anesthesia clearly showed that the diaphragm ascended into the chest by about 2 cm during anesthesia with or without paralysis, and this change accorded roughly with the decrease in FRC. It seems very likely that this is due to the loss of end-expiratory diaphragmatic tone described above.

Hedenstierna and his colleagues (1985) have used computerized tomography to measure changes in the volume of thorax and abdomen following induction of anesthesia and paralysis. Their results are summarized in Fig. 1, which shows the changes in the geometry of the thoracic cage and blood volume distribution, which interact to result in the observed changes in FRC.

Consequences of the Change in Functional Residual Capacity

In the supine position, the expiratory reserve of the conscious subject is usually less than 1 litre and induction of anaesthesia will bring the lung volume close to residual volume. This has major effects on lung function, particularly in respect to airway closure, airway calibre, compliance, and gas exchange.

Airway Closure

The reduction of FRC which occurs during anesthesia in the supine position will tend to reduce the end-expiratory lung volume below the closing capacity (CC), at least in older patients. This would be expected to result in compression atelectasis, airway closure, absorption collapse, shunting, and arterial hypoxaemia. The latter changes can very easily be demonstrated in older subjects who breathe at reduced lung volume in the supine position (Nunn et al. 1965).

Airway closure would not occur during anesthesia if the CC were to decrease by the same amount as the FRC, as has been suggested by Juno et al. (1978) and Bergman and Tien (1983). Nevertheless the discovery of compression atelectasis during anaesthesia (see below) strongly suggests that airway closure does occur during anesthesia. Furthermore, Dueck et al. (1988) have shown during anesthesia a very close relationship between the shunt and [FRC (anaesthesia) – CC (preanaesthesia)]/total lung capacity. This would appear to indicate that the shunt seen during anaesthesia is indeed related to the change in FRC and airway closure appears to be the likely cause.

Pulmonary Collapse

Whether or not pulmonary collapse occurs during anesthesia has been debated for many years, particularly since the classical study of Bendixen et al. (1963). A series of later studies failed to confirm this and it was never demonstrated by conventional radiography, except in the dependent lung in the lateral position. However, "compression atelectasis" in dependent lung areas following induction of anesthesia has now been unequivocally demonstrated by computerised tomography (Brismar et al. 1985; Tokics et al. 1987; Hedenstierna et al., 1989).

Airway Calibre

Changes in lung volume affect all components of the tracheobronchial tree and have a direct effect on airway calibre, particularly in the dependent parts of the lung. However, this effect of the reduction in lung volume which occurs during anesthesia, is to a large extent offset by the bronchodilator effect of the common inhalational anesthetics. As a result airway resistance is not greatly changed following induction of uneventful anesthesia.

Nevertheless, there are many other abnormal causes of increased airway resistance during anesthesia which may be serious and threaten life. Excessive resistance or obstruction may arise in apparatus such as breathing circuits, valves, connectors, and tracheal tubes. The pharynx is commonly obstructed as described above. The large airways may be blocked with foreign material such as blood, tumour, pus, or inhaled gastric contents. Bronchospasm may result from many causes.

Compliance

The effect of anesthesia on the pressure/volume relationship of the lung and chest wall, as shown in Fig. 2, is based on the work of Westbrook et al. (1973) and Butler and Smith (1957). There are major differences between the conscious state and anesthesia, and these contrast sharply with the surprisingly minor differences between anaesthesia with and without paralysis. In addition to the reduction of FRC and expiratory reserve already described, there is a reduction of total lung capacity and compliance. The major component of the

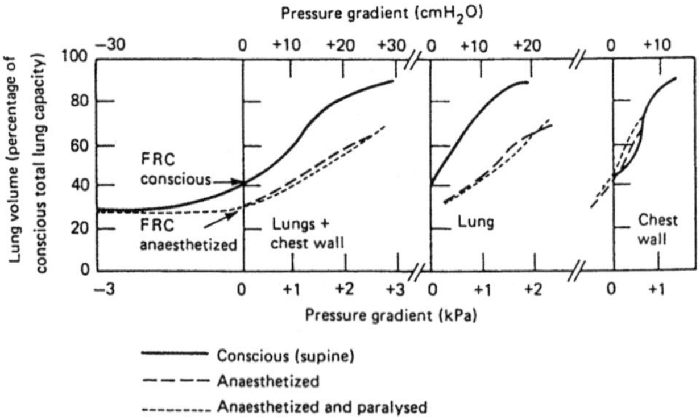

Fig. 2. Pressure/volume relationships in supine volunteers before and after induction of anesthesia and paralysis. [Redrawn from the data of Butler and Smith (1957) and Westbrook et al. (1973) with permission, and reproduced from Nunn (1987) with the permission of Butterworths]

change in compliance is in the lung rather than the chest wall, but there is no general agreement on the effect of anesthetics on the pulmonary surfactant. The reduced compliance may well be secondary to the reduced FRC. It will be clear from Fig. 2 that negative end-expiratory pressure can do little to increase the tidal volume during anaesthesia.

Control of Breathing

Anesthesia with preserved spontaneous breathing usally decreases the pulmonary ventilation and increases the PCO_2, commonly within the range 6–10 kPa. However, this overall statement conceals the fact that there are quite different and highly specific effects of anaesthesia on the various mechanisms controlling ventilation.

Effect on PCO_2/Ventilation Response Curve

The flat curve in Fig. 3 shows the effect of varying levels of ventilation on the alveolar PCO_2 in the absence of a carbon dioxide challenge. As anesthesia is deepened, the point representing the respiratory state of the patient usually moves along the curve to the right and downwards. If the respiratory system is challenged by increasing the inspired concentration of carbon dioxide, the resultant change in ventilation is shown as a function of alveolar PCO_2 by a family of approximately straight lines known as CO_2/ventilatory response curves. The slope of these lines is predominantly a function of the sensitivity of the central chemoreceptors. In Fig. 3, drawn from the data of Munson et al. (1966), it will be seen that progressive increases in the alveolar concentration of an inhalational anesthetic agent decreases the slope of the PCO_2/ventilation response curve and, at deep levels of anesthesia, there may be no response at all to an increase of PCO_2. This effect was originally thought to be

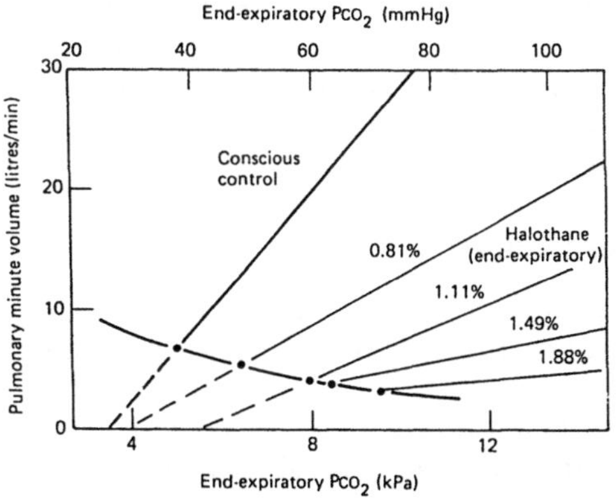

Fig. 3. Displacement of PCO_2/ventilation response curve resulting from various end-tidal concentrations of halothane. [Redrawn from the data of Munson et al. (1966) with permission, and reproduced from Nunn (1987) with the permission of Butterworth]

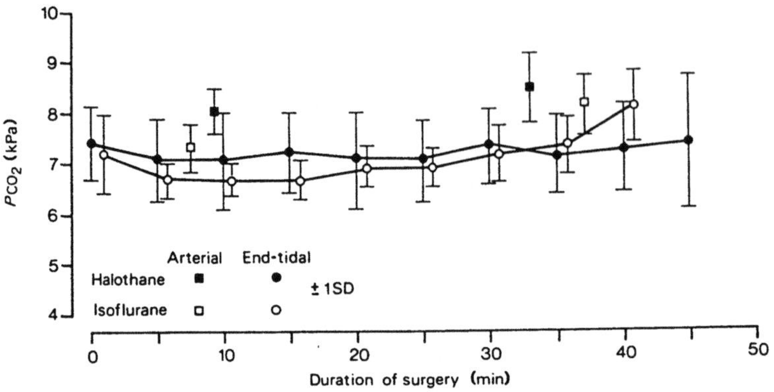

Fig. 4. Time course of changes in alveolar and arterial PCO_2 during routine anaesthesia and surgery, with preserved spontaneous breathing at a constant end-tidal concentration of halothane (or isoflurane) and nitrous oxide corresponding to 1.4 times the minimal alveolar concentration required for anesthesia [reproduced from Alagesan et al. (1987) with the permission of the editor and publishers of the *British Journal of Anaesthesia*]

exerted entirely in the medulla, but it now appears to be attributable in part to the effect of anaesthetics on the pattern of contraction of the inspiratory muscles (Tusiewicz et al. 1977).

Figure 3 also shows the extrapolation of the CO_2/ventilatory response curves to the axis of zero ventilation. The intersection on this axis corresponds to apnoea, and the PCO_2 at the point of intersection is known as the apnoeic PCO_2 threshold. Conscious subjects do not necessarily stop breathing when their PCO_2 is less than the apnoeic threshold. However, during anaesthesia, patients almost invariably become apnoeic when PCO_2 is less than the apnoeic threshold value.

Anesthetics differ quantitatively in their capacity to depress the response of ventilation to PCO_2, probably because of their differing capacity to release catecholamines. Surgical stimulation antagonizes the effect of anesthesia on the PCO_2/ventilation response curve. Surprisingly there is no evidence of significant progressive increase in PCO_2 when anaesthesia is maintained at constant depth during surgery (Fig. 4, from Alagesan et al. 1987).

Effect on PO_2/Ventilation Response Curve

It used to be thought that the hypoxic ventilatory drive was highly resistant to anaesthetics. However, it is now clear that the hypoxic ventilatory response is, in fact, extremely sensitive to inhalational anesthetics, even at 0.1 MAC (Fig. 5, drawn from the data of Knill and Gelb 1978). It seems likely that the effect is on the carotid body chemoreceptor itself (Davies et al. 1982; Knill and Clement 1984).

There are some important consequences of this effect which must be presumed to continue into the postoperative period, until the alveolar concentra-

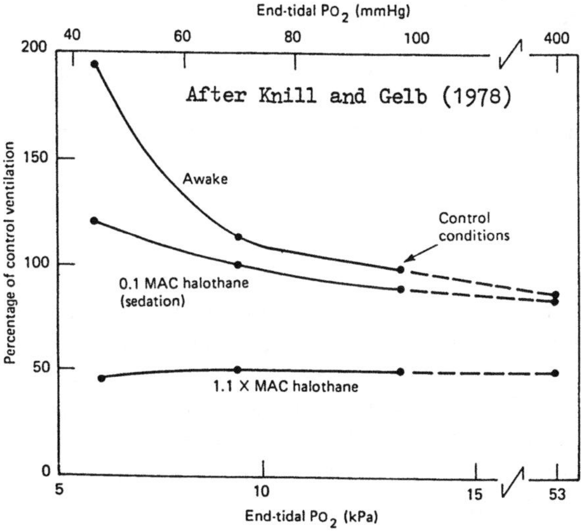

Fig. 5. Effect of halothane anesthesia and sedation on the ventilatory response to hypoxia. MAC is the minimal alveolar concentration required for anaesthesia. [Redrawn from the data of Knill and Gelb (1978) with permission, and reproduced from Nunn (1987) with the permission of Butterworths]

tion of the anesthetic has declined well below the level which causes loss of consciousness. First, the patient cannot act as his own hypoxia alarm by responding with hyperventilation. Second, the patient who has already lost his sensitivity to PCO_2 (e.g. "the blue bloater" category of patient with chronic bronchitis) may stop breathing after anesthesia has abolished his hypoxic drive. Finally, anesthesia may be dangerous at very high altitude or in other situations where survival depends on hyperventilation in response to hypoxia (Nunn 1989).

Response to Metabolic Acidemia

The ventilatory response to metabolic acidemia is also obtunded by anesthesia, and even by subanaesthetic concentrations of anaesthetics (Knill and Clement 1985).

Response to Added Resistance

In view of the very disturbing effects described above, it comes as a considerable surprise to find that the ability of a patient to increase his work of breathing in response to added resistance is remarkably well preserved during anesthesia (Nunn and Ezi-Ashi 1961; Moote et al. 1986). The anaesthetized patient responds to inspiratory loading by two mechanisms, one of which appears to be reflex and the other due to an increased PCO_2. The first is instantaneous and occurs during the first loaded breath. The second takes several minutes to develop and results in hyperventilation when the resistance is removed. This provides a very sensitive test of excess respiratory resistance.

Anesthetics and Pulmonary Stretch Receptors

The common inhalational anaesthetics, particularly trichloroethylene, sensitize the pulmonary stretch receptors in cats, but this is unlikely to be the full explanation of slowing of respiratory rate in man in whom the Hering-Breuer reflex is virtually absent.

Metabolic Rate

During anesthesia, the metabolic rate is reduced about 15% below basal according to the conventional standards, which do not stipulate sedation or any period of rest. A similar reduction in metabolic rate follows 3 h of rest, with or without sedation (Robertson and Reid 1952). The sub-basal metabolic rate during anaesthesia mitigates to some extent the adverse effects of anesthesia upon gas exchange. However, dramatic increases in metabolic rate may occur during hyperthermia, shivering, or convulsions.

Pulmonary Ventilation

During anesthesia with preserved spontaneous breathing, the minute volume may remain normal but is usually decreased because of interference with the control of breathing and the function of the respiratory muscles as described above. Sometimes the minute volume reaches very low levels and as little as 3 l/min has been recorded, with corresponding PCO_2 values up to about 10 kPa (Alagesan et al. 1987). This is particularly likely to occur in the absence of surgical stimulation. There are no outcome studies to indicate that this is harmful to a healthy patient.

Quite different conditions apply during anesthesia with artificial ventilation. The minute volume can then be set at almost any level which seems appropriate to the anesthetist. Hyperventilation is usual and values up to 15 l/min are commonplace. Observed values for arterial PCO_2 extend from the normal range down to about 2.5 kPa. Again, it has proved difficult to demonstrate that this does any significant harm to the healthy patient, although there is obvious concern for the cerebral circulation.

Distribution

In all except some very young and fit patients, even uncomplicated anesthesia causes abnormalities of distribution of pulmonary blood flow and inspired gas. These changes do not normally pose any major threat to the patient. However, they may be contrasted with a more serious range of pathological alterations in distribution due to such causes as bronchial intubation, tension pneumothorax, gross hypotension, or the combination of respiratory disease with anaesthesia. Under such conditions, maldistribution may be a potent cause of mortality and morbidity.

Although there is a continuous gradation of ventilation/perfusion ratios ($\dot{V}/\dot{Q}$) in different alveoli, it is often convenient and practical to consider the lung as a three-compartment model. In this model the alveoli are considered to fall into three groups – "ideally" ventilated and perfused alveoli, unperfused alveoli (alveolar dead space or infinite $\dot{V}/\dot{Q}$ ratio), and unventilated alveoli (shunt or zero $\dot{V}/\dot{Q}$ ratios). The advantages of this approach are twofold. First, the equipment for making the relevant measurements should be available in any department of anesthesia. Second, the results provide clear guidance for making physiological correction for the abnormality.

Dead Space

During anesthesia, the dead space/tidal volume ratio from carina downwards averages 32% during anesthesia, with either spontaneous or artificial ventilation, and over a wide range of tidal volume (Nunn and Hill 1960). This relationship still applies during hypoventilation (Fig. 6).

In practice, the apparatus dead space of the tracheal tube (or face mask) and its connections must be added for the purpose of calculating alveolar ventilation during anesthesia. As a roughguide, the total dead space is then about one-half of the tidal volume with a tracheal tube, and two-thirds of the tidal volume with a mask. Compensation for increased dead space may be made, during artificial ventilation, by increasing the minute volume to maintain the alveolar ventilation. During artificial ventilation, the high minute volumes usually employed, are generally more than adequate for carbon dioxide homeostasis. In the case of the hypoventilating patient (usually breathing spontaneously), the reduction in dead space (Fig. 6) offsets much of the expected diminution in alveolar ventilation.

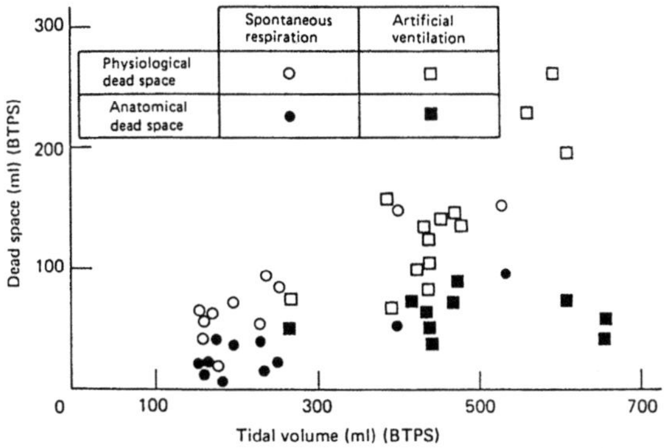

Fig. 6. Anatomical and physiological dead space as a function of tidal volume in anaesthetised patients with tracheal intubation, but excluding all apparatus dead space. [Redrawn from the data of Nunn and Hill (1960), and reproduced from Nunn (1987) with the permission of Butterworths]

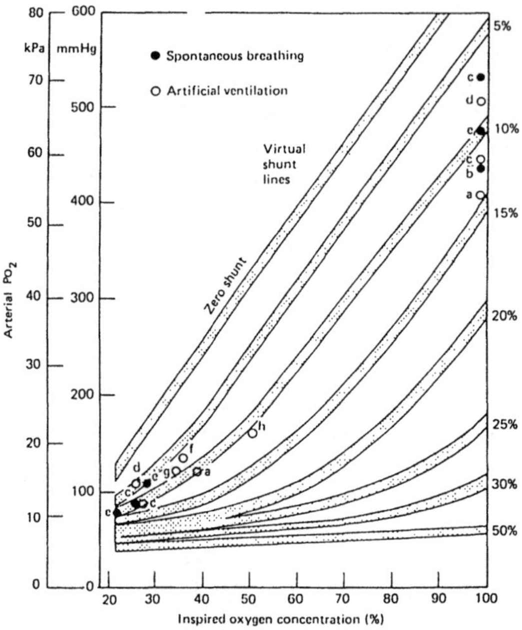

Fig. 7. Mean values for arterial PO_2 as a function of inspired oxygen concentration from 15 published studies of anaesthetised patients plotted on an iso-shunt diagram. References to the individual studies are contained in Nunn (1987) from which this diagram is reproduced with the permission of Butterworths

Shunt

During anesthesia, the alveolar/arterial PO_2 difference is usually increased to a value which corresponds to a shunt of about 10%. This provides an acceptable basis for calculating the concentration of oxygen in the inspired gas which will provide an acceptable arterial PO_2 during anesthesia, usually some 30%–40%. Figure 7 shows the iso-shunt diagram with the means of a large number of studies conducted during anesthesia with both spontaneous and artificial ventilation. References to individual studies were cited by Nunn (1987).

There now seems little doubt that the shunt is due to compression collapse of the lung (Hedenstierna et al. 1986, 1989. This in turn is explained by the reduction in lung volume (Dueck et al. 1988), which appears to be mainly due to loss of the end-expiratory tone in the diaphragm.

Ventilation/Perfusion ($\dot{V}/\dot{Q}$) Relationships

A more sophisticated approach to maldistribution is the analysis of distribution of pulmonary ventilation and perfusion in terms of $\dot{V}/\dot{Q}$ ratios. Rehder et al. (1979) found, in young fit subjects, that both ventilation and perfusion were distributed to a somewhat wider range $\dot{V}/\dot{Q}$ ratios after induction of anesthesia and paralysis but the true intrapulmonary shunt had a mean value of less than 1% during anaesthesia.

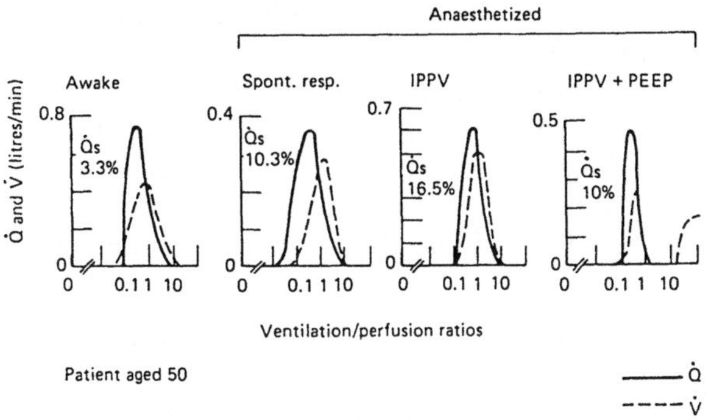

Fig. 8. Changes in pulmonary distribution of ventilation and perfusion from a typical patient in the study of Bindslev et al. (1981) from which this diagram is redrawn with permission, and reproduced from Nunn (1987) with the permission of Butterworths. IPPV, intermittent positive pressure ventilation; PEEP, positive end-expiratory pressure

Table 1. Changes in factors influencing gas exchange after induction of anaesthesia

	Awake	Anesthesia		
		Spontaneous ventilation	IPPV	IPPV+PEEP
F_{IO_2}	0.21	0.4	0.4	0.4
$\dot{Q}_S/\dot{Q}t$ (%)	1.6	6.2	8.6	4.1
V_D/V_T (%)	30	35	38	44
Cardiac output (l/min)	6.1	5.0	4.5	3.7
Pa_{O_2} (kPa)	10.5	17.6	18.8	20.5
$\dot{V}$ – mean $\dot{V}/\dot{Q}$	0.81	1.30	2.20	3.03
$\dot{Q}$ – mean $\dot{V}/\dot{Q}$	0.47	0.51	0.83	0.55

(Adapted from Bindslev et al. (1981) and reproduced from Nunn (1987) by permission of the publishers)
IPPV, intermittent positive pressure ventilation; PEEP, positive end-expiratory pressure;
F_{IO_2}, inspiratory oxygen concentration; PaO_2, O_2 partial pressure, arterial

Older surgical patients were studied by Bindslev et al. (1981) while awake, anesthetized and breathing spontaneously, anesthetized paralysed and ventilated artificially and finally with PEEP (Fig. 8 and Table 1). They found that the true intrapulmonary shunt was increased during anesthesia but not sufficiently to account for the increased alveolar/arterial PO_2 gradient, the difference being due to perfusion of areas of low $\dot{V}/\dot{Q}$ ratio. The dead space/tidal volume ratio was increased during anesthesia in spite of the tracheal tube bypassing the upper airway. PEEP reduced the shunt but also reduced the cardiac output and therefore the mixed venous oxygen content. The decreased admixture of more desaturated blood resulted in virtually no change in arterial PO_2. Dueck et al. (1980) studied elderly patients (mean age 60) who all had some deterioration in pulmonary function. They observed large increases in true shunt and also in perfusion of regions of very low $\dot{V}/\dot{Q}$ ratios.

These studies have greatly clarified our thinking and enabled us to draw firm conclusions when previously we relied heavily on deduction and inference. They have not, however, produced information leading to any radical reappraisal of our understanding of the effects of anesthesia on the respiratory system. We may now summarize the effect of anesthesia on gas exchange as follows:

1. Changes in alveolar/arterial PO_2 gradient are markedly dependent on age, being minimal in the young.
2. The increase in alveolar/arterial PO_2 gradient is due partly to an increase in true intrapulmonary shunt and partly to increased distribution of perfusion to areas of low (but not zero) $\dot{V}/\dot{Q}$ ratios.
3. The increase in alveolar dead space appears to be due to increased distribution of ventilation to areas of high (but not usually infinite) $\dot{V}/\dot{Q}$ ratios.
4. The major differences are between the awake and the anaesthetized states. Paralysis and artificial ventilation do not greatly alter the parameters of gas exchange in spite of the quite different spatial distribution of ventilation.
5. PEEP reduces the shunt but the beneficial effect on arterial PO_2 is offset by the decrease in cardiac output which reduces the mixed venous oxygen content.

Effect on Hypoxic Pulmonary Vasoconstriction (HPV)

It appears that all inhalational (but not intravenous) anesthetics inhibit HPV by a mechanism which is still unclear. A typical sigmoid dose/response curve has been demonstrated with an ED50 of slightly less than twice the minimal alveolar concentration (MAC) required for anesthesia and an ED90 of about 3 MAC (Marshall 1988). In the past, studies with inhalational anesthetics have given results which were apparently conflicting. This was due to the additional effect of anesthetics on cardiac output and thence on mixed venous PO_2, an important component in HPV (Marshall and Marshall 1985). It is now clear that inhalational anesthetics depress HPV in a predictable manner, provided that allowance is made for changes of cardiac output.

Interference with HPV is an important factor increasing pulmonary blood flow through the atelectatic areas of the lung during inhalational anesthesia. Similarly in one-lung anesthesia, inhalational anaesthetics cause a small but definite increase in the flow through the collapsed lung (Benumof 1989).

The Postoperative Period

It has been known for many years that both elevated PCO_2 and increased alveolar/arterial PO_2 gradient return to normal during the first few hours after minor operations (Nunn and Payne 1962). In the first few minutes of recovery, alveolar PO_2 may be reduced by elimination of nitrous oxide which dilutes alveolar oxygen and carbon dioxide. Shivering in the early postoperative period causes a large increase in oxygen consumption, which requires a corresponding increase in minute volume (Bay et al. 1968). Following major surgery, the restoration of a normal alveolar/arterial PO_2 gradient may take a few days and this is associated with a continued reduction in FRC (Alexander et al. 1973).

References

Alagesan K, Nunn JF, Feeley TW, Heneghan CPH (1987) Comparison of the respiratory depressant effects of halothane and isoflurane in routine surgery. Br J Anaesth 59:1070–1079

Alexander JL, Spence AA, Parikh RK, Stuart B (1973) The role of airway closure in postoperative hypoxaemia. Br J Anaesth 45:34–40

Bay J, Nunn JF, Prys-Roberts C (1968) Factors influencing arterial PO_2 during recovery from anaesthesia. Br J Anaesth 40:398–407

Bendixen HH, Hedley-Whyte J, Laver MB (1963) Impaired oxygenation in surgical patients during general anaesthesia with controlled ventilation. N Engl J Med 269:991–996

Benumof JL (1989) Anesthesia for thoracic surgery: pt II-management of one-lung ventilation. In: Stanley TH, Sperry RJ (eds) Anesthesia and the lung. Kluwer, pp 141–148

Bergman NA, Tien YK (1983) Contribution of the closure of pulmonary units to impaired oxygenation during anesthesia. Anesthesiology 59:395–401

Bindslev LG, Hedenstierna G, Santesson J, Gottlieb I, Carvalhas A (1981) Ventilation-perfusion distribution during inhalation anaesthesia. Acta Anaesthesiol Scand 25:360–371

Boidin MP (1985) Airway patency in the unconscious patient. Br J Anaesth 57:306–310

Brismar B, Hedenstierna G, Lundquist H, Strandberg A, Svenson L, Tokics L (1985) Pulmonary densities during anesthesia with muscular relaxation – a proposal of atelectasis. Anesthesiology 62:422–428

Butler J, Smith BH (1957) Pressure-volume relationships of the chest in the completely relaxed anaesthetised patient. Clin Sci 16:125–146

Davies RO, Edwards MW, Lahiri S (1982) Halothane depresses the response of carotid body chemoreceptors to hypoxia and hypercapnia in the cat. Anesthesiology 57:153–159

Dueck R, Young I, Clausen J, Wagner PD (1980) Altered distribution pulmonary ventilation and blood flow following induction of inhalational anesthesia. Anesthesiology 52:113–125

Dueck R, Prutow RJ, Davies JH, Clausen JL, Davidson TM (1988) The lung volume at which shunting occurs with inhalation anesthesia. Anesthesiology 69:854–861

Freund F, Roos A, Dodd RB (1964) Expiratory activity of the abdominal muscles in man during general anesthesia. J Appl Physiol 19:693–697

Froese AB (1985) Effects of anesthesia and paralysis on the chest wall. In: Covino BG, Fozzard HA, Rehder K, Strichartz G (eds) Effects of anesthesia. American Physiological Society, Bethesda MD

Froese AB, Bryan AC (1974) Effects of anesthesia and paralysis on diaphragmatic mechanics in man. Anesthesiology 41:242–255

Hedenstierna G, Standberg A, Brismar B, Lundquist H, Svenson L, Tokics L (1985) Functional residual capacity, thoracoabdominal dimensions and central blood volume during general anesthesia with muscle paralysis and mechanical ventilation. Anesthesiology 62:247–254

Hedenstierna G, Tokics L, Strandberg A, Lundquist H, Brismar B (1986) Correlation of gas exchange impairment to development of atelectasis during anaesthesia and muscle paralysis. Acta Anaesthesiol Scand 30:183–191

Juno P, Marsh M, Knopp TJ, Rehder K (1978) Closing capacity in awake and anesthetized-paralyzed man. J Appl Physiol 44:238–244

Kaul SU, Heath JR, Nunn JF (1973) Factors influencing the development of expiratory muscle activity during anaesthesia. Br J Anaesth 45:1013–1018

Knill RL, Clement JL (1984) Site of selective action of halothane on the peripheral chemoreflex pathway in humans. Anesthesiology 61:121–126

Knill RL, Clement JL (1985) Ventilatory responses in acute metabolic acidemia in humans awake, sedated and anesthetized with halothane. Anesthesiology 62:745–753

Knill RL, Gelb AW (1978) Ventilatory responses to hypoxia and hypercapnia during halothane sedation and anesthesia in man. Anesthesiology 49:244–251

Marshall BE (1988) Pulmonary blood flow and oxygenation. In: Marshall BE, Longnecker DE, Fairly HB (eds) Anesthesia for thoracic procedures. Blackwell, Oxford, pp 73–118

Marshall BE, Marshall C (1985) Anesthesia and pulmonary circulation. In: Covino BG, Fozzard HA, Rehder K, Strichartz G (eds) Effects of anesthesia. American Physiological Society, Bethesda MD

Moote CA, Knill RL, Clement J (1986) Ventilatory compensation for continuous inspiratory resistive and elastic loads during halothane anesthesia in humans. Anesthesiology 64:582–589

Muller N, Volgyesi G, Becker L, Bryan MH, Bryan AC (1979) Diaphragmatic muscle tone. J Appl Physiol 47:279–284

Munson ES, Larson CP, Bahad AA, Regan MJ, Buechel DR, Eger EI (1966) The effects of halothane, fluroxene and cyclopropane on ventilation: a comparative study in man. Anesthesiology 27:716–727

Nishino T, Honda Y, Kohchi T, Shirahata M, Yonezawa T (1985) Effects of increasing depth of anaesthesia on phrenic nerve and hypoglossal nerve activity during the swallowing reflex in cats. Br J Anaesth 57:208–213

Nunn JF (1987) Applied respiratory physiology, 3rd edn. Butterworths, London

Nunn JF (1989) Anaesthesia at altitude. In: Ward MP, Milledge JS, West JB (eds) High altitude medicine and physiology. Chapman and Hall, London, pp 481–486

Nunn JF, Ezi-Ashi TI (1961) The respiratory effects of resistance to breathing in anaesthetized man. Anesthesiology 22:174–185

Nunn JF, Hill DW (1960) Respiratory dead space and arterial to end-tidal CO_2 tension difference in anesthetized man. J Appl Physiol 15:383–389

Nunn JF, Payne JP (1962) Hypoxaemia after general anaesthesia. Lancet II:631–632

Nunn JF, Coleman AJ, Sachithanandan T, Bergman NA, Laws JW (1965) Hypoxaemia and atelectasis produced by forced expiration. Br J Anaesth 37:3–12

Rehder K (1985) Anesthesia and the mechanics of respiration. In: Covino BG, Fozzard HA, Rehder K, Strichartz G (eds) Effects of anesthesia. American Physiological Society, Bethesda MD

Rehder K, Knopp TJ, Sessler AD, Didier EP (1979) Ventilation-perfusion relationship in young healthy awake and anesthetized paralysed man. J Appl Physiol 47:745–753

Robertson JD, Reid DD (1952) Standards for the basal metabolism of normal people in Britain. Lancet I:940–943

Tokics L, Hedenstierna G, Standberg A, Brismar B, Lundquist H (1987) Lung collapse and gas exchange during general anesthesia – effects of spontaneous breathing, muscle paralysis and positive end-expiratory pressure. Anesthesiology 66:157–167

Tusiewicz K, Bryan AC, Froese AB (1977) Contribution of changing rib cage-diaphragm interactions to the ventilatory depression of halothane anesthesia. Anesthesiology 47:327–337

Westbrook PR, Stubbs SE, Sessler AD, Rehder K, Hyatt RE (1973) Effects of anaesthesia and muscle paralysis on respiratory mechanics in normal man. J Appl Physiol 34:81–86

Anesthesia for the Patients with Coronary Artery Disease

J. Tarnow

Patients with coronary artery disease (CAD) undergoing surgery, particularly those with previous myocardial infarction, are at increased risk. Several authors have documented a high incidence of myocardial ischemia during the preoperative period (42%), the day of surgery (24%–37%), and within the first 2–3 days of surgery (40%) [1–5]. Most of this ischemia is silent and unrelated to adverse hemodynamic changes such as tachycardia, hypertension, or hypotension leading to increased myocardial oxygen demand or decreased supply. Since a significant relationship between the incidence of new ischemic episodes and the occurrence of postoperative myocardial infarction has been demonstrated [1, 2], the primary anesthetic goal in managing patients with CAD is the prevention of ischemia. In any ischemic event, time elapses between the detection of the problem, the identification of the cause, and its correction. Delay in any of these phases increases the likelihood of injury. Therefore, efforts in the anesthetic management of patients with CAD should mainly be directed toward improved methods for either prevention or earlier diagnosis of perioperative myocardial ischemia.

Clinical Possibilities and Limitations to Detect Perioperative Myocardial Ischemia

Angina Pectoris

A number of publications demonstrate that approximately 70% of the ischemic episodes in patients with CAD are not associated with angina, and that about 10%–15% of acute myocardial infarctions are silent [6]. Moreover, pre- or postoperative angina pectoris may be obscured by premedicants and residual anesthetic or analgesic drug effects.

Electrocardiography

A multiple-lead ECG system consists of four electrodes on the extremities and a fifth electrode in the V_5 position, which allows for selection of any of seven different ECG leads (I, II, III, aVR, AVL, aVF, or V_5). Leads II and V_5 are usually displayed simultaneously, allowing for observation of both inferior wall and anterolateral ischemia. This system has become the standard way of monitoring patients with CAD. Sensitivity may be increased by the further addition of V_2–V_4 leads or by precordial mapping from multiple loci (16–72 leads) on the chest wall [4, 7]. However, many operating-room ECG monitors still have only a three-electrode system which can be adapted so that similar precordial ECG information can be obtained by using modified bipolar standard limb leads. For example, the CM_5 (central manubrium) lead is obtained by placing the negative (red) right arm electrode on the manubrium of the sternum, the positive (yellow) left arm electrode in the V_5 position, and the ground (black) electrode in the left leg position. Lead I is then selected. Alternatively, a CB_5 (central back) lead can be used by placing the right arm electrode over the center of the right scapula.

Accurate interpretation of the ECG – and in particular of the ST segment – requires the availability of a recorder. It is essential that the recorder is properly calibrated (1 mV = 10 mm) and that the ST segment is analysed at a sufficient paper speed (50 mm/s) 60 ms from the J-point. Changes in the ST segment indicative of ischemia may be evaluated visually or subjected to computer analysis.

In addition to recording the electrical potentials of the heart from the surface of the body, they may also be obtained from body cavities adjacent to the heart (i.e., esophagus and trachea) or from the heart itself (by using a multipurpose balloon-tipped PA catheter with two pairs of electrodes for atrial and ventricular electrograms). Esophageal ECG monitoring has been demonstrated to be particularly helpful in detecting posterior myocardial ischemia usually not present in leads II and V_5 [8].

PA Catheter Monitoring

The pulmonary artery catheter has been widely used in the operating room for almost 2 decades. Apart from the ability to obtain several measured and derived hemodynamic data the device can also be helpful in the early diagnosis of myocardial ischemia [9, 10]. Elevated PCWP and abnormal PCWP tracing (prominent a- and v-waves) frequently develop before the onset of ECG changes, or may represent the only sign of myocardial ischemia. However, Swan-Ganz catheters have raised major questions with regard to the benefit-to-hazard ratios, which are still unresolved [11–13].

To date there are no prospective, randomized, controlled studies which demonstrate improvement in perioperative morbidity or mortality as a direct result of PA-catheter monitoring in patients with CAD. Tuman et al. [45] have recently demonstrated that even high-risk patients undergoing coronary artery surgery may be safely managed without routine placement of a PA catheter.

Echocardiography

A promising use of echocardiography (preferably from the esophagus) is the detection of anesthesia-induced acute abnormalities of regional ventricular contraction which are highly sensitive and relatively specific indicators of myocardial ischemia [14, 15]. Although the superiority of echocardiography over electrocardiography for the detection of myocardial ischemia has been demonstrated [44], this technique suffers from the same problem as the ECG, because the signal must be aimed at the ischemic segment or the changes will be missed. In addition, transesophageal echocardiography can only be used after induction of anesthesia and the equipment is expensive, which may explain why anesthesiologists have been slow to adopt this method.

Cardiokymography

This technique uses alterations of an electromagnetic field to detect anterior wall motion abnormalities of the left ventricle [16–18]. Since cardiokymography (CKG) also records chest-wall motion, measurements must be performed during apnea at end-expiration. Another limitation is that CKG cannot be used to detect new anterior-wall motion abnormalities if dyskinesia is already present. It is insensitive to changes in motion of the inferior, posterior, and lateral left ventricular (LV) walls. Advantages of this method include safety, ease of interpretation, and its noninvasive nature.

Nuclear Stethoscope

Moderate to severe regional myocardial ischemia may be detected by an acute and persistent fall of the left ventricular ejection fraction [19, 20]. With the development of a computerized gamma camera of small size and true mobility (nuclear "stethoscope") a real-time left ventricular time-activity curve can be recorded after in vivo labeling of red blood cells with ^{99m}-technetium pertechnetate 15–20 mCi, so that LV ejection fraction (EF) can be obtained beat-to-beat [21].

Compensatory hyperfunction in normal regions can limit the sensitivity of the EF for detecting regional myocardial ischemia, and a normal global EF can be produced despite the presence of regional ischemic dysfunction [19]. Further problems include probe positioning over the left ventricle, recording of background activity, and radiation safety in the operating room.

Coronary Sinus and Great Cardiac Vein Catheterization

Because coronary blood flow is intimately coupled to myocardial oxygen demand, any specific measured values for global and/or regional blood flows per se cannot be interpreted as "normal" or "abnormal" unless these values are related to metabolic indices of myocardial ischemia.

Under aerobic conditions the healthy heart consumes lactate. Myocardial ischemia is characterized by a transition from lactate uptake to lactate production or a reduction of the global lactate extraction to less than 10% [22]. Sampling at the coronary sinus, however, causes dilution of metabolites because of the much larger volume of blood draining nonischemic muscle. Thus, ischemia within a regional portion of the heart may not be reflected by chemical analysis of coronary sinus blood. This limited degree of sensitivity may be improved by great cardiac vein sampling and flow measures. However, the perioperative possibilities of assessing myocardial blood flow and oxygenation are invasive and time consuming.

Some Principles in the Anesthetic Management of Patients with Coronary Artery Disease

Preoperative Considerations

The presence of definite or suspected CAD, its severity, the time of recent myocardial infarction (MI), the presence of additional risk factors such as peripheral vascular disease, hypertension or diabetes, and the treatment of the disease provide important information to the anesthesiologist. In patients who have a history of MI less than 0–6 months from the time of anesthesia and surgery, the risk of perioperative reinfarction is reported to be 2.3%–5.7%, whereas the incidence of MI without evidence of a previous infarction ranges from 0.1%–0.7% [23]. Since the overall reinfarction mortality is still high, elective noncardiac surgery should be postponed for patients who have had a MI less than 6 months earlier. After 6 months, the reinfarction rate stabilizes at 1%–1.7% and should be associated with a reduced perioperative mortality.

Most authors agree that chronic antianginal and/or antihypertensive drug therapy [e.g., nitrates, β-adrenoceptor blocking drugs, calcium entry blockers or, angiotensin-converting enzyme (ACE) inhibitors] should be continued with its regular dose regimen up to, and including, the day of surgery. The benefits of perioperative β-blocker therapy, as well as the consequences of preoperative withdrawal are well documented [21]. Untreated or not sufficiently treated hypertensive patients should receive oral doses of a beta-adrenergic blocking agent along with premedication [25]. Preoperative clonidine administration has also been shown to effectively suppress the hyperdynamic cardiovascular response to laryngoscopy and intubation by reducing sympathetic outflow via alpha-adrenergic stimulation [26]. The effectiveness of chronic treatment with calcium entry blocking drugs in preventing perioperative MI has recently been questioned [3, 27].

Prophylactic digitalization in CAD patients without failure is probably unnecessary and potentially dangerous because it may favor the development of dysrhythmias in the presence of perioperative hypokalemia, respiratory alkalosis, or MI [28]. Indications for digitalis include congestive heart failure, atrial fibrillation with rapid ventricular response, atrial flutter, paroxysmal atrial or nodal tachycardia, and Wolff-Parkinson-White tachyarrhythmias.

Premedication should be adequate to sedate the patient sufficiently to prevent the hemodynamic consequences of apprehension. The benzodiazepines used for overnight sedation and as oral premedicants have a high patient acceptance because they relieve anxiety and frequently produce amnesia [29]. Narcotic analgesics and anticholinergic drugs are rarely indicated and not favored by patients because of their unpleasant side effects and lack of relief from anxiety. Adequate premedication (i.e., benzodiazepines, antianginal medications) may contribute to reduce the reported high incidence of ischemia in the preinduction period.

Finally, preoperative planning should also consider the fact that physician selection (anesthesiologist and surgeon) may have an important influence on the incidence of ischemic events, perioperative MI, and probably patient outcome [1].

Anesthesia and Intraoperative Considerations

Since the induction of anesthesia is one of the most stressful periods for the CAD patient, all monitoring should be established before starting anesthesia. The extent of monitoring has to take account of the patient's preoperative condition and the extent of surgery. It is difficult at this time, however, to establish definitive guidelines as to exactly which patient should receive invasive monitoring such as the use of PA catheters. Thus, a major area for future investigation will be to determine which type of patient is a likely candidate for the cost-effective benefits of expensive and invasive monitoring techniques. Nevertheless, the most effective monitor continues to be the constant presence of a skilled and attentive clinician and, above all, it is necessary for the anesthetist to monitor him/herself.

The major goals of anesthesia and intraoperative care in CAD patients are to prevent or promptly treat myocardial ischemia while preserving or improving LV function. In patients with good LV function, hypertension and tachycardia as a result of inadequate attenuation of the responses to noxious stimuli are the most likely mechanisms for upsetting the myocardial oxygen balance. Conversely, in patients with poor LV function, tachycardia and increased ventricular filling pressure without hypertension are likely to accompany noxious stimulation. To date no single technique using one or multiple anesthetic drugs has been shown to be superior to any other technique. Therefore, the approach to these patients varies widely among major cardiovascular centers. The choice of volatile anesthetics is probably less critical than recent publications might suggest [30–31]. While isoflurane may cause a redistribution of coronary blood flow away from ischemic areas when using maintenance concentrations of more than 1% end-tidal in the absence of surgical stimulation, there is no evidence that lower concentrations of isoflurane which do not cause significant coronary vasodilation are harmful to patients with CAD [32, 33, 46, 48]. Thus, since isoflurane-associated coronary vasodilation is dose-dependent, concentrations of less than 1% end-tidal may well be used to supplement opioids for maintenance of anesthesia. The first large-scale (1012 patients) prospective and randomized outcome study recently published by Slogoff and Keats [47], clearly demonstrates that isoflurane (even when used as the primary anesthetic) was not different from halothane or enflurane with regard to the incidence of myocardial ischemia, postoperative myocardial infarction, and death.

In summary, the choice of specific anesthetic drugs appears to be far less important than the need for meticulous adjustments of anesthetic depth and prophylactic measures to prevent predictable autonomic responses by potent noxious stimuli such as laryngoscopy, tracheal intubation, skin incision, sternotomy, or aortic clamping. For example, low doses of opioids combined with i.v. anesthetics are effective in suppressing the hemodynamic response to laryngoscopy and intubation. The adrenergic responses can also be modified by β-adrenoceptor antagonists for the supplementation of nitroglycerin [34]. The anesthetist should ensure that these antianginal drugs and vasodilators are readily available.

The period from intubation to skin incision may sometimes be unnecessarily prolonged and often is associated with hypotension unless appropriate adjustments of anesthetic depth are made. Although more than 50% of ischemic episodes are not temporally related to hemodynamic abnormalities [1, 2], hypotension, high cardiac filling pressures, and, in particular, tachycardia continue to be important factors in precipitating MI, while hypertension per se may play a relatively minor role [1, 35]. In patients with a history of MI the incidence of perioperative reinfarction is significantly greater following intrathoracic or upper abdominal operations [23].

Patients undergoing major vascular sugery are also known to have a high frequency of cardiac complications. Even without selecting patients with previous MI, the infarction rate is high [36]. The duration of surgery per se, the urgency of the surgical intervention, patient age and sex do not affect reinfarction rate [23]. In patients undergoing coronary artery bypass grafting perioperative myocardial infarction (PMI) accounts for almost 50% of the mortality [36]. Variables associated with an increased risk of PMI include left main coronary artery stenosis, high LVEDP or a decreased ejection fraction, and a patient age of 70 years or older [36, 37].

Postoperative Considerations

Termination of the operative procedure and anesthesia is a period of increased stress, and the likelihood of the development of MI is increased. Rapid recovery may be appropriate for the healthy patient, but every effort should be made to ensure a smooth emergence from anesthesia for the patient with CAD. Maintenance of light anesthesia during extubation may be recommended for the severely compromised patient even if recovery is prolonged. Excessive suctioning and the use of opiate antagonists should be avoided [38–40]. If shivering occurs the administration of meperidine (25 mg i.v.) is advisable to reduce major increases in oxygen demand [41]. Avoidance of pain, hypoxia, and of Mueller maneuvers resulting from upper airway obstruction [42] may also contribute to prevent the development of MI during the period of emergence from anesthesia. Antianginal medications should be continued as soon as possible after operation. Since most postoperative MIs occur within 6 days after surgery (with a peak around the 3rd day after operation) Rao et al. [23] recommend prolongation of invasive monitoring for prompt recognition and therapy of hemodynamic abnormalities until the 4th postoperative day in all patients after thoracic and major upper abdominal surgery with and without a prior infarction in the past 6 months. At present, however, the data of Rao et al., which imply that extended ICU monitoring in selected patients decreases the incidence of MI, provide only a hypothesis that this is so.

The postoperative care of the patient with coronary artery disease should also consider the fact that at least 50% of postoperative myocardial infarctions are painless and many such infarctions present with otherwise unexplained alterations in vital signs or mental status [43].

References

1. Slogoff S, Keats AB (1985) Does perioperative myocardial infarction lead to postoperative myocardial infarction? Anesthesiology 62:107
2. Slogoff S, Keats AS (1986) Further observations on perioperative myocardial ischemia. Anesthesiology 65:539
3. Slogoff S, Keats AS (1988) Does chronic treatment with calcium entry blocking drugs reduce perioperative myocardial ischemia? Anesthesiology 68:676
4. London MJ, Hollenberg M, Wong MG et al. (1988) Intraoperative myocardial ischemia: localization by continuous 12 lead electrocardiography. Anesthesiology 69:232
5. Knight AA, Hollenberg M, London MJ et al. (1988) Perioperative myocardial ischemia: importance of the preoperative ischemic pattern. Anesthesiology 68:681
6. Epstein SE, Quyyumi AA, Bonow RO (1988) Myocardial ischemia – silent or symptomatic. N Engl J Med 318:1038
7. Maroko PR, Libby P, Covell JW et al. (1972) Precordial S-T segment elevation mapping: an atraumatic method for assessing alterations in the extent of myocardial ischemic injury. Am J Cardiol 29:223
8. Kates RA, Zaidan JR, Kaplan JA (1982) Esophageal lead for intraoperative electrocardiographic monitoring. Anesth Analg 61:781
9. Kaplan JA, Wells PH (1981) Early diagnosis of myocardial ischemia using the pulmonary artery catheter. Anesth Analg 60:798
10. Waller JL, Johnson SP, Kaplan JA (1982) Usefulness of pulmonary artery catheters during aortocoronary bypass surgery. Anesth Analg 61:221
11. Keefer JR, Barash PJ (1983) Pulmonary artery catheterization. A decade of progress? Chest 84:241
12. Gore JM, Goldberg RJ, Spodick DH et al. (1987) A community-wide assessment of the use of pulmonary artery catheters in patients with acute myocardial infarction. Chest 92:721
13. Sibbald WJ, Sprung CL (1988) The pulmonary artery catheter. The debate continues. Chest 94:899
14. Abel MD, Nishimura RA, Callahan MJ et al. (1987) Evaluation of intraoperative transesophageal two-dimensional echocardiography. Anesthesiology 66:64
15. Clements FM, de Bruijn NP (1987) Perioperative evaluation of regional wall motion by transesophageal two-dimensional echocardiography. Anesth Analg 66:249
16. Bellows WH, Bode RH, Levy JH et al. (1984) Noninvasive detection of periinduction ischemic ventricular dysfunction by cardiokymography in humans: preliminary experience. Anesthesiology 60:155
17. Silverberg RA, Diamond GA, Vas R et al. (1980) Noninvasive diagnosis of coronary artery disease: the cardiokymographic stress test. Circulation 61:579
18. Häggmark S, Hohner P, Östman M et al. (1980) Comparison of hemodynamic, electrocardiographic, mechanical, and metabolic indicators of intraoperative myocardial ischemia in vascular surgical patients with coronary artery disease. Anesthesiology 70:19
19. Ross R (1986) Assessment of ischemic regional myocardial dysfunction and its reversibility. Circulation 74:1186
20. Markham RV, Winniford MD, Firth BG et al. (1983) Symptomatic, electrocardiographic, metabolic, and hemodynamic alterations during pacing-induced myocardial ischemia. Am J Cardiol 51:1589
21. Giles RW, Berger HJ, Barash PG et al. (1982) Continuous monitoring of left ventricular performance with the computerized nuclear probe during laryngoscopy and intubation before coronary artery bypass surgery. Am J Cardiol 50:735
22. Waters D, Forrester JS (1978) Myocardial ischemia, detection and quantification. Ann Intern Med 88:239
23. Rao TL, Jacobs KH, El-Etr AA (1983) Reinfarction following anesthesia in patients with myocardial infarction. Anesthesiology 59:499

24. Slogoff S, Keats AS, Ott E (1978) Preoperative propranolol therapy and aortocoronary bypass operation. JAMA 240:1487
25. Stone JG, Foëx P, Sear JW et al. (1988) Myocardial ischemia in untreated hypertensive patients: effect of a single small oral dose of a beta-adrenergic blocking agent. Anesthesiology 68:495
26. Ghignone M, Quintin L, Duke PC et al. (1986) Effects of clonidine on narcotic requirements and hemodynamic response during induction of fentanyl anesthesia and endotracheal intubation. Anesthesiology 64:36
27. Chung F, Houston PL, Cheng DC et al. (1988) Calcium channel blockade does not offer adequate protection from perioperative myocardial ischemia. Anesthesiology 69:343
28. Morrison J, Killip T (1973) Serum digitalis and arrhythmia in patients undergoing cardiopulmonary bypass. Circulation 47:341
29. Kanto J (1981) Benzodiazepines as oral premedicants. Br J Anaesth 53:1179
30. Reiz S, Bålfors E, Sørensen MB et al. (1983) Isoflurane – a powerful coronary vasodilator in patients with coronary artery disease. Anesthesiology 59:91
31. Reiz S (1988) Myocardial ischaemia associated with general anaesthesia. A review of clinical studies. Br J Anaesth 61:68
32. Cucchiara RF, Sundt TM, Michenfelder JD (1988) Myocardial infarction in carotid endarterectomy patients anesthetized with halothane, enflurane, or isoflurane. Anesthesiology 69:783
33. Smith JS, Roizen MF, Cahalan MK et al. (1988) Does anesthetic technique make a difference? Augmentation of systolic blood pressure during carotid endarterectomy: effects of phenylephrine versus light anesthesia and of isoflurane versus halothane on the incidence of myocardial ischemia. Anesthesiology 69:846
34. Fusciardi J, Godet G, Bernard JM et al. (1986) Roles of fentanyl and nitroglycerin in prevention of myocardial ischemia associated with laryngoscopy and tracheal intubation in patients undergoing operations of short duration. Anesth Analg 65:617
35. Lieberman RW, Orkin FK, Jobes DR et al. (1983) Hemodynamic predictors of myocardial ischemia during halothane anesthesia for coronary artery revascularization. Anesthesiology 59:36
36. Haagensen R, Steen PA (1988) Perioperative myocardial infarction. Br J Anaesth 61:24
37. Acinapura AJ, Rose DM, Cunningham JN et al. (1988) Coronary artery bypass in septuagenarians. Analysis of mortality and morbidity. Circulation [Suppl I] 78:I–179
38. Michaelis LL, Hickey PR, Clark TA et al. (1974) Ventricular irritability associated with the use of naloxone hydrochloride. Ann Thorac Surg 18:608
39. Azar I, Turndorf H (1979) Severe hypertension and multiple atrial premature contractions following naloxone administration. Anesth Analg 58:524
40. Patschke D, Eberlein HJ, Tarnow J (1977) Antagonism of morphine with naloxone in dogs: cardiovascular effects with special reference to the coronary circulation. Br J Anaesth 49:525
41. MacIntyre PE, Pavlin EG, Dwersteg JF (1987) Effect of meperidine on oxygen consumption, carbon dioxide production, and respiratory gas exchange in postanesthesia shivering. Anesth Analg 66:751
42. Scharf SM, Bianco JA, Tow DE et al. (1981) The effects of large negative intrathoracic pressure on left ventricular function in patients with coronary artery disease. Circulation 63:871
43. Goldman L (1988) Assessment of the patient with known or suspected ischaemic heart disease for non-cardiac surgery. Br J Anaesth 61:38
44. Smith JS, Cahalan MK, Benefiel DJ et al. (1985) Intraoperative detection of myocardial ischemia in high risk patients: electrocardiography versus two-dimensional transesophageal echocardiography. Circulation 72:1015

|5. Tuman KJ, McCarthy RJ, Spiess BD et al. (1989) Effect of pulmonary artery catheterization on outcome in patients undergoing coronary artery surgery. Anesthesiology 70:199
|6. Tuman KJ, McCarthy RJ, Spiess BD et al. (1989) Does choice of anesthetic agent significantly affect outcome after coronary artery surgery? Anesthesiology 70:189
|7. Slogoff S, Keats AS (1989) Randomized trial of primary anesthetic agents on outcome of coronary artery bypass operations. Anesthesiology 70:179
|8. O'Young J, Mastrocostopoulos G, Hilgenberg A et al. (1987) Myocardial circulatory and metabolic effects of isoflurane and sufentanyl during coronary artery surgery. Anesthesiology 66:653

Isoflurane: Effects on Coronary Circulation and Clinical Implications

H.-J. Priebe

The effects of isoflurane (ISO) on the coronary circulation remain highly controversial [1–4]. Both coronary vasodilation [5–13] as well as little or unchanged coronary vascular resistance (CVR) [14–17] have been attributed to ISO in man [11–13, 17] and the experimental animal [5–10, 14–16]. To complicate the issue even further, beneficial [18], no adverse [16, 19–22], and detrimental effects [9, 11–13, 17, 23, 24] of ISO on the myocardial oxygen (O_2) supply/demand relationship in the presence of an abnormal coronary circulation have been reported in humans [11–13, 17–20] and animals [9, 16, 21–24]. Considering the remarkable differences in methodology, such discrepancies in results are to be expected. Proper interpretation of existing data thus requires individual analysis, including differentiation between experimental and clinical, and between data obtained in the absence or presence of an abnormal coronary circulation. This should enable us to better define the basis for the existing controversy surrounding this entire issue, and to subsequently formulate appropriate clinical implications.

Effects of ISO During Normal Coronary Circulation

In the experimental animal, increases (25%–30%) [6], no changes [5, 7], and decreases (15%–40%) [7, 14, 15] in myocardial blood flow (MBF) have been reported. These were accompanied by either little change [14, 15] or decreases (30%–50%) in CVR [5–7]. Investigations using quantitative coronary angiography have confirmed that ISO is a true dose-dependent coronary vasodilator [8]. Since ISO throughout a wide range of concentrations (0.75%–2.25%) and coronary perfusion pressures (50–110 mmHg) had no effect on epicardial coronary artery dimensions, the distal coronary arterioles must have constituted the site of ISO-induced coronary vasodilation.

An increase in coronary sinus O_2 saturation and a decrease in myocardial O_2 extraction during a decline in MVO_2 clearly imply uncoupling of myocardial O_2 demand and supply during ISO [5, 10], indicating interference with coronary autoregulation. In the chronically instrumented dog it has, in fact, been shown that 1 MAC (minimum alveolar concentration) ISO anesthesia blunts but in no way abolishes autoregulation [10]. This effect is more pronounced with ISO than with halothane (HAL) or enflurane. However, ISO (as HAL and enflurane) did not significantly affect maximum coronary conductance, coronary vascular reserve, or coronary zero-flow pressure (P_{zf}).

Despite convincing evidence of considerable coronary vasodilation, uncoupling of myocardial O_2 demand and cerebral blood flow (CBF), and interference with autoregulation during ISO, there is no indication of inadequate myocardial perfusion even at low perfusion pressures (55 mmHg) [7, 14] or high concentrations (3.3%) [14].

Detailed investigations of the effects of ISO on coronary hemodynamics in humans with a normal coronary circulation are, to my knowledge, not available. However, indirect evidence [25–28] would suggest that ISO at end-tidal concentrations as high as 2.4% [25] and mean arterial pressures as low as 45 mmHg [25] is tolerated without adverse cardiac effects. In summary, there is no evidence – neither in the experimental animal nor in man – that the effects of ISO on coronary hemodynamics (i.e., coronary arteriolar dilation) in the presence of a normal coronary circulation lead to any impairment in myocardial oxygenation.

Effect of ISO During Abnormal Coronary Circulation

Experimental Data

There are several recent investigations that have looked at the effects of ISO on coronary hemodynamics and cardiac performance in the presence of preexisting impairment of myocardial perfusion [9, 16, 22–24]. Results have been highly contradictory. Deleterious [9, 23, 24] as well as no detrimental effects on the myocardial O_2 supply-demand relationship [16, 22] and development [9] as well as no evidence [16] of coronary "steal" in seemingly similar models have been reported. Are those results mutually exclusive, or may there be, in fact, a common basis?

Severe regional myocardial dysfunction suggestive of myocardial ischemia developed when ISO was administered during critical stenoses (approximately 10% reduction of resting CBF) of the right and the left anterior descending (LAD) coronary artery [23]. However, it is likely that the observed regional myocardial ischemia occurred primarily on the basis of a localized decrease in blood supply due to a reduced pressure gradient across the stenosis.

The results of another study seem to contradict the above findings [22]. When a similar concentration of ISO (1.7% $\pm$ 0.1% end-tidal) was administered during critical stenosis of the left circumflex coronary artery, myocardial functional ischemia was not observed. However, a close look at the data reveals some degree of maldistribution of MBF across myocardial layers consistent with the development of transmural coronary steal [29].

The effects of ISO on coronary hemodynamics, myocardial flow distribution and metabolism, and regional myocardial performance have been studied in dogs 3–4 weeks after encasement of the proximal LAD in an ameroid constrictor [9]. At either a *constant flow rate* (equivalent to an amount observed at full autoregulation, a coronary pressure of 90 mmHg, a mean arterial pressure of 60 mmHg, and a ventricular pacing rate of 100/min), or at a *constant coronary pressure* of 90 mmHg, neither 0.94% (at constant flow) nor 1.46%

ISO (at constant coronary pressure) resulted in redistribution of MBF or regional myocardial dysfunction. In contrast, when left coronary artery perfusion was reduced initially by 16%–26% of the autoregulated flow value, subsequent administration of either ISO concentration then resulted in redistribution of blood flow from the collateral-dependent to the normally perfused area (intercoronary steal), from the endocardium to the epicardium (transmural coronary steal), and it resulted in a 60% decrease in systolic contraction (ISO 0.96%) or a practical cessation of any systolic thickening (ISO 1.46%) in the collateral-dependent zone. Such types of regional myocardial dysfunction very likely reflect severe myocardial ischemia [30].

It is of considerable clinical relevance that the initial reduction in autoregulated flow prior to the administration of ISO already caused considerable regional myocardial dysfunction suggestive of ischemia in the collateral-dependent area: flow reductions caused 28% and 43% decreases in regional systolic shortening or systolic wall thickening, respectively. Reductions in perfusion and contractile function in collateral-dependent regions to such a degree cannot typically be expected in patients [31, 32]. On the basis of the material presented one would, therefore, have to conclude that ISO caused transmural and intercoronary steal only when superimposed on preexisting myocardial ischemia. The fact, nevertheless, remains that HAL under identical experimental conditions did not induce maldistribution of MBF or worsen the underlying myocardial dysfunction.

These findings and conclusions are entirely consistent with results from another study [24]. Following the induction of a critical stenosis of the LAD, mean aortic pressure was reduced by either ISO or HAL from 97 to 55 mmHg. Subsequently, both anesthetics were substituted for each other at concentrations that would maintain mean aortic pressure at 55 mmHg. Substitution of HAL (mean end-tidal concentration, 1.9%; range, 1.3%–2.6%) for ISO (mean end-tidal concentration, 1.9%; range, 1.1%–3.0%) caused an approximately 20% increase in flow through the critically stenosed LAD, a 20% decrease in flow through the unconstricted left circumflex coronary artery, and an improvement in regional myocardial function in the area supplied by the stenosed LAD.

At first, it is not at all intuitively apparent why, with no change in external constriction, flow through the stenosed LAD fell following the substitution of ISO for HAL despite unchanged proximal perfusion pressure, HR, cardiac filling pressure, and presumably MVO_2 [24]. A possible explanation is that there had been dynamic changes in the severity of the stenosis itself. There is unequivocal experimental evidence that coronary stenoses induced by external constrictors of normal coronary arteries may become hydraulically worse after distal coronary bed vasodilation when associated with a reduction in distal coronary artery pressure [33–36]. With a decrease in distal pressure, intraluminal distending pressure at the site of the stenosis will decrease, and flow turbulence in the stenotic segment itself will increase. As a result, there can be a passive collapse of the wall of the stenotic segment which, in turn, may cause a seemingly paradoxical decrease in CBF despite an increase in pressure gradient ιcross the stenosis [37]. Thus, distal coronary arteriolar vasodilators may vorsen and proximal arterial large-vessel dilators may lessen the severity of tenosis by increasing or decreasing stenotic resistance. The net effect of a 'asodilating drug may thus depend on its relative potency as arteriolar vs arge-vessel dilator. The decrease in LAD flow following substitution of ISO or HAL could, in part, be explained on this basis. Whereas ISO is an arterio-ar-type vasodilator [8], HAL is more potent than ISO as a direct relaxant of arge, preconstricted, epicardial arterial segments [38].

In another study also using a canine model with a recent ameroid-induced AD occlusion, there was no evidence of development of coronary steal folowing the administration of 0.75% and 2.25% ISO, and in this regard there vas no difference to HAL at equianesthetic concentrations (i.e., 0.45% and .3%) [16]. There were, however, considerable discrepancies in methodology vhich can explain most if not all contrasting findings. Differences include distolic aortic pressure, CVR, degree of stenosis, and maturity of collaterals.

It has been shown that the addition of a critical coronary stenosis does not vorsen the fatal/anesthetic ratio of ISO [21]. However, this does not exclude he possibility that acute ischemia might have developed. It may simply imply hat regional ischemia is not necessarily reflected in global hemodynamic disurbances and that it may not result in acute mortality. The possibility thus emains that late mortality might have increased due to the development of peioperative myocardial infarction had the animals been resuscitated.

Iuman Data

)f the five investigations that have studied the effects of ISO on coronary heıodynamics in the presence of coronary artery disease (CAD), evidence of ıyocardial ischemia has been reported in four of them [11–13, 17]. One study id not report any incidence of myocardial ischemia [20].

Coronary hemodynamics and myocardial metabolism have been studied in en patients with 2- or 3-vessel CAD, stable angina, and normal LV function EF >0.55) who were about to undergo coronary artery bypass grafting CABG) [17]. Measurements were made awake, 20 min after intubation at a ıean end-tidal concentration of 0.4% ISO and 50% N_2O, and during sternoomy at 1.5% ISO (mean, end-tidal) and 50% N_2O. Lactate extraction fell rogressively. Actual lactate production was observed in one patient post inıbation, and in three during sternotomy in the absence of hemodynamic intability. Mean HR and arterial pressure remained between 62–70/min and 07–81 mmHg, respectively. There were decreases in MVO_2, myocardial O_2 xtraction, and arteriocoronary sinus O_2 difference, and increases in coronary inus O_2 saturation indicating "luxury perfusion."

The effects of ISO were evaluated in another, similar group of ten normoensive patients with CAD and preserved LV function (mean EF, 0.61; range, .50–0.83) scheduled for CABG [13]. Measurements were made at a mean inpired ISO concentration of 1.76% (range, 0.67%–3.8%). Immediately followıg induction, mean arterial pressure fell from 98 to 67 mmHg, and MVO_2 decreased by approximately 40%. This was accompanied by a decrease in CVR, unchanged CBF, and an increase in coronary sinus O_2 saturation, all consistent with coronary vasodilation out of proportion to myocardial O_2 requirements. There was no statistically significant change in mean myocardial lactate extraction at any time of the investigation. However, three patients produced lactate after induction, and lactate production was detectable in one or two patients throughout the study.

The clinical significance of these findings remains uncertain. One of the three patients had lactate production when still awake. Three patients had "stormy" inductions, and two of these patients showed myocardial lactate production. Therefore, it cannot be determined with certainty whether ISO or the "stormy" induction contributed primarily to the development of myocardial ischemia.

Evidence of myocardial ischemia was also present during an end-tidal concentration of 1% ISO in patients with a history of CAD undergoing major vascular surgery [11]. None of the 21 patients was on calcium entry blockers, only 11 patients received β-adrenergic receptor blockers and/or nitrates, and 13 patients were taking digitalis and/or diuretics. Such a regimen may reflect a higher incidence of congestive heart failure in this study population. On the other hand, the baseline (awake) values for systolic arterial pressure (178 mmHg), mean arterial pressure (113 mmHg), and HR (75/min) would suggest inadequate cardiac medication, or they reflect the lack of premedication (in patients about to undergo major surgery and catheterization for invasive monitoring).

Following induction with ISO, systolic and mean arterial pressure fell from 178 to 94 mmHg, and from 113 to 68 mmHg, respectively. Coronary sinus flow did not decrease significantly, CVR fell by 25%, myocardial O_2 extraction by 30%, and MVO_2 by 35%. This clearly indicates that 1% end-tidal ISO had a direct dilatory effect on coronary vessels in these patients with CAD. At the same time, one patient started to produce myocardial lactate, and ten patients (i.e., 48%) developed ST-T depression or T-wave inversion suggestive of myocardial ischemia.

In an attempt to differentiate between reductions in coronary perfusion pressure and redistribution of blood flow within the myocardium as the cause of ischemia, systemic arterial and pulmonary capillary wedge pressures, and HR were restored to preanesthetic levels by the combined use of phenylephrine, nitroglycerin, and pacing. Five out of ten patients studied this way had initial ECG and metabolic changes suggestive of regional myocardial ischemia during steady-state ISO anesthesia. Upon normalization of coronary perfusion pressure, LV filling pressure, and HR, signs of myocardial ischemia disappeared in two patients, but remained unchanged in the remaining three patients. This would suggest that mechanisms other than a decrease in coronary perfusion pressure contributed to the development of ischemia during ISO. A possible mechanism would be redistribution of CBF (i.e., coronary steal).

The effects of a combination of 1.5 MAC ISO and 70% N_2O were investigated in a group of patients with a similar history of CAD, on similar cardiac medication, similarly unpremedicated, and about to undergo major vascular surgery [12]. Seven of the 13 patients (i.e., 54%) developed ECG and metabolic indications of myocardial ischemia. This was, again, associated with marked coronary vasodilation despite a concomitant decrease in MVO_2 by 45%.

When looking at those four clinical studies [11–13, 17] as a whole it is noteworthy that myocardial ischemia seemed to occur in all of them despite differences in premedication, central hemodynamics, HR, concomitant use of N_2O, depth of anesthesia, and ISO concentrations. This could be taken as suggestive evidence that it is, in fact, a specific drug effect (i.e., coronary vasodilation) that compromises myocardial oxygenation in patients with CAD, rather than associated hemodynamic alterations. On the other hand, in all but one study [17] there were concomitant acute decreases in mean systemic arterial pressure between 35% and 45%.

In marked contrast to the above studies, there was no ECG or metabolic evidence of myocardial ischemia when an inspired concentration of 0.75%–1.0% ISO was administered to control intraoperative increases in systemic arterial pressure and systemic vascular resistance in response to sternotomy in patients undergoing elective CABG [20]. However, there were major differences between the two studies in HR (80 vs 48/min), the pressure-rate ratio (0.85 vs 1.46), preoperative cardiac medication (ineffective vs effective), premedication (absent vs present), and baseline anesthesia (none vs sufentanil). Effective premedication with calcium entry blockers, nitrates, β-blockers, and narcotics, and baseline anesthesia with a high-dose narcotic may have prevented or minimized the incidence of myocardial ischemia by reducing basal sympathetic activity, maintaining a low HR, and decreasing vasomotor tone of epicardial and collateral vessels, thus counteracting the development of coronary vasospasm and ISO-induced maldistribution of MBF. On the other hand, lack of such effective medication should facilitate the occurrence of coronary vasospasm and maldistribution of MBF (i.e., coronary steal), and may well be responsible for the high incidence of myocardial ischemia in Reiz's study [11]. Such differences in regional vasomotor tone may not at all be reflected in global hemodynamics. This, in turn, may explain the differences in the incidence of myocardial ischemia despite no obvious differences in global hemodynamics. Differences in baseline sympathetic tone become obvious when comparing hemodynamic values before induction of anesthesia. Baseline HR, mean arterial pressures, and systemic vascular resistances were 75 vs 47/min, 113 vs 71 mmHg (Reiz's study [11]) and 37 vs 27 units respectively, in Reiz [11] vs. (O'Young's study [20]). In addition, the fact that 60% of patients in Reiz's study were treated with digitalis and/or diuretics would imply a greater incidence of congestive heart failure and poorer cardiac function in this than in O'Young's population. Degree and distribution of CAD may thus also have differed considerably.

In conclusion, the results of these two studies [11, 20] are not necessarily mutually exclusive. Differences in results may reflect primarily differences in preexisting cardiac function, effectiveness of preoperative cardiac medication, and in baseline anesthesia.

Finally, a brief look at an investigation that is being quoted repeatedly for providing evidence that ISO may exert beneficial effects in patients with CAD [18]. Coronary hemodynamics, however, were not studied. In 14 premedicated patients with stable angina, no evidence of cardiac failure, and on cardiac medications who were scheduled for elective CABG, ISO (0.5% end-tidal) plus 50% N_2O improved the tolerance to pacing-induced ischemia. During ISO, first signs of ischemia (as defined by ECG changes, and/or abnormally high cardiac filling pressures and v-waves in pulmonary capillary wedge pressure tracings) occurred at a higher pacing rate (mean 11%) than in the awake patient. Similarly, at a pacing rate at which angina pectoris had been induced in the awake patient there was less pronounced ST segment depression during ISO. A few comments are required to put these findings into proper perspective.

First, only 0.5% ISO was used. Results might have been different at higher concentrations. Second, the pacing rate at which signs of myocardial ischemia first appeared was not different from awake in three (21%) patients, different by 10% in seven (50%) patients, and different by more than 10% in only four (29%) patients. Third, during ISO at pacing rates that had produced angina in the awake patient there was in fact *improvement* of ischemia in ten (71%) patients. However, ischemia resolved entirely in only four (19%) patients, and some degree of ischemia remained in 10 (71%) patients. In all patients, however, there was a considerable decrease in systemic arterial pressure and rate-pressure product (and thus presumably in MVO_2) during ISO. Therefore, the question needs to be raised (which, however, cannot be answered) whether the tolerance to pacing-induced myocardial ischemia should not have been greater considering the concomitant substantial decrease in MVO_2. Thus, I do not think that these data conclusively exclude the possibility that inadequate coronary perfusion or flow redistribution during ISO contributed to the persistance of myocardial ischemia despite lower MVO_2.

Clinical Implications

Studies in animals and humans have clearly documented that ISO is a coronary vasodilator, and that the distal arterioles constitute the site of dilation. Although drugs that dilate large, proximal coronary arteries are often beneficial for patients with CAD, those that cause distal arteriolar dilation may, paradoxically, provoke angina pectoris [39]. There is compelling experimental as well as clinical evidence that ISO can cause redistribution of MBF (i.e., intercoronary and transmural steal) under certain circumstances, and that such maldistribution of MBF may be a contributory factor for the development of myocardial ischemia in patients with CAD receiving ISO. Thus, the clinically relevant question that needs to be answered on the basis of existing experimental and clinical data is: What are the factors that predispose to the development of maldistribution of MBF? If they are definable, they may either be avoided or counteracted by appropriate measures which, in turn, might minimize the development of myocardial ischemia on the basis of redistribution of MBF during ISO.

There is no experimental or clinical evidence to suggest that ISO-induced coronary vasodilation will, in any way, adversely affect intramyocardial blood flow distribution or myocardial metabolism in the presence of a healthy coronary circulation event at very low coronary perfusion pressures. In addition, coronary vascular reserve may remain unaffected until considerably higher equianesthetic concentrations of ISO than HAL, and the fatal/anesthetic ratio, a measure of relative safety of an anesthetic agent, for ISO is almost twice that of HAL [21, 40]. Thus, adverse effects of ISO on coronary hemodynamics are only to be expected in the presence of an abnormal coronary circulation.

For intercoronary steal to develop in humans, a specific "steal-prone" coronary anatomy is required. This includes total occlusion of a major coronary artery branch with collateral flow into the vascular bed distal to the occlusion [41–43], and, in addition, a hemodynamically significant proximal stenosis of the coronary artery which supplies the collaterals (i.e., "jeopardized" collateral circulation) [29]. What are the chances for such steal-prone coronary anatomy to be present?

Of 16249 angiograms included in the Coronary Artery Surgery Study (CASS) registry, 15% to 19% met the criteria for steal-prone coronary anatomy (Buffington, personal communication). Administration of ISO in this setting can be expected to cause vasodilation of the vasculature and a pressure drop distal to the stenosis, sufficient to reduce flow across the high-resistance, pressure-dependent collaterals at the expense of increased flow to the normal area of myocardium, resulting in maldistribution of MBF (i.e., intercoronary steal). Considering the large number of patients with CAD who undergo anesthesia, quite a few patients will be at risk of developing myocardial ischemia on the basis of coronary steal. Although a history of a prior myocardial infarction may be a clue to the presence of steal-prone coronary anatomy [44], we have to realize that it can be identified or excluded with relative certainty by angiography only. It would, thus, seem prudent to assume presence of steal-prone coronary anatomy in any patient with CAD. Based on the anatomical findings it is to be expected that the majority of studies will continue to find no adverse effects of ISO in patients with CAD – simply, because approximately 80% of them will not have steal-prone coronary anatomy. The issue of whether or not ISO is capable of producing clinically relevant myocardial ischemia purely on the basis of coronary steal can ultimately only be settled if outcome data will differentiate between patients with or without steal-prone coronary anatomy.

Short of avoiding ISO altogether in patients with CAD, what can we do to reduce the likelihood for myocardial ischemia to develop during ISO? As with all anesthetic techniques, the ultimate goal in all patients with CAD is to maintain myocardial O_2 demand at a low level without compromising myocardial O_2 supply. Too light an anesthetic will result in sympathetic overactivity and an increase in MVO_2. On the other hand, too deep an anesthetic will decrease coronary perfusion pressure and myocardial O_2 supply. Since in the presence of a coronary stenosis flow becomes progressively pressure-dependent, any decrease in perfusion pressure by more than 20%–25% of awake must be expected to exert detrimental effects by decreasing O_2 supply out of proportion to any concomitant decrease in MVO_2. Subendocardial and subepicardial flows will vary directly with changes in mean coronary perfusion pressure below values of approximately 70 and 45 mmHg, respectively [45]. It has to be remembered that in the presence of a coronary stenosis diastolic coronary pressure may be lower than diastolic aortic pressure by as much as 45 mmHg [46, 47]. Conceivably, this pressure gradient across a stenosis may increase even further when a distal coronary vasodilator is administered. On the other hand, even greater than 20%–25% decreases in coronary perfusion pressure are likely to be tolerated or may even be beneficial provided this decrease results in normalization of a previously hyperdynamic circulation. In this case, MVO_2 will fall out of proportion to myocardial O_2 supply, and the myocardial O_2 supply/demand relationship will improve.

However, coronary perfusion pressure is only one of the determinants of myocardial O_2 supply. Particularly in patients with CAD, coronary vasomotor tone may be as important a factor as coronary perfusion pressure, especially in patients undergoing anesthesia. Inappropriate changes in proximal and distal coronary vasomotor tone may cause myocardial ischemia on the basis of coronary vasospasm or coronary steal. This may be of particular clinical relevance considering the isolated effect of ISO on arterioles.

Considering the crucial impact of large coronary artery vasomotor tone on myocardial O_2 supply, of distal arteriolar vasomotor tone on intramyocardial blood flow distribution, and that of HR on collateral flow [48, 49], MVO_2 [50], and diastolic filling time [51], on the one hand, and the coronary arteriolar vasodilating and positive chronotropic effects of ISO on the other, effective preoperative cardiac medication with calcium entry blockers, β-blockers and nitrates, adequate premedication, and a baseline anesthetic with narcotics may be of even greater importance during ISO than during other inhalational anesthetics. Effective baseline medication might help to reduce the incidence of tachycardia and coronary vasospasm, thus counteracting the potential development of coronary steal. The crucial importance of adequate baseline medication in reducing the incidence of myocardial ischemia during ISO unrelated to global hemodynamic disturbances seems to be supported by clinical evidence [20].

Because of the basic mechanism of ISO and the site of action it will never be possible to entirely eliminate the potential for the development of maldistribution of MBF. However, with optimal preoperative medical preparation and careful perioperative hemodynamic management it would appear that the added risk of potential development of myocardial ischemia on the basis of coronary steal can be reduced to such a degree that the ultimate outcome will not be essentially different from that seen with other anesthetic techniques and agents. Low HR and adequate systemic arterial pressure take on added importance during ISO anesthesia. For that matter, absolute values may be less important than the circumstances under which they come about. Clinical significance of a fall in perfusion pressure will depend on its initial value (normal vs abnormaly elevated), the speed of reduction (slow vs abrupt, thus acutely triggering compensatory mechanisms that lead to increases in sympathetic tone and catecholamine release), and it will depend on baseline conditions (presence vs absence of adrenergic receptor and Ca^{2+} entry blockade, with its resultant effects on sympathetic activity and large-vessel coronary vasomotor tone). Similarly, a pressure-rate ratio of >1 may be of greater significance than an absolute value for HR [52].

In addition to perfusion pressure and HR, CBF in patients with CAD is governed by a large variety of factors the most important ones being degree and kind of stenosis (fixed vs functional; single vs multivessel lesions; short vs long vessel segment; singular vs sequential; localized vs diffuse), status of collateral circulation (immature vs well developed), intramyocardial compressive forces, P_{zf}, MVO_2, and coronary vasomotor tone. Such a multitude of factors will create infinite flow conditions which will render any prediction on who will experience impaired myocardial perfusion under what exact global hemodynamic conditions practically impossible – independent of the anesthetic technique or agent employed.

The question has been raised: Is ISO dangerous for the patient with CAD [1–4]? The answer should be: Yes, it is *potentially* dangerous in *some* patients, under *some* conditions – an answer that can be applied to all anesthetic agents, and for that matter to all therapeutically efficacious drugs. A recent editorial comment may particularly apply to ISO: "It may not be sufficient to keep the determinants of MVO_2 as close to the unanesthetized angina-free value as possible while maintaining coronary perfusion pressure. Rather, such conditions may represent a necessary base fom which better clinical methods for detecting and effectively treating myocardial ischemia must be discovered and used for optimal patient care" [53].

References

1. Becker LC (1987) Is isoflurane dangerous for the patient with coronary artery disease (editorial)? Anesthesiology 66:259–261
2. Merin RG (1987) Is isoflurane dangerous for the patient with coronary artery disease? Another view. I (letter). Anesthesiology 67:284–286
3. Hamilton WK (1987) Is isoflurane dangerous for the patient with coronary artery disease? Another view. II (letter). Anesthesiology 67:286
4. Abramowitz J (1987) Is isoflurane dangerous for the patient with coronary artery disease? Another view. III (letter). Anesthesiology 67:286–287
5. Tarnow J, Eberlein HJ, Oser G, Patschke D, Schneider E, Schweichel E, Wilde J (1977) Hämodynamik, Myokardkontraktilität, Ventrikelvolumina und Sauerstoffversorgung des Herzens unter verschiedenen Inhalationsanästhetika. Anaesthesist 26:220–230
6. Gelman S, Fowler KC, Smith LR (1984) Regional blood flow during isoflurane and halothane anesthesia. Anesth Analg 63:557–565
7. Priebe H-J (1987) Differential effects of isoflurane on regional right and left ventricular performances, and on coronary, systemic, and pulmonary hemodynamics in the dog. Anesthesiology 66:262–272
8. Sill JC, Bove AA, Nugent M, Blaise GA, Dewey JD, Grabau C (1987) Effects of isoflurane on coronary arteries and coronary arterioles in the intact dog. Anesthesiology 66:273–279
9. Buffington CW, Romson JL, Levine A, Duttlinger NC, Huang AH (1987) Isoflurane induces coronary steal in a canine model of chronic coronary occlusion. Anesthesiology 66:280–292

10. Hickey RF, Sybert PE, Verrier ED, Cason BA (1988) Effects of halothane, enflurane, and isoflurane on coronary blood flow autoregulation and coronary vascular reserve in the canine heart. Anesthesiology 68:21–30
11. Reiz S, Bålfors E, Sørensen MB, Ariola S Jr, Friedman A, Truedsson H (1983) Isoflurane – a powerful coronary vasodilator in patients with coronary artery disease. Anesthesiology 59:91–97
12. Reiz S, Östman M (1985) Regional coronary hemodynamics during isoflurane – nitrous oxide anesthesia in patients with ischemic heart disease. Anesth Analg 64:570–576
13. Moffitt EA, Barker RA, Glenn JJ, Imrie DD, Delcampo C, Landymore RW, Kineley E, Murphy DA (1986) Myocardial metabolism and hemodynamic responses with isoflurane anesthesia for coronary arterial surgery. Anesth Analg 65:53–61
14. Merin RG, Basch S (1981) Are the myocardial functional and metabolic effects of isoflurane really different from those of halothane and enflurane? Anesthesiology 55:398–408
15. Manohar M, Parks C (1984) Regional distribution of brain and myocardial perfusion in swine while awake and during 1.0 and 1.5 MAC isoflurane anesthesia produced without or with 50% nitrous oxide. Cardiovasc Res 18:344–353
16. Cason BA, Verrier ED, London MJ, Mangano DT, Hickey RF (1987) Effects of isoflurane and halothane on coronary vascular resistance and collateral myocardial blood flow: their capacity to induce coronary steal. Anesthesiology 67:665–675
17. Larsen R, Hilfiker O, Philbin DM, Sonntag H (1986) Isofluran: Koronardurchblutung und Myokardstoffwechsel bei Patienten mit koronarer Herzkrankheit. Anaesthesist 35:284–290
18. Tarnow J, Markschies-Hornung A, Schulte-Sasse U (1986) Isoflurane improves the tolerance to pacing-induced myocardial ischemia. Anesthesiology 64:147–156
19. Hess W, Arnold B, Schulte-Sasse U, Tarnow J (1983) Comparison of isoflurane and halothane when used to control intraoperative hypertension in patients undergoing coronary artery bypass surgery. Anesth Analg 62:15–20
20. O'Young J, Mastrocostopoulos G, Hilgenberg A, Palacios I, Kyritsis A, Lappas DG (1987) Myocardial circulatory and metabolic effects of isoflurane and sufentanil during coronary artery surgery. Anesthesiology 66:653–658
21. Roberts SL, Gilbert M, Tinker JH (1987) Isoflurane has a greater margin of safety than halothane in swine with and without major surgery or critical coronary stenosis. Anesth Analg 66:485–491
22. Tatekawa S, Traber KB, Hantler CB, Tait AR, Gallagher KP, Knight PR (1987) Effects of isoflurane on myocardial blood flow, function, and oxygen consumption in the presence of critical coronary stenosis in dogs. Anesth Analg 66:1073–1082
23. Priebe H-J, Foëx P (1987) Isoflurane causes regional myocardial dysfunction in dogs with critical coronary artery stenoses. Anesthesiology 66:293–300
24. Priebe H-J (1988) Isoflurane causes more severe regional myocardial dysfunction than halothane in dogs with a critical coronary artery stenosis. Anesthesiology 69:72–83
25. Stevens WC, Cromwell TH, Halsey MJ, Eger EI II, Shakespeare TF, Bahlmann SH (1971) The cardiovascular effects of a new inhalation anesthetic, Forane, in human volunteers at constant arterial carbon dioxide tension. Anesthesiology 35:8–16
26. Cromwell TH, Stevens WC, Eger EI II, Shakespeare TF, Halsey MJ, Bahlman SH, Fourcade HE (1971) The cardiovascular effects of compound 469 (Forane) during spontaneous ventilation and CO_2 challenge in man. Anesthesiology 35:17–25
27. Tarnow J, Brückner JB, Eberlein HJ, Hess W, Patschke D, Weymar A (1975) Kreislaufwirkungen des neuen Inhalationsanaesthetikums Isofluran (Forane) beim Menschen. Anaesthesist 24:425–431
28. Tarnow J, Brückner JB, Eberlein HJ, Hess W, Patschke D (1976) Haemodynamics and myocardial oxygen consumption during isoflurane (Forane) anaesthesia in geriatric patients. Br J Anaesth 48:669–675
29. Gross GJ, Warltier DC (1981) Coronary steal in four models of single or multiple vessel obstruction in dogs. Am J Cardiol 48:84–92

30. Vatner SF (1980) Correlation between acute reductions in myocardial blood flow and function in conscious dogs. Circ Res 47:201–207
31. Levin DC (1974) Pathways and functional significance of the coronary collateral circulation. Circulation 50:831–837
32. Flameng W, Schwarz F, Hehrlein F, Boel A (1978) Functional significance of coronary collaterals in man. Basic Res Cardiol 73:188–199
33. Gould KL (1978) Pressure-flow characteristics of coronary stenoses in unsedated dogs at rest and during coronary vasodilation. Circ Res 43:242–253
34. Logan SE (1975) On the fluid mechanics of human coronary artery stenosis. IEEE Trans Biomed Eng 22:327–334
35. Schwartz JS, Carlyle PF, Cohn JN (1979) Effect of dilation of the distal coronary bed on flow and resistance in severely stenotic coronary arteries in the dog. Am J Cardiol 43:219–224
36. Walinsky P, Santamore WP, Wiener L, Brest AN (1979) Dynamic changes in the hemodynamic severity of coronary artery stenosis in a canine model. Cardiovasc Res 13:113–118
37. Santamore WP, Walinsky P (1980) Altered coronary flow responses to vasoactive drugs in the presence of coronary arterial stenosis in the dog. Am J Cardiol 45:276–285
38. Bollen BA, Tinker JH, Hermsmeyer K (1987) Halothane relaxes previously constricted porcine artery segments more than isoflurane. Anesthesiology 66:748–752
39. Brown BG, Josephson MA, Petersen RB, Pierce CD, Wong M, Hecht HS, Bolson EL, Dodge HT (1981) Intravenous dipyridamole combined with isometric handgrip for near-maximal acute increase in coronary flow in patients with coronary artery disease. Am J Cardiol 48:1077–1085
40. Gilbert M, Roberts SL, Mori M, Blomberg R, Tinker JH (1988) Comparative coronary vascular reactivity and hemodynamics during halothane and isoflurane anesthesia in swine. Anesthesiology 68:243–253
41. Rowe GG (1970) Inequalities of myocardial perfusion in coronary artery disease (coronary steal). Circulation 42:193–194
42. Patterson RE, Kirk ES (1983) Coronary steal mechanisms in dogs with one-vessel occlusion and other arteries normal. Circulation 67:1009–1015
43. Fam WM, McGregor M (1964) Effect of coronary vasodilator drugs on retrograde flow in areas of chronic myocardial ischemia. Circ Res 15:355–365
44. Nestico PF, Hakki AH, Meissner MD, Bemis CE, Kimbiris D, Mintz GS, Segal BL, Iskandrian AS (1985) Effect of collateral vessels on prognosis in patients with one vessel coronary artery disease. JACC 6:1257–1263
45. Guyton RA, McClenathan JH, Newman GE, Michaelis LL (1977) Significance of subendocardial ST-segment elevation caused by coronary stenosis in the dog. Am J Cardiol 40:373–380
46. Hoffman JIE (1984) Maximal coronary flow and the concept of coronary vascular reserve. Circulation 70:153–159
47. Gallagher KP, Folts JD, Shebuski RJ, Rankin JHG, Rowe GG (1980) Subepicardial vasodilator reserve in the presence of critical coronary stenosis in dogs. Am J Cardiol 46:67–73
48. Domenech RJ, Goich J (1976) Effect of heart rate on regional coronary blood flow. Cardiovasc Res 10:224–231
49. Heusch G, Yoshimoto N (1983) Effects of heart rate and perfusion pressure on segmental coronary resistances and collateral perfusion. Pflügers Arch 397:284–289
50. Weber KT; Janicki JS, Fishman AP (1980) Aerobic limit to the heart perfused at constant pressure. Am J Physiol 238:H118–H125
51. Hoffmann JIE (1978) Determinants and prediction of transmural myocardial perfusion. Circulation 58:381–391
52. Buffington CW (1985) Hemodynamic determinants of ischemic myocardial dysfunction in the presence of coronary stensosis in dogs. Anesthesiology 63:651–662
53. Merin RG, Lowenstein E, Gelman S (1986) Is anesthesia beneficial for the ischemic heart? III (editorial). Anesthesiology 64:137–140

Hepatic Oxygen Supply During Surgery and Anesthesia

S. Gelman

Postoperative liver dysfunction is observed relatively often after major surgical procedures [1]. Hepatic circulatory disturbances with a subsequent decrease in hepatic oxygen supply play an important role in the multifactorial etiology in perioperative liver injury.

Physiology of Hepatic Circulation

Hepatic blood flow equals approximately 100 $ml \cdot min^{-1} \cdot 100\ g^{-1}$ which represents about 25% of cardiac output. The liver is supplied by two large vessels: the hepatic artery brings arterial blood to the liver and represents approximately 25% of total hepatic blood flow and approximately 45% to 50% of hepatic oxygen supply, while the portal vein provides 75% of the total hepatic blood supply and only 50% to 55% of the hepatic oxygen supply. Portal venous blood is partially deoxygenated in the preportal organs and tissues (stomach, intestines, spleen, and pancreas). On the other hand, portal venous blood is rich with nutrients and other substances absorbed in the gastrointestinal tract. Portal venous blood flow is controlled primarily by the arterioles in the preportal splanchnic organs. This flow, combined with resistance to portal flow within the liver, determines portal pressure (7 to 10 mmHg). Presinusoidal (precapillary) sphincters determine the relatively uniform distribution of flow through the liver and play a certain, although rather limited role in the regulation of portal blood flow. There are data suggesting that the major site of venous resistance within the liver is postsinusoidal. The sinusoidal pressure is determined by the tone of presinusoidal and postsinusoidal sphincters and blood flow. Smooth muscles in the wall of the venules regulate venous compliance and blood volume. Both resistance and compliance are predominantly controlled by the sympathetic innervation mediated through alpha-adrenoceptors. Changes in hepatic venous compliance play an essential part in the overall regulation of cardiac output. The liver vasculature plays a vital role as a blood reservoir. An increase or a decrease in resistance in the hepatic veins is accompanied by rather dramatic changes in blood volume within the liver. This reservoir function is mainly mediated through the sympathetic nervous system. The myogenic and metabolic intrinsic regulation of hepatic venous compliance play a very little role, if any, in controlling the hepatic venous resistance. During hemorrhage the liver may squeeze out up to 500 ml of blood into the systemic circulation. Anesthetics that suppress the sympathetic nervous system function may interfere with such compensatory responses and lead to decompensation if blood is not replaced immediately. Patients with liver disease have a decreased sensitivity to catecholamines, probably due to an increase in blood glucagon concentration and, therefore, these patients may have a decreased ability to compensate for hemorrhage and hypovolemia by a mechanism related to the sympathetic nervous system, e.g., lack of ability to develop vasoconstriction to divert blood to the heart and brain from the muscles and splanchnic circulation, as well as the lack of ability to constrict the capacitance vasculature and to expel blood from the splanchnic reservoir into the systemic circulation.

The major site of resistance in the hepatic arterial vasculature is the arterioles. Regulation of the hepatic arteriolar tone is mainly achieved by local and intrinsic mechanisms that adjust hepatic arterial flow to compensate for changes in portal blood flow. This phenomenon is referred to as the arterial buffer response. The decrease in portal blood flow is usually associated with an increase in hepatic arterial blood flow [2–4]. This increase in hepatic arterial blood flow may be considered an attempt to maintain hepatic oxygen supply (which is essential for hepatocyte function) and/or total hepatic blood flow (which, in turn, is essential for clearance of exogenous and endogenous compounds with a high hepatic extraction. The mechanisms by which the described hepatic arterial blood flow autoregulation is achieved involve neural, myogenic, and metabolic controls, as well as content of portal blood and washout effect [2, 3]. It has been demonstrated that a decrease in portal blood pH and/or oxygen content is accompanied by an increase in hepatic arterial blood flow, even when portal blood flow is intentionally maintained unaltered [2]. The washout theory suggests that a substance, apparently adenosine, is generated within the liver tissue; when portal blood flow decreases, this vasodilating substance is not washed out, but accumulates and subsequently leads to hepatic arterial vasodilation. Increased portal blood flow leads to an effective washout of this substance and a reduction in the vasodilating effect on the hepatic arterial vasculature [3, 4].

Different anesthetics affect systemic and regional circulation, including the splanchnic vasculature, in various directions and to different degrees. The effects are related to both the extrinsic and intrinsic mechanisms of hepatic flow regulation. These mechanisms would include alterations in systemic hemodynamics, changes in sympathetic tone, the release of many hormones and other endogenous substances, changes in intestinal motility and intestinal wall tension, intraabdominal pressure, as well as alterations in fluid absorption, metabolism, oxygen requirements and tissue pressure. Anesthetics also affect the portal venous blood flow-hepatic arterial blood flow relationship which seems to be important for hepatic oxygen supply.

The combination of anesthesia with superimposed surgery affects the hepatic circulation, including the interaction of hepatic arterial and portal venous blood flows, and therefore is accompanied by different degrees of reduction in hepatic blood and oxygen supply. Anesthetics may be responsible for perioperative liver damage. However, it appears that surgical intervention per se plays a predominate role in splanchnic circulatory disturbances, while anesthesia may play a modifying protective role [5].

Effects of Surgical Stress on Hepatic Circulation

Surgical intervention induces certain disorders inhomeostasis, including alterations in hepatic circulation. The general response to stress has been studied rather well and certain responses to surgical stress such as an increase in circulating catecholamines, cortisol, growth hormone, antidiuretic hormone, aldosterone, and activation of the renin-angiotensin systems are very well known. However, specific effects of stress on hepatic circulation have been studied to a much lesser degree. Available data strongly suggest that laparotomy per se reduces blood flow through the gut and the liver [5, 6].

A study devoted specifically to the separate roles played by anesthesia and surgical intervention in liver circulation showed that anesthesia alone can be accompanied by different degrees of liver blood flow reduction. When a surgical procedure is superimposed with anesthesia, liver blood flow is further decreased. The degree of the decrease depends on the type of surgical intervention. Minor peripheral procedures are accompanied by a small degree of blood flow reduction, while major procedures such as laparotomy are associated with a substantial decrease in liver blood flow [5]. Moreover, when standard surgical stress (laparotomy) was applied under different types of anesthesia, the degree of reduction in splanchnic blood flow varied greatly. The data demonstrate that (a) surgical intervention, rather than anesthesia, is the main determinant of the alterations in the splanchnic circulation, and that (b) anesthesia can play a modifying role for circulatory disturbances developing during surgical stress.

It has been demonstrated that laparotomy is accompanied by a decrease in portal blood flow with associated increase in hepatic arterial blood flow [7]. What is the mechanism of splanchnic circulatory disturbances developing during surgical stress? Apparently, unavoidable tractions and manipulations on the splanchnic organ play a certain role in these disturbances [8]. However, a general biological response to surgical stress seems to be important. It has been shown that laparotomy per se causes marked mesenteric vasoconstriction and a reduction in gstrointestinal blood flow which could be abolished by acute hypophysectomy [9]. The results of this study indicate that both the renin-angiotensin system and antidiuretic hormone play important roles in the control of the mesenteric vascular resistance during laparotomy. Catecholamine release, which always accompanies surgery, also plays a notable role in decreasing splanchnic blood volume and flow [10, 11]. Liver function is apparently compromised when splanchnic blood flow is reduced; it has been shown that major surgery was associated with a significant increase in serum concentration of liver enzymes. The degree of increase was similar, regardless of the anesthesia provided. This increase was not observed when the same kind of anesthesia was administered during minor surgery [12, 13]. It is important to realize that splanchnic circulatory disturbances can affect systemic hemodynamics and reduce the clearance of drugs and hormones with high hepatic extraction ratios [14].

The effect of surgical stress on hepatic function seems to be particularly harmful in patients with advanced liver disease. Relatively mild surgical stress (only laparotomy and liver biopsy) was accompanied by a 10% immediate postoperative mortality, with another 10% of life-threatening complications [15]. Recent developments in modern anesthesia and life-supporting techniques have not improved the outcome. In one study, exploratory laparotomy in patients with advanced liver disease was associated with a 31% mortality within 1 month of operation; all patients with viral or alcoholic hepatitis died [16]. Another similar study reported a 67% 30-day mortality rate in patients with advanced cirrhosis; 83% of the patients with ascites and 91% of the patients with an elevated prothrombin time greater than 2.5 s died [17]. Obviously, there are many reasons for such a high mortality rate. The role of hepatic circulatory disorders with concomitant hepatic ischemia might be quite prominent.

Effects of General Anesthetics on Hepatic Circulation and Oxygen Regimen

Anesthetics can alter the splanchnic circulation by different mechanisms acting on the various factors controlling splanchnic blood flow. Systemic hemodynamics (cardiac output, blood volume, vascular resistance, blood pressure), and neural and humoral mechanisms (including the release of "stress" hormones and mediators such as ACTH, cortisol, catecholamines, and antidiuretic hormones), direct influence of anesthetics on the splanchnic vasculature, and changes in oxygen and blood requirements appear to be the main factors directly and indirectly affecting the splanchnic and hepatic circulation during anesthesia. The mechanisms involved in the development of splanchnic circulatory disturbances depend on the baseline state and essential characteristics of an anesthetic per se, as well as the dose and method of administration. The majority of anesthetics decrease total splanchnic blood flow [18]. Many anesthetics also decrease total splanchnic and hepatic oxygen consumption, however, usually to a lesser extent than total splanchnic blood flow.

A decrease in hepatic blood flow is usually accompanied by an increased oxygen extraction and maintained or slightly decreased oxygen uptake [19, 20]; therefore, the safety margin, determined by the difference between oxygen supply and demand, or, in other words, the difference between values of oxygen supply to the liver and values of "critical" oxygen supply (oxygen supply at which oxygen uptake starts to decrease) during anesthesia seems to be rather important. Oxygen supply to the liver depends to a large extent on hepatic arterial blood flow. Total hepatic blood flow equals 100–130 $mL \cdot min^{-1} \cdot 100\ g^{-1}$. Twenty to forty percent is delivered via the hepatic artery [21, 22]. Hepatic oxygen uptake equals 2–7 $mL\ O_2 \cdot min^{-1} \cdot 100\ g^{-1}$ of the liver [19, 20, 22]. Calculations show that if hepatic arterial blood flow is 20% of total hepatic blood flow, the hepatic arterial blood would contribute

27% of the hepatic oxygen uptake; however, if the arterial flow proportion is taken as 30%, arterial blood would contribute 65% of the consumed oxygen [22]. It is clear that the ratio of hepatic arterial blood flow to portal blood flow might play a much more important role in hepatic oxygen supply than changes in total hepatic blood flow per se.

Inhalational Anesthetics

In the isolated liver, halothane, chloroform, and ether perfused through the hepatic artery and portal vein at constant rates did not change perfusion pressure significantly, suggesting that vascular resistances within the liver are not affected by these inhalational agents [23]. These data probably mean that changes in liver circulation during anesthesia are mainly related to the effect of anesthetics on the circulation in other splanchnic organs, and to other indirect influences such as changes in systemic cardiovascular function, and neural and humoral control.

Halothane

Halothane is apparently the best studied inhalational anesthetic with respect to influence on the hepatic circulation. The majority of studies, regardless of the species used and methodology employed, has shown that portal blood flow (or blood flow through the preportal organs and tissues – stomach, intestines, pancreas, and spleen – is decresed during halothane anesthesia [24]. The decrease more or less parallels the decrease in blood pressure and particularly cardiac output [25–27]. During halothane anesthesia, cardiac output is the main determinant of portal blood flow [27]. In sheep, portal venous oxygen tension decreased from 46 mmHg in the awake state to 39 mmHg with 1.5% halothane. Hepatic venous oxygen tension was also reduced by 25% [28].

The changes in hepatic arterial blood flow during halothane anesthesia vary tremendously in different studies. A few angiographic studies in humans, mainly children, demonstrated a severe vasoconstriction in the hepatic arterial vasculature [29–31]. However, there have been no reports to quantitate these changes. The incidence of such response of the hepatic arterial vasculature to halothane is also unknown. Some authors observed an increased fraction of cardiac output to the liver via the hepatic artery [32] and an actual increase in hepatic arterial blood flow that was rather substantial according to the mean values. However, owing to high standard deviations, the differences in values of flow between anesthetic and control states did not reach statistically significant levels [33, 34]. Careful analysis of the available data shows that in all studies where laparotomy was performed and/or a barbiturate was used as a baseline anesthetic, hepatic arterial blood flow decreased. On the other hand, in the majority of studies where the methodology employed did not require a laparotomy, hepatic arterial blood flow increased or did not change, provided halothane anesthesia did not reduce blood pressure and/or cardiac output by more than 30% [27, 34, 35–38]. Even in experiments employing laparotomy and electromagnetic flowmeters, low concentrations of halothane increased hepatic arterial blood flow by 49%, while concentrations of halothane, which reduced mean arterial pressure to 80 mmHg, decreased hepatic arterial flow by 37%; portal blood flow decreased by 49% and 45%, respectively [39]. It appears that the discrepancy between studies employing and not employing laparotomy depends on this particular characteristic of the experiment.

Halothane, as well as other inhalational anesthetics, decreases total body oxygen uptake to a larger extent than splanchnic oxygen uptake, which usually follows a decrease in splanchnic blood flow [40, 41]. Oxygen uptake in the preportal area was not changed under halothane anesthesia in the majority of studies, while the hepatic oxygen uptake also was not changed or was slightly decreased [42]. In one study, hepatic oxygen consumption decreased under halothane anesthesia by only 10% from control values, whereas hepatic blood flow decreased by 30% [28]. It appears that the development of circulatory hypoxia in the liver during halothane anesthesia is mainly related to a substantial decrease in portal blood flow and oxygen content in the portal blood, which results from an increase in oxygen extraction in the preportal tissues [43]. This reduction in oxygen delivery to the liver is compensated predominantly by an increase in oxygen extraction, mainly from hepatic arterial blood flow because oxygen content in portal blood flow is usually decreased during halothane anesthesia. The second mechanism of compensation is an increase in, or at least a preservation of, hepatic arterial blood flow.

All these data were obtained in experiments with different, normal, healthy animals. However, it is important to realize that the ability of hepatic arterial blood flow to increase is extremely limited in animals with induced liver damage [44, 45].

Enflurane

In the intact animal, enflurane reduces portal blood flow [34, 46, 47]. This reduction is apparently related to changes in the systemic circulation (mainly to a decrease in cardiac output), and possibly to a decrease in oxygen requirement in the preportal area. The fraction of cardiac output to the hepatic arterial flow is usually increased during enflurane anesthesia [32, 34]. It is worth noting that in greyhounds (where the methodology employed is laparotomy and electromagnetic flowmeters), enflurane, in a dose which reduced blood pressure by 55% and cardiac output by 33%, did not change hepatic arterial blood flow. Only when blood pressure decreased to 25% and cardiac output to 50% of control, hepatic arterial blood flow decreased [47]. Enflurane anesthesia decreased total body oxygen uptake to a lesser extent than cardiac output, leading to an increase in arteriovenous oxygen difference [46). Oxygen uptake in the preportal tissues was unchanged and hepatic oxygen uptake was not significantly altered, although there were decreases in hepatic oxygen uptake in some of the individual experiments. Hepatic and preportal tissue oxygen consumption was maintained by increased oxygen extraction [46]. Analysis of the available data suggests, and two comparative studies confirm, that enflurane preserves splanchnic blood flow and liver oxygen supply better than halothane when used in equipotent doses [47, 48].

Isoflurane

In intact animals, isoflurane, as other inhalational agents, decreases blood flow through the preportal areas [27, 36, 49]. This decrease in blood flow through the preportal area is related probably to both a reduction in cardiac output [27] and a reduction in oxygen requirement [50]. Hepatic arterial blood flow was substantially increased at two levels of isoflurane anesthesia used [27, 49]. This increase can reflect the preserved autoregulatory ability of the hepatic arterial vasculature to increase in response to reduction in portal blood flow, including the hepatic arterial buffer response. On the other hand, this increase in hepatic arterial blood flow may result from a profound vasodilating effect of isoflurane on the hepatic arterial vasculature. Seyde and Longnecker [51] suggested an interesting coefficient characterizing hepatic arterial blood flow autoregulation ability. The ratio of change in hepatic arterial resistance to change in portal flow multiplied by 10^2 was equal to $+3.2$ in the awake state, -2.7 during halothane, $+3.3$ during enflurane, and $+2.9$ during isoflurane anesthesia in rats [51[9]. Hypovolemia was used to alter portal flow, and both portal flow and hepatic arterial resistance were determined before and after hemorrhage.

Nitrous Oxide

Inhalation of nitrous oxide per se is usually not accompanied by substantial changes in blood pressure and cardiac output. Hepatic circulation was not disturbed significantly when nitrous oxide was used in trained animals without any baseline anesthesia or surgical preparation [49]. However, a significant decrease in both portal and hepatic artery blood flows by 15% and 24%, respectively, was observed when nitrous oxid was used in conditions of barbiturate anesthesia and laparotomy [52]. In rats, nitrous oxide decreased cardiac output, intestinal blood flow, splenic blood flow, and total hepatic blood flow [53].

Thus, comparing inhalational agents, it appears that all dilate the intestinal vasculature (direct and centrally mediated effects). However, in the intact animals, portal blood flow is reduced. This reduction is apparently associated with a decrease in cardiac output and partially with a reduction in intestinal oxygen requirement. It also appears that isoflurane and enflurane facilitate oxygen delivery to the liver much better than halothane, mainly by a more effective preservation of hepatic arterial blood flow.

Intravenous Anesthetics

The effects of intravenous anesthetics on the hepatic circulation are difficult to compare because the end results depend on the anesthetic per se and its influence on the systemic and regional circulation, as well as on the dose of the drug.

Barbiturates

Barbiturates did not dramatically affect the splanchnic circulation in some studies (except a slight decrease in flow through the preportal area) [54–57]. However, other investigators observed a substantial decrease in splanchnic blood flow by almost 50% [58, 59]. Thiopental, in a dose which was not accompanied by statistically significant changes in cardiac output and blood pressure, led to a significant decrease in hepatic arterial, portal venous, and total hepatic blood flows [60]. A decrease in portal blood flow is often accompanied by an increase in hepatic arterial blood flow during pentobarbital anesthesia [61–63]. It has also been demonstrated that barbiturates induce short-lasting but substantial vasodilation in the preportal area, reflected in a temporary increase in mesenteric arterial blood flow [64, 65]. Similarly, a temporary increase in portal blood flow was observed during anesthesia with one of the benzodiazepines, midazolam [66].

Ketamine

There are some contradicting reports regarding the changes in the splanchnic circulation during ketamine administration in rats. Some studies did not reveal any significant changes in systemic or hepatic circulation under different doses of ketamine [67]. Compared with pentobarbital, rats anesthetized with ketamine had lower cardiac outputs without significantly different values of blood flow through the gut, spleen, and hepatic artery [68]. Other investigators observed a 28% reduction in cardiac output with an apparently corresponding decrease in splanchnic blood flow [32]. A 33% increase in cardiac output under ketamine anesthesia with an associated similar increase in hepatic arterial blood flow and blood flow through the small intestines with unchanged blood flow through the stomach, large intestine, and spleen has also been observed [69]. Many different circumstances are obviously responsible for these discrepancies. Surgical preparation might be one of them. A decrease in cardiac output and blood pressure with unchanged hepatic arterial and portal blood flows was observed during ketamine administration in dogs under barbiturate anesthesia and laparotomy, while an increase in cardiac output and blood pressure, with an accompanied increase in hepatic arterial blood flow without changes in portal blood flow, was observed in dogs with implanted electromagnetic flowmeters [70]. This study clearly shows that the effect of an anesthetic on the splanchnic circulation can be changed by surgical preparation and baseline anesthesia.

Opioids

It has been shown that morphine in a dose of 0.2 $mg \cdot kg^{-1}$ increases splanchnic blood flow by 19% without significant changes in wedged hepatic venous pressure. The study was performed in humans; total splanchnic blood flow was measured using indocyanine green infusion technique [71]. Somewhat similar results were observed earlier in monkeys: morphine in a dose of 2 $mg \cdot kg^{-1}$

led to a slight decrease in blood pressure with maintained cardiac output and a 23% increase in portal and hepatic arterial blood flows [72]. In dogs with implanted electromagnetic flowmeters, morphine in doses of 1 $mg \cdot kg^{-1}$ did not cause any significant changes in blood pressure or cardiac output, but led to a significant increase in blood flow through the mesenteric artery by 55% (a 30% decrease in the mesenteric artery resistance). Doses of 3 $mg \cdot kg^{-1}$ were associated with a decrease in mesenteric arterial blood flow by 40% (a 12% increase in resistance) [73].

The mechanisms by which morphine exerts its effect on the splanchnic circulation are rather complex. Smaller doses may produce a central sympathetic withdrawal action with an associated release of splanchnic vasoconstriction, and/or morphine-induced histamine release with subsequent preportal vasodilation, while larger doses of morphine may increase catecholamine concentrations by increasing their release from the adrenal medulla and/or from sympathetic nerve endings [74].

Fentanyl, another widely used opioid, has not attracted much attention. In a study involving pigs, a rather large dose of fentanyl (20 and 50 $\mu g \cdot kg^{-1}$ followed by 0.17 and 0.42 $\mu g \cdot kg^{-1} \cdot min^{-1}$, respectively) was associated with no significant change in hepatic arterial blood flow or portal blood flow [24]. However, the experiments also demonstrated that hepatic oxygen uptake during fentanyl administration increased significantly. This was not observed during inhalation anesthesia with halothane or isoflurane. These changes in hepatic oxygen supply and uptake resulted in a well-maintained, but unimproved, hepatic oxygen supply/uptake relation.

Effects of Surgical Stress and Anesthesia on the Hepatic Oxygen Supply-Demand Relationship

All anesthetics, particularly inhalational anesthetics, decrease total hepatic blood flow in a relatively dose-related fashion, to different degrees and even in different ways. On the other hand, when surgical intervention is superimposed with anesthesia, hepatic blood flow is further decreased [5]. The degree of this reduction depends on the specific type of surgical intervention. Minor peripheral procedures are accompanied by a relatively small reduction in hepatic blood flow, while major procedures, especially upper laparotomy, are associated with a much larger decrease in hepatic blood flow [5]. These data also demonstrate that anesthesia may play a modifying role in the complex of surgery and anesthesia: similar surgical interventions are associated with different degrees of hepatic circulatory disturbances when different types of anesthesia are administered. Therefore, the modifying role of anesthesia in the development of hepatic circulatory disorders, as well as hepatic dysfunction during surgery, can be clinically more important than the effect of one or another anesthetic per se. Probably a question of paramount importance in this regard is, what kind of anesthesia administered for similar surgical procedures would be accompanied by minimal hepatic circulatory disturbances and hepatic dysfunction?

During surgical stress, even a 30% reduction in mean arterial pressure induced by isoflurane is not associated with a deterioration in hepatic oxygen supply, while a similar degree of arterial hypotension achieved by halothane reduces the hepatic oxygen supply and supply-uptake ratio during severe surgical stress (thoracotomy, laparotomy, and extensive surgical preparation) in pigs [24]. It is interesting to note that anesthesia using fentanyl, also in pigs, does maintain hepatic oxygen supply at baseline levels or even higher, but is accompanied by hepatic oxygen requirements somewhat higher than observed during isoflurane or halothane anesthesia and, therefore, the hepatic oxygen supply-uptake relationship during anesthesia with fentanyl is maintained rather than increased. The reasons for the increase in hepatic oxygen uptake during fentanyl administration are not clear. It seems conceivable that the stress response to surgical intervention is accompanied by an increased metabolism within the liver, yielding a subsequent increase in hepatic oxygen demand. This increase in demand, followed by an increase in supply, was not blocked by fentanyl, but was substantially modified by isoflurane as well as halothane. One way or the other, regarding the hepatic oxygen supply-demand relationship during surgery, halothane is certainly less desirable than isoflurane or fentanyl anesthesia [24].

Thus, the concept of the oxygen supply-demand relationship seems to be rather important, not only for the heart and brain, but also for the liver. It appears that surgical stress and anesthetics are generally decreasing hepatic oxygen supply. Whether anesthetics are able to sufficiently decrease hepatic oxygen demand is questionable at present.

References

1. Cahalan MK, Mangano DT (1982) Liver function and dysfunction with anesthesia and surgery. In: Zakim D, Boyer TD (eds) Hepatology, a textbook of liver disease. Saunders, Philadelphia, pp 1250–1261
2. Gelman S, Ernst E (1977) Role of pH, PCO_2, O_2 and content of portal blood in hepatic circulatory autoregulation. Am J Physiol 233:E255–E262
3. Lautt WW (1983) Relationship between hepatic blood flow and overall metabolism: the hepatic arterial buffer response. Fed Proc Fed Am Soc Exp Biol 42:1662–1666
4. Lautt WW (1985) Mechanism and role of intrinsic regulation of hepatic arterial blood flow: hepatic arterial buffer response. Am J Physiol 249:G549
5. Gelman S (1976) Disturbances in hepatic blood flow during anesthesia and surgery. Arch Surg 111:881–883
6. Gelman S (1986) Effects of anesthetics on splanchic circulation. In: Altura BM, Halevy S (eds) Cardiovascular action of anesthetics and drugs used in anesthesia. Karger, Basel, pp 126–161
7. Bohrer SL, Rogers EL, Koehler RC, Traystman RJ (1981) Effect of hypovolemic hypotension and laparotomy on splanchnic and hepatic arterial blood flow in dogs. Curr Surg 38:325–328
8. Seltzer JL, Ritter DE, Starsnic MA, Marr AT (1985) The hemodynamic response to traction on the abdominal mesentery. Anesthesiology 63:96–99
9. McNeill JR, Pang CC (1982) Effect of pentobarbital anesthesia and surgery on the control of arterial pressure and mesenteric resistance in cats: role of vasopressin and angiotensin. Can J Physiol Pharmacol 60:363–368

10. Donald DE (1983) Splanchnic circulation. In: Sheperd JT, Abbound FM, Geiger ST (eds) Handbook of physiology, vol 3. American Physiological Society, Bethesda, pp 219–240
11. Greenway CV (1983) Role of splanchnic venous system in overall cardiovascular homeostasis. Fed Proc Fed Am Soc Exp Biol 42:1678–1684
12. Clarke RSJ, Doggart JR, Lavery T (1976) Changes in liver function after different types of surgery. Br J Anaesth 18:119–128
13. Viegas O, Stoelting RK (1979) LDH5 changes after cholecystectomy or hysterectomy in patients receiving halothane, enflurane, or fentanyl. Anesthesiology 51:556–558
14. Wilkinson GR, Schenker S (1975) Drug disposition and liver disease. Drug Metab Rev 4:139–175
15. Harville DD, Summerskill HJ (1963) Surgery in acute hepatitis. Causes and effects. JAMA 184:257–261
16. Powell-Jackson P, Greenway B, William R (1982) Adverse effects of exploratory laparotomy in patients with unsuspected liver disease. Br J Surg 69:449–451
17. Aranha GV (1986) Intra-abdominal surgery in patients with advanced cirrhosis. Arch Surg 121:275–277
18. Gelman S (1987) General anesthesia and hepatic circulation. Can J Physiol Pharmacol 65:1762–1779
19. Lutz J, Henrich H, Bauereisen E (1975) Oxygen supply and uptake in the liver and the intestine. Pfluegers Arch 360:7–15
20. Gelman S, Dillard E (1985) Hepatic oxygen supply-demand relationship during anesthesia in the dog. Anesthesiology 63:A504
21. Richardson PDI, Withrington PG (1981) Liver blood flow. Gastroenterology 81:159–173, 356–375
22. Greenway CV, Stark RD (1971) Hepatic vascular bed. Physiol Rev 51:23–65
23. Bombeck CT, Aoki T, Smuckler EA, Nyhus LM (1969) Effects of halothane, ether, and chloroform on the isolated, perfused, bovine liver. Am J Surg 117:91–106
24. Gelman S, Dillard E, Bradley EL Jr (1987) Hepatic circulation during surgical stress and anesthesia with halothane, isoflurane, or fentanyl. Anesth Analg 66:936–943
25. Ahlegren I, Aronsen F, Bjorkman I, Wetterlin S (1978) Hemodynamics during superficial thiopental anesthesia in the dog. Acta Anaesthesiol Scand 22:76–82
26. Juhl B, Einer-Jensen N (1974) Hepatic blood flow and cardiac output during halothane anesthesia: an animal study. Acta Anaesthesiol Scand 18:114–122
27. Gelman S, Fowler KC, Smith LR (1984) Liver circulation and function during isoflurane and halothane anesthesia. Anesthesiology 61:726–730
28. Runciman WB, Mather LE, Ilsley AH, Carapetis RJ, Upton RN (1984) A sheep preparation for studying interactions between blood flow and during drug disposition. III. Effects of general and spinal anaesthesia on regional blood flow and oxygen tensions. Br J Anaesth 56:1247–1258
29. Berger PE, Culham JA, Fitz CR, Harwood-Nash DC (1976) Slowing of hepatic blood flow by halothane: angiographic manifestations. Radiology 118:303–306
30. Benumof ND, Bookstein JJ, Saidman LJ, Harris R (1976) Diminished hepatic arterial flow during halothane administration. Anesthesiology 45:545–551
31. Mortensson W, Nilsson J (1977) Effect of halothane on arterial hepatic flow as reflected at coeliac angiography. Pediatr Radiol 17:183–185
32. Miller ED, Kistner JR, Epstein RM (1980) Whole body distribution of radioactively labelled microspheres in the rat during anesthesia with halothane, enflurane, or ketamine. Anesthesiology 52:296–302
33. Ross WT Jr, Daggy BP (1981) Hepatic blood flow in phenobarbital-pretreated rats during halothane anesthesia and hypoxia. Anesth Analg 60:306–309
34. Tranquilli WJ, Manohar M, Parks CM, Thurmon JC, Theodorakis MC, Benson CGJ (1982) Systemic and regional blood flow distribution in unanesthetized swine and swine anesthetized with halothane + nitrous oxide, halothane, or enflurane. Anesthesiology 56:369–379

35. Gelman S (1975) The effect of enteral oxygen administration on the hepatic circulation during halothane anaesthesia: experimental investigations. Br J Anaesth 47:1253–1259
36. Gelman S, Fowler KC, Smith LR (1984) Regional blood flow during isoflurane and halothane anesthesia. Anesth Analg 63:557–565
37. Lees MH, Hill H, Ochsner AJ, Thomas C (1971) Regional blood flows of the rhesus monkey during halothane anesthesia. Anesth Analg 50:270–281
38. Wyler F (1974) Effect of general anesthesia on distribution of cardiac output and organ blood flow in the rabbit: halothane and chloralose-urethane. J Surg Res 17:381–386
39. Matsumoto N, Hori T, Miyazzaki T et al. (1982) Effects of halothane anesthesia with various fractions of inspired oxygen and halothane concentrations on splanchnic circulation and serum enzymes leakage. Masui to Sosei 18:39–43
40. Theye RA, Michenfelder JD (1975) Individual organ contributions to the decrease in whole-body $\dot{V}O_2$ with isoflurane. Anesthesiology 42:35–40
41. Theye RA, Michenfelder JD (1975) Whole-body and organ $\dot{V}O_2$ changes with enflurane, isoflurane, and halothane. Br J Anaesth 47:813–817
42. Andreen M, Irestedt L, Zetterstrom B (1977) The different responses of the hepatic arterial bed to hypovolaemia and to halothane anaesthesia. Acta Anaesthesiol Scand 21:457–469
43. Andreen M (1982) Inhalation versus intravenous anaesthesia. Effects on the hepatic and splanchnic circulation. Acta Anaesthesiol Scand [Suppl] 75:25–31
44. Takenchi J, Jubo T, Yoshida H, Kitagawa T, Tuneo T (1972) Hemodynamics in the dog liver after carbon tetrachloride injury. J Appl Physiol 32:320–324
45. Gelman S, Ernst E (1982) Hepatic circulation during sodium nitroprusside infusion in the carbon tetrachloride-treated dog. Ala J Med Sci 19:371–374
46. Irestedt I, Andreen M (1979) Effects of enflurane on haemodynamics and oxygen consumption in the dog with special reference to the liver and preportal tissues. Acta Anaesthesiol Scand 23:13–26
47. Hughes RL, Campbell D, Fitch W (1980) Effects of enflurane and halothane on liver blood flow and oxygen consumption in the greyhound. Br J Anaesth 52:1079–1086
48. Mizukami S, Hori T, Matsumoto N, Miyazaki T, Goto I, Aikawa K, Sato I (1984) Effects of enflurane and halothane anesthesia on hepatic circulation and hepatic metabolism. Masui 33:1213–1217
49. Lundeen G, Manohar M, Parks C (1983) Systemic distribution of blood flow in swine while awake and during 1.0 and 1.5 MAC isoflurane anesthesia with and without 50% nitrous oxide. Anesth Analg 62:499–512
50. Tverskoy M, Gelman S, Fowler KC, Bradley EL (1985) Intestinal circulation during inhalation anesthesia. Anesthesiology 62:462–469
51. Seyde WC, Longnecker DE (1984) Effect of halothane, enflurane, or isoflurane on the regulation of total hepatic blood flow in rats. Anesthesiology 61:A277
52. Thomson IA, Fitch HW, Campbell D (1982) Effects of nitrous oxide on liver haemodynamics and oxygen consumption in the greyhound. Anesthesia 37:548–553
53. Ellis JE, Longnecker DE (1984) Nitrous oxide decreases renal and splanchnic blood flow in rats. Anesthesiology 61:A26
54. Galindo A (1965) Hepatic circulation and hepatic function during anaesthesia and surgery: II. The effect of various anaesthetic agents. Can Anaesth Soc J 12:337–348
55. Ericsson BF (1971) Effect of pentobarbital sodium anesthesia, as judged with aid of radioactive carbonized microspheres, on cardiac output and its fractional distribution in the dog. Acta Chir Scand 137:613–620
56. Becker H, Manganaro A, Lazar H, Mulder DG, Buckberg GD (1979) Limitations of studying splanchnic blood flow during anesthesia. Surg Forum 30:347–349
57. Bond JH, Prentiss RA, Levitt MD (1980) The effect of anesthesia and laparotomy on blood flow to the stomach, small bowel, and colon of the dog. Surgery 87:313–318

58. Forsyth RP, Hoffbrand BI (1970) Redistribution of cardiac output after sodium pentobarbital anesthesia in the monkey. Am J Physiol 218:214–217
59. Svanvik J, Lundgren O (1977) Gastrointestinal circulation. Int Rev Physiol 12:1–34
60. Ahlgren I, Aronsen F, Bjorkman I, Wetterlin S (1978) The hemodynamic effect of halothane in the normovolemic dog. Acta Anaesthesiol Scand 22:83–92
61. Katz ML, Bergman EN (1969) Simultaneous measurements of hepatic and portal venous blood flow in the sheep and dog. Am J Physiol 216:946–952
62. Sjostrom B, Wulff KE (1975) Influence of long-term anesthesia on regional blood flow distribution and hemodynamics in the dog. Eur Surg Res 7:1–9
63. Tuma RF, Irion GL, Vasthaire US, Heinel LA (1985) Age-related changes in regional blood flow in the rat. Am J Physiol 249:H485–H491
64. Manders WT, Vatner SF (1976) Effects of sodium pentobarbital anesthesia on left ventricular function and distribution of cardiac output in dogs, with particular reference to the mechanism for tachycardia. Circ Res 39:512–517
65. Kawaue Y, Iriuchijima J (1984) Changes in cardiac outout and peripheral flows on pentobarbital anesthesia in the rat. Jpn J Physiol 34:283–294
66. Gelman S, Reves JG, Harris D (1983) Circulatory responses to midazolam anesthesia: emphasis on canine splanchnic circulation. Anesth Analg 62:135–139
67. Dhasmana KM, Prakash O, Saxena PR (1982) Effects of fentanyl, and the antagonism by naloxone, on regional blood flow and biochemical variables in conscious rabbits. Arch Int Pharmacodyn Ther 260:115–129
68. Bell GJ, Hiley CR, Yates MS (1977) The effects of four general anaesthetic agents on the regional distribution of cardiac output in the rat. Br J Pharmacol 61:126P–127P
69. Idvall J, Aronsen KF, Stenberg P (1980) Tissue perfusion and distribution of cardiac output during ketamine anesthesia in normovolemic rats. Acta Anaesthesiol Scand 24:257–263
70. Gelman S, Mardis M (1980) Splanchnic circulatory response to ketamine in stressed and unstressed dogs. Anesthesiology 53:S53
71. Leaman DM, Levenson L, Zelis R, Shiroff R (1978) Effect of morphine on splanchnic blood flow. Br Heart J 40:569–571
72. Miller RL, Forsyth RP, Melon KL (1972) Morphine-induced redistribution of cardiac output in the unanesthetized monkey. Pharmacology 7:138–148
73. Priano LL, Vatner SF (1981) Morphine effects on cardiac output and regional blood flow distribution in conscious dogs. Anesthesiology 55:236–243
74. Tverskoy M, Gelman S, Fowler KC, Bradley EL (1985) Influence of fentanyl and morphine on intestinal circulation. Anesth Analg 64:577–584

Cardiopulmonary Resuscitation and Cardiac Transplantation

Cerebral Metabolism in Hypoxia and Ischemia – Therapeutic Implications

B. K. Siesjö

Cerebrovascular disease is one of the major causes of death. In the United States, for example, stroke exacts a greater toll than that of all other diseases except heart disease and cancer. Thus, close to 500 000 persons are affected by the disease each year, the estimated number of fatal cases being around 150 000 (Hachinski and Norris 1985). At present, the number of survivors are about 2 million. Figures are comparable in most other countries.

Although stroke is the dominant form of cerebrovascular disease, many patients die of cerebrovascular complications to resuscitation following myocardial infarction, and others are left neurologically and neuropsychologically disabled (Safar 1986). It now also emerges that neuropsychological sequalae are common after open-heart surgery, probably because the bypass operations lead to microembolization of cerebral vessels.

In view of these facts, it is understandable that intense efforts are being made to unravel the pathophysiology of ischemic brain damage. Progress within this field is now rapid, and it seems likely that effective therapy will soon be feasible, at least in stroke. It is my purpose with this chapter to review recent advances in cerebral metabolism during ischemia, with particular emphasis on factors and mechanisms contributing to irreversible brain damage, and to describe how these advances relate to current therapeutic avenues. Further details are given in recent review articles, some of which cover the general topic of the pathophysiology of ischemic brain disease (Siesjö 1984, 1988 a; Hossmann 1985; Kaplan et al. 1987; Krause et al. 1988), while others are centered on calcium metabolism (Choi 1988 a, Siesjö 1988 b; Siesjö and Bengtsson 1989; Siesjö et al. 1989), acid-base metabolism (Siesjö 1989), and excitotoxic mechanisms of neuronal necrosis (Rothman and Olney 1986; Choi 1988 a and 1988 b).

Forms of Cerebral Ischemia

When considering the pathophysiology of ischemic brain damage, it is necessary to distinguish between complete and incomplete, and between permanent and transient ischemia. For most practical purposes, one may consider ischemia due to cardiac arrest as being complete, or as one leaving only a trickle of flow to the ischemic tissue. It is also usually of brief duration and, if resuscitation is successful, it is always transient. These characteristics (brief, dense ischemia followed by reperfusion) make the condition hard to treat and, at present, the only really effective preventive measure is a reduction in body (and brain) temperature. However, this does not mean that the condition invites therapeutic nihilism. Thus, following transient ischemia optimal recovery requires that measures be taken to prevent a secondary ischemic insult to the metabolically perturbed tissue. Such a secondary insult may be incurred if the perfusion pressue is inadequate, either because blood pressure is low or the intracranial pressure is high. Conditions favoring complications of this kind are loss of vascular autoregulation and edema. This means that resuscitative measures following cardiac arrest much be directed towards maintaining perfusion pressure, improving blood rheology, and combatting tissue edema. However, as will be discussed in more detail below, it is widely felt that even if reperfusion is adequate, brain damage is nonetheless incurred during the recirculation/reoxygenation period, perhaps triggered by the formation of toxic oxygen radicals.

An entirely different type of ischemia is that due to stroke. In this disease, the ischemia is often permanent, but dissolution or recanalizatioin of an embolus can terminate the ischemia and achieve reperfusion. In the latter case, though, the duration of ischemia is usually long. Another feature is that the severity of the ischemia varies between regions. When an artery such as the middle cerebral artery (MCA) is occluded there is usually a densely ischemic core (the "focus") in the distribution territory of the artery. However, this is surrounded by an area which, although having a reduced flow, is less severely affected (the "penumbra"). The difference between the focus and the penumbra is pathogenetically and therapeutically important. Thus, the penumbra zone may be viable for many hours but, unless optimal conditions prevail or are created, it may eventually suffer dense ischemic damage. Essentially, the original stroke lesions may gradually be extended into the penumbra zone ("stroke in evolution"). It seems very likely that a clinically efficacious treatment of stroke mainly serves to preserve cell viability in the penumbra zone and/or to prevent reperfusion damage, should the occluded vessel be reopened.

Energy Failure in Ischemia

As emphasized elsewhere (Siesjö 1988 a; Siesjö et al. 1989) ischemic damage is not likely to be incurred unless energy failure develops. However, as soon as the ATP stores are depleted, cell viability is threatened. This is because ATP is required for resynthesis of macromolecules and macromolecular assemblies which are spontaneously broken down during the normal "wear and tear" of cells, and because ATP failure sets in motion a series of reactions which are potentially harmful. To take only one example, depletion of the ATP stores disrupts ion homeostasis. This disruption encompasses a rise in intracellular calcium concentration (Ca_i^{2+}) which, by activating lipases, proteases, and endonucleases, hastens breakdown of cell structure. At a certain point, such breakdown becomes irreversible.

I will discuss two aspects of energy failure during ischemia: the rate of depletion of cerebral energy stores during complete ischemia (anoxia) and the flow thresholds for energy failure.

Energy Failure During Anoxia

The metabolic events during complete ischemia have been described in some detail (Lowry et al. 1964; Ljunggren et al. 1974a, 1974b; Folbergrová et al. 1974). Figure 1 summarizes the following findings. First, interruption of oxygen supply leads to a noticeable reduction in tissue PCr and ATP contents within 10–20 s. Second, whereas the PCr stores are depleted already within 1 min, the ATP content is tapped off more gradually. Simultaneously, the glucose and glycogen contents are reduced to zero (not shown), and tissue lactate content rises by corresponding amounts. Figure 2 illustrates, on another time scale, how the depletion of ATP is accompanied by accumulation of ADP and AMP. The sum of adenine nucleotides (ATP+ADP+AMP) is gradually decreased, with accumulation of degradation products of AMP, such as adenosine, inosine, IMP, and hypoxanthine (not shown). This is because accu-

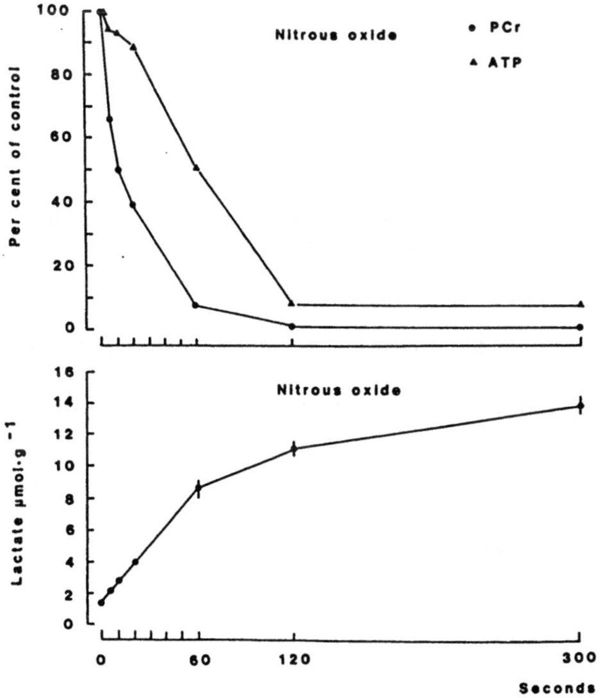

Fig. 1. Rate of depletion of cerebral cortical concentrations of phosphocreatine (PCr) and ATP, and rate of accumulation of lactate, during total ischemia in rats. Note that the energy reserves are essentially depleted after 2 min. (Modified after Nordström and Siesjö 1978)

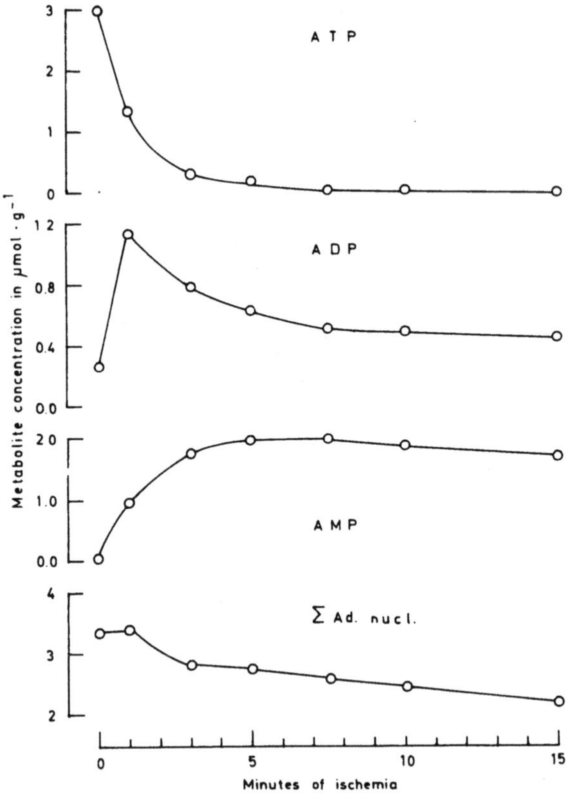

Fig. 2. Changes in tissue concentrations of ATP, ADP, and AMP, and in the sum of these concentrations (Ad.nucl.) during 15 min of ischemia in rats. Sustained ischemia leads to a gradual decrease in the sum of adenine nucleotides, reflecting breakdown of AMP by dephosphorylation and deamination. One of the main breakdown products is hypoxanthine (not shown in figure). (Reproduced with permission from Siesjö 1978)

mulation of AMP triggers its own degradation by dephosphorylation and deamination.

The reactions elicited (excluding the degradation of AMP) can be described by the following four equations

$$\text{ATP} + \text{HOH} \rightarrow \text{ADP} + \text{P}_i + \text{H}^+ \quad (1)$$

$$\text{PCr} + \text{ADP} + \text{H}^+ \rightarrow \text{Cr} + \text{ATP} \quad (2)$$

$$\text{ADP} + \text{ADP} \rightarrow \text{ATP} + \text{AMP} \quad (3)$$

$$\text{Glucose} \rightarrow 2\ \text{lactate}^- + 2^+ \quad (4)$$

Reactions (2) and (3) are, in reality, equilibrium reactions but reaction (2) is driven to the right (as written) because ADP and H^+ accumulate, and ATP falls, and reaction (3) is driven in the same direction because ADP rises and

ATP falls. Glycolysis is stimulated because phosphofructokinase, the main regulatory step in glycolysis, is stimulated by a fall in PCr, and by rises in ADP, AMP, and P_i concentrations. The net result of glycolysis is production of lactate$^-$ plus H^+. This does not mean that H^+ is produced in the lactate dehydrogenase reaction (see Alberti and Cuthbert 1982; Hochachka and Mommsen 1983). However, if ATP concentration remains constant (which may be normal or zero) lactate$^-$ accumulates with a stoichiometrical amount of H^+. Other sources of H^+ production are the ATPase reaction (Eq. 1), and the hydrolysis of phospholipids to free fatty acids (FFAs; see below). However, at the massive amounts of lactate which are usually formed during ischemia, glycolysis is the dominating source of H^+. As a first approximation, therefore, the severity of the acidosis is proportional to the amount of lactate accumulated during the ischemia (see below).

Flow Thresholds for Energy Failure

The brain tolerates a considerable decrease in cerebral perfusion pressure (CPP) before energy metabolism is perturbed. This is because of two defense mechanisms: vascular autoregulation and increased oxygen extraction. At CPP values of about 30 mm Hg, the cerebral energy state is affected. It is noteworthy that when this occurs, the change is sudden and extensive (Fig. 3). This

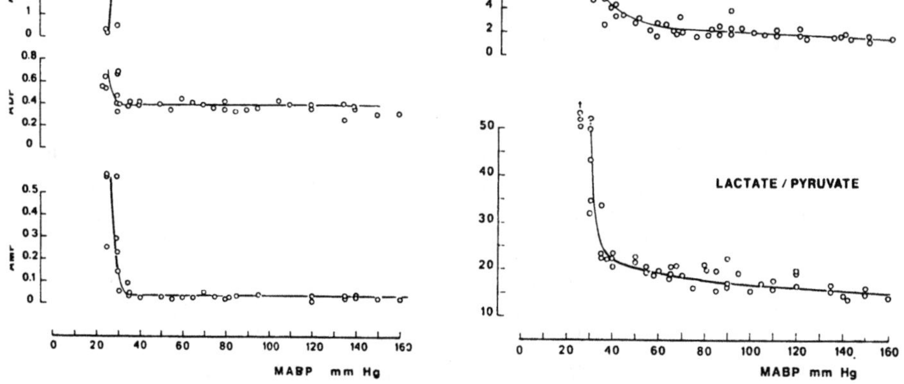

Fig. 3. changes in rat brain concentrations of PCr, ATP, ADP, AMP, and lactate, as well as changes in the lactate/pyruvate ratio, during progressive reductions in the mean arterial blood pressure (MABP) induced by bleeding. Note abrupt deterioration of cerebral energy state at a MABP of about 30 mmHg. (Reproduced with permission from Siesjö 1978)

"all-or-none" response suggests that once energy failure develops events are triggered which enhance energy consumption (see below).

Experiments in which blood flow was gradually reduced have shown a threshold for maintenance of electrical functions (at about 0.20 $ml \cdot ^{-1} \cdot min^{-1}$), and another one below which ion homeostasis is lost (at about 0.10–0.15 $ml \cdot g^{-1} \cdot min^{-1}$); when the latter is transgressed extracellular K^+ concentration (K_e^+) rises, and Ca^{2+} concentration is reduced (Branston et al. 1977; Harris et al. 1981; Harris and Symon 1984). It seems very likely that this threshold for preservation of membrane functions is identical to that at which energy homeostasis is lost (see below). Probably, though, anaerobic glycolysis is stimulated at somewhat higher CBF values, and pH_e is observed to decrease before K_e^+ and Ca_e^{2+} are affected. An even clearer difference between the thresholds for stimulation of glycolysis and for a decrease in energy charge is observed in hypoxia. Thus, whereas tissue (and CSF) lactate contents increase below a PaO_2 of about 45 mmHg, a decrease in ATP and increase in ADP and AMP concentrations are not observed until the PO_2 is reduced below 20 mmHg (Siesjö and Nilsson 1971). This suggests that glycolysis is stimulated at degrees of tissue hypoxia which do not elicit the cascade of events which encompass gross energy failure and loss of ion homeostasis.

Loss of Ion Homeostasis

There is now considerable information on the coupling of energy failure and loss of ion homeostasis. As mentioned, these two events seem to occur simultaneously when CBF is reduced to the threshold for "membrane failure." I will describe how they are coupled during complete ischemia and use data on hypoglycemia to discuss coupling mechanisms. In ischemia, the primary event is energy failure, while loss of ion homeostasis is secondary. In hypoglycemia, this relationship is less obvious.

Ion Fluxes and Energy Failure

Ion gradients across nerve and glial cells are upheld at the expense of energy in the form of ATP. This is because the uphill transport of Na^+, K^+, Ca^{2+}, and H^+ either is acieved by the appropriate ATPases, or is coupled to the downhill flux of Na^+, at the expense of the energy stored in the Na^+ gradient (Fig. 4). Inevitably, therefore, energy failure leads to dissipation of the ionic gradients, with efflux of K^+ from cells, and influx of Na^+, Cl^-, and Ca^{2+} (Nicholson 1980; Hansen 1985; Siesjö 1988 b). However, the changes in ionic gradients following induction of anoxia (as evidenced by measurements of the extracellular concentrations) have a time course which is somewhat unexpected since the initial 70- to 90-s period is dominated by a slow increase in K_e^+, and a gradual fall in pH_e (Fig. 5). At the end of this period (phase 1) K^+ rapidly leaves cells, while Na^+, Cl^-, and Ca^{2+} enter (phase 2). The entry of Na^+ and Cl^- seems to occur with osmotically obliged water since the ECF volume rapidly decreases to about 50% of control, and the rapid ionic fluxes are

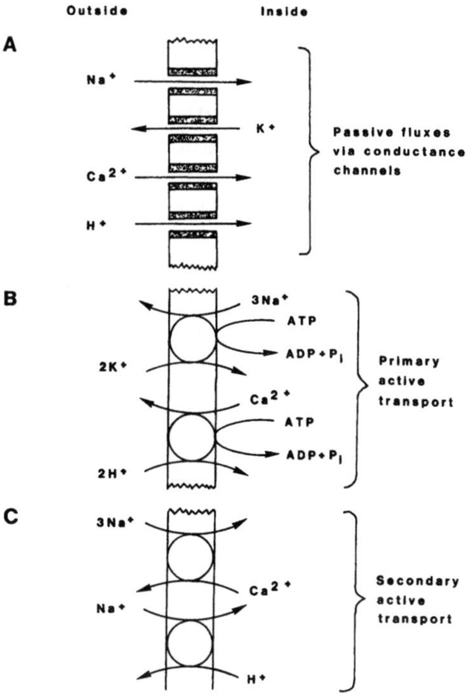

Fig. 4 A–C. Passive and energy-dependent fluxes of Na^+, K^+, Ca^{2+}, and H^+ across cell membranes. Active transport is depicted to occur by primary active transport, directly fuelled by ATP energy, and by secondary active transport, in which Ca^{2+} and H^+ are exported in exchange for Na^+, i.e., at the expense of the energy stored in the Na^+ gradient. (Modified after Siesjö 1984)

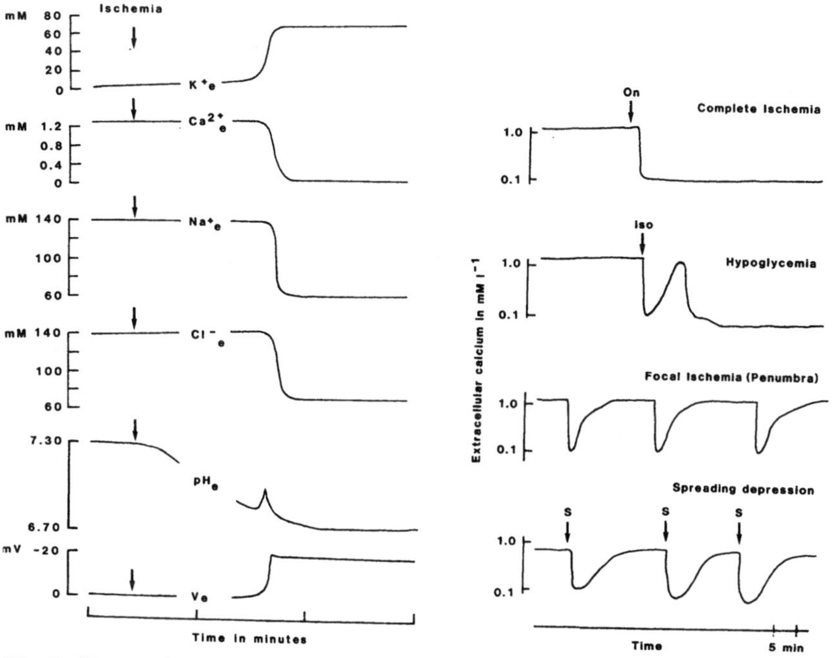

Fig. 5. Changes in extracellular concentrations of K^+, Ca^{2+}, Na^+, and Cl^-, as well as in extracellular pH (pH_e) and DC-potential between brain and an extracerebral site (V_e) during complete ischemia *(left panel)*, and changes in Ca_e^{2+} during complete ischemia, hypoglycemic coma, focal ischemia, and electrically induced spreading depressions. (Reproduced with permission from Siesjö et al. 1989)

accompanied by a change in DC potential, the brain becoming negative to an extracranial site. At the time when this occurs, pH_e transiently shifts in the alkaline direction. In other words, the sudden collapse of ion gradients encompasses efflux of K^+, and influx of Na^+, Cl^-, Ca^{2+}, and H^+ (note, though, that the pH_e change can be caused by efflux of HCO_3^- rather than by influx of H^+).

Phase 1 is the period during which tissue ATP concentration rapidly decreases towards zero (see above). Since preischemic hyperglycemia prolongs and hypoglycemia shortens phase 1 (Hansen 1985), it is tempting to assume that the phase 2 ionic fluxes occur when the preischemic ATP stores have been used up, and when no more ATP can be formed by glycolysis. However, although energy failure is what precipitates loss of ion homeostasis, the phase 2 ionic fluxes do not simply reflect leakage of ions through preexisting pores in the membrane, unmatched by uphill, ATP-dependent transport. Rather, it is necessary to assume that the rapid downhill ion fluxes reflect the activation of a large ion conductance, i.e., that they represent energy failure *plus* a sudden increase in membrane permeability to ions. In order to grasp the importance of the latter, it seems justified to consider ion fluxes during spreading depression and hypoglycemia (see Nicholson 1980; Hansen 1985; Siesjö 1988b; Siesjö and Bengtsson 1989). Figure 5 (right panel) illustrates calcium fluxes in these conditions, as they can be assessed by extracellular recordings.

Spreading depression (SD), a propagated disturbance in brain electrical activity which can be elicited by high K_e^+, strong electrical stimulation, or a stab wound, leads to changes in extracellular ion concentrations, in ECF volume, and in DC potential, which are identical to those observed in ischemia, except for the lack of a preceding (phase 1) rise in K_e^+; yet, the condition is not accompanied by compromised energy production. Obviously, we have to conclude that the phase 2 type of ionic changes can occur in the absence of a fall in ATP concentration. A similar conclusion can be drawn from results obtained in hypoglycemia which, if severe enough to abolish spontaneous EEG activity ("coma"), is accompanied by a marked rise in K_e^+, and fall in Ca_e^{2+}. At the onset of hypoglycemic coma, the tissue ATP concentration decreases to 20%–40% of control, and remains depressed as long as coma prevails (see Siesjö 1988c). However, the decrease in ATP concentration seems to be the consequence of the activation of ion conductances, rather than its direct cause (Wieloch et al. 1984). In fact, one can make the reasonable assumption that, at least in the rat, the sudden loss of ion homeostasis represents a SD, or a similar depolarization event (elicited somewhere in the tissue by local energy failure), which then spreads to involve the rest of the brain. However, in contrast to SD elicited in a normal subject, the depolarization arising in a hypoglycemic one cannot be reversed; instead, the activation of ion conductances consumes a large fraction of the energy stores, and provides an ionic leak which exceeds the capacity of the ionic pumps in the energetically compromised tissue.

Changes in Membrane Permeability

As discussed elsewhere (Siesjö and Bengtsson 1989; Siesjö et al. 1989), changes in extracellular ion concentrations during ischemia are best explained if one assumes that the phase 2 type of ionic fluxes occur in response to a massive presynaptic release of excitatory amino acids, chiefly glutamate. Following the induction of anoxia, the slow increase in K_e^+ may represent K^+ efflux through a channel which is opened in response to a rise in intracellular calcium concentration (Ca_i^{2+}). Since efflux of K^+ carries positive charge from the inside to the outside of the cell, it may hyperpolarize the membrane containing the K^+ channels, perhaps explaining the block in synaptic function which is observed after 15–20 s of anoxia. However, a rise in K_e^+ is apt to depolarize other membranes of glial and neuronal origin, and a rise in K_e^+ to about 15 $mM \cdot l^{-1}$ could well be the stimulus to massive release of transmitters, i.e., what triggers the phase 2 ionic fluxes.

Figure 6 gives a schematic illustration of the major ionic channels which may be involved in the ionic changes discussed. For reasons which will be discussed below, I will confine the description to agonist-operated channels, particularly to those linked to receptors activated by glutamate and related excitatory amino acids (EAAs, henceforth discussed as glutamate). Glutamate ac-

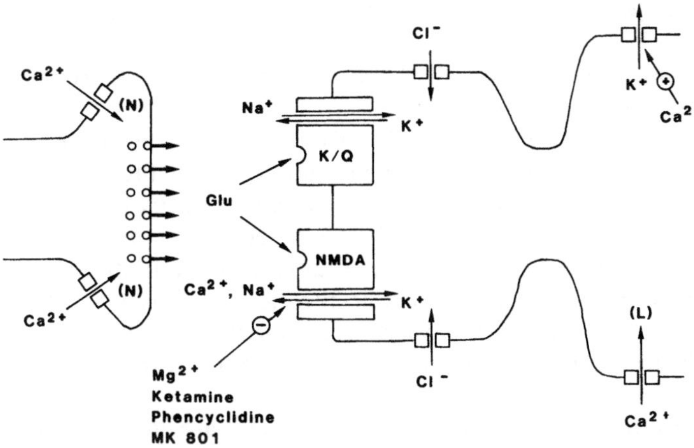

Fig. 6. Schematic diagram illustrating ionic fluxes in presynaptic and postsynaptic structures. Presynaptic release of transmitter is assumed to be triggered by calcium, entering by an *N* type of voltage-sensitive calcium channel (VSCC). Postsynaptic calcium entry may in part occur via an L type of VSCC, perhaps localized more centrally on dendrites and soma. However, major contributors to postsynaptic calcium entry are agonist-operated calcium channels (AOCCs), assumed to be gated by glutamate receptors. These are of two main types: kainate (K)/quisqualate (Q)-preferring, and *N*-methyl-D-aspartate (NMDA)-preferring. The former is linked to a channel which allows monovalent cations to pass, while the latter has a permeability to calcium as well. By allowing Na^+ and calcium to enter, glutamate excites postsynaptic elements. Inhibition is shown to occur by activation of Cl^- and K^+ conductances which are, at least in part, calcium-dependent. NMDA-linked channel is blocked by Mg^{2+} in physiological concentrations, by ketamine, and by phencyclidine, and related compounds

tivates two types of membrane receptors, presumably localized mainly to dendrites and dendritic spines (Fagg et al. 1986; Ascher and Nowak 1987; Foster and Fagg 1987; MacDermott and Dale 1987; Mayer and Westbrook 1987; Miller 1987; Choi 1988a; Reynolds and Miller 1988). The first receptor, which is selectively activated by the glutamate analogues kainate (K) and quisqualate (Q), is linked to a channel which is permeable to monovalent cations, i.e., to Na^+ and K^+ (and to H^+). Thus, this channel provides a route for the rapid efflux of K^+ and influx of Na^+ during the phase 2 ionic shifts (and for the transient influx of H^+). The second receptor, selectively activated by *N*-methyl-D-aspartate (NMDA), is linked to a channel which is permeable to both the monovalent cations K^+ and Na^+, and to the divalent ion Ca^{2+}. The activation of the NMDA receptor is potentiated by very low concentrations of glycine and antagonized by Zn^{2+}. Apart from contributing to the downhill K^+ and Na^+ fluxes, the NMDA-linked channel provides a major entry route for calcium. This channel is thus a typical agonist-operated calcium channel (AOCC). Interestingly, the channel is blocked by physiological concentrations of Mg^{2+} in a voltage-dependent manner. The Mg^{2+} block is relieved when the membrane depolarizes. Glutamate, being a mixed agonist, activates both receptors, and their sequential activation may be what provides a massive leak for Ca^{2+}. Thus, by allowing Na^+ influx the activation of K/Q receptors leads to depolarization. The latter, by relieving the Mg^{2+} block, is a requirement for influx of Ca^{2+} in response to glutamate activation of the receptor. Clearly, though, since depolarization also activates voltage-sensitive calcium channels (VSCCs), these may contribute substantially to calcium influx, particularly at pronounced degrees of depolarization.

As described elsewhere (e.g., Mayer and Westbrook 1987; Watkins and Olverman 1987; Choi et al. 1988), there are some broad-spectrum antagonists which block both the K/Q and the NMDA type of receptors. One of these is kynurenate, which also blocks the site at which glycine acts. At present, the competitive NMDA antagonists are too poorly soluble in the lipid phase to penetrate the blood-brain barrier in sufficient concentrations. This is why considerable interest is now being directed towards noncompetitive NMDA antagonists which block the receptor-gated channel, rather than the receptor itself (see Fig. 6).

The glutamate receptors discussed are ionotropic, i.e, they are linked to ion channels, thereby triggering fluxes of ions along their thermodynamic gradients. Recent results demonstrate that glutamate also activates metabolotropic receptors, i.e., receptors which give rise to a metabolic response, rather than to fluxes of ions. Of particular interest is the fact that these are linked to phospholipase C, an enzyme which triggers breakdown of membrane-bound PIP_2 to DG and IP_3, the latter serving as a stimulus to intracellular calcium release (see below). The subtype of glutamate receptors involved is quisqualate-preferring. Clearly, release of glutamate gives rise to both influx and intracellular release of calcium.

The ionic fluxes described are, especially if massive, potentially harmful since they constitute the molecular basis for the so-called excitotoxic hypothesis of neuronal necrosis (Olney 1978; Rothman and Olney 1986). One adverse effect is related to Na^+ influx which, as we have discussed, may occur via both K/Q- and NMDA-linked channels. Since Na^+ entry involves influx of positive charge, large amounts of Na^+ can only enter in exchange for K^+, or if the Na^+ current is short-circuited by cotransport of an anion, such as Cl^-. However, entry of Na^+ and Cl^- must be accompanied by osmotically obliged water, and thus results in cellular edema. This is the mechanism behind the osmolytic damage which is supposed to mediate at least part of the toxicity of EAAs. The second adverse effect of excessive stimulation of glutamate receptors is the influx of calcium (see below). Both osmolytic damage and calcium-related damage are prone to particularly affect dendrites and dendritic spines, probably explaining why excitotoxic damage has the characteristics of dendrosomatic, axon-sparing lesions. The reasons are probably twofold: glutamate receptors are mainly localized to these structures, and ions entering them may be physical constraint be prevented from leaving the sites of entry by convection and diffusion. I will discuss in more detail the pathophysiological background of calcium-related damage, but postpone the corresponding discussion of acidosis-related damage until tissue acid-base metabolism has been considered.

Cell Calcium Metabolism: the Achilles Heel of Metabolic Perturbation

Intracellular calcium is a ubiquitous second messenger and regulator of metabolic pathways, serving to purposefully transform external messages into intracellular responses (Berridge 1984, 1987; Carafoli 1982; 1987; Rasmussen 1986). These functions fulfilled by calcium impose a load on mechanisms regulating Ca^{2+}, especially since markedly raised Ca_i^{2+} values are potentially harmful.

Influx of calcium through AOCCs and VSCCs during activity is normally balanced by energy-dependent outflux via ATP-driven transport, catalyzed by a Ca^{2+}-ATPase, and by $3Na^+/Ca^{2+}$ exchange. This exchange is electrogenic, carrying positive charge into the cell; accordingly, it is driven both by the Na^+ gradient and by the membrane potential. It follows from this that if the sodium gradient and/or the membrane potential are reduced the flux catalyzed by the exchanger may be reversed, i.e., Na^+ efflux may be coupled to Ca^{2+} entry. Normally, the two membrane devices maintain Ca_i^{2+} at about 10^{-7} *M*, i.e., at a concentration which is 10000-fold lower than Ca_e^{2+}. When large amounts of calcium enter, the high-capacity $3Na^+/Ca^{2+}$ exchanger may extrude the bulk of the calcium load, the low capacity ATPase serving to regulate Ca_i^{2+} at moderately raised levels. The cell calcium content, as opposed to the free concentration, is about $10^{-3}\ M \cdot kg^{-1}$. This means that close to 100% of the calcium of the cell is bound or sequestered. Binding occurs to proteins (some of which may primarily serve to bind calcium, like calcibindin, and others which are effector proteins, like calmodulin), to phospholipids, and to a host of compounds of lower molecular weight. In this way, calcium binding resembles the buffering of H^+, which exists at a similar intracellular concentration

(10^{-7} *M*). In fact, Ca^{2+} and H^+ may be bound to common sites, and thus compete for occupancy at these sites.

Binding serves to dampen the increase in Ca_i^{2+} for a given calcium load. Another mechanism achieving the same purpose is the sequestration of calcium in endoplasmic reticulum (ER), mitochondria, and other subcellular organelles. Sequestration either requires ATP (ER) or an oxygen-dependent electromotive force (mitochondria). Probably, ER and related structures regulate Ca_i^{2+} at moderate calcium loads, while mitochondria (which have a large capacity to sequester calcium) come into play only when Ca_i^{2+} exceeds the physiological range.

Probably, neither ER nor the mitochondria serve the primary purpose of regulating Ca_i^{2+} (e.g., Berridge 1984; Denton and McCormack 1985; Hansford 1985). Thus, the primary purpose of calcium sequestration in the ER may be to keep a pool of calcium which can be released in response to receptor stimulation, and IP_3 formation, the calcium then serving a role as an intracellular messenger. Similarly, calcium cycling across the mitochondrial membrane could primarily serve to transmit changes in Ca_i^{2+} to the intramitochondrial space, with the purpose of regulating the dehydrogenases which form rate-limiting steps in citric acid metabolism. However, under adverse conditions these functions may be upset, since massive receptor stimulation may further raise Ca_i^{2+} in a situation in which influx is enhanced, and since a pathologically raised Ca_i^{2+} can cause sequestration in the mitochondria to the extent that ATP formation is inhibited and structural mitochondrial damage becomes imminent.

Clearly, since ischemia (and hypoglycemia) leads to release of EAAs, to energy failure, and to membrane depolarization, one would expect both enhanced calcium entry and release of calcium from intracellular stores in a situation in which both extrusion of calcium and its intracellular sequestration are compromised. In theory, such events could be prevented (or delayed/attenuated) by blockers of AOCCs and VSCCs. However, the situation is complicated by the cellular influx of Na^+, and the accompanying depolarization, since these can reverse calcium transport via the $3Na^+/Ca^{2+}$ exchanger (see below).

Calcium-Related Damage

In the original hypothesis of calcium-related damage, advanced to explain ischemic damage to heart muscle and dystrophic damage to skeletal muscle, it was assumed that calcium enters through voltage-sensitive calcium channels (Fleckenstein et al. 1974; Wrogemann and Pena 1976). It was later proposed that increased calcium permeability for any reason (e.g., the unspecific permeability change caused by a variety of toxins) could trigger calcium-related damage, also that such damage encompassed overactivation of lipases and proteases (e.g., Leonard and Salpeter 1979; Farber 1981; Chien et al. 1981), or even endonucleases (Nicotera et al. 1986; Orrenius et al. 1988). A schematic diagram depicting such events is shown in Fig. 7. The results of such overac-

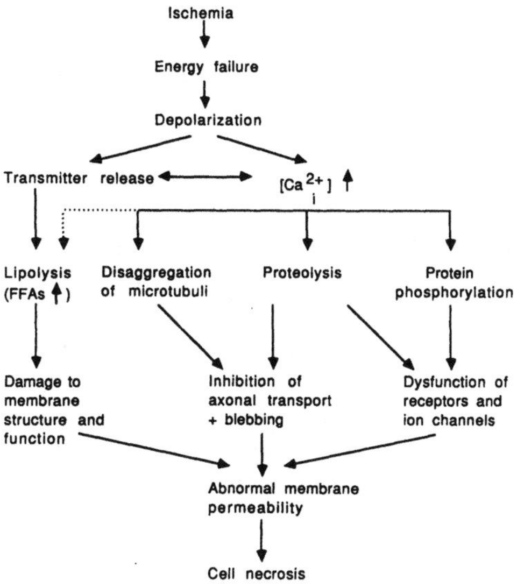

Fig. 7. Schematic diagram illustrating the coupling between ischemia, energy failure, depolarization, loss of calcium homeostasis, and calcium-related, pathological events. (Reproduced with permission from Siesjö 1988 b)

tivation are breakdown of phospholipids and proteins, important constituents of membranes, and DNA fragmentation.

Probably, energy failure and calcium accumulation both contribute to degradation of cell structure during ischemia, the rise in Ca_i^{2+} serving to hasten processes which are set in motion by ATP depletion per se. Since proteolysis affects cytoskeletal components such as neurofilaments, and severs the proteins which anchor the plasma membrane to the cytoskeleton, it may seriously disturb cytoskeletal functions such as axoplasmic transport and cause "blebbing" of the plasma membrane, the latter leading to an unspecific increase in membrane permeability.

Loss of calcium homeostasis also contributes to a derangement of phospholipid metabolism (see Bazan 1976). As Fig. 7 shows, lipolysis is enhanced by several of the consequences of ischemia: depletion of energy stores, presynaptic release of agonists, and calcium accumulation. Accumulation of fatty acids (FFAs) per se may be harmful since some of them are membrane-active and may serve as ionophores and initiators of cellular and vasogenic edema (Chan et al. 1984; Chan and Fishman 1985). Possibly, though, the adverse effects of the accumulation of polyenoic fatty acids such as arachidonic acid become manifest first during recirculation (see below).

Acidosis

Obviously, energy failure triggers loss of ion homeostasis, a potential cause of ischemic (and hypoglycemic) brain damage. Another consequence of energy failure is acidosis.

Lactate Content Versus Intracellular pH

Complete ischemia converts the tissue into a closed system. In this situation, the amount of lactate accumulated closely corresponds to the preischemic tissue stores of glycogen and glucose (Ljunggren et al. 1974c). Since the latter is increased during hyperglycemia, and decreased during hypoglycemia, the severity of the tissue acidosis during ischemia varies with the nutritional state (i.e., the plasma glucose concentration). For example, at preischemic plasma glucose concentrations of 4, 8, and 20 $\mu M \cdot l^{-1}$ the ischemic tissue lactate concentrations are 10, 14, and 20 $\mu mol \cdot g^{-1}$. It was predicted (Ljunggren et al. 1974c) and later verified (Smith et al. 1986) that increasing lactate concentrations are associated with progressively lower intracellular pH (pH_i). For example, for the three lactate concentrations given, estimated pH_i values were 6.35, 6.15, and 5.95, respectively (Smith et al. 1986). Figure 8 illustrates the time course of changes in pH_e and pH_i during and following 15 min of ischemia in moderately hypoglycemic and in hyperglycemic animals.

Additional lactate can be formed during incomplete ischemia, i.e., when a trickle of flow can deliver additional glucose to the energy-compromised tissue (for reviews, see Siesjö 1981, 1989). Under those conditions, hyperglycemic animals can accumulate lactate in excess of 30 $\mu mol \cdot g^{-1}$. Clearly, such values must be associated with excessive degrees of intracellular acidosis. Another condition in which large amounts of lactate can accumulate in the tissue is arterial hypoxia, especially if complicated by a fall in cerebral perfusion pressure (Siesjö and Nilsson 1971; Salford et al. 1973; Gardiner et al. 1982). However, in hypoxia the severity of the tissue lactic acidosis correlates to the reduction in adenylate energy charge, rather than to plasma glucose concentration (Gardiner et al. 1982). This is to say that when the tissue is adequately supplied with

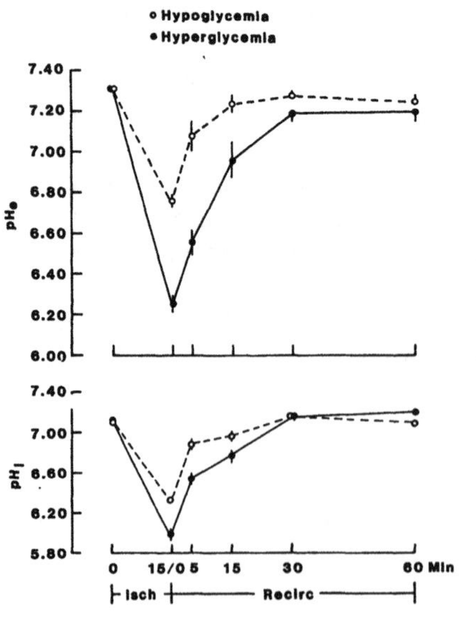

Fig. 8. Changes in extra- and intracellular pH in rat cerebral cortex during and following 15 min of near-complete ischemia in moderately hypoglycemic and in hyperglycemic animals. Values for pH_i were calculated on the assumption that the intracellular fluids represent a homogenous compartment (see text). (Reproduced with permission from Smith et al. 1986)

glucose, accumulation of lactate depends on the severity of the fall in cellular energy state. In other words, hyperglycemia is detrimental only under the conditions of severe incomplete ischemia (in which glucose supply is upheld and energy failure is dense).

Extracellular pH and Compartmentation of H^+

Two unexplained findings complicate interpretation of tissue acid-base changes in ischemia. One is the remarkable changes in extracellular pH (pH_e) during complete ischemia with varying tissue lactate concentrations (Kraig et al. 1985, 1986). Measurements of pH_e in ischemia with lactate values varying between about 8 and 30 $\mu mol \cdot g^{-1}$ have shown two plateau values, with Δ pH_e values of about 0.5 and 1.1, with a transition zone at tissue lactate contents of 15–17 $\mu mol \cdot g^{-1}$ (Kraig et al. 1986). This is to say that tissue lactate can increase from about 8 to 16, and from about 18 to 30 $\mu mol \cdot g^{-1}$, at constant pH_e values of about 6.8 and 6.2, respectively.

The behavior of pH_e, and the associated changes in tissue PCO_2, have led Kraig et al. (1985, 1986) to suggest that H^+ is compartmentalized during ischemia. Their assumption is that above lactate concentrations of 15–17 $\mu mol \cdot g^{-1}$, any additional lactate is formed in a compartment whose HCO_3^- content has already been reduced to zero. This compartment, assumed to represent glial cells, will thus become excessively acid (about 5), while neurons are assumed to maintain a pH close to that of ECF (about 6.2). The predictions made by the authors have later been substantiated by direct intracellular pH measurements, and the proposal has been made that the low pH_i is what destryos glial cells, predisposing to ischemic infarction (Kraig et al. 1987; Kraig and Chesler 1989). However, ^{31}P-NMR measurements have so far failed to support the suggestion of major H^+ compartmentation during ischemia (Boris-Möller et al. 1988). This suggests that if such compartmentation is at hand, it may affect a smaller volume of the tissue than that usually assumed to be occupied by glial cells.

Acidosis-Related Brain Damage

Preischemic hyperglycemia is known to enhance ischemic brain damage. Typically, this enhancement encompasses infarction, edema, and postischemic seizures which, especially following brief periods of ischemia, occur after a free interval (Myers 1979a and 1979b; Siesjö 1981, 1989; Plum 1983; Siesjö et al. 1987). The mechanisms have not been defined but three major ones can be envisaged, the first two of which are likely to operate *during* an ongoing ischemia.

When pH falls, the respiratory functions of isolated mitochondria decline and, below pH values of about 6, oxidative phosphorylation ceases (e.g., Hillered et al. 1984). This suggests that severe acidosis strongly inhibits ATP production in vivo. Very likely, failure of mitochondrial function prevents recovery in a severely acidotic, ischemic tissue, and hastens irreversible breakdown of cell structure. One can also envisage that, following reperfusion of such tissue, normalization of pH_i is a requirement for ATP synthesis and, thereby, for metabolic and functional recovery.

How is recovery of pH_i achieved? In all probability, pH_i is normalized by two mechanisms: by oxidation of the lactate accumulated with removal of a stoichiometrical amount of H^+ and, as shown in Fig. 4, by extrusion of H^+ via Na^+/H^+ exchange (e.g., Roos and Boron 1981; Grinstein and Rothstein 1986; Mahnensmith and Aronsen 1985). The latter mechanism requires that the transmembrane Na^+ gradient is restored by resumed Na^+, K^+-ATPase activity. However, another requirement is that pH_e be not too low. This is because H^+ and Na^+ compete for the same binding site on the external site of the Na^+/H^+ exchanger (e.g., Grinstein et al. 1984; Jean et al. 1986). Clearly, recovery after ischemia is critically dependent on normalization of pH_i and pH_e and, since the latter depends on resumption of ATP production, in itself influenced by pH_i, one can envisage a situation in which recovery is prevented by retention of H^+, and inability to produce ATP, two interdependent events.

The second mechanism is a more speculative one in which regulation of pH_i by a Na^+/H^+ exchanger is assumed to occur at the expense of volume regulation (e.g., Siesjö 1985, 1989). This could occur if both Na^+/H^+ and Cl^-/HCO_3^- exchangers are activated since the concerted action of the two antiporters would be influx of both Na^+ and Cl^-, with osmotically obliged water. Essentially, since the H^+ pumped out by Na^+/H^+ exchange leaks back via the Cl^-/HCO_3^- exchanger (as HCO_3^- efflux) the coupled antiporters would achieve futile cycling of H^+ (and HCO_3^-), with accumulation of Na^+, Cl^-, and H_2O. We do not know, though, if brain cells contain such coupled antiporters, nor do we know under what conditions they would be simultaneously activated.

None of these mechanisms can explain delayed brain damage, and delayed edema since these occur when acidosis is no longer present. Perhaps the most fruitful hypothesis is one which assumes that acidosis exerts part of its detrimental effect by enhancing free radical reactions, especially since these may well yield damage which matures after an interval. Although one can envisage that permanent ischemia, e.g., that affecting the penumbra zone of a stroke lesion, leads to free radical damage to vascular and nonvascular cells, I will discuss this mechanism under the assumption that it is primarily a reperfusion event.

Reperfusion Damage

The literature abounds in hypotheses which predict that part, if not all, of the final damage incurred after transient ischemia is caused by mechanisms which come into play first when blood and oxygen supply is restored. It is clear that the calcium-dependent events discussed, particularly the degradation of membrane and cytoskeletal components, can yield a lingering dysfunction of membranes and lead to cell damage which "matures" first after some period of recirculation. For example, if the ischemia leaves the membranes with an enhanced calcium permeability, delayed calcium-dependent damage may occur. However, the concept of reperfusion damage is a different one, since it implies that new, potentially devastating reactions are set into motion by reperfusion/reoxygenation. We are left with the question, therefore, wheter delayed damage reflects failure of repair of metabolic and/or structural damage incurred during the ischemia, or the consequences of new, adverse reactions.

Experiments with postischemic administration of drugs which ameliorate ischemic damage leave some, albeit not consistent, support for the second possibility. However, the strongest support is received from results with post-insult cooling of the brain (Busto et al. 1987; Boris-Möller et al. 1989). Previous data suggested that such cooling may be beneficial, but it was only very recently that the potentiality of this treatment modality was realized. For example, out of seven animals subjected to 20 min dense forebrain ischemia at a brain temperature of 37 °C, and subjected to postischemic cooling (27 °C) for 1 h, one had virtually no brain damage and two others very moderate damage (Boris-Möller et al. 1989). Similar results have recently been obtained by Buchan and Pulsinelli (personal communication). If animals are subjected to similar ischemia with recovery temperature maintained at 37 °C, *all* animals show extensive brain damage. The results demonstrate that postinsult hypothermia inhibits events which are initiated during recirculation, events which otherwise trigger injurious reactions in the metabolically perturbed tissue. It seems highly justified to define these reactions, and to find out why only some animals are protected by the hypothermia. One can, at present, speculate about two adverse reactions which are set into motion by recirculation/reoxygenation.

Delayed Calcium-Related Damage

One may envisage two types of calcium-related damage during recirculation: immediate and delayed. Immediate mitochondrial damage could occur when reoxygenation restores the ability of mitochondria to sequester the calcium which has accumulated during the insult. However, unless additional calcium enters the cell, or membrane devices for calcium extrusion fail, it is difficult to envisage that the mitochondria remain calcium-loaded. Delayed calcium-related damage is possible if the initial insult increases membrane leakage, allowing increased futile cycling of calcium, and slow mitochondrial overload (see Rasmussen and Waisman 1983; Deshpande et al. 1987; Siesjö 1988b).

If we assume that reperfusion damage is, at least in part, calcium-dependent we have to enquire into the routes of entry. Excitotoxic damage in vitro is calcium-dependent (Choi 1985, 1987; Garthwaite et al. 1986; Clark and Rothman 1987). An intriguing finding is that addition of NMDA antagonists to cell cultures *after* they have been exposed to NMDA prevents or ameliorates the damage (Rothman et al. 1987; Choi et al. 1987, 1988b). It seems justified to explore whether seepage of EEAs from presynaptic endings continues during recirculation, or if activation of conductance mechanisms for calcium entry shows hysterisis, i.e., if calcium channels in vulnerable cell structures remain open for some time during recirculation. Recent results by Andiné et al. (1988) provide an elegant demonstration of a lingering derangement of cell calcium metabolism following transient ischemia. Whether they reflect enhanced release of EAAs from presynaptic endings, or postsynaptic facilitation of calcium entry, the results underscore the possibility that postinsult treatment may ameliorate the final lesion.

Free Radical Damage: a Role for Fe^{2+} and H^{+}?

The hypothesis of reperfusion damage caused by production of free radicals, overwhelming the antioxidative defense of the tissue, was advanced more than 10 years ago (Demoupolos et al. 1977; Flamm et al. 1978). It was originally assumed that free radicals, formed either during or after ischemia, gave rise to membrane damage by the autocatalytic reactions of lipid peroxidation, with secondary damage to membrane-bound proteins. However, it proved difficult to demonstrate the presence of peroxidative damage in vivo, and the therapeutic effects of antioxidants and free radical scavengers were undramatic, if at all demonstrable (see e.g. Siesjö 1981; Siesjö and Wieloch 1985).

The situation has now changed. Thus, it has been realized, or at least suggested, that the primary targets are proteins and DNA rather than lipids, that the damage is site-specific rather than diffuse, and that catalysis by iron is involved (Aust et al. 1985; Halliwell and Gutteridge 1985; White et al. 1985; Komara et al. 1986; Halliwell 1987; Krause et al. 1988). It has often been assumed that the extremely toxic hydroxyl radical species ($\cdot OH$) is formed from the less toxic superoxide anion ($+\cdot O_2^-$) and hydrogen peroxide in the so-called Haber-Weiss reaction:

$$\cdot O_2^- + H_2O_2 \rightarrow \cdot OH^- + OH^- + O_2 \qquad (5)$$

However, this reaction only proceeds as written if catalyzed by iron according to the reactions

$$Fe^{3+} + \cdot O_2^- \rightarrow Fe^{2+} + O_2 \qquad (6)$$

$$Fe^{2+} + H_2O_2 \rightarrow Fe^{3+} + \cdot OH + {}^-OH \qquad (7)$$

We observe that the net result of reactions (6) and (7) is reaction (5). Thus, if $\cdot O_2^-$ and H_2O_2, normal products of some enzymatic and nonenzymatic cellular reactions, are formed in increased amounts in the presence of "free" iron, damage due to $\cdot OH$ or a similar oxidation product can result. Furthermore, diffusion of H_2O_2 and/or $\cdot O_2^-$ to the site where iron is normally bound in proteins and DNA can result in site-specific damage, i.e., damage which is strictly localized to the site where the iron-catalyzed Haber-Weiss reaction occurs.

The first question which arises is: Why are free radicals formed in increased amounts during reperfusion? Probably, reoxidation of many compounds which have been reduced during ischemia gives rise to free radical formation. Furthermore, enzymes are activated which generate free radicals. Two such enzymes are cyclooxygenase and lipoxygenase, which degrade the arachidonic acid accumulated during ischemia, once oxygen supply is restored (for review, see Siesjö 1981, 1988 a). Another free radical forming enzymes is xanthine oxidase which converts hypoxanthine, accumulated during ischemia, to uric acid, with the production of $\cdot O_2^-$ and H_2O_2. Interestingly, the enzyme normally occurs in the dehydrogenase form (which does not form free radicals), but this can be converted into the oxidase form by a calcium-dependent protease (McCord 1985). Thus, since accumulation of arachidonic acid is, at least in part, also a calcium-dependent event, there is an obvious link between loss of calcium homeostasis and free radical formation.

The second question is: What leads to the formation of "free" iron? This question is related to another one: Is there a role for acidosis in the sequence of events which involves iron release and free radical damage? As discussed elsewhere (Siesjö 1985, 1989), acidosis may aggravate damage by one of two mechanisms. According to one suggestion (Gebicki and Bielski 1981), acidosis acts by converting the anion $\cdot O_2^-$ to its acid form $H \cdot O_2$ ($pK' = 4.7$), which is not only more lipid soluble but also a stronger prooxidant than $\cdot O_2^-$. The other possibility is that acidosis acts by releasing iron from transferrin (see below). An effect of this type was suggested already by Barber and Bernheim (1967), and it was later shown that a reduction in pH to 6.5–6.2 in brain homogenates was accompanied by enhanced lipid peroxidation, which was inhibited by the iron chelator desferrioxamine (Siesjö et al. 1985; Rehncrona et al. 1989). Thus, acidosis may be detrimental by providing prooxidative iron to catalyze reaction [7], or a similar reaction yielding a toxic radical species.

Iron, an essential component of respiratory and other enzymes, is transported to cells bound to transferrin, and mainly stored in cells bound to ferritin (e.g., Aisen 1979; Crichton 1979). In these forms, iron is not prooxidative, i.e., it cannot catalyze free radical reactions. However, iron stored in ferritin in the Fe^{3+} form can be released by reducing agents, particularly $\cdot O_2^-$ and, as discussed, iron stored in transferrin in the form of a Fe^{3+}-HCO_3-protein complex is released by a decrease in pH. Clearly, since ischemia leads to the accumulation of H^+ and since reoxidation gives rise to a spurt of formation of $\cdot O_-$, iron is apt to be released from its binding sites in proteins (see Babbs 1985). This is illustrated in Fig. 9. The iron released is chelated by low-molecular weight compounds such as ADP, AMP, citrate, etc. In these forms, the iron is prooxidative and, provided that $\cdot O_2^-$ and H_2O_2 are available, it can give rise to the production of $\cdot OH$. One can thus envisage a web of interrelated reactions, dependent on loss of Ca^{2+}, H^+, and Fe^{2+} homeostasis, which ultimately causes free radical damage.

Yet another fact has emerged, pertaining to free radical damage to brain tissues: the damage is apt to occur after relatively long periods of ischemia, and it may preferentially (but probably not exclusively) affect the vasculature, thereby predisposing to edema. In support, administration of free radical scavengers has clearly proved to ameliorate brain damage due to sustained focal ischemia (see below).

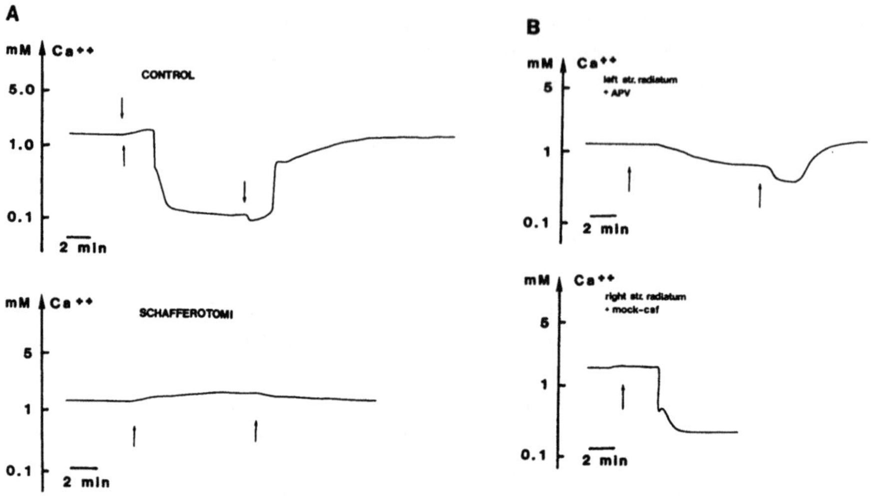

Fig. 9 A. Extracellular Ca^{2+} concentrations (Ca_e^{2+}) in the CA1 sector of the rat hippocampus during ischemia. *Arrows* indicate start and end of the ischemic period in a control rat *(top)* and in a rat with denervated CA1 region ("Schafferotmi"; *bottom*). Virtually no changes in Ca_e^{2+} are observed on the deafferentated side. **B** Ca_e^{2+} concentrations in the CA1 sector during ischemia in a rat pretreated with APV in the left CA1 *(top)*, and in its control right CA1 sector *(bottom)*. Injection of APV delays and curtails the decrease in Ca_e^{2+} during ischemia. (Reproduced with permission from Benveniste et al. 1989)

Therapeutic Implications

At present, and with available information, one can envisage the participation of EAAs, calcium, acidosis, iron, and free radicals in the pathogenesis of ischemic brain damage. Dense, transient ischemia of the type seen in cardiac arrest may well be an excitotoxic lesion, leading to osmolytic and calcium-related damage. Following long periods of less dense ischemia, free radicals are conceivably involved, particularly in causing vascular damage with vasogenic edema. However, such sweeping statements represent little more than assumptions, and the ultimate test is provided by experiments in which attempts are made to ameliorate ischemic brain damage by drugs specifically blocking the effects of the putative mediators.

Excitatory Amino Acids: Effect of NMDA Antagonists

For several years, noncompetitive NMDA antagonists have provided the most promising pharmacological tool in ameliorating ischemic brain damage due to experimental stroke, and the drugs have proved efficacious even when given a few hours after MCA occlusion (see Oyzert et al. 1988; Park et al. 1988; Gotti et al. 1988; Carter et al. 1988). Both competitive and noncompetitive NMDA antagonists have also been found to reduce hypoglycemic damage to the caudoputamen (Wieloch 1985; Westerberg et al. 1988). It is widely held that the NMDA antagonists act by preventing an extension of the infarct into the penumbra zone, while they lack effect on the ischemic core, usually comprising the caudoputamen and part of the overlying neocortex. Since noncompetitive NMDA antagonists block the ionic channel which provides a conductance mechanism for calcium, it has seemed likely that their principal effect is to impede calcium influx into those structures which abound in NMDA receptors.

This interpretation is put in question by a series of discrepant and seemingly contradictory results (for literature, see Siesjö and Bengtsson 1989; Siesjö et al. 1989). For example, several groups have found that NMDA antagonists fail to ameliorate ischemic brain damage caused by severe global or forebrain ischemia. Furthermore, MK-801, a noncompetitive NMDA antagonist with a pronounced antiischemic effect in experimental stroke, could not prevent influx of calcium during forebrain ischemia, or during hypoglycemic coma. Finally, some results obtained with electrically induced spreading depression (SD) have been difficult to interpret. In this context SD is an interesting phenomenon, since it leads to ionic shifts similar to the phase 2 ionic changes seen in ischemia and hypoglycemia. The calcium hypothesis of ischemic cell damage has been hard to reconcile with the fact that, in the normal brain, repeated SDs can be elicited over several hours, with no untoward effects on cell viability. Furthermore, both competitive and noncompetitive NMDA antagonists block the phase 2 ionic changes during SD (including the calcium influx).

We have recently attempted to integrate available information in this field into a unifying hypothesis which has the dual purpose of explaining the discrepant results, and predicting under what conditions NMDA antagonists will be efficacious (Siesjö and Bengtsson 1989; Siesjö et al. 1989). This interpretation was furthered by recent results reported by Benveniste et al. (1988), who reported that deafferentation of CA1 cells by prior Schafferotomi completely prevented calcium influx into CA1 dendrites during 10 min of dense ischemia, while local injection of AP5 delayed and attenuated calcium influx. This is illustrated in Fig. 10, which also recalls the lack of effect of systemically injected MK-801 on anoxic calcium fluxes.

On the basis of these and other results, we assume that the initial ionic fluxes are precipitated by a sudden release of glutamate, or a related EAA. This will have the effect of opening channels for K^+, Na^+, and Ca^{2+}. In the first version of our hypothesis (Siesjö and Bengtsson 1989), we assumed that the rise in Ca_i^{2+} above a certain threshold value activated a nonselective cation conductance (NSCC), explaining the "shock opening" of ionic gates in ischemia, hypoglycemia, and spreading depression. This assumption allowed us to make certain predictions. First, an NMDA antagonist will prevent a SD from being elicited, simply because any calcium entering by non-NMDA routes will be extruded or sequestered by the energetically uncompromised tissue, preventing Ca_i^{2+} from reaching the threshold value. Since the Ca^{2+} entering will be promptly extruded, and/or efficiently bound/sequestered, Ca_i^{2+} will not reach values which will trigger destructive events.

The NMDA antagonists will be predictably inefficacious in complete or near-complete ischemia, simply because multiple mechanisms exist for raising

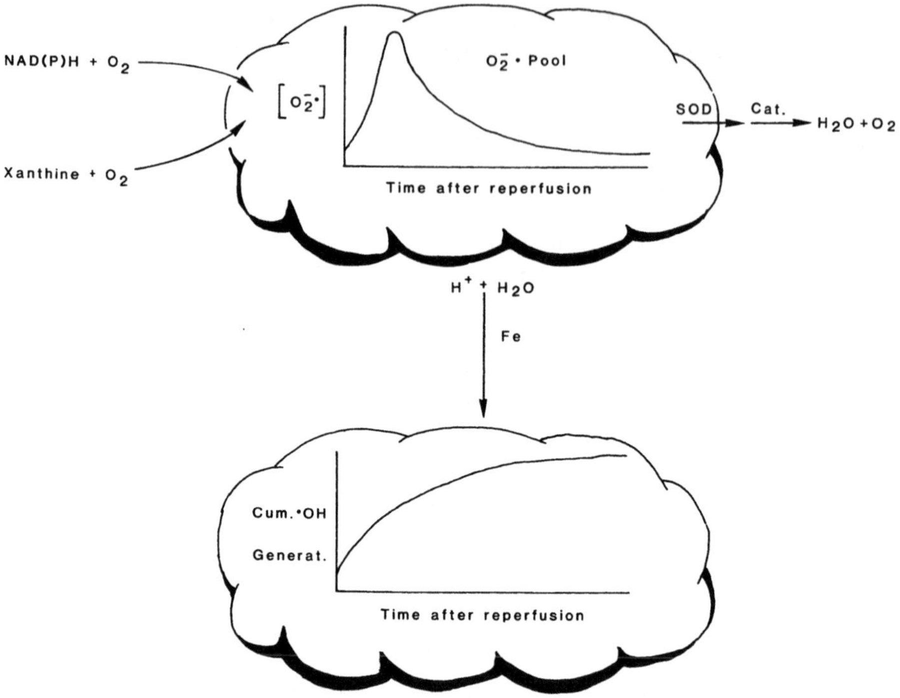

Fig. 10. A conceptual model for the role of iron in causing reperfusion damage following transient brain ischemia. Reperfusion enhances $\cdot O_2^-$ formation, e.g., by oxidation of NADH (and NADPH). In the presence of increased concentrations of $\cdot O_2^-$ and H^+, iron can become decompartmentalized and trigger the production of the very toxic $\cdot OH$ species. (Reproduced with permission from Babbs 1985)

Ca^{2+}. I wish to recall that glutamate release will activate the K/Q receptor-gated ion channel, causing Na^+ influx and depolarization, as well as of metabolotropic glutamate receptors, causing intracellular calcium release. Mechanisms for raising Ca_i^{2+} encompass entry through VSCCs or reversal of the $3Na^+/Ca^{2+}$ exchanger and release of Ca^{2+} from intracellular binding sites by acidosis and by formation of IP_3. Under these conditions, Ca_i^{2+} will rapidly reach the threshold value for activating the NSCC. Clearly, since glutamate release is what initiates depolarization and activation of calcium conductances, deafferentation will block calcium influx. Furthermore, since the NMDA-gated channel represents the major entry channel for calcium, it is not surprising that local injection of an NMDA antagonist can delay and curtail calcium entry. Probably, systemically injected MK-801 does not block NMDA-linked channels as efficiently, explaining its lack of effect in preventing calcium influx.

In moderately severe ischemia, or in hypoglycemia, calcium extrusion may be able to balance calcium influx, especially if the latter is prevented from increasing. In these situations, NMDA antagonists are probably efficacious because they reduce calcium influx through the major route of entry, in a situation in which ATP production may be sufficient to extrude calcium entering via non-NMDA-dependent channels. In this way, NMDA antagonists may prevent phase 2 ionic shifts from occurring, or reduce their incidence. Essentially, this could prevent extension of the infarct into the penumbra zone, or help in maintaining Ca_i^{2+} during ischemia and hypoglycemia from reaching concentrations precipitating adverse reactions.

In a subsequent version of the unifying hypothesis we concluded that it was not necessary to assume the activation of a NSCC, but that VSCCs and reversal of the $3Na^+/Ca^{2+}$ exchanger could provide the calcium leak in a situation in which the NMDA channel was blocked, or partially blocked (Siesjö et al. 1989). The essential feature of the hypothesis is that it is the presence or absence of a remaining energy source which determines whether or not NMDA antagonists can ameliorate brain damage. Thus, if no energy remains the cell will be flooded with calcium by non-NMDA-dependent routes. However, if some energy is produced this may be enough to extrude or sequester the calcium entering, thereby preventing calcium-related damage.

Antagonists of VSCCs

When dihydropyridines and other blockers of VSCCs were tested for their efficacy in ameliorating ischemic brain damage, it was tacitly assumed that massive entry of calcium mainly occurred via VSCCs. The results did not live up to the expectations. Thus, although pretreatment of animals with a dihydropyridine antagonist (nimodipine) reduced infarction size following MCA occlusion in rats (Mohamed et al. 1985), the effect was nil if the drug was given after the occlusion (Gotoh et al. 1986). Furthermore, although brain damage was ameliorated by posttreatment with nimodipine following global ischemia in monkeys (Steen et al. 1985), or with flunnarizine following forebrain ischemia in rats (Deshpande and Wieloch 1986), the literature abounds in reports showing either no, or only a moderate effect of such treatment. Possibly, this may be because of poor bioavailability of the drugs, since recent data demonstrate marked effects of one calcium antagonist, which is also a serotonin antagonist (Nakayama et al. 1988). It may be that blockade of VSCCs per se is not a very efficient way of preventing excessive calcium entry into cells, in a situation in which AOCCs remain patent. However, since VSCCs must provide one route of calcium entry, one can foresee the therapeutic advantage of combining blockers of AOCCs and VSCCs.

Free Radical Scavengers – Iron Chelators

As stated above, it has now been realized that free radical damage, perhaps mainly affecting the vasculature, is likely to occur after long periods of ischemia. Some promising results have been reported with a novel class of 21-aminosteroids, lipid-soluble drugs which probably exert their effects as chain breakers in free radical reactions. For example, one of these drugs was shown to reduce infarct volume to 15% of control in a model with 1 h of MCA occlusion, followed by 6 h of recovery (Silvia et al. 1987; see also Hall et al. 1988; Young et al. 1988). Results supporting the participation of free radicals in brain damage due to stroke are those showing that edema formation following long-lasting ischemia in gerbils is reduced by the free radical scavenger dimethyl thiourea, or by measures which reduce xanthine oxidase activity (Patt et al. 1988), and those showing that similar measures reduce infarct volume in permanent MCA occlusion in rats (Martz et al. 1989).

Other therapeutic attempts have been directed against the release of prooxidant iron, mainly by administration of free or conjugated desferrioxamine, an iron chelator (Michelson et al. 1988; Chan et al. 1987). Available results are promising, but not yet conclusive.

In general, results obtained with measures specifically directed towards iron-triggered production of free radicals suggest that it would be a gross simplification to assume that only one of the mediators discussed (EAAs, calcium, acidosis, and free radicals) are involved in ischemic (or hypoglycemic) and epileptic brain damage. Probably, efficient therapy of brain damage will be multimodal.

References

Aisen P (1979) Some physiochemical aspects of iron metabolism. In: CIBA Foundation Symposium, No. 51: Iron metabolism. Elsevier, Amsterdam, pp 1–17

Alberti KGMM, Cuthbert C (1982) The hydrogen ion in normal metabolism: a review. In: Porter R, Lawrenson G (eds) Metabolic acidosis. CIBA Foundation Symposium 87. London, Pitman Books Ltd, pp 1–19

Andiné P, Jacobson I, Hagberg H (1988) Calcium uptake evoked by electrical stimulation is enhanced postischemically and precedes delayed neuronal death in CA1 of rat hippocampus: involvement of *N*-methyl-D-aspartate receptors. J Cereb Blood Flow Metab 8:799–807

Ascher P, Nowak L (1987) Electrophysiological studies of NMDA receptors. TINS 10(7):284–288

Aust SD, Morehorse LA, Thomas CE (1985) Role of metals in oxygen radical reactions: hypothesis paper. J Free Radic Biol Med 1:3–25

Babbs CF (1985) Role of iron ions in the genesis of reperfusion injury following successful cardiopulmonary resuscitation: preliminary data and a biochemical hypothesis. Ann Emerg Med 14:777–783

Barber AA, Bernheim F (1967) Lipid peroxidation: its measurement, occurrence, and significance in animal tissues. Adv Gerontol Res 2:355–403

Bazan (1976) Free arachidonic acid and other lipids in the nervous system during early ischemia and after electroshock. Adv Exp Med Biol 72:317–335

Benveniste H, Jørgensen MB, Diemer NH, Hansen AJ (1988) Calcium accumulation by glutamate receptor activation is involved in hippocampal cell damage after ischemia. Acta Neurol Scand 78:529–536

Berridge MJ (1984) Inositol triphosphate and diacylglycerol as second messengers. Biochem J 221:345–360

Berridge MJ (1987) Inositol triphosphate and diacylglycerol: two interacting second messengers. Ann Rev Biochem 56:159–193

Boris-Möller F, Drakenberg T, Elmdén K, Forsén S, Siesjö BK (1988) Evidence against major compartmentalization of H^+ in ischemic rat brain tissue. Neurosci Lett 85:113–118

Boris-Möller F, Smith M-L, Siesjö BK (1989) Effects of hypothermia on brain ischemia: a comparison of intraischemic and postischemic hypothermia. J Cereb Blood Flow Metab 9(Suppl):5276
Branston NM, Strong AJ, Symon L (1977) Extracellular potassium activity, evoked potential and tissue blood flow. Relationships during progressive ischaemia in baboon cerebral cortex. J Neurol Sci 32:305–321
Busto R, Dietrich WD, Globus MY-T, Valdés I, Scheinberg P, Ginsberg M (1987) Small differences in intraischemic brain temperature critically determine the extent of ischemic neuronal injury. J Cereb Blood Flow Metab 7:729–738
Carafoli E (1982) The regulation of intracelular calcium. Adv Exp Med Biol 151:461–472
Carafoli E (1987) Intracellular calcium homeostasis. Annu Rev Biochem 56:395–433
Carter C, Benavides J, Legendre P, Vincent JD, Noel F, Thuret F, Lloyd KG, Arbilla S, Zivkovic B, MacKenzie ET, Scatton B, Langer SZ (1988) Ifenprodil and SL 82.0715 as cerebral anti-ischemic agents. II. Evidence for *N*-methyl-D-aspartate receptor antagonist properties. J Pharmacology and Experimental Therapeutics 247(3):1222–1232
Chan PH, Fishman RA (1985) Brain edema. In: Lajtha A (ed) Handbook of neurochemistry, vol 10. Plenum, New York, NY, pp 153–174
Chan PH, Schmidley JW, Fishman RA, Longar SM (1984) Brain injury, edema, and vascular permeability changes induced by oxygen-derived free radicals. Neurology 34:315–320
Chan PH, Longar S, Fishman RA (1987) Protective effects of liposome-entrapped superoxide dismutase on posttraumatic brain edema. Ann Neurol 21:540–547
Chien KR, Reeves JP, Buja LM, Bonte F, Parkey RW, Willerson JT (1981) Phospholipid alterations in canine ischemic myocardium. Temporal and topographical correlations with Tc-99m-PPi accumulation and in vitro sarcolemmal Ca^{2+} permeability defect. Circ Res 48:711–719
Choi DW (1985) Glutamate neurotoxicity in cortical cell culture is calcium dependent. Neurosci Lett 58:293–297
Choi DW (1987) Ionic dependence of glutamate neurotoxicity. J Neurosci 7:369–379
Choi DW (1988 a) Glutamate neurotoxicity and diseases of the nervous system. Neuron 1:623–634
Choi DW (1988 b) Calcium-mediated neurotoxicity: relationship to specific channel types and role in ischemic damage. TINS 11:465–469
Choi DW, Koh J-Y, Peter S (1988) Pharmacology of glutamate neurotoxicity in cortical cell culture: attenuation by NMDA antagonists. J Neurosci 8(1):185–196
Clark GD, Rothman SM (1987) Blockade of excitatory amino acid receptors protects anoxic hippocampal slices. Neurosci 21:665–761
Crichton RR (1979) Interactions between iron metabolism and oxygen activation. In: Oxygen free radicals and tissue damage. Ciba Foundation Symposium 65. New York, Excerpta Medica, pp 57–72
Demoupolos H, Flamm E, Seligman M, Power R, Pietronigro D, Ransohoff J (1977) Molecular pathology of lipids in CNS membranes. In: Jöbsis FF (ed) Oxygen and physiological function. Dallas, Texas, Professional Information Library, pp 491–508
Denton RM, McCormack JG (1985) Ca^{2+} transport by mammalian mitochondria and its role in hormone action. Am J Physiol 249:E543–E554
Deshpande JK, Wieloch T (1986) Flunarizine, a calcium entry blocker, ameliorates ischemic brain damage in the rat. Anesthesiology 64:215–224
Deshpande JK, Siesjö BK, Wieloch T (1987) Calcium accumulation and neuronal damage in the rat hippocampus following cerebral ischemia. J Cereb Blood Flow Metab 7:89–95
Fagg GE, Foster AC, Ganong AH (1986) Excitatory amino acid synaptic mechanisms and neurological function. TIPS – September: 357–363
Farber JL (1981) The role of calcium in cell death. Life Sci 29:1289–1295

Flamm ES, Demopoulos HB, Seligman ML et al. (1978) Free radicals in cerebral ischemia. Stroke 9:445–447

Fleckenstein A, Janke J, Doring HJ, Leder O (1974) Myocardial fiber necrosis due to intracellular Ca overload – a new principle in cardiac hypertrophy. Rec Adv Stud Cardiac Struct Metab 4:563–568

Folbergrová J, Ljunggren B, Norberg K, Siesjö BK (1974) Influence of complete ischemia on glycolytic metabolites, citric acid cycle intermediates, and associated amino acids in the rat cerebral cortex. Brain Res 80:265–279

Foster AC, Fagg GE (1987) Taking apart NMDA receptors. Nature (London) 329:395–396

Gardiner A, Smith M-L, Kågström E, Shohami E, Siesjö BK (1982) Influence of blood glucose concentration on brain lactate accumulation during severe hypoxia and subsequent recovery of brain energy metabolism. J Cereb Blood Flow Metab 2:429–438

Garthwaite G, Hajos F, Garthwaite J (1986) Ionic requirements for neurotoxic effects of excitatory amino acid analogues in rat cerebellar slices. Neurosci 18:437–447

Gebicki JM, Bielski BHJ (1981) Comparison of the capacities of the perhydroxyl and the superoxide radicals to initiate chain oxidation of linoleic acid. J Am Chem Soc 103(23):7020–7022

Gotoh O, Mohamed AA, McCulloch J, Graham DI, Harper AM, Teasdale GM (1986) Nimodipine and the haemodynamic and histopathological consequences of middle cerebral artery occlusion in the rat. J Cereb Blood Flow Metab 6:321–331

Gotti B, Duverger D, Bertin J, Carter C, Dupont R, Frost J, Gaudilliere B, MacKenzie ET, Rousseau J, Scatton B, Wick A (1988) Ifenprodil and SL 82.0715 as cerebral anti-ischemic agents. I. Evidence for efficacy in models of focal cerebral ischemia. J Pharmacology and Experimental Therapeutics 247(3):1211–1221

Grinstein S, Rothstein A (1986) Mechanisms of regulation of the Na^+/H^+ exchanger: topical review. J Membrane Biol 90:1–12

Grinstein S, Cohen S, Rothstein A (1984) Cytoplasmic pH regulation in thymic lymphocytes by an amiloride-sensitive Na^+/H^+ antiport. J Gen Physiol 83:341–369

Hachinski V, Norris JW (1985) The acute stroke. FA Davis Company, Philadelphia

Hall ED, Pazara KE, Braughler JM (1988) 21-Aminosteroid lipid peroxidation inhibitor U74006F protects against cerebral ischemia in gerbils. Stroke 19:997–1002

Halliwell B (1987) Oxidants and human disease: some new concepts. FASEB J 1:358–364

Halliwell B, Gutteridge JMC (1985) Oxygen radicals and the nervous system. TINS 8:22–26

Hansen AJ (1985) Effects of anoxia on ion distribution in the brain. Physiol Rev 65:101–148

Hansford RG (1985) Relation between mitochondrial calcium transport and control of energy metabolism. Rev Physiol Biochem Pharmacol 102:1–72

Harris RJ, Symon L (1984) Extracellular pH, potassium, and calcium activities in progressive ischaemia rat cortex. J Cereb Blood Flow Metab 4:178–186

Harris RJ, Symon L, Branston NM, Bayhan M (1981) Changes in extracellular calcium activity in cerebral ischaemia. J Cereb Blood Flow Metab 1:203–209

Hillered L, Ernster L, Siesjö BK (1984) Influence of in vitro lactic acidosis and hypercapnia on respiratory activity of isolated rat brain mitochondria. J Cereb Blood Flow Metab 4:430–437

Hochachka PW, Mommsen TP (1983) Protons and anaerobiosis. Science 219:1391–1397

Hossmann K-A (1985) Post-ischemic resuscitation of the brain: selective vulnerability versus global resistance. In: Kogure K, Hossmann K-A, Siesjö BK et al. (eds) Progress in brain research, vol 63. Elsevier, pp 3–17

Jean T, Frelin C, Vigne P, Lazdunski M (1986) The Na^+/H^+ exchange system in glial cell lines. Properties and activation by an hyperosmotic shock. Eur J Biochem 160(2):211–219

Kaplan J, Dimlich RVW, Biros MH, Hedges J (1987) Mechanisms of ischemic cerebral injury. Resuscitation 15:149–158
Komara JS, Nayini NR, Bialick HA, Indrieri RJ, Evans AT, Garritano AM, White BC, Aust SD (1986) Brain iron delocalization and lipid peroxidation following cardiac arrest. Ann Emerg Med 15:384–389
Kraig RP, Chesler M (1989) Astrocytic acidosis in hyperglycemia and complete ischemia. J Cereb Blood Flow Metab (in press)
Kraig RP, Pulsinelli WA, Plum F (1985) Hydrogen ion buffering during complete brain ischemia. Brain Res 342:281–290
Kraig RP, Pulsinelli WA, Plum F (1986) Carbonic acid buffer changes during complete brain ischemia. Am J Physiol 250 (Regulatory Integrative Comp Physiol 19):R348–R357
Kraig RP, Petito CK, Plum F, Pulsinelli WA (1987) Hydrogen ions kill brain at concentrations reached in ischemia. J Cereb Blood Flow Metab 7:379–386
Krause GS, White BC, Aust SD, Nayini NR, Kusum Kumar MBBS (1988) Brain cell death following ischemia and reperfusion: a proposed biochemical suquence. Crit Care Med 16:714–726
Leonard JP, Salpeter MM (1979) Agonist-induced myopathy at the neuromuscular junction is mediated by calcium. J Cell Biol 82:811–819
Ljunggren B, Schutz H, Siesjö BK (1974a) Changes in energy state and acid-base parameters of the rat brain during complete compression ischemia. Brain Res 73:277–289
Ljunggren B, Ratcheson RA, Siesjö BK (1974b) Complete metabolic state following complete compression ischemia. Brain Res 73:291–307
Ljunggren B, Norberg K, Siesjö BK (1974c) Influence of tissue acidosis upon restitution of brain energy metabolism following total ischemia. Brain Res 77:173–186
Lowry OH, Passonneau JV, Hasselberger FX, Schultz DW (1964) Effect of ischemia on known substrates and cofactors of the glycolytic pathway in brain. J Biol Chem 239:18–30
MacDermott AB, Dale N (1987) Receptors, ion channels and synaptic potentials underlying the integrative actions of excitatory amino acids. TINS 10(7):280–284
Mahnensmith RL, Aronsen PS (1985) The plasma membrane sodium-hydrogen exchanger and its role in physiological and pathophysiological processes. Circ Res 57:773–788
Martz D, Rayos G, Schielke GP, Betz AL (1989) Allopurinol and dimethylthiourea reduce brain infarction following middle cerebral artery occlusion in the rat. Stroke, in press
Mayer ML, Westbrook GL (1987) The physiology of excitatory amino acids in the vertebrate central nervous system. Prog Neurobiol 28:197–276
McCord JM (1985) Oxygen-derived free radicals in postischemic tissue injury. The New England Journal of Medicine 312(3):159–163
Michelson AM, Jadot G, Puget K (1988) Treatment of brain trauma with liposomal superoxide dismutase. Free Rad Res Comms 4(4):209–224
Miller RJ (1987) Multiple calcium channels and neuronal function. Science 235:46–52
Mohamed AA, Gotoh O, Graham DI, Osborne KA, McCulloch JM, Mendelow AD, Teasdale GM, Harper AM (1985) Effect of pretreatment with the calcium antagonist nimodipine on local cerebral blood flow and histopathology after middle cerebral artery occlusion. Ann Neurol 18:705–711
Myers RE (1979a) Lactic acid accumulation as cause of brain edema and cerebral necrosis resulting from oxygen deprivation. In: Korobkin R, Guilleminault G (eds) Advances in perinatal neurology. Spectrum, New York, pp 85–114
Myers RE (1979b) A unitary theory of causation of anoxic and hypoxic brain pathology. In: Fahn S, Davis JN, Rowland LP (eds) Cerebral hypoxia and its consequences. Adv Neurol 26, Raven Press, New York
Nakayama H, Ginsberg MD, Dietrich WD (1988) Emopamil, a novel calcium channel blocker and serotonin S_2 antagonist markedly reduces infarct size following middle cerebral artery occlusion in the rat. Neurology 38:1667–1673

Nicholson C (1980) Dynamics of the brain cell microenvironment. Neurosci Res Program Bull 18:177–322
Nicotera P, Harzell P, Davis G, Orrenius S (1986) The formation of plasma membrane blebs in hepatocytes exposed to agents that increase cytosolic Ca^{2+} is mediated by the activation of a non-lysosomal proteolytic system. FEBS Lett 209:139–144
Nordström C-H, Siesjö BK (1978) Effects of phenobarbital in cerebral ischemia. Part I: Cerebral energy metabolism during pronounced incomplete ischemia. Stroke 9:327–335
Olney J (1978) Neurotoxicity of excitatory amino acids. In: McGeer EG, Olney JW, McGeer PL (eds) Kainic as a tool in neurobiology. Raven Press, New York, pp 95–121
Orrenius S, McConkey DJ, Jones DP, Nicotera P (1988) Ca^{2+}-activated mechanisms in toxicity and programmed cell death. ISI Atlas Sci: Pharmacology 2:319–324
Oyzuart E, Graham DI, Woodruff GN, McCulloch J (1988) Protective effect of the glutamate antagonist, MK-801 in focal cerebral ischemia in the cat. J Cereb Blood Flow Metab 8:138–143
Park CK, Nehls DG, Graham DI, Teasdale GM, McCulloch J (1988) The glutamate antagonist MK-801 reduces focal ischemic brain damage in the rat. Ann Neurol 24:543–551
Patt A, Harken AH, Burton LK, Rodell TC, Piermattei D, Schorr WJ, Parker NB, Berger EM, Horesh IR, Terada LS, Linas SL, Cheronis JC, Repine JE (1988) Xanthine oxidase-derived hydrogen peroxide contributes to ischemia reperfusion-induced edema in gerbil brains. J Clin Invest 81:1556–1562
Plum F (1983) What causes infarction in ischemic brain? The Robert Wartenberg Lecture. Neurology 33:222–233
Rasmussen H (1986) The calcium messenger system. N Engl J Med 314:1094–1101
Rasmussen H, Waisman DM (1983) Modulation of cell function in the calcium messenger system. Rev Physiol Biochem Pharmacol 95:111–148
Rehncrona S, Nielsen Hauge H, Siesjö BK (1989) Enhancement of iron-catalyzed free radical formation by acidosis in brain homogenates: difference in effect by lactic acid and CO_2. J Cereb Blood Flow Metab 9:65–70
Reynolds IJ, Miller RJ (1988) Multiple sites for the regulation of the *N*-methyl-D-aspartate receptor. Mol Pharmacol 33:581–584
Roos A, Boron WF (1981) Intracellular pH. Physiol Rev 61:296–434
Rothman SM, Olney JW (1986) Glutamate and the pathophysiology of hypoxic-ischemic brain damage. Ann Neurol 19:105–111
Rothman SM, Thurston JH, Hauhart RE (1987) Delayed neurotoxicity of excitatory amino acids in vitro. Neurosci 22(2):471–480
Safar P (1986) Cerebral resuscitation after cardiac arrest: a review. Circulation 74 (suppl IV):138–153
Salford LG, Plum F, Siesjö BK (1973) Graded hypoxia-oligemia in rat brain. I. Biochemical alterations and their implications. Arch Neurol 29:227–233
Siesjö BK (1978) Brain energy metabolism. John Wiley, Chichester
Siesjö BK (1981) Cell damage in the brain: a speculative synthesis. J Cereb Blood Flow Metab 1:155–185
Siesjö BK (1984) Cerebral circulation and metabolism. J Neurosurg 60:883–908
Siesjö BK (1985) Acid-base homeostasis in the brain: physiology, chemistry, and neurochemical pathology. In: Kongure K, Hossmann K-A, Siesjö BK, Welsh FA (eds) Progress in brain research. Elsevier Science Publishers B.V. (Biomedicial Division), vol 63, pp 121–154
Siesjö BK (1988a) Mechanisms of ischemic brain damage. Crit Care Med 16:954–963
Siesjö BK (1988b) Historical overview. Calcium, ischemia, and death of brain cells. Ann NY Acad Sci 522:638–661
Siesjö BK (1988c) Hypoglycemia, brain metabolism, and brain damage. Diabetes/Metabolism Reviews 4(2):113–144
Siesjö BK (1988) Acidosis and ischemic brain damage. Neurochem Pathol 9:31–88

Siesjö BK, Nilsson L (1971) The influence of arterial hypoxemia upon labile phosphates and upon extracellular and intracellular lactate and pyruvate concentration in the rat brain. Scand J Clin Lab Invest 27:83–96

Siesjö BK, Wieloch T (1985) Cerebral metabolism in ischemia: neurochemical basis for therapy. Br J Anaesth 57:47–62

Siesjö BK, Bengtsson F (1989) Calcium fluxes, calcium antagonists, and calcium-related pathology in brain ischemia, hypoglycemia, and spreading depression: a unifying hypothesis. J Cereb Blood Flow Metab. 9:127–140

Siesjö BK, Bendek G, Koide T, Westerberg E, Wieloch T (1985) Influence of acidosis on lipid peroxidation in brain tissues in vitro. J Cereb Blood Flow Metab 5:253–258

Siesjö BK, Smith M-L, Warner DS (1987) Acidosis and ischemic brain damage. In: Raichle ME, Powers WJ (eds) Cerebrovascular diseases. Raven Press, New York, pp 83–95

Siesjö BK, Bengtsson F, Grampp W, Theander S (1989) Calcium, excitotoxins and neuronal death in the brain. Ann NY Acad Sci, in press

Silvia RC, Piercey MF, Hoffmann WE, Chase RL, Braughler JM, Tang AH (1987) U-74006F, an inhibitor of lipid peroxidation, protects against lesion development following experimental stroke in the cat: histological and metabolic analysis. Soc Neurosci Abst 13:1495

Smith M-L, van Hanwehr R, Siesjö BK (1986) Changes in extra- and intracellular pH in the brain during and following ischemia in hyperglycemic and in moderately hypoglycemic rats. J Cereb Blood Flow Metabol 6:574–583

Steen PA, Gisvold SE, Milde JH, Newberg LA, Scheithauer BW, Lanier WL, Michenfelder JD (1985) Nimodipine improves outcome when given after complete cerebral ischemia in primates. Anesthesiology 62:406–414

Watkins JC, Olverman HJ (1987) Agonists and antagonists for excitatory amino acid receptors. TINS 10(7):265–272

Westerberg E, Kehr J, Ungerstedt U, Wieloch T (1988) The NMDA-antagonist MK-801 reduces extracellular amino acid levels during hypoglycemia and prevents striatal damage. Neurosci Res Commun 3:151–158

White BC, Hildebrand JF, Evans AT, Aronson L, Indrieri RJ, Hoehner T, Fox L, Huang R, Johns D (1985) Prolonged cardiac arrest and resuscitation in dogs: brain mitochondrial function with different artificial perfusion methods. Ann Emerg Med 14(5):383–388

Wieloch T (1985) Hypoglycemia-induced neuronal damage is prevented by a *N*-methyl-D-aspartate receptor antagonist. Science 230:681–683

Wieloch T, Harris RJ, Symon L, Siesjö BK (1984) Influence of severe hypoglycemia on brain extracellular calcium and potassium activities, energy and phospholipid metabolism. J Neurochem 43:160–168

Wrogemann K, Pena SDJ (1976) Mitochondrial calcium overload: a general mechanism for cell-necrosis in muscle diseases. Lancet I:672–674

Young W, Wojak JC, DeCrescito V (1988) 21-Aminosteroid reduces ion shifts and edema in the rat middle cerebral artery occlusion model of regional ischemia. Stroke 19:1013–1019

Cardiopulmonary Resuscitation – State of the Art

F. W. Ahnefeld and K. H. Lindner

Clinical practice and new experimental evidence have brought changes to the technique of cardiopulmonary resuscitation with respect to both the mechanical measures, drug therapy, and the technique of defibrillation. We would like to discuss this topic in three separate sections: (1) Basic principles of cardiopulmonary resuscitation; (2) advanced principles of cardiopulmonary resuscitation; and (3) the potentials and limits of cardiopulmonary resuscitation. The following summary refers only to the more important changes recently made, and does not include the basic essentials of the procedures which are already well known.

Basic Principles of Cardiopulmonary Resuscitation

Diagnosis of Cardiocirculatory Arrest

Cardiopulmonary resuscitation should only be started when the carotid pulse is absent. When carotid artery pulsation is only weak, cardiac massage should not be used because cardiac massage hinders the spontaneously beating heart, and thus reduces cardiac output.

Precordial Thump

As a first step, the precordial thump is only employed when cardiocirculatory arrest is witnessed, when the heart has not been arrested for longer than 30 s, and when there is severe bradycardia going into asystole or ventricular tachycardia leading into ventricular fibrillation [4, 43, 58]. Under these circumstances, a forcible thump with the fist to the center of the sternum from a height of about 30 cm can evoke electrical activity which produces a myocardial contraction. In isolated cases, repeated thumps at intervals of 1–2 s can induce effective myocardial contractions (pacing). The precordial thump is not without its hazards, because it can convert bradycardia and ventricular tachycardia into ventricular fibrillation [61].

The precordial thump is an attempt to convert mechanical energy into an organized electrical impulse, which is followed by a myocardial contraction. Electromechanical coupling must be intact in order for the thump to be effective. For this reason, the precordial thump is not a routine procedure at the beginning of every cardiopulmonary resuscitation, and should only be performed when cardiopulmonary arrest is witnessed.

Bolus Obstruction

Recommendations for the management of foreign body aspiration have changed. Aspiration usually occurs suddenly, while the victim is eating. Asphyxia develops very quickly, and is followed by unconsciousness after a few minutes, which in turn is followed by cardiac arrest. When the upper airways are completely blocked, the victim wretches, grasps his neck in panic (choking sign) and can neither breath nor speak. In most cases the foreign body is in the hypopharynx, lying over the entrance to the larynx.

If the patient is still conscious, he should be urged to cough and spit the foreign body out. If he does not manage to do this, use of the abdominal thrust is recommended [23, 24]; this should be done while standing behind the victim. Intermittent thrusts are applied between the navel and the xiphoid, which are repeated either until the foreign body is expelled, or until the patient becomes unconscious.

When the victim becomes unconscious, he should be laid flat on his back. Manual removal of the foreign body should be attempted (finger sweep), and ventilation applied. With a strong slow insufflation, one can often still bring a certain amount of air into the lungs. If ventilation is nevertheless not possible, the abdominal thrusts should be performed up to 6–10 times. If you have no success try again to reach the foreign body with your fingers and attempt ventilation.

Abdominal thrusts have potential complications [7, 11, 46, 56]. They can cause regurgitation of gastric contents, gastric rupture, liver rupture, or even aortic injury.

Blows applied between the shoulder blades, so-called back blows, as formerly recommended for the removal of a foreign body from the upper airways, have been found to occasionally cause the offending bolus to pass more deeply [12, 13]. Use of abdominal thrusts is also still a matter for argument, the efficacy of this procedure is based on individual observations [46]. Through the rise in intraabdominal pressure, an artificial cough is produced. The results of recent investigations indicate, however, that neither abdominal nor chest thrusts, nor blows between the shoulder blades can cause as high an air flow and pressure as that of a natural cough [49].

Abdominal thrusts should not be applied in infants – here the combination of back blows and chest thrusts is recommended – and in grossly obese persons or women in advanced stages of pregnancy – here chest thrusts are recommended.

As an alternative to the use of abdominal or chest thrusts, a doctor with appropriate equipment and training can visualize the larynx with a laryngoscope and attempt to remove the foreign body with Magill forceps. As an ultimate measure, coniotomy can be carried out.

External Cardiac Compression

Two different mechanisms can contribute to the blood flow during cardiopulmonary resuscitation (CPR) when external cardiac massage is applied. It was

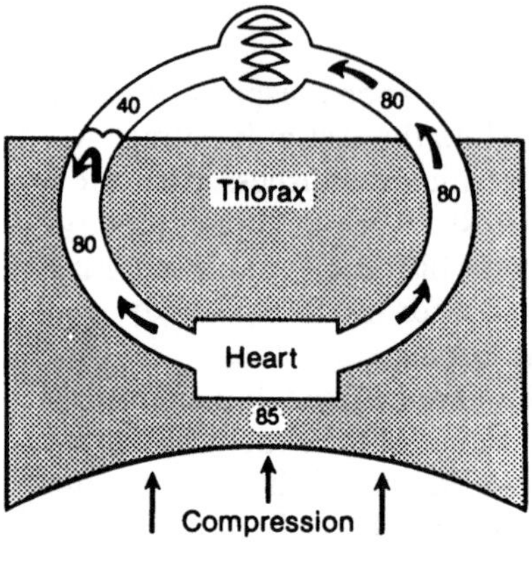

Fig. 1. Thoracic pump mechanism: Generalized changes in intrathoracic pressure lead to the circulation of blood and the direction of flow is determined by collapse of the greater veins of the upper thoracic inlet and the valves in the jugular and subclavian veins

initially thought that the forward flow of blood was caused by compression of the heart between the sternum and the vertebral column [1, 29]. More recent studies indicate that generalized changes in intrathoracic pressure lead to the circulation of blood, and that the direction of flow is determined by collapse of the greater veins at the upper thoracic inlet and the valves in the jugular and subclavian veins [10, 40, 50, 60] (Fig. 1). It appears that in the adult, blood flow is generated by both cardiac compression and the thoracic pump mechanism. It seems probable that during the course of a single compression, the primary mechanism alters in that an effective direct cardiac compression only occurs at the point of maximal compression between the sternum and vertebral column. Even under optimal conditions, cardiac minute volume during external cardiac massage is only 20%–40% of the normal resting level.

Various modifications of the mechanical measures applied have been tested in order to improve on this. These include:

1. Simultaneous ventilation and chest compression at a rate of 40/min [6]
2. Increased depth of compression and increased compression rate to 150/min
3. The continuous application of abdominal compression either manually or with an abdominal binder [3, 41], and interposed abdominal compression [45], i.e., abdominal compression only during the cardiac relaxation phase

To date, none of these modifications could be shown, either in animal experiments or in clinical practice, to increase survival rates or to improve the cerebral outcome of resuscitation, and are therefore not recommended for general use.

It is particularly important to ensure that the compression and the relaxation phase of external cardiac massage are both of equal duration. The compression phase should not be too short, as this would result in poor functioning of the thoracic pump mechanism. On the other hand, it must not be too long, as this would reduce the time available for coronary perfusion.

Ventilation

With respect to ventilation, in 1980 the American Heart Association recommended the following [51]:

1. Cardiopulmonary resuscitation should always begin with four quick, full insufflations without waiting for full lung deflation between breaths.
2. In one-rescuer cardiopulmonary resuscitation two full breaths, without allowing time for full lung deflation between breaths, are delivered after each cycle of 15 compressions.
3. In two-rescuer cardiopulmonary resuscitation, one interposed breath is delivered after five compressions without a pause between.

Recent investigations have revealed a number of flaws in these guidelines:

1. During cardiac arrest and resuscitation, pathological pulmonary changes which are somewhat similar to pulmonary edema develop, with a reduction in compliance, and a marked hypoxemia and hypercapnia. The cause of the changes is not clear, but it seems probable that as in the case of cardiogenic shock, these pulmonary changes result from a combination of a reduced cardiac minute volume and an increased pulmonary artery pressure.
2. During resuscitation the closing pressure of the lower esophageal sphincter is below 15 cm of water.
3. During two rescuer cardiopulmonary resuscitation with a compression rate of 60/min and a compression to relaxation of 1 : 1, there is only 0.5 s left for the interposed ventilation.

New recommendations have been formulated as a result of these observations [52]:

1. Start CPR with two slow lung inflations.
2. Wait for full expiration before beginning second inflation.
3. Pause for ventilation between compressions.
4. Consider use of cricoid pressure.

Resuscitation should no longer be started with four "quick," but with two "slow" insufflations. In order to avoid an unnecessary increase in ventilation pressure, the second insufflation should not be applied until full passive deflation has occurred. Between the series of compressions a pause of 1–1.5 s for one insufflation should be kept, because inspiratory flow rate and ventilation pressure are reduced by prolonging the inspiratory time. In this way, gastric insufflation, regurgitation, and aspiration are avoided, or at least reduced.

Head-tilt/chin-lift is the only open-the-airway technique recommended for the lay public. For the sake of simplicity, and effectiveness, it is recommended that only one airway management technique be taught to the lay rescuer. Other groups can and should be taught the jaw-thrust.

Slightly different techniques are recommended for one- and two-rescuer cardiopulmonary resuscitation. There is no doubt, however, that two-rescuer cardiopulmonary resuscitation is technically easier and more effective, but, the two-rescuer procedures should only be taught to health care providers and professional rescuers, while lay rescuers may be taught this procedure, the likelihood of their using this technique is limited. Instructional time may well be better spent practicing the one-rescuer procedure rather than learning an additional method.

The mechanical measures for cardiopulmonary resuscitation should be applied in stages. Place the victim supine and horizontal, then clear the airway.

In one-rescuer cardiopulmonary resuscitation:

1. Ventilate two times at 1–1.5 s per inspiration
2. Feel carotid pulse (5–10 s)
3. If no pulse, begin chest compression
4. Compression rate: 80–100/min (15 compressions in approximately 10 s)
5. Compression/ventilation ratio: 15 compressions to two ventilations per cycle
6. Two ventilations in approximately 5 s
7. Do four cycles of 15 compressions and two ventilations (for four cycles you need approximately 60 s)
8. Feel for the carotid pulse (5 s)
9. If no pulse, resume compression/ventilation for a further four cycles

The first three stages of two-rescuer cardiopulmonary resuscitation are the same as for one-rescuer cardiopulmonary resuscitation:

1. The compression rate is 80–100/min (five in 3–4 s).
2. The compression/ventilation ratio is five compressions to one ventilation per cycle.
3. Ventilation is performed in a pause of 1–1.5 s between compressions; compression should be started immediately at the end of inspiration.
4. Do a minimum of ten cycles of five compressions and one ventilation.
5. If you can feel no pulse, resume compression/ventilation for a further ten cycles.

Child cardiopulmonary resuscitation parallels adult cardiopulmonary resuscitation with one exception. The ratio of compression to ventilation for children is 5:1 in both one- and two-rescuer cardiopulmonary resuscitation. In infants, compressions are performed one fingerbreadth below an imaginary line between the nipples. The compression rate is at least 100/min, the compression/ventilation ratio is five compressions to one slow ventilation per cycle.

Advanced Principles of Cardiopulmonary Resuscitation

Before more specific measures (drug application, defibrillation) can be taken, an ECG diagnosis of the type of cardiac arrest is necessary. This diagnosis can broadly be defined as:

1. Ventricular fibrillation
2. Asystole
3. Electromechanical dissociation

Modes of Drug Application

The following four routes of drug application can be used: In most cases a peripheral vein can be cannulated after mechanical cardiopulmonary resuscitation has been started. Peripheral circulation is not very adequate during cardiopulmonary resuscitation, however, and the injection of all drugs must always be followed by a few milliliters of saline in order to flush the substance into the central circulation. One of the large lumen veins of the lower arm or at the elbow should be selected. The external jugular vein can also be punctured. The veins at the back of the hand are usually difficult to find under these conditions.

Central Venous Route

The routine introduction of a central venous line during cardiopulmonary resuscitation is not recommended – cardiac massage has to be interrupted, working conditions are usually not sterile, and the complication rate is higher than that during routine clinical use.

Endobronchial Application

If there is difficulty in placing an intravenous line within a relatively short space of time, epinephrine, lidocaine, and atropine can be given at up to double the intravenous dose when diluted to 10 ml with saline and injected via an endotracheal tube as far as possible into the bronchial tree [18]. Under these conditions the action of these drugs is almost as rapid as when given intravenously.

Intracardiac Injection

Intracardiac injection should no longer be used as a routine procedure for drug application during CPR. It is not without its dangers because injury of the surrounding tissues and of the heart itself can occur. Mechanical cardiopulmonary resuscitation must be interrupted during the procedure, and each injection requires renewed puncture.

Substances and Dosages

The following drugs are used during cardiopulmonary resuscitation: oxygen, adrenaline, sodium bicarbonate, lidocaine, and occasionally calcium.

Oxygen

The earliest possible ventilation using manual breathing devices with high oxygen concentration either by mask or after intubation can reduce the extent of hypoxemia in the presence of minimum circulation. Although ventilation is usually adequate in mouth-to-nose ventilation, the expired air of the rescuer contains only about 16%–17% oxygen. The alveolar partial oxygen pressure does not exceed 80 mmHg in this case. Since the stroke volume achieved with external cardiac compression is only about 20%–40% of normal, mixed venous blood is maximally desoxygenated. Additional ventilation-perfusion disorders, aspiration or pulmonary edema reduce the arterial partial oxygen pressure to a critical level shunt formation, in this situation. Due to the impaired organ perfusion during reanimation, an attempt should be made to avoid additional hypoxemia by ventilation with a high oxygen concentration (over 80%).

Adrenaline

Adrenaline is the drug of choice in improving the effectivity of mechanical measures during all forms of cardiac arrest (Fig. 2). Success rates are improved when asystole and electromechanical dissociation are present. The drug therapy of ventricular fibrillation is somewhat different, however. It has previously been stated that adrenaline converts fine ventricular fibrillation to slower, coarser fibrillation which is more easily defibrillated by stimulation of the $beta_1$-receptors. This assumption has not as yet been experimentally proved. It may be that noradrenaline is a good alternative drug, because we were able to show, using an electrically induced ventricular fibrillation model, that restoration of spontaneous circulation is possible in a significantly shorter time than with adrenaline [31]. This is probably because noradrenaline improves the balance between myocardial oxygen delivery and consumption during CPR [33].

The desired effect of adrenaline during cardiopulmonary resuscitation is caused by the stimulation of alpha-receptors [27, 37]. At the same time, beta-receptors are also stimulated, however. In some cases this can lead to an increase in myocardial oxygen requirements during resuscitation immediately after a spontaneous circulation has been established, and also to malignant tachyarrhythmias, and to a recurrence of cardiac arrest [34, 44, 62]. Therefore, adrenaline should not be given routinely before every attempt at defibrillation.

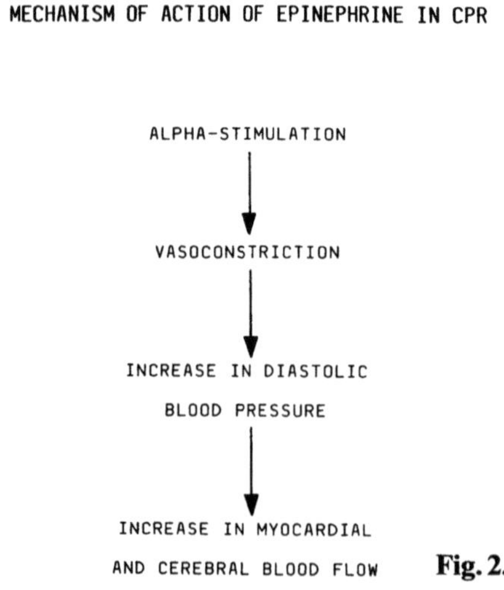

Fig. 2. Mechanism of action of epinephrine in CPR

Until further evidence can be presented, the use of adrenaline should only be considered, when three consecutive DC shocks have failed to convert ventricular fibrillation.

The recommended dosage of adrenaline in all three forms of cardiac arrest is 0.5–1.0 mg given undiluted or diluted to 10 ml with saline intravenously. This same dose is repeated at intervals of 5 min as necessary. This dosage has been established on an empirical basis. It may well be that depending on the duration of hypoxia a higher dose of up to 3 mg adrenaline as a bolus injection can improve the results of cardiac resuscitation. It must be borne in mind, however, that the incidence of a severe neurologic deficit may be higher.

Sodium Bicarbonate

The success of resuscitation is probably not improved with sodium bicarbonate even after prolonged times of hypoxia [20, 38]. Bicarbonate should, if at all, only be used after other measures such as defibrillation, adrenaline injection, and endotracheal intubation have been implemented. Thus, bicarbonate is no longer recommended as a routine drug for cardiopulmonary resuscitation.

The too rapid, or too generous infusion of bicarbonate into the minimal circulation achieved by external cardiac compression leads to a metabolic alkalosis which in turn can induce a state of tonic myocardial concentration and to a reduction in peripheral oxygen release. When arrest is secondary to, or complicated by disturbances in pulmonary function, as, for example, by massive aspiration or by pulmonary edema, too high a dose of bicarbonate will also lead to a rise in partial pressure of carbon dioxide in arterial and venous blood [59].

Finally, and again because of the reduced circulation during cardiopulmonary resuscitation, the serum sodium concentration, and hence the serum osmolality rise rapidly and to such a degree that cerebral recovery may be jeopardized [2, 32, 36].

The following dosage should never be exceeded: 1 mmol = 1 ml/kg body weight i.v. of 8.4% sodium bicarbonate solution during 10 min of resuscitation, with a repeat dosage of 0.5 mmol = 0.5 ml/kg body weight i.v. every 10 min.

After restoration of spontaneous circulation an arterial blood gas analysis should determine whether to carry out buffer therapy. It should be remembered that a pH value of as low as 7.2 improves cardiac contractility.

Lidocaine

Following successful defibrillation, lidocaine is given prophylactically in order to prevent renewed ventricular fibrillation and to treat ventricular premature beats [15, 28, 30]. A further indication for use is the treatment of resistant ventricular fibrillation, but here the role of lidocaine is as yet unproven [22]. Nevertheless, if repeated defibrillation is without success despite having given epinephrine, lidocaine can be given 30–120 s before further attempts of defibrillation.

Larger amounts, and more frequent injections rapidly lead to toxic blood levels in the minimal circulation present during cardiopulmonary resuscitation [8]. Lidocaine can also cause a peripheral vasodilation and raise the defibrillation threshold [16, 25].

The recommended dosage is 1.0 mg/kg body weight i.v. of the 2% solution (1 ml = 200 mg), with a repeat dosage of 0.5 mg/kg body weight after 8–10 min up to a total dose of 3 mg/kg body weight.

Calcium

Electromechanical dissociation was previously considered an indication for the additional injection of calcium salts to improve electromechanical coupling. More recent studies have raised doubts as to the therapeutic value of calcium salts in cardiopulmonary resuscitation [5, 14]. Calcium is definitely indicated for the treatment of simultaneous hyperkalemia, hypocalcemia (e.g., after mass transfusion), and overdose of calcium-blocking agents. These conditions are at present the only indications for calcium treatment.

Precautions. Excessive dosage and repeated injections within short periods of time during external cardiac compression can elevate the level of ionized calcium and lead to sinus node depression and coronary spasms which may produce systolic cardiac arrest.

Interactions. Due to precipitation of calcium carbonate, calcium salts should not be administered together with a sodium bicarbonate infusion.

The dosage recommended is calcium chloride 10% 2 ml/70 kg body weight i.v. (2–4 mg/kg body weight) and calcium gluconate 10% 5–8 ml/70 kg body weight i.v., with a repeat dosage same as the initial dose, after 10 min at the earliest.

Potassium Chloride

An injection of potassium chloride (20 mmol i.v. maximum), in the absence of data on serum electrolyte levels, should only be considered for resistant ventricular fibrillation. There are as yet no adequate study results concerning its effectiveness.

Electrotherapy

Ventricular fibrillation should be treated as early as possible with electrical defibrillation which causes the instantaneous depolarization of a large number of myocardial cells. If the electrodes are placed too close together, the electrical current does not reach an adequate amount of the myocardium. For this reason, one electrode should be placed on the right side of the chest wall, beneath the clavicle, and next to the sternum, while the second electrode is placed at the apex beat in order that the current may pass through the longitudinal axis of the heart. It is not the amount of energy applied for defibrillation that is important, but the amount of current which flows through the heart.

The recommendations shown in Fig. 3 are aimed at providing a sufficient flow of current through the heart in order to improve the success of defibril-

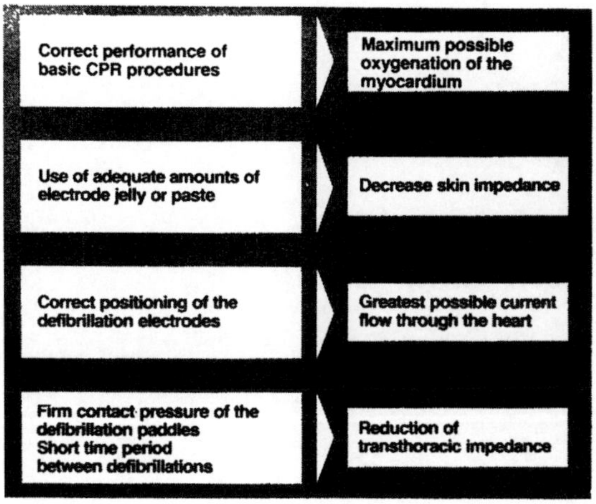

Fig. 3. Optimal electrical defibrillation

ation. When repeated defibrillation is necessary this should be carried out as quickly as possible.

Defibrillation may remain without success despite maximal energy application and an optimal current flow. This can be because cardiac arrest is already of long duration and/or the myocardium is already irreversibly damaged. It can also be because of an imbalance between myocardial oxygen requirements and reduced oxygen supply during cardiopulmonary resuscitation. Thus, causes of unsuccessful defibrillation include:

1. Inadequate current flow through the heart.
2. Disparity between myocardial oxygen need and myocardial oxygen supply during external cardiac compression.
3. Prolonged duration of cardiac circulatory arrest and thus irreversible damage to the myocardium.

In general, it can be said that observed ventricular fibrillation should be defibrillated as quickly as possible. Should the first defibrillation not result in a stable cardiac rhythm, the further chances of success depend largely on the quality of cardiopulmonary resuscitation which in turn determines whether myocardial oxygen supply is adequate. In these cases mechanical measures are necessary in order to ensure the success of defibrillation.

Practical Procedures According to ECG Criteria

The ECG diagnosis of cardiac arrest can be differentiated as follows: (1) Ventricular fibrillation, pulseless ventricular tachycardia; (2) asystole; and (3) electromechanical dissociation. The further procedure, which depends on the diagnosis made, is shown in the following descriptions.

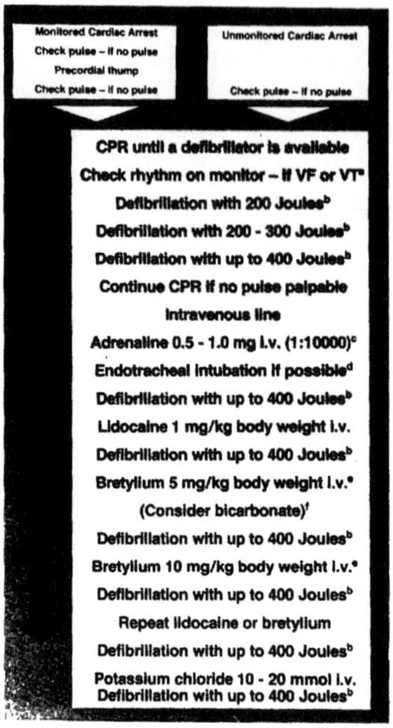

Fig. 4. Ventricular fibrillation and pulseless ventricular tachycardia

Ventricular Fibrillation and Pulseless Ventricular Tachycardia

In Fig. 4 it is assumed that there is continuing ventricular fibrillation after each step in the procedure. In addition:

1. Ventricular tachycardia (VT) without a palpable carotid pulse is treated like ventricular fibrillation (VF).
2. Check pulse and rhythm after each defibrillation. If there is renewed ventricular fibrillation, the energy level with which defibrillation was successfully achieved should be chosen for the next defibrillation.
3. Adrenaline should be repeated every 5 min at the dose indicated.
4. Endotracheal intubation should be instituted as soon as possible parallel to the other measures. However, if the patient can be adequately ventilated without intubation, defibrillation and adrenaline administration should not be delayed by time-consuming attempts at intubation.
5. The antiarrhythmic agent, bretylium tosylate, which can be used as a primary agent in the treatment of therapy-resistant ventricular fibrillation, is not permitted in some countries (e.g., FRG). Its cardiovascular action is complex and initially leads to a release of catecholamines after injection, followed by a postganglionic adrenergic blocking action with concomitant arterial hypotension. Although a so-called chemical defibrillation has been observed with bretylium, direct comparison does not show this agent to be superior to lidocaine in the treatment of resistant ventricular fibrillation. Since there is a hypotensive effect even under external cardiac compression,

repeated injections of lidocaine at 0.5 mg/kg body weight in intervals of 10 min up to a total dose of 3 mg/kg body weight are also recommended in this stage of the algorithm.

6. The routine use of sodium bicarbonate is not recommended. If it is used at all, it should first be given at this stage by i.v. infusion at a dosage of 1 mmol/kg body weight over a period of 10 min.

Asystole

In Fig. 5 it is assumed that asystole persists. Asystole should be demonstrated in two ECG leads. If the type of rhythm present cannot be differentiated, and if there is a possibility that ventricular fibrillation is present, the patient should first be defibrillated.

1. Adrenaline should be repeated every 5 min in the indicated dose.
2. Endotracheal intubation should be instituted as soon as possible parallel to the other measures. However, if the patient is adequately ventilated without intubation, the injection of adrenaline should not be delayed by possibly unsuccessful attempts at intubation.
3. The routine use of sodium bicarbonate is not recommended. If at all, this drug should be given in an i.v. infusion over 10 min at a dose of 1 mmol/kg body weight.

Certain modifications must be applied to these recent recommendations of the use of atropine for cardiac asystole. There is no doubt that parasympathetic hyperexcitation can cause sinus arrest.

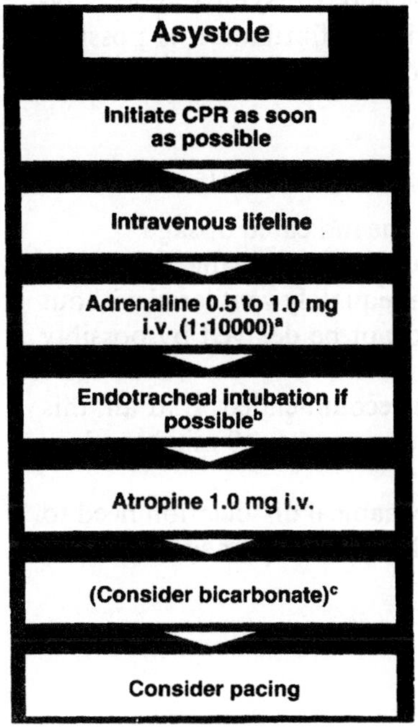

Fig. 5. Asystole

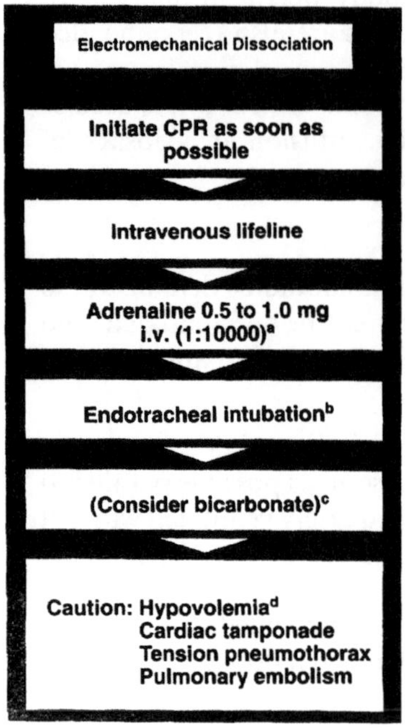

Fig. 6. Electromechanical dissociation

In certain instances, such as carotid sinus stimulation, the administration of atropine may well be beneficial, but in the majority of arrest victims it is impossible to predict the relationship of sympathetic and parasympathetic activity. If the rhythm can be elucidated, and ventricular fibrillation is possibly present, defibrillation should be undertaken as for VF.

Electromechanical Dissociation

In Fig. 6 it is assumed that electromechanical dissociation persists.

1. Adrenaline should be repeated every 5 min in the indicated dosage.
2. Endotracheal intubation should be initiated as soon as possible parallel to the other measures. However, if the patient is adequately ventilated without intubation, the injection of adrenaline should not be delayed by possibly unsuccessful attempts at intubation.
3. The routine use of sodium bicarbonate is not recommended. If at all, this drug should be given at this stage in an i.v. infusion over 10 min at a dose of 1 mmol/kg body weight.
4. Any possible extracardiac causes of electromechanical dissociation need to be considered and treated directly in order to lay the basis for successful resuscitation.

The Potentials and Limits of Cardiopulmonary Resuscitation

We would first like to define the facts which determine the success of resuscitation in order to achieve conclusions for an improvement in the management of the cardiac arrest victim.

The success of resuscitation is determined by individual factors depending on the patient, but also on the time lapse until resuscitative measures have been started. The results are poor when cardiac arrest is caused by severe chronic lung disease or chronic cardiac failure. On the other hand, up to 60% of those patients who developed cardiac arrest after acute myocardial infarction could be discharged when resuscitation was started immediately [54].

In 70% of cases of sudden cardiac arrest, ventricular fibrillation is present, which has an overall good prognosis when mechanical measures and early defibrillation are performed [42]. If no therapeutic interventions are taken ventricular fibrillation usually deteriorates to asystole or electromechanical dissociation, and the rate of hospital discharge is only about 6%, as in cases of primary asystole [19, 26, 39, 47, 48, 57].

Neurological recovery from cardiac arrest is mainly determined by the duration and extent of hypoxia. If mechanical measures are started within 1 min after the development of cardiac arrest only 6% of patients show minor neurological damage, the remainder none at all. If resuscitation is delayed 1 to 5 min, 13% of the patients have neurological damage, and after 5 to 10 min 50% of the patients have severe neurological deficits [35]. Even advanced cardiopulmonary resuscitation measures, such as drugs or defibrillation meet with no success, if they are not started within a critical time limit. A large number of investigations show that mechanical measures must be started within 4 min after cardiac arrest develops [9, 17, 19, 21, 47, 53, 55]. It must be borne in mind, however, that this is a median value, and that the cause and type of cardiac arrest is not taken into account in these results. Clinical practice demonstrates that in the majority of cases mechanical measures are not sufficient to restore spontaneous circulation. In many instances advanced techniques are necessary in order to correct the metabolic disturbances.

Despite the alterations in cardiopulmonary resuscitation methods, it must nevertheless be stressed that neither these improvements in technique nor in drug therapy can alter the outcome when resuscitation has been started too late.

References

1. Babbs CF (1980) New versus old theories of blood flow during CPR. Crit Care Med 8:191–195
2. Bishop RL, Weisfeldt ML (1976) Sodium bicarbonate administration during cardiac arrest. Effect on arterial pH, pCO_2, and osmolality. JAMA 235:506–509
3. Bircher N, Safar P, Steward R (1980) A comparison of standard "MAST"-augmented, and open-chest CPR in dogs: preliminary investigation. Crit Care Med 8:147–152

4. Caldwell G, Millar G, Quinn E et al. (1985) Simple mechanical methods of cardioversion: a defense of the precordial thump and cough version. Br Med J 291:627–630
5. Carlon GC, Howland WS, Kahn RC et al. (1980) Calcium chloride administration in normocalcemic critically ill patients. Crit Care Med 8:209–213
6. Chandra N, Rudikoff M, Weisfeldt M (1980) Simultaneous chest compression and ventilation at high airway pressure during cardiopulmonary resuscitation. Lancet i:175–178
7. Chapman JH, Menapace FJ, Howell RR (1983) Ruptured aortic valve cusp: a complication of the Heimlich maneuver. Ann Emerg Med 12:446–452
8. Chow MS, Ronfeld RA, Hamilton RA, Helmink R, Fieldman A (1983) Effect of external cardiopulmonary resuscitation on lidocaine pharmacokinetics in dogs. J Pharmacol Exp Ther 224:531–537
9. Copley DP, Mantle JA, John AM, Rogers WJ, Russel RO, Rackley CE (1977) Improved outcome for prehospital cardiopulmonary collapse with resuscitation by bystanders. Circulation 56:901–905
10. Criley JM, Blaufuss AH, Kissel GL (1976) Cough-induced cardiac compression. Self-induced form of cardiopulmonary resuscitation. JAMA 236:1246–1250
11. Croom EW (1983) Rupture of stomach after attempted Heimlich maneuver. JAMA 250:2602–2608
12. Day R (1983) Differing opinions on the emergency treatment of choking. Pediatrics 71:976–983
13. Day R, Crelin ES, DuBois AB (1982) Choking: the Heimlich abdominal thrust vs back blows. An approach to measurement of inertial and aerodynamic forces. Pediatrics 70:113–119
14. Dembo DH (1981) Calcium in advanced life support. Crit Care Med 9:358–360
15. DeSilva RA, Hennekens CH, Lown B, Casscells W (1981) Lignocaine prophylaxis in acute myocardial infarction. An evaluation of randomized trials. Lancet ii:855–858
16. Dorian P, Fain ES, Davy JM, Winkle RA (1986) Lidocaine causes a reversible, concentration-dependent increase in defibrillation energy requirements. J Am Coll Cardiol 8:327–332
17. Eisenberg MS, Bergner L, Hallstrom AP (1984) Sudden cardiac death in the community. Praeger, New York
18. Elam JO (1977) The intrapulmonary route for CPR drugs. In: Safar P, Elam JO (eds) Advances in cardiopulmonary resuscitation. Springer, Berlin Heidelberg New York, pp 132–137
19. Gudjonsson H, Baldvinsson E, Oddson G (1982) Results of attempted cardiopulmonary resuscitation of patients dying suddenly outside the hospital in Reykjavik and the surrounding area. Acta Med Scand 212:247–251
20. Guerci AD, Chandra N, Johnson E, Hayburn B, Wurmb E, Tsitlik J, Halperin HR, Siu C, Weisfeldt ML (1986) Failure of sodium bicarbonate to improve resuscitation from ventricular fibrillation in dogs. Circulation 74 [Suppl IV]:IV75–IV79
21. Guzy PM, Pearce ML, Greenfield S (1983) The survival benefit of bystanders cardiopulmonary resuscitation in a paramedic-served metropolitan area. Am J Public Health 73:766–769
22. Harrison EE (1981) Lidocaine in prehospital countershock refractory ventricular fibrillation. Ann Emerg Med 10:420–430
23. Heimlich HJ, Uhtley MH (1979) The Heimlich maneuver. Clin Symp 31:22–30
24. Heimlich HJ, Hoffman KA, Canestri FR (1975) Food-choking and drowning deaths prevented by external subdiaphragmatic compression: physiological basis. Ann Thorac Surg 20:188–195
25. Kerber RE, Pandian NG, Jensen SR, Constantin L, Kieso RA, Melton J, Hunt M (1986) Effect of lidocaine and bretylium on energy requirement for transthoracic defibrillation. Experimental studies. J Am Coll Cardiol 7:397–405

26. Kloess T, Roewer N, Wischhusen F (1985) Prognose der präklinischen kardiopulmonalen Reanimation. Anaesth Intensivther Notfallmed 20:237–248
27. Koehler RC, Michael JR, Guerci AD, Chandra N, Schleien CL, Dean JM, Rogers MC, Weisfeldt ML, Trystman RJ (1985) Beneficial effect of epinephrine infusion on cerebral and myocardial blood flows during CPR. Ann Emerg Med 14:744–749
28. Koster RW, Dunning AJ (1985) Intramuscular lidocaine for prevention of lethal arrhythmias in the prehospitalization phase of acute myocardial infarction. N Engl J Med 313:1105–1110
29. Kouwenhoven WB, Jude JR, Knickerbocker GG (1960) Closed-chest cardiac massage. JAMA 173:1064–1067
30. Lie KI, Wellens HJ, van Capelle FJ (1974) Lidocaine in the prevention of primary ventricular fibrillation. A double-blind, randomized study of 212 consecutive patients. N Engl J Med 291:1324–1326
31. Lindner KH, Ahnefeld FW (1986) Vergleichende tierexperimentelle Untersuchungen zur Wiederherstellung der spontanen Zirkulation mit Adrenalin und Noradrenalin nach asphyktisch bzw. elektrisch ausgelöstem Kreislaufstillstand. Anaesthesist 35:126 (abstr)
32. Lindner KH, Ahnefeld FW, Dick W, Lotz P (1985) Natriumbikarbonatgabe während der kardiopulmonalen Reanimation. Ergebnisse einer tierexperimentellen Untersuchung. Anaesthesist 34:37–45
33. Lindner KH, Ahnefeld FW, Schürmann W, Pfenninger EG, Bowdler IM (1988) A comparison of epinephrine and norepinephrine on myocardial oxygen delivery and consumption during cardiopulmonary resuscitation. Anesthesiology 69:96 (abstr)
34. Livesay JJ, Follette DM, Fey KH, Nelson RL, DeLand EC, Barnard J, Buckberg GD (1978) Optimizing myocardial supply/demand balance with alpha-adrenergic drugs during cardiopulmonary resuscitation. J Thorac Cardiovasc Surg 76:244–251
35. Lund I, Skulberg A (1976) Cardiopulmonary resuscitation by lay people. Lancet II:702–704
36. Mattar JA, Weil MH, Shubin H, Stein L (1974) Cardiac arrest in the critically ill. II. Hyperosmolal states following cardiac arrest. Am J Med 56:162–168
37. Michael JR, Guerci AD, Koehler RC, Shi AY, Tsitlik J, Chandra N, Niedermeyer E, Rogers MC, Traystman RJ, Weisfeldt ML (1984) Mechanisms by which epinephrine augments cerebral and myocardial perfusion during cardiopulmonary resuscitation in dogs. Circulation 69:822–835
38. Minuck M, Sharma GP (1977) Comparison of THAM and sodium bicarbonate in resuscitation of the heart after ventricular fibrillation in dogs. Anesth Analg 56:38–45
39. Myerburg RJ, Kessler KM, Zaman L, Conde CA, Castellanos A (1982) Survivors of prehospital arrest. JAMA 247:1485–1490
40. Niemann JT, Rosborough J, Hausknecht M, Ung S, Criley JM (1981) Blood flow without cardiac compression during closed-chest CPR. Crit Care Med 9:380–381
41. Niemann JT, Rosborough JP, Ung S (1984) Hemodynamic effects of continuous abdominal binding during cardiac arrest and resuscitation. Am J Cardiol 53:269–274
42. Ornato JP, McNeill SE, Smith RG, Carenborough FA (1984) Limitation on effectiveness of rapid defibrillation by emergency medical technicians in a rural setting. Ann Emerg Med 13:1097–1108
43. Pennington JE, Taylor J, Lown B (1970) Chest thump for reverting ventricular tachycardia. N Engl J Med 283:1192–1195
44. Ralston SH (1984) Alpha agonist drug usage during CPR. Ann Emerg Med 13:786–788
45. Ralston SH, Babbs CF, Niebauer MJ (1982) Cardiopulmonary resuscitation with interposed abdominal compression in dogs. Anesth Analg 61:645–651

46. Redding JS (1979) The choking controversy: critique of evidence on the Heimlich maneuver. Crit Care Med 7:745–748
47. Ritter G, Wolfe RA, Goldstein S, Landis JR, Vasu CM, Acheson A, Leighton R, VanderBrug Medendrop S (1985) The effect of bystander CPR on survival of out-of-hospital cardiac arrest victims. Am Heart J 110:932–937
48. Roth R, Stewart RD, Rogers K, Cannon GM (1984) Out-of-hospital cardiac arrest: factors associated with survival. Ann Emerg Med 13:237–243
49. Ruben H, MacNaughton FI (1978) The treatment of food-choking. Practitioner 221:725–736
50. Rudikoff MT, Maughan WL, Effron M, Freund P, Weisfeldt ML (1980) Mechanism of blood flow during cardiopulmonary resuscitation. Circulation 61:345–352
51. Standards and guidelines for cardiopulmonary resuscitation (CPR) and emergency cardiac care (ECC) (1980) JAMA 244:453–509
52. Standards and guidelines for cardiopulmonary resuscitation (CPR) and emergency cardiac care (ECC) (1986) JAMA 255:2905–2989
53. Stueven HA, Troiano P, Thompson B, Mateer JR, Kastenson EH, Tonsfeld D, Hargarten K, Kowalski R, Aprahamian C, Darin J (1986) Bystander/first responder CPR: ten years experience in a paramedic system. Ann Emerg Med 15:707–710
54. Thimme W, Schäfer JH, Tönnesmann U (1977) Ergebnisse der „Reanimation." Intensivmed 14:398–403
55. Tweed WA, Bristow G, Donen N (1980) Resuscitation from cardiac arrest: assessment of a system providing only basic life support outside of hospital. Can Med Assoc J 122:297–300
56. Visintine RE, Baick CH (1975) Ruptured stomach after Heimlich maneuver. JAMA 234:415–422
57. Weaver WD, Cobb LA, Thompson RG (1985) Enhancing survival after cardiac arrest – the effect of initial rhythm and a new strategy in emergency care. Ann Emerg Med 14:79–88
58. Wei JY, Green HL, Weisfeldt ML (1980) Cough facilitated cardioversion of ventricular tachycardia. Am J Cardiol 45:174–176
59. Weil MH, Rackow EC, Trevino R, Grundler W, Falk JL, Griffel MI (1986) Difference in acid-base state between venous and arterial blood during cardiopulmonary resuscitation. N Engl J Med 315:153–156
60. Werner JA, Greene HL, Janko CL, Cobb LA (1981) Visualization of cardiac valve motion in man during external chest compression using two-dimensional echocardiography. Implications regarding the mechanism of blood flow. Circulation 63:1417–1421
61. Yakaitis RW, Redding JS (1973) Precordial thumping during cardiac resuscitation 1:22–26
62. Yakaitis RW, Otto CW, Blitt CD (1979) Relative importance of alpha- and beta-adrenergic receptors during resuscitation. Crit Care Med 7:293–296

O_2 Transport in Low Flow States of Circulatory Shock and Cardiac Arrest

D. M. Shah, M. H. Weil, R. J. Gazmuri, and E. C. Rackow

Introduction

Oxygen is the most critical substrate for cellular metabolism [1, 2]. Decreases in oxygen availability to cells may result from impairment in arterial oxygenation, reduction in hemoglobin, decrease in forward blood flow, or due to a primary defect at the tissue level (Table 1). This contribution addresses the pathophysiology, clinical measurements, and therapeutic implications of oxygen deficit associated with the low flow state of circulatory shock and the extreme low flow states of cardiac arrest and cardiopulmonary resuscitation.

Table 1. Tissue oxygen deficit[a]

Type	Primary defect	Clinical examples
Anoxic:	↓ Arterial oxygen saturation	● ARDS ● Asphyxiation
Anemic:	↓ In functional hemoglobin	● Anemia ● CO intoxication
Stagnant:	↓ In cardiac output	● Intravascular volume depletion ● Heart failure ● Pulmonary embolism
Histotoxic:	Primary cellular injury	● Cyanide intoxication ? Sepsis

[a] Three basic mechanisms of tissue oxygen deficit, i. e., anoxic, anemic, and stagnant, were first proposed by Barcroft [3] in 1920. Histotoxic was subsequently added by Peters and Van Slyke [4] in 1931

Physiology and Pathophysiology of Tissue Oxygenation

Once oxygen reaches the capillary level, it diffuses passively across the capillary endothelium, the interstitium, and the cell membrane. Its destiny is the mitochondria in which oxygen is utilized as an electron acceptor of the reduced nucleotides NADH and NADPH [5]. The driving force for oxygen diffusion is the partial pressure gradient of oxygen from the capillary to mitochondria.

Under normal physiological conditions, the PO_2 of the blood entering the capillaries averages 95 mmHg and the PO_2 of blood leaving the capillaries averages 40 mmHg. The interstitial PO_2 ranges from 20 to 40 mmHg. In the cells, PO_2 is further reduced to approximately 15 to 20 mmHg. Oxygen then diffuses into the mitochondria. The oxygen tension of the tissues largely exceeds the physiologic requirements and serves as a protective buffer. Accordingly, a substantial decrease in tissue PO_2 is well tolerated. Remarkably, mitochondria may operate normally with a PO_2 tension as low as 1 mmHg. However, a further decrease in oxygen tension precludes aerobic metabolism. With the onset of anaerobiosis, there is lactate generation [2]. Oxygen diffusion is also diminished when there is an increase in the distance between the capillaries and the cell. This may result from accumulation of excess of fluid in the interstitial compartment and may augment the oxygen deficit which evolves during the early stages of sepsis, heart failure, and the later stages of circulatory shock [6–9].

It is estimated that a mixed venous PO_2 ($P\bar{v}O_2$) of 28 mmHg represents the critical threshold level below which oxygen diffusion is not adequate for sustaining aerobic metabolism [10, 11]. Such decrease in $P\bar{v}O_2$ during cardiogenic shock in patients correlates with both increases in systemic lactate content of blood and decreases in survival. When mixed venous PO_2 is decreased to levels of less than 18 mmHg, there is impairment of consciousness. Decreases to less than 15 mmHg over intervals exceeding 10 min are likely to produce irreversible brain damage [12]. However, such estimates may not apply when decreases in oxygen demand moderate the effects of decreases in oxygen supply [13–15].

Relationship Between Oxygen Delivery ($\dot{D}O_2$), Oxygen Consumption ($\dot{V}O_2$) and Lactate Generation

Under basal conditions, oxygen transport is approximately 600 $ml/min \cdot m^2$ and oxygen consumption 150 $ml/min \cdot m^2$. Accordingly, only 25% of the available oxygen is extracted by the tissues. A reduction in oxygen delivery triggers compensatory responses by which oxygen availability to cells is increased. These include activation of the sympathoadrenal axis with both neurogenic and humoral catecholamine release which may augment blood flow to vital organs [16, 17]. This also triggers increases in oxygen extraction [10, 11], and decreases in the affinity of hemoglobin for oxygen. Accordingly, more oxygen is released to tissues [18–22).

When these compensatory mechanisms fail, a critical oxygen deficit results in progressive impairment of mitochondrial function. The regeneration of high energy phosphates is decreased and excess of lactic acid accumulates [23, 24]. These are the hallmarks of anaerobic metabolism and the associated tissue injury which culminates in potentially fatal outcome of the low flow states.

Circulatory Shock

In the setting of circulatory shock, the primary defect is a decrease in effective cardiac output and therefore decreases in $\dot{D}O_2$. As the $\dot{D}O_2$ decreases, there is an initial increase in oxygen extraction such that $\dot{V}O_2$ is preserved. However, further curtailment in $\dot{D}O_2$ compromises $\dot{V}O_2$ such that $\dot{V}O_2$ becomes flow ($\dot{D}O_2$) dependent [21, 22, 25, 26]. Nevertheless, under most clinical circumstances, the absolute $\dot{D}O_2$ and $\dot{V}_2$ levels do not predict the presence or absence of tissue oxygen deficits [10, 11, 27, 28].

The severity of oxygen deficits is contingent on the duration and severity of the low flow state in relation to the overall oxygen needs. This, commonly referred to as oxygen debt, correlates directly with the onset of anaerobic metabolism and ultimate outcome [2, 29, 30]. Crowell and Lewis [1] demonstrated in dogs that when oxygen deficit increased from 100 ml to 150 ml/kg during hemorrhagic shock, survival declined from 100% to 0%. Similar studies by Weil et al. [2] in a rodent model of hemorrhagic shock demonstrated that both oxygen debt and survival were correlated with arterial lactate. These observations were subsequently confirmed in human patients during circulatory shock of diverse etiologies [2, 31].

Following the onset of septic shock, the cardiac output is likely to be normal or increased. The oxygen deficit in this setting stems primarily from a deficit of oxygen availability at the tissue level. Early during sepsis, an increase in tissue oxygen demands which may exceed 50% of normal values accentuate this failure of oxygen availability to tissues [32]. This represents primarily abnormal distribution of blood flow. The capability for maintaining microcirculatory flow is reduced either by arteriovenous shunting or by failure of substrate exchange at capillary levels. Notwithstanding tissue oxygen deficits, the arterial-venous oxygen difference is decreased [27, 33]. Accordingly, there may be an increased $\dot{D}O_2$ and $\dot{V}O_2$ despite critical reduction in tissue oxygenation [34, 35].

When cardiac output is reduced during septic shock, it is typically associated with an absolute or a relative volume deficit [36–38]. However, such may also indicate myocardial depression [39–42].

Increases in lactic acid, despite "normal" $\dot{V}O_2$ indicate inadequate oxygen delivery. Recent studies have consistently demonstrated that lactate signals the state in which $\dot{V}_2$ is limited because of reduced $\dot{D}O_2$ [43–45]. The effectiveness of therapeutic interventions are monitored by the extent to which they augment oxygen delivery and oxygen consumption with concurrent reduction in blood lactate concentration [44, 46].

Progressive increases in blood lactate during circulatory shock, regardless of the primary mechanism or etiology, correlate closely with survival. Increases in lactate from 2 to 8 mmol/l are associated with a decrease in survival from approximately 90% to only 10% [47]. Similar relationships have been independently confirmed by other investigators in the setting of myocardial infarction associated with cardiogenic shock, in septic shock, and during hemorrhagic shock states [48, 49].

Cardiac Arrest

Cardiopulmonary resuscitation [CPR) after cardiac arrest represents an extreme low flow state in which peripheral tissue perfusion is severely compromised. Systemic flow generated by conventional closed-chest CPR rarely exceeds 25% of normal [50–54]. During CPR, the critical determinant of resuscitation and ultimate survival relates to myocardial and cerebral blood flow, rather than systemic oxygen delivery and oxygen consumption. Accordingly, the primary goal is that of maintaining adequate flow to these two critical organs, rather than securing perfusion of peripheral tissues. This may explain why initial measurements of blood lactate may not predict outcome in this setting. However, measurements indicative of myocardial and cerebral perfusion are highly predictive of initial resuscitation and long-term outcome [55–57].

Clinical and Laboratory Assessment

Physical Signs and Hemodynamic Parameters During Low Flow States

Cold clammy skin, collapse of superficial veins, alteration of mental status, peripheral cyanosis of distal extremities, ear lobes and tip of the nose, and suppression of the formation of urine, usually indicate poor organ perfusion and oxygenation [58]. Conventional blood pressure measurements may be misleading because of extremes of peripheral vasoconstriction in association with decreased arterial blood flow. Intraarterial pressure measured in a large artery or in the aorta and cardiac output which may be clinically measured with ease by the thermodilution technique are useful bedside hemodynamic measurements for both diagnosis and quantitation of the severity of the low flow states which occur in the setting of circulatory shock.

Blood Lactate

Blood lactate is an independent indicator of tissue oxygen deficit with prognostic and therapeutic implications [2, 23, 29, 30, 39, 59, 60]. The techniques for blood lactate measurements have evolved in the past 20 years from a technically cumbersome chemical method [61], to the enzymatic methods [62], and finally to a simple electrode technique which allows rapid measurement of blood lactate at the bedside [63–65]. Accordingly, lactate measurement may now be incorporated into the routine stat blood analysis on a par with blood gases.

Arterial and large vein lactate levels are highly correlated and there is no significant venoarterial gradient of lactate during low-flow states. Accordingly, venous blood which has been sampled from either a central venous or pulmonary artery catheter has the same lactate content as arterial blood [66].

Although increases in lactate must be interpreted in the context of the physiological conditions which prevail at the time of sampling, it has been a very useful clinical guide. For instance, marked increases in oxygen requirements and blood lactate concentrations accompany intense muscular activity, such as extreme exercise, convulsive seizures, or shaking chills [67, 68]. However, such increases are usually transient and the mechanism thereof is usually obvious to the bedside clinician. Moreover, sequential measurements of lactate indicate that such "physiological" increases in lactate concentration under extreme exercise conditions are quite rapidly cleared in comparison with pathophysiological increases. Accordingly, the lactate concentration is reduced to one-half of its maximum measured value (i.e., t_{50}) in less than 1 h after "physiological" anaerobiosis, which contrasts to more prolonged lactacidemia associated with circulatory shock states in which t_{50} is protracted for 2 or more h [66, 69, 70].

Mixed Venous Oxygen Tension ($P\bar{v}O_2$) and Oxygen Saturation ($S\bar{v}O_2$)

Although there is currently no "gold standard" for evaluation of global or regional balances of oxygen supply and demand, the measurement of mixed venous PO_2 ($P\bar{v}O_2$) appears to be a reasonable physiologic indicator. More specifically, the $P\bar{v}O_2$ in most instances reflects systemic supply/demand balance. Accordingly, decrease in supply or increase in demands for oxygen will correspondingly decrease $P\bar{v}O_2$. Simultaneous measurement of mixed venous oxygen saturation ($S\bar{v}O_2$) also incorporates oxyhemoglobin dissociation and more accurately reflects the quantity of oxygen released from hemoglobin.

Although a decrease in $P\bar{v}O_2$ to less than 28 mmHg correlates with the onset of anaerobic metabolism and lactate generation, normal or increased $P\bar{v}O_2$ does not exclude an oxygen deficit [10, 11, 71]. Reference has already been made to septic shock in which maldistribution of microcirculatory flow, rather than decreases in cardiac output, are implicated. Whether such maldistribution is due to arteriovenous communication or impaired oxygen utilization which Peter and Van Slyke [4] designated as histotoxic anoxia is as yet unresolved. For purposes of diagnosis, however, a disproportionately high cardiac output and $P\bar{v}O_2$ in patients who present with physical signs of circulatory shock pinpoint the likelihood of septic shock [46].

Measurement of $S\bar{v}O_2$ in the pulmonary artery using a fiberoptic catheter system provides a continuous assessment of the overall balance between $\dot{D}O_2$ and $\dot{V}O_2$ [72–74]. Decreases in $S\bar{v}O_2$ usually constitute an early indication of decreased oxygen availability. A low or decreasing $S\bar{v}O_2$, like cardiac output, refractory to therapeutic interventions typically prognosticates poor outcome. This also applies in the settings of respiratory failure, myocardial infarction, and traumatic shock [10, 75–77]. However, there is as yet no consensus as to whether the routine use of such fiberoptic systems is cost redeeming when interval measurements of cardiac output and noninvasive hemodynamic or blood gas measurements are available.

Noninvasive Monitoring of Arterial and Tissue Oxygenation

Noninvasive options for monitoring oxygenation include fingertip and ear oximeters [78, 79], and transcutaneous and conjunctival oxygen electrodes [80, 81]. These correlate well with arterial blood oxygenation in hemodynamically stable patients [82]. However, during circulatory shock and especially during cardiac arrest, blood flow is reduced to the skin and conjunctiva to the extent that these measurements lose reliability. More specifically, failure of tissue perfusion precludes reliability and accuracy of such measurements. Although there are anecdotal reports of parallel changes in cardiac output and transcutaneous oxygen tension during circulatory shock, such is not theoretically or objectively supported [22].

Therapeutic Implications

The fundamental defect during low flow states of circulatory shock is poor tissue perfusion and decreased oxygen delivery to the cellular and subcellular levels. Therefore, interventions which would improve tissue perfusion such as to fulfill the systemic and regional oxygen requirements constitute basic therapeutic goals [46, 83, 84]. However, we also propose increasing awareness that the issue is that of oxygen supply vs demand. Accordingly, interventions by which oxygen demands are reduced are likely to improve the balance between oxygen supply and demand [13–15]. Such may also be accomplished by extracorporeal support of either or both the circulation [85–89] and ventilation [90–94]. The potential of reducing energy requirements and therefore the shortfall between oxygen supply and demand has been less extensively investigated than options for increasing cardiac output and oxygen content and therefore oxygen delivery.

Fluids

The assessment of volume status and subsequent volume expansion is the single most important intervention for treatment of shock states regardless of cause [95]. Volume expansion increases the preload, i.e., venous return, and thereby augments cardiac output. However, invasive monitoring may be needed to guide volume repletion, such as to minimize the risk of volume overload with heart failure [96].

The specific prescription of colloid, crystalloid, and electrolyte fluids by the clinician is best based on an understanding of the cause of fluid loss and the severity of the hemodynamic defect in relation to the cardiorespiratory status of the patient. We have for many years favored a formal protocol of "fluid challenge" under conditions when large volumes of fluid are required. The risk of hypervolemic heart failure is substantially decreased if changes in filling pressure are objectively monitored as part of the fluid challenge routine [83, 95, 96].

Colloids and Crystalloids

Both colloids and crystalloids effectively reverse the hypovolemic state. However, we believe that colloids pose advantages in that they do not rapidly diffuse out of the intravascular compartment. Crystalloid and electrolyte fluids decrease colloid osmotic pressure and thereby increase the risk of pulmonary and interstitial edema. Accordingly, they may increase the risk of anoxic anoxia [8, 9, 97, 98].

Approximately three- or fourfold larger volumes of crystalloid fluid are required to achieve hemodynamic effects equivalent to those of isooncotic colloids such as 5% human serum albumin [99]. In conjunction with a fluid challenge protocol, isooncotic colloids, such as 5% albumin and 6% hydroxyethyl starch, allow for more precise titration of volumes [95, 96].

Finally, a greater increase in $\dot{V}O_2$ has been experimentally documented when colloid fluids were compared with noncolloid fluids for therapy of hypovolemic shock [100, 101]. Nevertheless, the benefits of colloid for routine management of patients with hypovolemic or septic shock have not been securely established [44–46, 102, 103]. However, for patients with critically reduced cardiopulmonary function, current evidence does favor the use of colloids in our judgement.

Blood and Its Derivatives

Red cell transfusion augments transport of oxygen to peripheral tissue by not only increasing intravascular volume and therefore preload and cardiac output, but also by increasing oxygen carrying capacity. However, there are theoretical and practical disadvantages. In stored blood, 2,3 diphosphoglycerate (2,3DPG) is reduced, the P_{50} is decreased, and hence the affinity of hemoglobin for oxygen is increased [104–106]. An increase in the hematocrit to supernormal levels increases blood viscosity and thereby reduces velocity and volume of blood flow [107]. Clinical studies in various disease states suggest that optimal oxygen availability and survival in critically ill patients are in the hematocrit range from 30% to 45% [108–110]. Acellular solutions of hemoglobin such as stroma free hemoglobin (SFH) and synthetic solutions, especially fluorocarbons, increase $\dot{D}O_2$ and $\dot{V}O_2$ [111–119]. However, at the time of this writing, the evidence of their benefit does not allow us to conclude that they will improve outcome.

Vasoactive and Inotropic Agents

Cardiac output and therefore $\dot{D}O_2$ may be augmented by pharmacologic interventions. Drugs which increase myocardial contractility [120–128] or decrease afterload [129–131] provide two major options at the present time. Though increased risks of digitalis toxicity are recognized in the hyperacute setting and titration of dose is more difficult, digitalis glycosides remain a therapeutically effective option for inotropic treatment and especially so in patients with preexisting heart failure [132–134]. β-Adrenoreceptor agonists may increase both contractility and heart rate. Consequently, their benefits are contingent on the extent to which they augment cardiac output and coronary blood flow in relation to increases in myocardial oxygen requirements. The risk of increasing myocardial oxygen requirements is greater when isoproterenol [135, 136] or (low dose) dopamine is utilized [121, 124, 137], but less with dobutamine [124]. Phosphodiesterase inhibitors augment cardiac output, increase myocardial contractility, and decrease arterial resistance without significant changes in heart rate or myocardial oxygen consumption [127, 138–142]. However, such agents require loading doses and, like other phosphodiesterase inhibitors, have increased risks of toxicity. Vasodilator agents, such as nitroprusside, effectively increase cardiac performance and forward blood flow, especially in the setting of primary pump failure in which ventricular afterload is increased [143, 144]. However, they may reduce arterial pressure and thereby compromise coronary perfusion pressure and consequently coronary blood flow in patients with borderline or overt hypotension. Vasodilator agents, like nitroglycerin, decrease preload predominantly. Accordingly, they reduce the workload on the heart. In the setting of myocardial ischemia, they have the additional advantage of reversing coronary spasm. However, increases in venous capacitance and therefore decreases in preload may reduce rather than augment cardiac output.

Alpha-adrenergic vasopressor agents, like levarterenol and high dose dopamine, increase vasoconstriction which may compromise already reduced arterial blood flow and therefore potentiate the shock state [145]. This increase in arterial resistance also augments the work load of the heart and constitutes therapy which is directly opposite that of vasodilator drugs [146]. Moreover, increases in small vein resistance provoke increases in capillary hydrostatic pressure and therefore extravasation of plasma water. This, in turn, reduces intravascular volume and potentially preload and cardiac output [36–38, 147]. Accordingly, the routine use of vasopressor agents in shock states is no longer recommended [83].

Assisted Circulation

Intraaortic balloon counterpulsation [85–87, 148, 149] and initiation of extracorporeal pumping (ECPO) [88, 89] may strikingly increase blood flow and oxygen delivery to the vital circuits and especially the coronary and cerebral arteries. This may revert myocardial and cerebral oxygen deficits. However, the ultimate benefits of balloon counterpulsation with respect to survival are limited to patients with cardiogenic shock associated with mechanical defects which are suitable for surgical correction, including acute valvular malfunction, acquired ventricular defects, or myocardial aneurysms. Experimentally, ECPO has been useful in the setting of cardiac arrest. ECPO increases myocardial blood flow and thereby facilitates the restoration of spontaneous cardiac contraction and circulation [88, 89]. We believe it to be a promising option for advanced life support when conventional resuscitative efforts fail. Such patients may now be identified by monitoring end-tidal CO_2 [150–152].

Decreased Oxygen Requirements

Analgesia and sedation moderate oxygen requirements and especially adrenergically mediated cardiovascular responses to pain and stress [13]. With such interventions, both regional and systemic oxygen demands are reduced. In patients with heart failure and angina, anesthesia reduces myocardial oxygen needs by one-third or more [14, 153–154]. Myocardial oxygen consumption (MvO_2) is also reduced by treatment with beta adrenoreceptor blockers [155–157] and calcium entry blockers [158–159] in patients with angina. Bilateral section or cooling of the cervical vagi and systemic atropinization [160–161] reduce the risks of coronary ligation. Thoracic epidural analgesia reversed hypotension in patients with cardiogenic shock who failed to respond to other measures on the basis of anecdotal reports [162]; however, controlled clinical trials are needed. Though the precise role of such interventions is not securely established in the setting of low flow states, except during cardiovascular surgery, investigations which should better expose the potential benefits of reducing oxygen demand are regarded by us as an important commitment.

In patients with inflammatory diseases and in patients in hypermetabolic states and especially hyperthyroidism or pheochromocytoma, oxygen consumption, ventilation, and the oxygen cost of breathing may be strikingly increased in parallel with increased metabolic rates [163–167]. Moreover, respiratory muscle fatigue may be a limiting factor in hypermetabolic patients who are physically unable to fulfill the need for such increases in oxygen requirements. Accordingly, mechanical ventilation may be an option for reducing oxygen demands [90–94]. A similar rationale applies to the use of assisted circulation [85–89].

Conclusion

O_2 delivery is reduced during low flow states. The oxygen deficit triggers anaerobic metabolism and generation of excesses of lactic acid. Initial therapeutic interventions are aimed at increasing cardiac output and thereby oxygen delivery such that perfusion failure and the oxygen deficit are reversed. This is usually accomplished by increasing the oxygen supply by vigorous fluid repletion, judicious use of inotropic and vasoactive drugs, and selective use of extracorporeal support systems. We are also alerted to the option of reducing oxygen demand so as to obviate the gap between oxygen requirements and oxygen availability, but appreciate the need of substantially greater insight into such and therefore the potential value of more intensive investigations.

References

1. Crowell JW, Smith EE (1964) O_2 deficit and irreversible haemorrhagic shock. Am J Physiol 206:313–316
2. Weil MH, Afifi AA (1970) Experimental and clinical studies on lactate and pyruvate as indicators of the severity of acute circulatory failure (shock). Circulation 41:989–1001

3. Barcroft J (1920) On anoxaemia. Lancet II:485–489
4. Peters JP, Van Slyke DD (1931) Quantitative clinical chemistry. Baltimore, Williams and Wilkins Co.
5. Robin ED (1980) Of men and mitochondria: coping with hypoxic dysoxia. Am Rev Respir Dis 122:517–531
6. Shah DM, Newell JC, Saba TM (1981) Defects in peripheral oxygen utilization following trauma and shock. Arch Surg 116:1277–1281
7. Shah DM, Gottlieb ME, Rahm RL et al. (1982) Failure of red blood cell transfusion to increase oxygen transport or mixed venous PO_2 in injured patients. Crit Care Med 22:741–746
8. Heughan C, Niinikowski J, Hunt JK (1972) Effect of excessive infusion of saline solution on tissue oxygen transport. Surg Gynecol Obstet 135:257–260
9. Weil MH, Rackow EC (1988) Pulmonary edema. In: Parmely WW, Chatterjee K (eds) Cardiology, vol 1. Physiology, pharmacology, diagnosis. Philadelphia J.B., Lippincott Company, Chapter 10:1–12
10. Kastniz P, Druger GL, Yorra F, Simmons DH (1976) Mixed venous oxygen tension and hyperlactatemia. Survival in severe cardiopulmonary disease. JAMA 236:570–574
11. Simmons DH, Alpas AP, Tashkin DP, Coulson A (1978) Hyperlactatemia due to arterial hypoxemia or reduced cardiac output or both. J Am Physiol Soc 45:195–198
12. Lenox WG, Gibbs FA, Gibbs EL (1935) Relationship of unconsciousness to cerebral blood flow and to anoxemia. Arch Neurol Psychiatry 34:1001–1013
13. Rouby JJ, Eurin B, Glaser P, Guillosson JJ, Nafziger J, Guesde R, Viras P (1981) Hemodynamic and metabolic effects of morphine in the critically ill. Circulation 64:53–59
14. Reiz S, Balfors E, Gustavasson B, Haggmark S, Nath S, Rydvall A, Truedsson H (1982) Effects of halothane on coronary haemodynamics and myocardial metabolism in patients with ischemic heart disease and heart failure. Acta Anaesthesiol Scand 26:133–138
15. Bursztein S, Taitelman U, De Myttenaere S, Michalson M, Dahan E, Gepstein R, Edelman D, Melamed Y (1978) Reduced oxygen consumption in catabolic states with mechanical ventilation. Crit Care Med 6:162–164
16. Heistad DD, Abboud FM (1980) Circulatory adjustments to hypoxia. Circulation 61:463–470
17. Finch CA, Lenfant C (1972) Oxygen transport in man. N Engl J Med 1286:407–415
18. Woodson RD, Torrance JD, Shappell SD, Lenfount C (1970) The effect of cardiac disease on hemoglobin-oxygen binding. J Clin Invest 49:1349–1356
19. Metcalfe J, Dhindsa DS, Edwards MJ et al. (1969) Decreased affinity of blood for oxygen in patients with low output heart failure. Circ Res 25:47–51
20. Kostuk W, Suwa K, Bernstein EF et al. (1973) Altered hemoglobin oxygen affinity in patients with acute myocardial infarction. Am J Cardiol 31:295–299
21. Da Luz PL, Cavanilles JM, Michaels S, Weil MH, Shubin H (1975) Oxygen delivery, anoxic metabolism and Hb-O_2 affinity (P50) in patients with acute myocardial infarction and shock. Am J Cardiol 36:148–154
22. Yang SC, Puri VK, Raheja R (1986) Oxygen delivery and consumption and P50 in patients with acute myocardial infarction. Circulation 73:1183–1185
23. Broder G, Weil MH (1964) Excess lactate: an index of reversibility of shock in human patients. Science 143:1457–1460
24. Bland RD, Shoemaker WC, Abraham E, Coho JC (1985) Hemodynamic and oxygen transport patterns in surviving and nonsurviving postoperative patients. Crit Care Med 13:85–90
25. Mohsenifar S, Amin D, Jasper AC et al. (1987) Dependence of oxygen consumption on oxygen delivery in patients with chronic congestive heart failure. Chest 92(3):447–450

26. Chappell TR, Rubin LJ, Markham RV Jr, Firth BG (1985) Independence of oxygen consumption and systemic oxygen transport in patients with either stable pulmonary hypertension or refractory left ventricular failure. Am Rev Respir Dis 128:30–38
27. Astiz ME, Rackow EC, Weil MH (1986) Oxygen delivery and utilization during rapidly fatal septic shock in rat. Circ Shock 20:281–290
28. Gutierrez G, Waxley AR, Dantzker DR (1986) Oxygen delivery and utilization in hypothermic dogs. J Appl Physiol 60:751–757
29. Huckabee WE (1961) Relationship of pyruvate and lactate during anaerobic metabolism. V. Coronary adequacy. Am J Physiol 200:1169–1176
30. Afifi AA, Change PC, Liu VY, da Luz PL, Weil MH, Shubin H (1974) Prognostic indexes in acute myocardial infarction complicated by shock. Am J Cardiol 33:826–833
31. Bihari D, Smithies M, Gimson A, Tinker J (1987) The effects of vasodilation with prostacyclin on oxygen delivery and uptake in critically ill patients. N Engl J Med 317:397–403
32. Gump FE, Price JB, Kinney JM (1970) Whole body and splanchnic blood flow and oxygen consumption measurements in patients with intraperitoneal infection. Ann Surg 171:321–328
33. Rackow EC, Falk JL, Fein IA, Siegel JS, Packman MI, Haupt MT, Kaufman BS, Putnam D (1983) Fluid resuscitation in circulatory shock. Crit Care Med 11:839–850
34. Hiller C, Bone R, Hill D et al. (1979) Mixed venous oxygen tension compared to tissue oxygen tension as a measure of oxygen delivery in endotoxin shock. Clin Res 399A:27 (Abstract)
35. Astiz ME, Rackow EC, Kaufman B, Falk JL, Weil MH (1988) Relationship of oxygen delivery and mixed venous oxygenation to lactic acidosis in patients with sepsis and acute myocardial infarction. Crit Care Med 16:656–658
36. Udhoji VN, Weil MH (1965) Hemodynamic and metabolic studies on shock associated with bacteremia: observations on 16 patients. Ann Intern Med 62:966–978
37. Kwaan M, Weil MH (1969) Differences in the mechanism of shock caused by bacterial infections. Surg Gynecol Obstet 128:37–45
38. Vincent JL, Weil MH, Puri V et al. (1981) Circulatory shock associated with purulent peritonitis. Am J Surg 142:262–270
39. Weisel RD, Vito L, Dennis RC, Valeri CR, Hechtman HB (1977) Myocardial depression during sepsis. Am J Surg 133:512–521
40. Parker MM, Shelhamer JH, Barcharach SL et al. (1984) Profound but reversible myocardial depression in patients with septic shock. Ann Intern Med 100:483–490
41. Parillo JE, Burch C, Shelhamer JH et al. (1985) A circulating myocardial depressant substance in humans with septic shock. J Clin Invest 76:1539–1553
42. Rackow EC, Kaufman BS, Falk JL et al. (1987) Hemodynamic response to fluid repletion in patients with septic shock: evidence for early depression of cardiac function. Circ Shock 22:11–22
43. Haupt MT, Gilbert EM, Carlson RW (1985) Fluid loading increases $\dot{V}O_2$ in septic patients with lactic acidosis. Am Rev Respir Dis 131:912–916
44. Kaufman BS, Rackow EC, Falk JL (1984) The relationship between oxygen delivery and $\dot{V}O_2$ during fluid resuscitation of hypovolemia and septic shock. Chest 85:336–340
45. Wolf YG, Cotev S, Perel A, Manny J (1987) Dependance of oxygen consumption on cardiac output in sepsis. Crit Care Med 15:198–203
46. Rackow EC, Astiz ME, Weil MH (1988) Cellular oxygen metabolism during sepsis and shock. The relationship of oxygen consumption to oxygen delivery. JAMA 259:1989–1993
47. Shubin H, Weil MH, Afifi AA et al. (1974) Selection of hemodynamic, respiratory and metabolic variables for evaluation of patients in shock. Crit Care Med 2:326–336

48. Vitek V, Cowley RA (1971) Blood lactate in the prognosis of various forms of shock. Ann Surg 173:308–313
49. Peretz DI, McGregor H, Dossetor B (1964) Lactic acidosis: a clinically significant aspect of shock. Can Med Assoc J 90:673–675
50. Del Guercio LRM, Coomaraswamy RP, Slate D (1963) Cardiac output and other hemodynamic variables during internal cardiac massage in man. N Engl J Med 289:1398–1403
51. Fitzgerald KR, Babbs CF, Frissova HA et al. (1981) Cardiac output during cardiopulmonary resuscitation at various compression rates and duration. Am J Physiol 241:H442–H448
52. Babbs CF, Voorhees WD, Fitzgerald KR et al. (1988) Relationship of blood pressure and flow during CPR to chest compression amplitude: evidence for an effective compression threshold. Ann Emerg Med 12:527–532
53. Bellamy RF, De Guzman LR, Pedersen DC (1984) Coronary blood flow during cardiopulmonary resuscitation in swine. Circulation 69:174–180
54. Wolfe JA, Maier GW, Newton JR et al. (1988) Physiologic determinant of coronary blood flow during internal cardiac massage. J Thorac Cardiovasc Surg 95:523–532
55. Sanders AB, Atlas M, Ewy GA et al. (1985) Expired PCO_2 as an index of coronary perfusion pressure. Am J Emerg Med 3:147–149
56. Gazmuri RJ, von Planta M, Weil MH, Rackow EC (1989) Arterial PCO_2 as an indicator of systemic perfusion during cardiopulmonary resuscitation. Crit Care Med 17(3):237–240
57. von Planta I, Weil MH, von Planta M et al. (1988) Cardiopulmonary resuscitation in the rat. J Appl Physiol 65(6):2641–2647
58. Weil MH, Shubin H (1967) Diagnosis and treatment of shock. Baltimore, Williams and Wilkins Co, p 10
59. Cady LD, Weil MH, Afifi AA (1973) Quantitation of severity of critical illness with special reference to blood lactate. Crit Care Med 1:75–80
60. Henning RJ, Weil MH, Weiner F (1982) Blood lactate as a prognosticator of survival in patients with acute myocardial infarction. Circ Shock 9:310–315
61. Barker SB, Summerson WH (1941) The colorimetric determination of lactic acid in biological material. J Biol Chem 138:535–538
62. Marbach EP, Weil MH (1967) Rapid enzymatic measurement of blood lactate and pyruvate. Clin Chem 13:314–325
63. Boycks E, Michaels S, Weil MH, Shubin H, Marbach EP (1975) Continuous-flow measurement of lactate in blood: a technique adapted for use in the emergency laboratory. Clin Chem 21:113–118
64. Clark LC Jr, Noyes LK, Grooms TA, Moore MS (1984) Rapid micromeasurement of lactate in whole blood. Crit Care Med 12:461–464
65. Weil MH, Leavy JA, Rackow EC et al. (1986) Validation of a semiautomated technique for measuring lactate in whole blood. Clin Chem 32:2175–2177
66. Weil MH, Michaels S, Rackow EC (1987) Comparison of blood lactate concentrations in central venous, pulmonary artery, and arterial blood. Crit Care Med 15:489–490
67. Oliva PB (1970) Lactic acidosis. Am J Med 48:209–225
68. Orringer CE, Eustace JC, Wunsch CD, Gardner LB (1977) Natural history of lactic acidosis after grand-mal seizure. A model for the study of an anion gap acidosis not associated with hyperkalemia. N Engl J Med 297:796–799
69. Michaels S, Weil MH (1980) Measurement of blood lactate on central venous and pulmonary artery blood for estimating severity and prognosis. Crit Care Med 8:263
70. Vincent JL, Dufaye P, Berre J et al. (1983) Serial lactate determination during circulatory shock. Crit Care Med 11:449–451
71. De La Roche AG, Edmonds JF, Williams WG et al. (1978) Importance of mixed venous oxygen saturation in the care of critically ill patients. Can J Surg 21:227–233

72. Gore J (1984) Use of continuous monitoring of mixed venous oxygen saturation in the CCU. Chest 86:757–761
73. Baele PL, McMichan JC, Marsh JM, Sill JC, Southorn PA (1982) Continuous monitoring of mixed venous oxygen saturation in critically ill patients. Anesth Analg 61:513–517
74. Nelson LD (1987) Continuous venous oximetry in surgical patients. Ann Surg 203:329–333
75. Lee J, Wright F, Barber R et al. (1972) Central venous oxygen saturation in shock. Anesthesiology 36:472–478
76. Kazarian KK, Del Guercio LRM (1980) The use of mixed venous blood gas determination in traumatic shock. Ann Emerg Med 9:179–182
77. Krauss XH, Verdouw PD, Hugenholtz PG et al. (1975) On-line monitoring of mixed venous oxygen saturation after cardiothoracic surgery. Thorax 30:636–641
78. Chaudhry BA, Burki NK (1978) Ear oximetry in clinical practice. Am Rev Respir Dis 117:173–175
79. Kim SK, Baidwan BS, Petty TL (1984) Clinical evaluation of a new finger oximeter. Crit Care Med 12:910–912
80. Fatt I, Deutsch TA (1983) The relationship of conjunctival PO_2 to capillary bed PO_2. Crit Care Med 11:445–448
81. Abraham E, Smith M, Silver L (1984) Continuous monitoring of critically ill patients with transcutaneous oxygen and carbon dioxide and conjunctival oxygen sensors. Ann Emerg Med 13:1021–1026
82. Tremper KK, Shoemaker WC (1981) Transcutaneous oxygen monitoring of critically ill adults, with and without low flow shock. Crit Care Med 9:706–709
83. Weil MH, Shubin H, Carlson R (1975) Treatment of circulatory shock. JAMA 231:1280–1286
84. Weil MH, Henning RJ (1979) New concepts in the diagnosis and fluid treatment of circulatory shock. Anaesth Analg 58:124–132
85. Scheidt S, Wilner G, Mueller H, Summers D et al. (1973) Intraaortic balloon counterpulsation in cardiogenic shock. N Engl J Med 288:979–984
86. Williams DO, Korr KS, Gewirtz H, Most AS (1982) The effect of intraaortic balloon counterpulsation on regional myocardial blood flow and oxygen consumption in the presence of coronary artery stenosis in patients with unstable angina. Circulation 66:593–597
87. Gewirtz H, Ohley W, Williams DO, Sun Y, Most AS (1982) Effect of intraaortic balloon counterpulsation on regional myocardial blood flow and oxygen consumption in the presence of coronary artery stenosis: observations in an awake animal model. Am J Cardiol 50:829–837
88. Gazmuri RJ, Weil MH, van Planta M, Bisera J, Erickson S, Rackow EC (1989) Cardiac resuscitation by extracorporeal pump oxygenator (ECPO) after failure of precordial compression. J Am Coll Cardiol 13(2):220A (Abstract)
89. Levine R, Gorayeb M, Safar P, Abramson N, Stezoski W, Kelsey S (1986) Cardiopulmonary bypass after cardiac arrest and prolonged closed-chest CPR in dogs. Ann Emerg Med 16:620–627
90. Aubier M, Viires N, Syllie G, Mozes R, Roussos C (1982) Respiratory muscle contribution to lactic acidosis in low cardiac output. Am Rev Respir Dis 126:648–652
91. Hussain SNA, Simkus G, Roussos G (1985) Respiratory muscle fatigue: a cause of ventilatory failure in septic shock. J Appl Physiol 58:2033–2040
92. Aubier M, Trippenbach T, Roussos C (1981) Respiratory muscle fatigue during cardiogenic shock. J Appl Physiol 51:499–508
93. Bjork VO, Grenvik A, Holmdahl MH et al. (1964) Cardiac output and oxygen consumption during respirator treatment. Acta Anaesth Scand 15:158–160
94. Viires N, Sillye G, Aubier M et al. (1983) Regional blood flow distribution in dogs during induced hypotension and low cardiac output. Spontaneous breathing versus artificial ventilation. J Clin Invest 72:935–947

95. Weil MH, Shubin H (1969) Critical care medicine. I. The "VIP" approach to the bedside management of shock. JAMA 207:337–340
96. Weil MH, Shubin H, Rosoff L (1965) Fluid repletion in circulatory shock: central venous pressure and other practical guides. JAMA 192:668–674
97. Haupt MT, Rackow EC (1982) Colloid osmotic pressure and fluid resuscitation with hetastarch, albumin and saline solutions. Crit Care Med 10:159–162
98. Haljamae H (1985) Rationale for the use of colloids in the treatment of shock and hypovolemia. Acta Anaesth Scand 29:48–54
99. Lamke LO, Liljedahl SO (1976) Plasma volume changes after infusion of various plasma expanders. Resuscitation 5:93–98
100. Dawidson I, Gelin LE, Haglind E (1980) Plasma volume, intravascular protein content, hemodynamic and oxygen transport changes in dogs. Comparison of the relative effectiveness of various plasma expanders. Crit Care Med 8:73–80
101. Nees JE, Hauser CJ, Shippy C et al. (1978) Comparison of cardiorespiratory effects of crystalline hemoglobin, whole blood, albumin and Ringer's lactate in the resuscitation of hemorrhagic shock in dogs. Surgery 83:639–647
102. Hauser CJ, Shoemaker WC, Turpin I, Goldberg SJ (1980) Oxygen transport responses to colloids and crystalloids in critically ill surgical patients. Surg Gynecol Obstet 150:811–816
103. Shoemaker WC, Schluchtre M, Hopkins JA, Appel PL, Schwartz S, Chang PC (1981) Comparison of the relative effectiveness of colloids and crystalloids in emergency resuscitation. Am J Surg 142:73–81
104. Aberman A, Cavanilles JM, Michaels SS, Shubin H, Weil MH (1976) In vitro changes in blood P50 and erythrocyte 2,3 diphosphoglycerate concentration. Clin Chem 22:1073–1077
105. Woodson RD (1979) Physiological significance of oxygen dissociation curve shifts. Crit Care Med 9:368–373
106. Dennis RC, Hechtman HB, Berger RL et al. (1978) Transfusion of 2,3 DPG-enriched red blood cells to improve cardiac function. Ann Thorac Surg 26:17–26
107. Dawidson I, Gelin LE, Haglind E (1980) Blood viscosity and red cell aggregation changes after hemodilution in vivo and in vitro: a comparison between different plasma substitutes. Biorheology 17:9–16
108. Laks H, O'Connor NE, Pilson FN et al. (1973) Acute normovolemic hemodilution effect on hemodynamics, oxygen transport and lung water in anesthetized man. Surg Forum 24:201
109. Czer LSC, Shoemaker WC (1978) Optimal hematocrit value in critically ill postoperative patients. Surg Gynecol Obstet 147:363
110. Wilson RF, Walt AF (1975) Blood replacement. In: Walt AF, Wilson RF (eds) Management of trauma: practices and pitfalls. Philadelphia, Lea and Febiger, pp 136–148
111. Peskin GW, O'Brien K, Rabiner SF (1969) Stroma-free hemoglobin solution: The "ideal" blood substitute? Surgery 66:185–193
112. Hauser CJ, Shoemaker WC (1982) Hemoglobin solutions in the treatment of hemorrhagic shock. Crit Care Med 10:283–287
113. De Venuto F (1982) Hemoglobin solutions as oxygen-delivering resuscitation fluids. Crit Care Med 10(4):238–245
114. Hoyt DB, Greenberg AG, Peskin GW et al. (1981) Resuscitation with pyridoxalated stroma free hemoglobin: tolerance to sepsis. J Trauma 21:938–942
115. Jesch FJ, Peters W, Hobbhahn J, Schoenberg M, Messmer K (1982) Oxygen transporting fluids and oxygen delivery with hemodilution. Crit Care Med 10:270–274
116. Gould SA, Rosen AL, Sehgal LR et al. (1981) Fluorocarbon emulsions: How good as oxygen carriers? Surg Forum 23:299–301
117. Gould SA, Rosen AL, Sehgal LR et al. (1982) Red cell substitutes: hemoglobin solutions or fluorocarbon? J Trauma 22:736–740

118. Sehgal LR, Gould SA, Rosen AL et al. (1983) Appraisal of red cell substitutes: hemoglobin solution and perfluorochemical emulsions. Lab Med 14:545–548
119. Chen HS, Yang ZH (1988) Perfluorocarbon as blood substitute in clinical applications and in war casualties. Biomater Artif Cells Artif Organs 16:403–409
120. Maccanell KL, Mc Nay JL, Meyer MB et al. (1966) Dopamine in the treatment of hypotension and shock. N Engl J Med 275(25):1389–1398
121. Mueller HS, Evans R, Ayres SM (1977) Effect of dopamine on hemodynamics and myocardial metabolism in shock following acute myocardial infarction in man. Circulation 57(2):361–365
122. Loeb HS, Khan M, Sandye A et al. (1976) Acute hemodynamic effects of dobutamine and isoproterenol in patients with low output cardiac failure. Circ Shock 1976; 3:55–63
123. Francis GS, Sharma B, Hodges M (1982) Comparative hemodynamic effects of dopamine and dobutamine in patients with acute cardiogenic circulatory collapse. Am Heart J 1982; 103:995–1000
124. Richard C, Ricome JL, Rimailho A, Bottineau G, Auzepy P (1983) Combined hemodynamic effects of dopamine and dobutamine in cardiogenic shock. Circulation 67:620–626
125. Fisher CJ, Horowitz Z, Albertson TE (1985) Cardiorespiratory failure in toxic shock syndrome. Effect of dobutamine. Crit Care Med 13:160–165
126. Vincent JL, Van der Linden P, Domb M, Blecic S, Azimi G, Bernard A (1987) Dopamine compared with dobutamine in experimental septic shock relevance to fluid administration. Anesth Anal 66:565–571
127. Vincent JL, Domb M, Van der Linden P, Motte S, de Boelpaepe C, Contempre B, Cantraine F (1988) Amrinone administration in endotoxin shock. Circ Shock 25:75–83
128. Ruiz CE, Weil MH, Carlson RW (1979) Treatment of circulatory shock with dopamine. JAMA 242:165–168
129. Henning RJ, Shubin H, Weil MH (1977) Afterload reduction with phentolamine in patients with acute pulmonary edema. Am J Med 63:568–572
130. Da Luz PL, Shubin H, Weil MH (1973) Effectiveness of phentolamine for reversal of circulatory failure (shock). Crit Care Med 1:135–138
131. Guiha NH, Cohen JN, Mikulie E et al. (1974) Treatment of refractory heart failure with infusion of nitroprusside. N Engl J Med 291:587
132. Nasraway SA, Rackow EC, Astiz ME, Karras G, Weil MH (1989) Inotropic response to digoxin and dopamine in patients with severe sepsis, cardiac failure and systemic hypoperfusion. Chest 95:612–615
133. Rackow EC, Packman MI, Weil MH (1987) Hemodynamic effects of digoxin during acute cardiac failure: a comparison in patients with and without acute myocardial infarction. Crit Care Med 15:1001–1005
134. Braunwald E (1985) Effects of digitalis on the normal and the failing heart. J Am Coll Cardiol 5:51A–59A
135. Weil MH, Shubin H (1969)Isoproterenol for the treatment of circulatory shock. Ann Intern Med 70:639–641
136. Mueller HS, Ayers SM, Gregory JJ et al. (1970) Hemodynamics, coronary blood flow and myocardial metabolism in coronary shock: response to 1-norepinephrine and isoproterenol. J Clin Invest 49:1885–1902
137. Crexells C, Bourassa MG, Bison P (1973) Effects of dopamine on myocardial metabolism in patients with ischemic heart disease. Cardiovasc Res 7:438
138. Vincent JL, Van Reeth O, Van Bogaert E et al. (1986) Use of the new inotropic agent ARL-115 BS to treat severe myocardial depression in septic shock. Crit Care Med 14:661–662
139. Jentzer JH, Lejemtel TH, Sonnenblick EH, Kirk ES (1981) Beneficial effect of amrinone on myocardial oxygen consumption during acute left ventricular failure in dogs. Am J Cardiol 48:75–83

140. Monrad ES, Baim DS, Smith HS, Lanoue A, Braunwald E, Grossman W (1985) Effects of milrinone on coronary hemodynamics and myocardial energetics in patients with dongestive heart failure. Circulation 71:972–979
141. Goenen M, Pedemonte O, Baele P, Col J (1985) Amrinone in the management of low cardiac output after open heart surgery. Am J Cardiol 56:33–38
142. Benotti JR, Grossman W, Braunwald E et al. (1980) Effects of amrinone on myocardial energy metabolism and hemodynamics in patients with severe congestive heart failure treated with milrinone. Circulation 62:28–34
143. Cohn JN (1972) Improved left ventricular function during nitroprusside infusion in acute myocardial infarction. Lancet 1:650–655
144. Chatterjee K, Swan HJC, Kaushik VS et al. (1976) Effects of vasodilator therapy for severe pump failure in acute myocardial infarction on short term and late prognosis. Circulation 53:797–801
145. Nickersson M (1955) Factors of vasoconstriction and vasodilation in shock. J Mich Med Soc 54:45–49
146. Goldberg LI, Bloodwell RD, Braunwald U et al. (1960) The direct effects of norepinephrine, epinephrine and methoxamine on myocardial contractile force in man. Circulation 22:1125–1132
147. Wilson RF, Sarver EJ, LeBlanc PL (1971) Factors affecting hemodynamics in clinical shock with sepsis. Ann Surg 174(6):939–943
148. Bregman D (1975) Assessment of intraaortic balloon counterpulsation in cardiogenic shock. Crit Care Med 3:90–94
149. Sanfelippo PM, Baker NH, Ewy HG et al. (1986) Experience with intraaortic balloon counterpulsation. Ann Thorac Surg 41:36–41
150. Weil MH, Bisera J, Trevino RP, Rackow EC (1985) Cardiac output and end-tidal carbon dioxide. Crit Care Med 13:907–909
151. Falk JL, Rackow EC, Weil MH (1988) End-tidal carbon dioxide concentration during cardiopulmonary resuscitation. N Engl J Med 318:607–611
152. Garnett RA, Ornato JP, Gonzalez ER, Johnson EB (1987) End-tidal carbon dioxide monitoring during cardiopulmonary resuscitation. 257:512–515
153. Reiz S, Balfors E, Friedman A, Haggmark S, Peter T (1981) Effects of thiopentone on cardiac performance, coronary haemodynamics and myocardial oxygen consumption in chronic ischemic heart disease. Acta Anaesthesiol Scand 25:103–110
154. Reiz S, Balfors S, Haggmark S, Nath S, Rydcall A, Truedsson H (1981) Myocardial oxygen consumption and coronary haemodynamics during fentanyl-droperidol-nitrous oxide anaethesia in patients with ischemic heart disease. Acta Anaesthesiol Scand 25:286–292
155. Subramanium VB, Bowles MJ, Davies AB, Raftery EB (1982) Calcium channel blockade as primary therapy for stable angina pectoris: a double-blind placebo-controlled comparison of verapamil and propranolol. Am J Cardiol 50:1158–1163
156. Grover GJ, Kostis JB, Weiss HR et al. (1988) Effect of beta adrenoceptor stimulation or blockade on regional myocardial function and regional O_2 consumption during myocardial ischemia. Arch Int Pharmacodyn Ther 291:68–87
157. Maroko P, Kjekshus JK, Sobel BE, Watanabe T, Covell JW, Ross J Jr, Braunwald E (1971) Factors influencing infarct size following experimental coronary artery occlusions. Circulation 63:67–82
158. DeServi S, Ferrario M, Ghio S et al. (1986) Effects of diltiazem on regional coronary hemodynamics during atrial pacing in patients with stable exertional angina: implications for mechanisms of action. Circulation 73:1248–1253
159. Emanuelsson H, Holmberg S (1983) Mechanisms of angina relief after nifedipine: a hemodynamic and myocardial metabolic study. Circulation 68:124–130
160. Guzman SV, Swenson E, Mitchell R (1962) Mechanisms of cardiogenic shock. Circ Res 10:746–752
161. Costantin L (1963) Extracardiac factors contributing to hypotension during coronary occlusion. Am J Cardiol 11:205–217

162. Agress CM, Binder MJ (1957) Cardiogenic shock. Am Heart J 54:458–477
163. Gump EF, Price JB Jr, Kinney JM (1970) Whole body flow and oxygen measurements in patients with intraperitoneal infection. Ann Surg 171:321–329
164. Gump EF, Price JB Jr, Kinney JM (1970) Blood flow and oxygen consumption in patients with severe burns. Surg Gynecol Obstet 130:23–28
165. McKerrow CB, Otis AB (1956) Oxygen cost of hyperventilation. J Appl Physiol 9:375–379
166. Bartlett RG, Brubach HF, Specht H (1958) Oxygen cost of breathing. J Appl Physiol 12:413–424
167. Roussos C, Macklem P (1982) The respiratory muscles. N Engl J Med 307:786–797

Perspectives in Cardiopulmonary Resuscitation

D. H. Shaffner and M. C. Rogers

Cardiopulmonary resuscitation (CPR) represents methods used to restore oxygen delivery and tissue oxygenation during cardiac arrest. Cardiac arrest is the ultimate deterioration in oxygen delivery. The restoration of oxygen delivery by cardiopulmonary resuscitation begins with the return of ventilation. Once ventilation is restored, circulation must be resumed. The resumption of ventilation and circulation provides oxygen delivery and tissue oxygenation. The goal of this paper is to review the perspectives of cardiopulmonary resuscitation related to oxygen delivery and tissue oxygenation.

This paper describes both ventilation and circulation during cardiopulmonary resuscitation. Circulation during CPR has been broken down into subtopics which include the mechanism of blood flow, the distribution of blood flow, the efficacy of blood flow during CPR, and methods used to augment conventional closed-chest CPR. This last group – methods to augment CPR – includes many of the new techniques being used in CPR research.

Ventilation During Cardiopulmonary Resuscitation

The clinical application of CPR begins with the reestablishment of ventilation. Ventilation is reestablished by regaining the airway and reinstituting breathing. The original description of closed-chest CPR in 1960 stated that compression of the chest alone provided adequate ventilation [1]. While this might have been true in dogs, soft tissue obstruction in humans prevented adequate ventilation [2]. When endotracheal intubation was used to relieve soft tissue obstruction, it was discovered that relief of the obstruction alone did not cause adequate ventilation and intermittent positive pressure breaths were recommended [2]. The type of breath was studied for optimal gas content and delivery pattern. While the optimal breath contained 100% inspired oxygen, exhaled air was found to contain sufficient oxygen to produce adequate oxygenation (90% saturation) [3]. The optimal pattern of ventilation was subsequently investigated. Five patterns of ventilation were compared: simultaneous ventilation with compression, ventilation independent of compression, ventilations interposed between compressions, no ventilation, and continuous positive airway pressure. All five patterns allowed adequate oxygenation but differed in terms of ventilation and hemodynamic effects. Patterns in which more than a few breaths per minute were given had beneficial hemodynamic effects. Simultaneous ventilations with compressions had the greatest improvement in blood flow and survival [4]. The discovery of the benefit of simultaneous ventilations (interposed ventilation had been the standard of care) led to further research into the mechanism of blood flow during closed chest CPR.

The Mechanism of Blood Flow During Cardiopulmonary Resuscitation

An increase in femoral artery pressure was observed when heavy paddles were placed on the chest of dogs during defibrillation experiments [5]. This observation led to the use of chest compressions to produce a rise in arterial pressure which led to the development of closed-chest CPR. The mechanism responsible for the increased arterial pressure was thought to be blood forced out of the heart which was squeezed between the sternum and spine [1]. This mechanism of producing blood flow and arterial pressure by compression of the heart, either internally or between the sternum and spine, is referred to as the cardiac pump. The cardiac pump, until recently, was believed to be the dominant mechanism for the generation of arterial pressure and blood flow during closed-chest CPR.

A second mechanism for the generation of arterial pressure and blood flow has been proposed. This mechanism causes an increase in intrathoracic pressure which squeezes blood out and increases intravascular pressures and blood flow without cardiac compression. This mechanism of producing blood flow by increasing intrathoracic pressure is called the thoracic pump. The significance of the thoracic pump mechanism for blood flow became evident as inconsistencies in the cardiac pump theory occurred. These inconsistencies included:

1. All the intrathoracic pressures are elevated during closed-chest CPR while the cardiac pump predicts that only intracardiac pressures should be elevated [6].
2. Coughing alone during ventricular fibrillation caused increased intrathoracic pressure which produced blood flow and maintained consciousness. This production of blood flow without cardiac compression is inconsistent with the cardiac pump mechanism [7].
3. Elevations of intrathoracic pressure simultaneous with compression during closed-chest CPR augment arterial pressure and blood flow [4]. This benefit of noncardiac compression and intrathoracic pressure elevation is inconsistent with the cardiac pump mechanism.
4. Patients with flail sternums, which allow direct cardiac compression, received ineffective CPR. When the integrity of the thorax was restored, with external binding, compressions became effective [8].
5. The rate of compressions had little effect on blood flow during closed-chest CPR [9]. This minimal rate effect is inconsistent with the cardiac pump mechanisms which predicts that the heart has a fixed stroke volume and increasing compression rate should increase the cardiac output.

6. The duty cycle length has a significant effect on blood flow [9, 10]. This duty cycle effect is also inconsistent with the cardiac pump mechanism which predicts that the heart should be emptied early and that prolonging the duty cycle should not contribute to cardiac output.
7. Cardiac atrioventricular valves stay open during compression [11] and blood moves from pulmonary veins to aorta and from venacava to lungs during a single compression relaxation cycle [12, 13]. This conduit-like action of the heart is consistent with the thoracic rather than cardiac pump mechanism of how blood flows.
8. Aortic diameter decreases while left ventricular (LV) size does not change during compression [11, 12]. The cardiac pump predicts that the left ventricle would decrease and aorta would increase during compression.

The contention that one blood flow mechanism alone is responsible for blood flow during closed-chest CPR remains controversial. Despite acceptance of the thoracic pump mechanism, direct cardiac compression is suspected in certain closed-chest CPR models. Studies utilizing high impulse compressions [14], compressions on small animals [15], and compressions in an infant model [16] have suggested direct cardiac compression in those situations. The interaction between these blood flow models in humans remains to be clarified.

The Distribution of Blood Flow During Cardiopulmonary Resuscitation

Information gained while studying the mechanism of blood flow during closed-chest CPR has increased our understanding of the distribution of that flow. The distribution of blood flow during CPR is definitely altered from the normal physiologic state. The total blood flow is decreased and the distribution is changed to maximize heart and brain flows. This alteration in distribution should have beneficial effect on outcome. Eventual outcome after CPR depends on the maintenance of myocardial blood flows. The quality of that outcome depends on the maintenance of cerebral blood flows.

The distribution of blood flow to the brain occurs at three levels. First is the flow of blood from the chest to upper extremities and head. This suprathoracic blood flow requires a pressure gradient from intrathoracic to suprathoracic vessels. Direct cardiac compression supplied this gradient by generating an upstream pressure. Hypothetically applying intrathoracic pressure would not supply a gradient because both upstream (arterial) and downstream (venous) pressures are elevated. Fortunately the downstream or venous pressure is not transmitted and a suprathoracic venous gradient exists. This venous gradient is produced by a combination of venous collapse, secondary to the elevated intrathoracic pressure, and closure of anatomic valves in the jugular system [12, 18]. That these barriers prevent retrograde flow has been demonstrated in humans [8]. Arterial collapse does not occur and elevated intrathoracic pressure results in a gradient that promotes suprathoracic blood flow. The type of CPR influences suprathoracic flow. Models which increase intrathoracic pressure or cause cardiac compression should increase the gradient and increase suprathoracic blood flow. Models of CPR which decrease subthoracic flow mechanically or pharmacologically will increase suprathoracic flow.

The second level of flow distribution to the brain involves movement away from the extracranial suprathoracic vessels and toward the intracranial vessels. Vasoconstrictors have litle effect on the intracranial vessels and when used will constrict the extracranial vessels, increasing blood flow intracranially. Use of the vasoconstrictor epinephrine increased brain blood flow while decreasing cephalic skin, muscle, and tongue flows [16].

The third level of distribution of blood flow occurs within the intracranial vessels. CPR alone seems to result in greater percentages of flow to caudal areas of the brain. Ischemia preceding CPR significantly increases the distribution of flow to caudal areas [19]. This greater caudal distribution of flow has also been seen in other models of global ischemia [20].

Myocardial blood flow does not have the advantage of the large extrathoracic pressure gradient that augments cerebral flow. The thoracic pump generates equal increases in all intrathoracic structures; this lack of gradient results in poor myocardial blood flows. Many studies show much lower blood flows for the myocardium during closed-chest CPR compared with cerebral flows [16, 19, 21].

The type of CPR used has an effect on myocardial blood flow. Methods which cause more direct cardiac compression, such as high impulse CPR, report unusually high myocardial blood flows [21, 22]. Some studies demonstrated myocardial flow only during diastole [22] and a correlation between diastolic pressure and perfusion [13]. Other studies implied that myocardial flow may also occur during systole and relate a correlation between systolic pressures and perfusion [16, 19].

Vasoactive agents effect myocardial blood flow [24]. Pure alpha and pure beta agents have little effect on myocardial blood flow. A significant effect was found when the combined alpha and beta agonist, epinephrine, was administered during CPR.

Regional flows within the heart appear to be altered by CPR. A shift in the ratio of subendocardial to subepicardial blood flow occurs during CPR. This ratio shifts from 1.5 to 0.8 during CPR [16]. This ratio reverts to normal with epinephrine administration.

Blood flow to organs other than the heart or brain is greatly reduced during CPR. The lack of valves in the intrathoracic veins leads to retrograde transmission of venous pressure and decreases the gradient for blood flow below the diaphragm [25]. Regional flows have been reported for several subthoracic organs: small intestine 5%–25%, pancreas 1.5%–25%, liver 1%–20%, kidney 1%–12%, adrenals 12%, extremity muscle 1%–5%, and spleen 0%–3% of prearrest flows [19, 27, 28, 29]. The addition of abdominal compressions on simultaneous ventilations during closed-chest CPR does not alter the subthoracic organ blood flows [27, 29]. The addition of epinephrine during closed-chest CPR almost eliminates flow in these organs except for the adrenal (flow increase with epinephrine).

Little data are available regarding pulmonary flow during CPR. It has been demonstrated that pulmonary blood flow occurs primarily during periods of low intrathoracic pressure during closed-chest CPR [13]. High extrathoracic venous pressure builds up during compression and results in pulmonary filling after compression release as intrathoracic pressure falls.

Efficacy of Blood Flow During Cardiopulmonary Resuscitation

Blood flows produced during conventional closed-chest CPR without pharmacologic support are disappointingly low. The range reported for cerebral blood flow is 3%–14% of prearrest levels in dogs [29–33]. Cerebral perfusion pressures are less commonly reported and are also low, 4%–24% of prearrest [29–31]. Myocardial blood flows in this basic CPR mode are also disapointinly low, 1%–15% [9, 27, 30, 33, 34] of prearrest levels in dogs. Myocardial perfusion pressures have been shown to correlate with myocardial blood flow. Plotting myocardial blood flow in ml/min/g versus myocardial perfusion pressure in mmHg gives a slope of 0.01–0.015 [23, 27].

Several factors affect cerebral and myocardial blood flows in the conventional closed-chest CPR model. Factors that improve blood flow during CPR will be discussed individually in the next section. Factors that seem to have a negative effect on blood flow during CPR include age, intracranial pressure, duration of CPR, and duration of preresuscitation ischemia.

Age appears to have an effect on cerebral blood flow during closed-chest CPR. Two-week old piglets have substantially higher cerebral blood flows (50% of prearrest) and slightly better myocardial flows (17% of prearrest) than those reported for adults [16]. Two studies on slightly older piglets gave opposing results. Cerebral blood flow values in these two studies are 26%–95% and 1%–4% of prearrest values with corresponding myocardial values of 2%–8% and 1%–6% [25, 28]. The cerebral flows in the first of these two studies are substantially higher than in adults during closed-chest CPR and neither of the myocardial flows are different from adult models.

Intracranial pressure can represent the downstream pressure for cerebral blood flow and if elevated inhibits cerebral perfusion. The intracranial pressure has been observed to increase in response to increasing intrathoracic pressure with closed-chest CPR [35]. This relationship is linear and the value for the ratio of the change in intracranial pressure to change in intrathoracic pressure is 0.33 [36]. The transmission of intrathoracic pressure to the intracranial contents is unrelated to carotid or jugular pressures. The transmission can be partially blocked by occluding the cerebrospinal fluid or vertebral vein flow. The rise in intracranial pressure with chest compressions becomes more significant in the setting of baseline increased intracranial pressure and abdominal binding.

Increased duration of CPR has a negative effect on cerebral blood flow and seems to be most bothersome in an infant preparation [16, 28]. The length of the ischemic period before CPR is started has a negative effect on cerebral blood flow [38]. It seems obvious that a minimal ischemic period and quick resuscitation would improve eventual outcome, but the cause of the effect on cerebral blood flow is less obvious.

There appear to be thresholds for minimal vital organ blood flow during CPR. The inability to maintain blood flow during CPR above these thresholds results in organ malfunction. In the case of the heart, myocardial blood flows of 20 ml/min/100 g or greater are necessary for successful defibrillation in dogs [36, 39]. Regarding the brain, cerebral blood flow of greater than 15–20 ml/min/100 g are necessary to maintain normal brain electrical activity during CPR [19].

Experimental Models of Cardiopulmonary Resuscitation

Abdominal Binding/MAST Application

Abdominal binders and military antishock trousers (MAST) have been used to augment closed-chest CPR. Both methods apply continuous compression below the diaphragm. Three mechanisms have been proposed for the augmentation of closed-chest CPR by these binders. First, binding the abdominal contents decreases the compliance of the diaphragm and raises intrathoracic pressure. Second, squeezing blood out of the subthoracic structures increases the circulating blood volume. Third, constricting the subdiaphragmatic vasculature, thus increasing the resistance, should improve suprathoracic blood flow.

The above proposed mechanisms have been supported by available studies. Intrathoracic pressure is elevated during compression by the addition of abdominal binding [40]. Increased aortic systolic pressure is produced in most studies and represents increased circulating blood volume [40–43]. Suprathoracic blood flow often measured as carotid flow, is increased in several studies [8, 40, 41, 44].

Despite the above favorable findings some concerns remain about the application of abdominal binding. First, there remains the possibility of causing abdominal injuries. Hepatobiliary injuries were reported in 33% of animals in one study [40]. Second, an increase in right atrial diastolic pressure may exceed the increase in aortic diastolic pressure. These increased diastolic pressures lead to decreased coronary perfusion pressure [40, 44]. Lastly, binding failed to contribute to blood flows in more effective methods of CPR. No significant hemodynamic improvement was found when binding was employed during vest or simultaneous compression ventilation CPR [31, 45]. Cerebral oxygenation and perfusion gradients were decreased in one study [31].

Interposed Abdominal Compressions

Interposed abdominal compressions (IAC) have been used to augment closed-chest CPR. Compression of the abdomen is delivered during the relaxation phase of chest compression and released at the initiation of the following chest compression. IAC CPR can be done with the addition of a second rescuer, requiring only a slight modification of conventional closed-chest CPR.

There are two proposed mechanisms for the augmentation of CPR by IAC. First, IAC increases the gradient for blood flow to the thorax during the relaxation phase of chest compression. This increased return "primes the pump," thereby augmenting the output delivered by the subsequent chest compression. This pump priming of the thorax by the abdomen has been compared to the atria priming the ventricles [46]. Second, the flow generated by abdominal compression may reach the head and brain during chest diastole, thus adding a second pump providing vital organ perfusion.

Hemodynamic improvements have been shown in several studies. Increased cardiac output and aortic pressures have been seen in human and in dog studies [46–49]. Coronary perfusion pressures have been improved compared with conventional closed-chest CPR [47, 48, 50]. Increased cerebral blood flow with IAC CPR has been shown in dogs [51].

Outcome studies with this method of CPR augmentation are scarce. A study which compared IAC CPR with conventional closed-chest CPR showed no difference in resuscibility, survival, or trauma produced [52]. This same study showed no hemodynamic benefits produced by IAC CPR. These results raise the possibility that either hemodynamic benefits reported in earlier studies were insignificant, or that IAC CPR was performed less effectively or conventional closed-chest CPR more effectively than previously. A study showing possibly detrimental effects from IAC CPR exists [53]. This study proposed that IAC CPR produced inadequate flows and thus compromised mitochondrial oxygen utilization more than both no flow and adequate flow.

Vest CPR

A vest has been designed to deliver chest compressions during closed-chest CPR. This vest consists of an inflatable bladder wrapped around the chest and inflated pneumatically (resembling a blood pressure cuff). This method of delivering CPR is itself interesting because it eliminates the possibility of direct cardiac compression. This diffuse method of applying compression force is the ideal model for the thoracic pump mechanism of CPR. This diffuse application of pressure also decreases the amount of thoracic trauma in CPR.

Hemodynamic improvements with vest CPR have been shown in several studies. The increase in cerebral blood flow appears to be more impressive than the myocardial flow with vest CPR. Cerebral blood flows from 21%–165% of prearrest values have been reported [9, 30, 54]. Myocardial blood flows have been 4%–100% of prearrest values in these same studies. Adding simultaneous ventilations further improved both blood flows [9]. Contradictory results regarding myocardial perfusion pressures are reported [45, 55].

Survival data in two separate studies showed very significantly improved survival when vest CPR or vest-binder CPR were compared with conventional closed-chest CPR [54, 56].

Simultaneous Compression Ventilation CPR

Simultaneous compression ventilation (SCV) CPR has been employed to augment closed-chest CPR. The elucidation of the thoracic pump mechanism for blood flow during CPR led to the realization that increasing intrathoracic pressure augmented/produced blood flow during CPR. The addition of ventilation simultaneously with chest compression, as opposed to interposed between compressions, adds to the intrathoracic pressure generated. This increased intrathoracic pressure should augment blood flows produced by closed-chest CPR.

Hemodynamic data indicate an increase in carotid blood flow in most SCV CPR studies when compared with conventional CPR [15, 31, 34, 59, 60]. The increase in flow was not significant in two of these studies [59, 60]. Cerebral blood flows produced during SCV CPR were 32%–60% of prearrest flows [19, 29, 30, 33]. Myocardial blood flows produced by SCV CPR were 5%–25% of the prearrest values [19, 29, 30, 33]. The addition of epinephrine produced even higher flows when added to this technique [19]. The myocardial and cerebral flows produced by SCV CPR appear higher than flows generated by vest CPR with interposed ventrilations [30].

Models that contain a component of direct cardiac compression received less hemodynamic benefit from SCV CPR [15, 57, 58, 59]. Sustained use of SCV CPR failed to prevent deterioration of blood flow in individual models [30, 58, 59]. It has been proposed that the augmented intrathoracic pressures increase the likelihood of arterial collapse during prolonged CPR [19, 59]. Coronary perfusion pressures have been adversely affected by SCV CPR in humans [45] and significantly decreased with the addition of abdominal binders in dogs [13, 44]. Survival was significantly impaired when SCV with abdominal binder was compared with conventional closed-chest CPR [44]. An additional concern regarding SCV CPR has been the production of pneumothoraces in an infant model [58].

High Impulse CPR

High impulse CPR refers to the application of greater than usual force during chest compression. This increase in force can be in the form of greater mass, velocity, or both. It has been hypothesized that the greater impulses result in greater chest deflection causing more contact with the heart. Direct cardiac compression is more likely with this form of closed-chest CPR. Direct cardiac compression results in the technique being more rate and less duty cycle dependent, as predicted by the cardiac pump mechanism of blood flow. This rate dependence has been demonstrated in high impulse CPR, thus supporting the cardiac pump hypothesis [22, 52].

Hemodynamic improvement is seen when this CPR technique is used to augment conventional closed-chest CPR. Dog studies demonstrate significant improvements in myocardial and cerebral blood flow with high impulse, compared with low impulse, CPR [21]. High impulse CPR can generate myocardial blood flows as high as 60%–75% of prearrest values [22]. In humans high impulse CPR generated increased aortic pressure (of undetermined clinical significance) [45]. An outcome study in dogs compared high impulse CPR with conventional closed-chest CPR and found no significant improvement in resuscitation, survival, or neurologic outcome [52].

Pharmacologic Augmentation of CPR

Epinephrine has emerged as the pharmacologic means of improving closed-chest CPR blood flow. Epinephrine has historically been used in the arrest situation for its chronotropic and inotropic effects. The vasoconstrictive effects of epinephrine appear to be its most important pharmacologic action during CPR. The vasoconstriction produced by epinephrine seems to be selective for noncardiac and noncerebral vessels. This selective vasoconstriction results in increased cerebral and myocardial blood flow. This vasopressor effect also bolsters the intrathoracic arteries against collapse secondary to high intrathoracic pressure.

Hemodynamically the use of epinehrine produces myocardial blood flows of 10%–90% and cerebral blood flows of 24%–95% of prearrest values during conventional closed-chest CPR [16, 23, 25, 32, 33]. The addition of epinephrine to SCV CPR produces myocardial blood flows of 28%–44% and cerebral blood flows of 75% of prearrest values [19, 33]. The myocardial and cerebral bloods flows with epinephrine were significantly greater in all models than without epinephrine in the identical model [16, 19, 23–25, 32, 33]. The doses employed in these studies for boluses were 10–2000 mcg/kg [16, 19, 23–25, 33] and for constant infusions were 4–30 mcg/kg/min [16, 19, 32, 33].

The increased blood flow generated by the addition of epinephrine during closed-chest CPR had additional clinical benefits. Resuscitation was improved [19], electroencephalographic activity was better [19], and cerebral oxygenation was improved [16]. The regional blood flow in the heart was shifted away from the endocardium during closed-chest CPR, the addition of epinephrine had no further effect [16]. While epinephrine prevented collapse of intrathoracic arteries in most models, it failed to do so in the infant model of CPR [16].

Attempts to further understand the effects of epinephrine on blood flow have focused on its alpha- and beta-adrenergic activity. The hemodynamic effects of epinephrine, with mixed alpha and beta effects, were compared with methoxamine, a pure alpha agent [61]. Pigs receiving 200 mcg/kg boluses had significantly greater cerebral blood flow and cardiac output than any methoxamine group (100, 1000, 10000 mcg/kg). These results indicate that the increased cerebral blood flow may be secondary to both alpha and beta effects.

Outcome studies have compared epinephrine with pure alpha and pure beta agents [62, 63]. Epinephrine above 80 mcg/kg produced excellent resuscitation and survival following closed-chest CPR (80%–100%). Phenylephrine, a pure alpha agent at 800 mcg/kg produced survival and resuscitation rates identical with epinephrine [62, 63]. Isoproterenol, a pure beta agent, resulted in significantly decreased survival compared with alpha agents [63]. Although some differences appeared in hemodynamic effects between epinephrine and methoxamine, both produced similar survival rates; beta agents gave a poor survival ratio compared with alpha agents. These bad outcome results with a beta agent may be related to vasodilation shunting blood away from the heart and brain, increasing myocardial wall tension, and increasing oxygen consumption.

Open-Chest Cardiopulmonary Resuscitation

Open-chest CPR involves a thoracotomy and results in direct compression of the heart generating blood flow. The application of this technique requires a high level of sophistication and training as well as special equipment and facilities. These requirements limit open-chest CPR to certain hospital settings.

Open-chest CPR represents a model of the cardiac pump mechanism for generation of blood flow. Theoretically this model eliminates the production of intrathoracic pressure which if transmitted could reduce the gradients for blood flow. This enhanced gradient combined with directly applied compression should result in near normal blood flows.

Hemodynamic data for open-chest CPR reveal cardiac outputs 25%–61% of prearrest values [31, 64, 65]. These studies and others show cardiac outputs two to three times larger than with conventional closed-chest CPR [31, 64–67]. Increases in cerebral perfusion pressure have been significant in some studies [66] and not in others [31, 67]. Myocardial perfusion pressures were significantly increased compared with closed-chest CPR [66, 68]. In dogs cerebral blood flows 150% of prearrest values could be produced with open-chest CPR [32]. Cross clamping the descending aorta during open-chest CPR further increases carotid blood flow.

Survival in dogs can be improved by use of open-chest CPR following inadequate closed-chest CPR [68]. Dogs with myocardial perfusion pressure less than 30 mmHg after 15 min of closed-chest CPR received 2–4 min of either open-chest or closed-chest external CPR and defibrillation was attempted. The dogs receiving open-chest CPR had significantly greater myocardial perfusion pressures and survival rates.

The length of time that closed-chest CPR was performed affected the success of subsequent open-chest CPR [69]. After 20 and 25 min of closed-chest CPR, the success rate of open-chest CPR dropped to 38% and 0% respectively. This implies that the benefits from open-chest CPR are time limited and are most beneficial when applied early.

Cardiopulmonary Bypass

Cardiopulmonary bypass (CPB) represents one of the newest and most sophisticated models of resuscitation. Animal studies show that CPB increases 72-h survival, recovery of consciousness, and causes less myocardial damage than closed-chest CPR. There was definite improvement, compared with conventional closed-chest CPR, in neurologic outcome with short ischemic times (approx. 4 min). Neurologic outcome was dismal in either group with a long (12 min) period of ischemia. When CPB followed 20 min of conventional closed-chest CPR 100% of animals were resuscitated. This compares favorably with a study of open-chest CPR which resuscitated zero dogs after 25 min of closed-chest CPR [69].

Experience with CPB in humans is limited. Implementation of CPB in an uncontrolled study in adults resulted in 15 of 39 patients with long-term survival [72]. The patients with the greatest benefit in this study were already hospitalized and had an acute pulmonary embolism (13 of 19). Survival was less likely with this CPB when used for trauma, drug overdose, myocardial infarction, or cardiac arrest of unknown etiology (2 of 20).

Conclusion

Attempts to restore oxygen delivery and tissue oxygen to adequate levels with CPR have met with limited success. Noninvasive mechanical methods can generate improved blood flows, but have less effect on survival and have had minimal experience in humans. Pharmacologic augmentation appears effective and pending further research epinephrine remains the agent of choice. Invasive resuscitation measures (open-chest CPR, CPB) appear to be more successful than conventional closed-chest CPR but because of lack of experience, indications and guidelines have not yet been established.

References

1. Kouwenhoven WB Ing, Jude JR, Knickerbocker GG (1960) Closed-chest cardiac massage. JAMA 173:1064–1067
2. Safar P, Brown TC, Holtey WJ, Wilder RJ (1961) Ventilation and circulation with closed-chest cardiac massage in man. JAMA 176:574–576
3. Elam JO, Brown ES, Elder JD (1954) Artificial respiration by mouth-to-mask method. NEJM 250:749–754
4. Wilder RJ, Weir D, Rush BF, Ravitch MM (1963) Methods of coordinating ventilation and closed chest cardiac massage in dogs. Surg 53:186–194
5. Sladen A (1984) Closed-chest massage, Kouwenhaven, Jude, Knickerbocker. JAMA 251:3137–3140
6. Weale FE, Lond MS, Rothwell-Jackson RL (1962) The efficiency of cardiac massage. Lancet I:990–992
7. Criley JM, Blaufuss AH, Kissel GL (1976) Cough-induced cardiac compression. JAMA 236:1246–1250
8. Rudikoff MT, Maughan WL, Effron M, Freund P, Weisfeldt ML (1980) Mechanisms of blood flow during cardiopulmonary resuscitation. Circulation 61:345–352
9. Halperin HR, Tsitlik JE, Guerci AD, Mellits ED, Levin HR, Shi AY, Chandra N, Weisfeldt ML (1986) Determinants of blood flow to vital organs during cardiopulmonary resuscitation in dogs. Circulation 73:539–550

10. Taylor GJ, Tucker WM, Greene HL, Rudikoff MT, Weisfeldt ML (1977) Importance of prolonged compression during cardiopulmonary resuscitation in man. NEJM 296:1515–1517
11. Werner JA, Greene HL, Janko CL, Cobb LA (1981) Visualization of cardiac valve motion in man during external chest compression using two-dimensional echocardiography. Circulation 63:1417–1421
12. Niemann JT, Rosborough JP, Hausknecht M, Garner D, Criley JM (1981) Pressure-synchronized cineangiography during experimental cardiopulmonary resuscitation. Circulation 64:985–991
13. Cohen JM, Chandra N, Alderson PD, Van Aswegen A, Tsitlik JE, Weisfeldt ML (1982) Timing of pulmonary and systemic blood flow during intermittent high intrathoracic pressure cardiopulmonary resuscitation in the dog. Am J Cardiol 49:1883–1889
14. Feneley MP, Maier GW, Gaynor JW, Gall SA, Kisslo JA, Davis JW, Rankin JS (1987) Sequence of mitral valve motion and tansmitral blood flow during manual cardiopulmonary resuscitation in dogs. Circulation 76:363–375
15. Babbs CF, Tacker WA, Paris RL, Murphy RJ, Davis RW (1982) CPR with simultaneous compression and ventilation at high airway pressures in 4 animal models. Crit Care Med 10:501–504
16. Schleien CL, Dean JM, Koehler RC, Michael JR, Chantarojanasiri T, Traystman RJ, Rogers MC (1986) Effect of epinephrine on cerebral and myocardial perfusion in an infant animal preparation of cardiopulmonary resuscitation. Circulation 73:809–817
17. Krause GS, Kumar K, White BC, Aust SD, Wiegenstein JG (1986) Ischemia, resuscitation and reperfusion: mechanisms of tissue injury and prospects for protection. Am Heart J 111:768–780
18. Fisher J, Vaghairwalla F, Tsitlik JE, Levin H, Brinker J, Weisfeldt ML, Yin F (1982) Determinants and clinical significance of jugular venous valve competence. Circulation 65:188–196
19. Michael JR, Guerci AD, Koehler RC, Shi AY, Tsitlik JE, Chandra N, Niedermeyer E, Rogers MC, Traystman RJ, Weisfeldt ML (1984) Mechanisms by which epinephrine augments cerebral and myocardial perfusion during cardiopulmonary resuscitation in dogs. Circulation 69:822–835
20. Jackson DL, Dole WP, McGloin J, Rosenblatt JI (1981) Total cerebral ischemia: application of a new model system to studies of cerebral microcirculation. Stroke 12:66–72
21. Ditchey RV, Winkler JV, Rhodes CA (1982) Relative lack of coronary blood flow during closed-chest resuscitation in dogs. Circulation 66:297–302
22. Maier GW, Tyson GS, Olsen CO, Kernstein KH, Davis JW, Conn EH, Sabiston DC, Rankin JS (1984) The physiology of external cardiac massage: high-impulse cardiopulmonary resuscitation. Circulation 70:86-101
23. Ralston SH, Voorhees WD, Babbs CF (1984) Intrapulmonary epinephrine during prolonged cardiopulmonary resuscitation: improved regional blood flow and resuscitation in dogs. Ann Emerg Med 13:79–86
24. Holmes HR, Babbs CF, Voorhees WD, Tacker WA, De Garavilla B (1980) Influence of adrenergic drugs upon vital organ perfusion during CPR. Crit Care Med 8:137–140
25. Brown CG, Werman HA, Davis EA, Hobson J, Hamlin RL (1987) The effects of graded doses of epinephrine on regional myocardial blood flow during cardiopulmonary resuscitation in swine. Criculation 75:491–497
26. Weisfeldt ML, Halperin HR (1986) Cardiopulmonary resuscitation: beyond cardiac massage. Circulation 74:443–448
27. Voorhees WD, Ralston SH, Babbs CF (1983) Regional blood flow during cardiopulmonary resuscitation with abdominal counterpulsation in dogs. Am J Emerg Med 2:123–128

28. Sharff JA, Pantley G, Noel E (1984) Effect of time on regioinal organ perfusion during two methods of cardiopulmonary resuscitation. Ann Emerg Med 13:649–656
29. Koehler RC, Chandra N, Guerci AD, Tsitlik JE, Traystman RJ, Rogers MC, Weisfeldt ML (1983) Augmentation of cerebral perfusion by simultaneous chest compression and lung inflation with abdominal binding after cardiac arrest in dogs. Circulation 67:266–275
30. Luce JM, Ross BK, O'Quin RJ, Culver BH, Sivarajan M, Amory DW, Niskanin RA, Alferness CA, Kirk WL, Pierson LB, Butler J (1983) Regional blood flow during cardiopulmonary resuscitation in dogs using simultaneous and nonsimultaneous compression and ventilation. Circulation 67:258–265
31. Bircher N, Safar P (1981) Comparison of standard and "new" closed-chest CPR and open-chest CPR in dogs. Crit Care Med 9:384–385
32. Jackson RE, Joyce K, Danosi SF (1984) Blood flow in the cerebral cortex during cardiac resuscitation in dogs. Ann Emerg Med 13:657–659
33. Koehler RC, Michael JR, Guerci AD, Chandra N, Schleien CL, Dean JM, Rogers MC, Weisfeldt ML, Traystman RJ (1985) Beneficial effect of epinephrine infusion on cerebral and myocardial blood flows during CPR. Ann Emerg Med 14:744–749
34. Chandra N, Weisfeldt ML, Tsitlik JE, Vaghaiwalla F, Synder LD, Hoffecker M, Rudikoff MT (1981) Augmentatiion of carotid blood flow during cardiopulmonary resuscitation by ventilation at high airway pressure simultaneous with chest compression. Am J Card 48:1053–1063
35. Rogers MC, Nugent SK, Stidham GL (1979) Effects of closed-chest cardiac massage on intracranial pressure. Crit Care Med 7:454–456
36. Guerci AD, Shi AY, Levin H, Tsitlik JE, Weisfeldt ML, Chandra N (1985) Transmission of intrathoracic pressure to the intracranial space during cardiopulmonary resuscitation in dogs. Circ Res 56:20–30
37. Guerci AD, Chandra N, Levin H, Koehler RC, Tsitlik JE, Traystman RJ, Rogers MC, Weisfeldt ML (1981) Hemodynamic determinants of intracranial pressure during resuscitation. Circulation 64:304
38. Lee K, Vaagenes P, Safar P, Stezoski SW, Scanlon M (1984) Impact of cardiac arrest time on the cortical cerebral blood flow generated by subsequent standard external CPR in rabbits. Ann Emerg Med 13:385
39. Sanders AB, Kern KB, Atlas M, Bragg S, Ewy GA (1985) Importance of the duration of inadequate coronary perfusion pressure on resuscitation from cardiac arrest. JACC 6:113–118
40. Niemann JT, Rosborough JP, Ung S, Criley JM (1984) Hemodynamic effects of continuous abdominal binding during cardiac arrest and resuscitation. Am J Cardiol 53:269–274
41. Lee HR, Wilder RJ, Downs P, Massion W, Blank WF (1981) MAST augmentation of external cardiac chest compression: role of changing intrapleural pressure. Ann Emerg Med 10:560–565
42. Lilja BP, Long RS, Ruiz E (1981) Augmentation of systolic blood pressure during external cardiac compression by use of the MAST suit. Ann Emerg Med 10:182–184
43. Chandra N, Snyder LD, Weisfeldt ML (1981) Abdominal binding during cardiopulmonary resuscitation in man. JAMA 246:351–353
44. Sanders AB, Ewy GA, Alferness CA, Taft T, Zimmerman M (1982) Failure of one method of simultaneous chest compression, ventilation, and abdominal binding during CPR. Crit Care Med 10:509–513
45. Swenson RD, Weaver WD, Niskanen RA, Martin J, Dahlberg S (1988) Hemodynamics in humans during conventional and experimental methods of cardiopulmonary resuscitation. Circulation 78:630–639
46. Ralston SH, Babbs CF, Neibauer MJ (1982) Cardiopulmonary resuscitation with interposed abdominal compression in dogs. Anesth Analg 61:645–651

47. Redding JS (1971) Abdominal compression in cardiopulmonary resuscitation. Anesth Analg 50:668–675
48. Berryman CR, Phillips GM (1984) Interposed abdominal compression-CPR in human subjects. Ann Emerg Med 13:226–229
49. Voorhees WD, Neibauer MJ, Babbs CF (1983) Improved oxygen delivery during cardiopulmonary resuscitation with interposed abdominal compressions. Ann Emerg Med 12:128–135
50. Howard M, Carrubba C, Guiness M, Foss F, Hogan B (1984) Interposed abdominal compression CPR: its effects on coronary perfusion pressure in human subjects. Ann Emerg Med 13:989–990
51. Walker JW, Bruestle JC, White BC, Evans AT, Indreri R, Bialek H (1984) Perfusion of the cerebral cortex by use of abdominal counterpulsation during cardiopulmonary resuscitation. Am J Emerg Med 2:391–393
52. Kern KB, Carter AB, Showen RL, Voorhees WD, Babbs CF, Tacker EA, Ewy GA (1986) Twenty-four hour survival in a canine model of cardiac arrest comparing three methods of manual cardiopulmonary resuscitation. JACC 7:859–867
53. White BC, Hildebrandt JF, Evans AT, Aronson L, Indrieri RJ, Hoehner T, Fox L, Huang R, Johns D (1985) Prolonged cardiac arrest and resuscitation in dogs: brain mitochondrial function with different artificial perfusion methods. Ann Emerg Med 14:383–388
54. Halperin HR, Guerci AD, Chandra N, Herskowitz A, Tsitlik JE, Niskanen RA, Wurmb E, Weisfeldt ML (1986) Vest inflation without simultaneous ventilation during cardiac arrest in dogs: improved survival from prolonged cardiopulmonary resuscitation. Circulation 74:1407–1415
55. Niemann JT, Rosborough JP, Niskanen RA, Alferness C, Criley JM (1985) Mechanical "cough" cardiopulmonary resuscitation during cardiac arrest in dogs. Am J Cardiol 55:199–204
56. Criley JM, Niemann JT, Rosborough JP, Hausknecht M (1986) Modifications of cardiopulmonary resuscitation based on the cough. Circulation 74:42–50
57. Babbs CF, Fitzgerald KR, Voorhees WD, Murphy RJ (1982) High-pressure ventilation during CPR with 95% O_2:5% CO_2. Crit Care Med 10:505–508
58. Berkowitz ID, Chantarojanasiri T, Koehler RC, Schleien C, Dean JM, Michael JR, Rogers MC, Traystman RJ (1988) Simultaneous compression and ventilation cardiopulmonary resuscitation doses not enhance cerebral and myocardial perfusion in an infant model of cardiopulmonary resuscitation. Anesthesiology 65:108
59. Chandra N, Rudikoff M, Weisfeldt ML (1980) Simultaneous chest compression and ventilation at high airway pressure during cardiopulmonary resuscitation. Lancet I:175–178
60. Harris LC, Kirimli B, Safar P (1967) Ventilation-cardiac compression rates and ratios in cardiopulmonary resuscitation. Anesthesiology 28:806
61. Brown CG, Davis EA, Werman HA, Hamlin RL (1987) Methoxamine versus epinephrine on regional cerebral blood flow during cardiopulmonary resuscitation. Crit Care Med 15:682–686
62. Brillman JA, Sanders AB, Otto CW, Fahmy H, Bragg S, Ewy GA (1985) Outcome of resuscitation from fibrillatory arrest using epinephrine and phenylephrine in dogs. Crit Care Med 13:912–913
63. Yakaitis RW, Otto CW, Blitt CD (1979) Relative importance of α and β adrenergic receptors during resuscitation. Crit Care Med 7:293–296
64. Bartlett RL, Stewart NJ, Raymond J, Anstadt GL, Martin SD (1984) Comparative study of three methods of resuscitation: closed-chest, open-chest manual, and direct mechanical ventricular assistance. Ann Emerg Med 13:773–777
65. Weiser FM, Adler LN, Kuhn LA (1962) Hemodynamic effects of closed and open chest cardiac resuscitation in normal dogs and those with acute myocardial infarction. Am J Cardiol 10:555–561
66. Bircher N, Safar P, Stewart R (1980) A comparison of standard, "MAST"-augmented, and open-chest CPR in dogs. Crit Care Med 8:147–152

67. Del Guercio LRM, Feins NR, Cohn JD, Coomaraswamy RP, Woolman SB, State D (1965) Comparison of blood flow during external and internal cardiac massage in man. Circulation 31:1-171-180
68. Sanders AB, Kern KB, Ewy GA, Atlas M, Bailey L (1984) Improved resuscitation from cardiac arrest with open-chest massage. Ann Emerg Med 13:672–675
69. Sanders AB, Kern KB, Ewy GA (1985) Time limitations for open-chest cardiopulmonary resuscitation from cardiac arrest. Crit Care Med 13:897
70. Levine R, Gorayeb M, Safar P, Abramson N, Stezoski W, Kelsey S (1987) Cardiopulmonary bypass after cardiac arrest and prolonged closed-chest CPR in dogs. Ann Emerg Med 16:620–627
71. Pretto E, Safar P, Saito R, Stezoski W, Kelsey S (1987) Cardiopulmonary bypass after prolonged cardiac arrest in dogs. Ann Emerg Med 16:611–619
72. Mattox KL, Beall AC (1976) Resuscitation of the moribund patient using portable cardiopulmonary bypass. Ann Thor Surg 22:436–442

Cardiorespiratory Adjustment to Exercise After Cardiac Transplantation

M. Meyer, P. Cerretelli, C. Marconi, M. Rieu,
and Ch. Cabrol

Introduction

Over the past two decades cardiac transplantation has evolved as an accepted therapeutic option for terminal heart failure in man. Successful transplantation can considerably improve the patient's quality of life and actuarial survival statistics of 78% for the first 2 years and greater than 60% for the first 5 years after surgery have been reported (Evans et al. 1984; Buxton et al. 1985; Macoviak et al. 1985). Evaluation of the chronically denervated heart has provided evidence for adequate overall performance to meet the circulatory and metabolic demands under basal conditions and during dynamic exercise (Shaver et al. 1969; Carleton et al. 1969; Campeau et al. 1970; Griepp et al. 1971; Stinson et al. 1972; Clark et al. 1973; Stinson et al. 1975; McLaughlin et al. 1978; Schroeder et al. 1976; Schroeder 1979; Pope et al. 1980; Savin et al. 1980; Borow et al. 1985; Degre et al. 1987; Kavanagh et al. 1988). Hemodynamic adjustment of the denervated heart early in exercise, i.e., in the absence of a significant sympathetic stimulation associated with lack of increase in heart rate, is brought about by an increased stroke volume secondary to augmented preload and the Frank-Starling mechanism (Donald 1968; Clark et al. 1973; Pope et al. 1980). Later in exercise or at higher work loads the increase of cardiac output adequate for the individual's metabolic demand is mediated by the chronotropic and inotropic effects of circulating catecholamines. Thus, unlike the normally innervated heart, the mechanisms effective for the cardiovascular response to exercise appear sequentially in the denervated heart.

The cardiac output during submaximal exercise measured under steady state conditions in relation to oxygen uptake is normal or slightly reduced (Mertens et al. 1987; Kavanagh et al. 1988). Recent evidence suggests that the healthy transplanted heart when tested pharmacologically maintains normal left ventricular contractility and contractile reserve (Borow et al. 1985; Reid and Yacoub 1988), and, moreover, develops an increased sensitivity to circulating catecholamines (Dempsey and Cooper 1968; Lurie et al. 1983; Yusuf et al. 1987). Notwithstanding, human physical work performance is impaired after cardiac transplantation as reflected by the average peak power output which is less than about one-half that attained by normal subjects (Pope et al. 1980; Theodore et al. 1987; Banner et al. 1988; Kavanagh et al. 1988; Cerretelli et al. 1988; Banner et al. 1989). Since the contribution of heart rate towards the increase of cardiac output at the onset of exercise is negligible, the delayed time course of readjustment of cardiac output and the lower peak heart rates achieved have been invoked as important factors limiting the individual's physical performance. Failure of adjustment of stroke volume and cardiac output compensating for the lack of heart rate response may in turn reduce the kinetics of adjustment of respiratory gas exchange at the onset of exercise.

Objectives

The aim of the present study was to get a better insight into the limiting factors of physical performance and exercise capacity in heart transplant recipients. The role of central and peripheral mechanisms limiting the maximal rate of gas exchange at steady state and in the transition from rest to rectangular exercise was studied in a group of heart transplant recipients and normal control subjects. Since heart transplant patients are frequently obligated to invasive reassessments instantaneous non-invasive techniques were employed for the assessment of gas exchange dynamics at the lungs and cardiovascular responses to exercise.

Subjects

The studies were performed in the Department of Cardiovascular Surgery of La Pitié-Salpétrière Hospital at Paris. Twenty-one short-term and long-term (over one year) recipients of an orthotopic heart transplant ranging in age from 28 to 59 years (means $\pm$ SD: 44.5 ± 8.1) were investigated (Table 1). Before surgery their clinical status had deteriorated with causes compiled in Table 1 to class IV disability (New York Heart Association classification). The patients were assessed from 1.3 to 137.1 (means $\pm$ SD: 24.2 ± 30.0) months after operation at the time of their routine evaluation. They had been free from suffering major episodes of graft rejection (for at least 3 months in the long-term patients) as documented by clinical, laboratory, electrocardiographic and endomyocardial biopsy findings. All patients were treated with cyclosporine A and low quantities of oral prednisone as routine immunosuppressive therapy but none were taking β-blocking agents. They were considered fully rehabilitated but were not engaged in any specific physical rehabilitation program. They performed only light spontaneous physical activity pursuing their pre-transplantation vocation or had retired and were only recreationally active. Informed consent was obtained from all patients and no complications resulted from any of the exercise testing procedures (see below).

Ten normal subjects were recruited as controls (mean age $\pm$ SD: 36.6 ± 9.6) but it had been impossible to organize a strictly age-matched control group (Table 1). The normal volunteers were sedentary untrained individuals and none were taking medication of any type.

Table 1. Physical characteristics of cardiac transplant patients and normal subjects

HTR Subj. ID	Age (yr)	Height (cm)	Body mass (kg)	Pre-transplant-diagnosis	Time of study (mo postop.)
A	40	162	66	IHD	1.3
B	50	175	66	RHD	11.5
D	41	169	65	IHD	1.9
E	43	170	74	CCM	19.4
F	59	175	62	IHD	1.7
G	33	162	58	RVF	4.3
H	38	167	58	CCM	14.9
I	53	176	81	CCM	14.8
J	43	165	83	CCM	26.9
K	44	169	77	CCM	44.0
L	36	175	80	ICM	21.4
M	36	173	72	IHD	137.1
N	52	172	65	CCM	29.7
O	36	172	61	CCM	63.2
P	49	165	58	CCM	4.6
Q	52	175	71	ICM	13.2
R	51	172	57	IHD	2.6
S	48	181	88	IHD	25.6
T	55	180	77	AVD	26.7
U	47	166	66	RHD	24.8
W	28	173	56	CCM	17.7
$\bar{x}$ ($n=21$)	44.5	171	68.6		24.2
SD	8.1	5	9.6		30.0
CTL					
$\bar{x}$ ($n=10$)	36.6	177	74.9		
SD	9.6	6	12.7		

IHD = ischemic heart disease. RHD = rheumatic heart disease. RVF = right ventricular failure. CCM = congestive cardiomyopathy. ICM = ischemic cardiomyopathy. AVD = aortic valve disease. All but one were male in the patient (HTR) and control (CTL) group

Methodology and Techniques

Breath-by-Breath Analysis of Gas Exchange

Continuous monitoring on a breath-by-breath basis of ventilation ($\dot{V}_E$), O_2 uptake ($\dot{V}_{O_2}$), CO_2 output ($\dot{V}_{CO_2}$), gas exchange ratio (RQ), and end-tidal O_2 and CO_2 partial pressures ($P_{E'O_2}$ and $P_{E'CO_2}$) was performed by a Sensor Medics 4400tc analyzer. Tidal volume and ventilation were calculated from instantaneous flow at the mouth determined from a turbine-type flowmeter. Metabolic parameters were determined from continuous monitoring of P_{O_2} and P_{CO_2} throughout the respiratory cycle and from established mass balance equations. A typical example of the data obtained in a heart transplant recipient during upright rectangular 50 W cycloergometric exercise (two 5 min 50 W bouts separated by 5 min recovery, see below) is presented in Fig. 1.

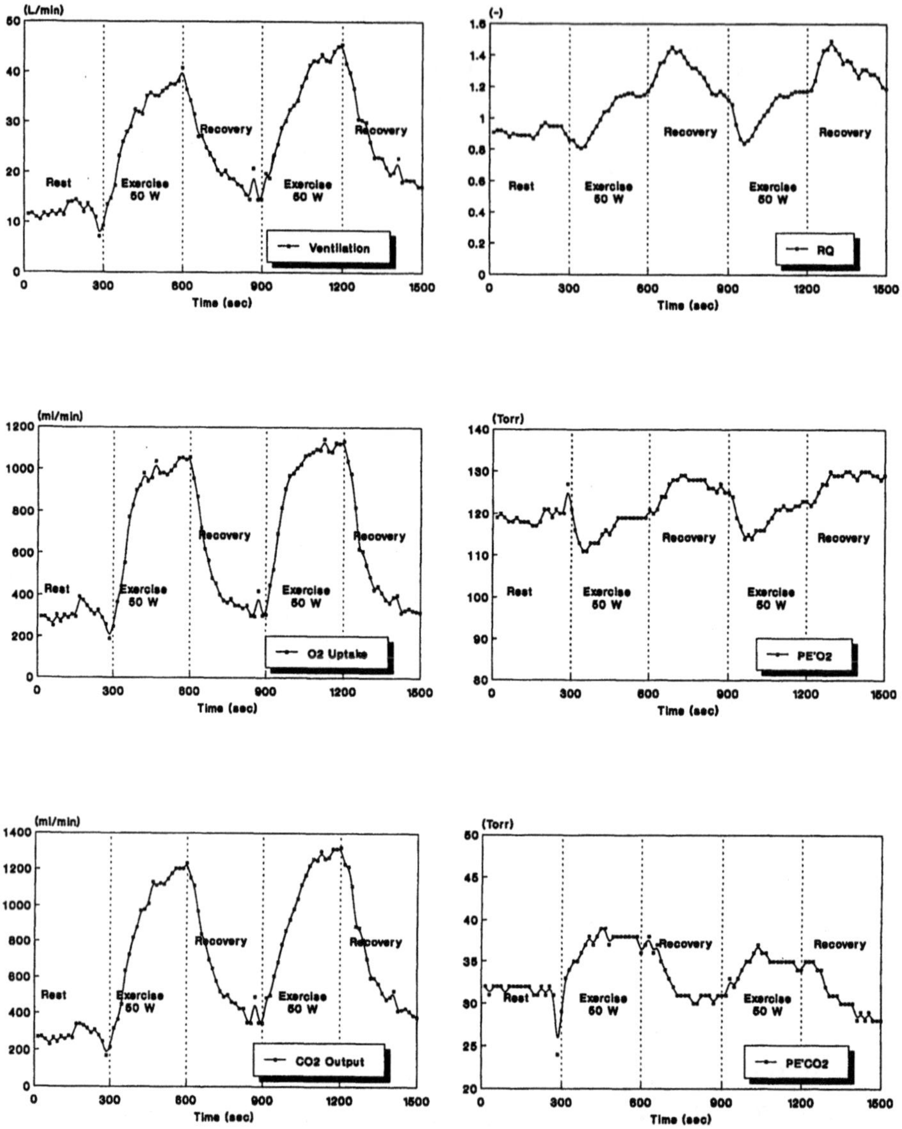

Fig. 1. Breath-by-breath analysis of pulmonary gas exchange in a heart transplant recipient during repetitive 50 W cycloergometric exercise

Impedance Cardiography

Impedance cardiography has gained attraction as a non-invasive method for estimation of beat-by-beat changes of stroke volume (SV), cardiac output ($\dot{Q}$) and systolic time intervals (STI) in patients and normal subjects during rest and exercise. The method and its potential applications have recently been re-

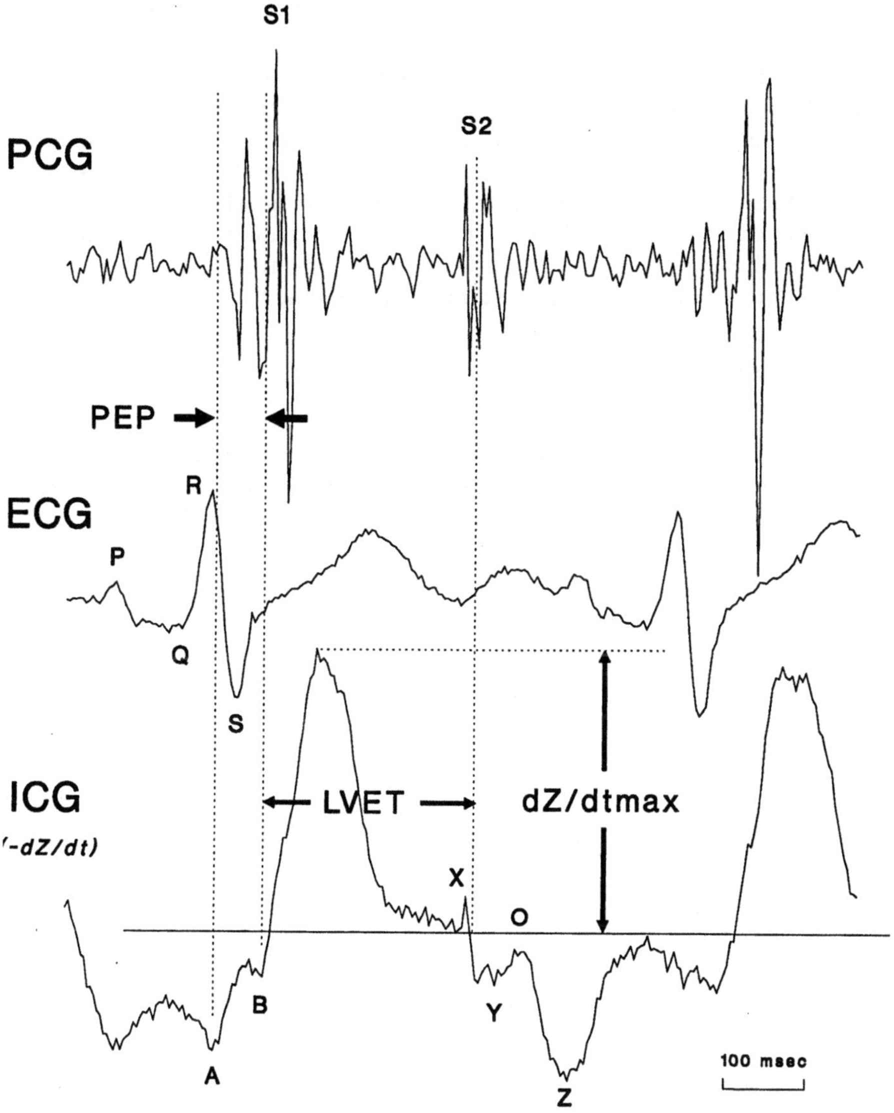

Fig. 2. Phonocardiogram (PCG), electrocardiogram (ECG) and impedance cardiogram (ICG) of a heart transplant recipient. PEP = pre-ejection period. LVET = left ventricular ejection time. dZ/dt_{max} = maximum of impedance derivative (see Methodology and Techniques)

viewed (Mohapatra 1981; Lamberts et al. 1984). Impedance cardiograms were obtained with an impedance cardiograph designed at the Department of Biomedical Engineering, University of Stuttgart. A constant current of 4 mA rms at a frequency of 100 kHz is introduced by two disposable self-adhesive electrodes. Two separate electrodes were used to measure changes of voltage resulting from variations in impedance within the segment under consideration.

The four-spot electrode array was placed according to Kubicek's scheme (Kubicek et al. 1966) with two electrodes 3 cm apart at the neck, the third at the level of the xiphisternal joint, and the fourth 3 cm below the third. Baseline thoracic impedance (Z_0), change of impedance (dZ/dt) and maximum of impedance derivative (dZ/dt_{max}) were automatically derived along with estimates of pre-ejection period (PEP), left ventricular ejection time (LVET), and heart rate (HR) facilitated by simultaneous recording of the electrocardiogram (ECG) and phonocardiogram (PCG). The impedance cardiogram (ICG) along with ECG and PCG recorded from a heart transplant recipient is shown in Fig. 2. The stroke volume is calculated according to the formula of Kubicek et al. (1966)

$$SV = \varrho\,(L/Z_0)^2\,(dZ/dt_{max})\,LVET$$

where, L is the distance between the inner electrodes, and ϱ is the resistivity of blood at 100 kHz. Continuous recording of heart rate, stroke volume and cardiac output (= SV · HR) in a heart transplant recipient undergoing exercise testing over 25 min (same protocol as in Fig. 1) is shown in Fig. 3.

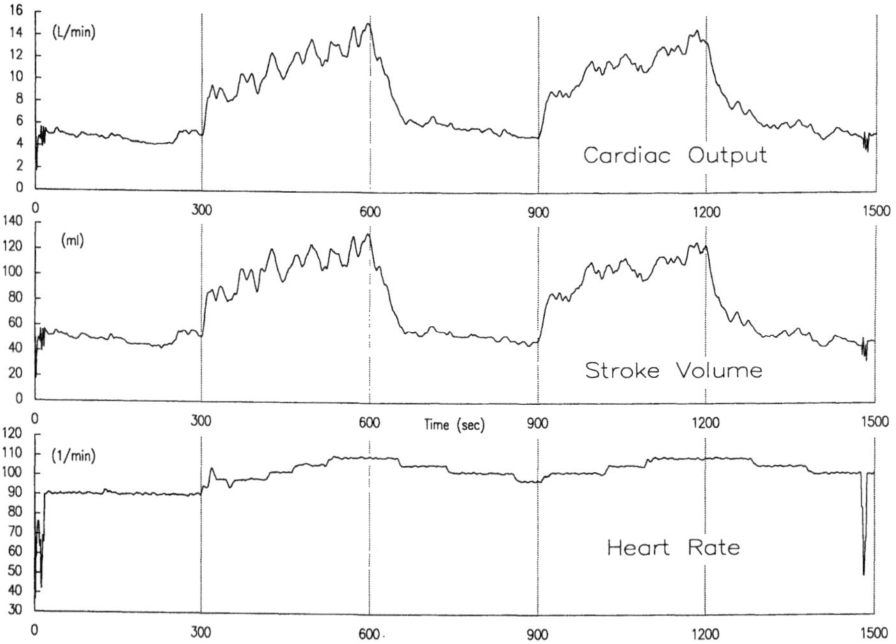

Fig. 3. Continuous recording of heart rate *(lower panel)*, stroke volume *(middle panel)* and cardiac output *(upper panel)* by impedance cardiography in a heart transplant patient during repetitive exercise testing (two-stage sequential rectangular 50 W work load over 5 min separated by 5 min recovery; same protocol as in Fig. 1). The recording demonstrates the rapid rate of adjustment of cardiac output at the onset of exercise brought about by an increased stroke volume secondary to augmented preload and the Frank-Starling mechanism. Similarly, during recovery from exercise cardiac output rapidly decelerates to pre-exercise levels while heart rate remains elevated

Catecholamines and Lactate

In 10 out of the 21 transplant patients blood samples were obtained from an indwelling external jugular vein catheter (inserted for routine endomyocardial biopsy) for analysis of circulating catecholamines. Plasma epinephrine and norepinephrine were assessed by high-pressure liquid chromatography, the sum of which was considered as total catecholamines. Similarly, blood lactate concentration ([LA]) was determined by a standard enzymatic assay.

Experimental Protocol

Exercise testing was performed on an electromagnetically braked cycle ergometer (Monark 818). Before performing any work load the subject sat on the bicycle for at least 10 min during which period resting respiratory, metabolic and cardiovascular parameters were recorded over 5 min prior to the onset of the square-wave exercise. The exercise protocol consisted of two 50 W bouts performed sequentially while separated by 5 min recovery. Similarly, recovery from the 2nd bout of exercise was followed over 5 min. On-line data acquisition of pulmonary and cardiovascular parameters (*cf.* Figs. 1 and 3) was performed over a period of 25 min. Arterial blood pressure was measured at 30 sec intervals by sphygmomanometry and blood samples were taken at designated points throughout the protocol. Due to bounds of time (volume loading experiments and other obligations of patients in the course of their routine exploration) the subject's symptom-limited maximum power output (generally expected at 70 to 100 W) could not be determined. In order to enable all patients to comply with the imposed load and to complete the test protocol the work load was arbitrarily set at a submaximal level of 50 W. Eight patients who claimed that they would easily go for higher work loads were tested at 75 W for 5 min after 7–10 min recovery from the first session while remaining seated on the ergometer.

The data obtained in the present series were analyzed by conventional statistical techniques. A breakdown of the information generally yielded no significant differences for any of the parameters between short-term and long-term heart transplant recipients. Therefore, the entire group forms the basis for the conclusions drawn. Moreover, given the inherent heterogeneity by history in the heart transplant group and the sizeable inter-individual variability particularly observed in untrained normal subjects when subjected to low-level exercise, some of the differences between groups exhibited borderline significance and should be interpreted as indicative of trends rather than taken as clear-cut evidence in favour of or against a particular difference or effect.

Pulmonary Gas Exchange

Cardiopulmonary parameters during rest and steady state submaximal 50 W exercise have collectively been summarized in Table 2 for heart transplant recipients (HTR) and normal control subjects (CTL).

Table 2. Cardiopulmonary parameters in heart transplant recipients (HTR) and normal control subjects (CTL) during rest and 50 W cycloergometric exercise

	Rest		50 W	
	HTR	CTL	HTR	CTL
$\dot{V}_E$ (L/min)	10.6±1.7	8.1±1.7	33.9±8.5	22.3±2.7
$\dot{V}_{O_2}$ (L/min)	0.27±0.05	0.28±0.04	0.96±0.1	0.95±0.08
$\dot{V}_{CO_2}$ (L/min)	0.24±0.04	0.22±0.03	1.02±0.19	0.82±0.06
RQ (−)	0.89±0.09	0.80±0.06	1.07±0.16	0.87±0.05
$P_{E'O_2}$ (Torr)	115±4	106±7	117±7	104±3
$P_{E'CO_2}$ (Torr)	34±3	39±4	34±3	39±4
HR (min^{-1})	102±12	72±9	120±12	98±16
$BP_s/_d$ (Torr)	145/105±15/10	120/85±20/10	175/95±20/15	150/80±25/15
SV (ml)	71±26	94±16	130±39	137±50
$\dot{Q}$ (L/min)	7.2±2.4	6.8±1.5	15.6±5.3	12.8±3.6

$\dot{V}_E$=expired ventilation. $\dot{V}_{O_2}=O_2$ uptake. $\dot{V}_{CO_2}=CO_2$ output. RQ=respiratory quotient. $P_{E'O_2}$=end-tidal O_2 partial pressure. $P_{E'CO_2}$=end-tidal CO_2 partial pressure. HR=heart rate. BP=arterial blood pressure; $_s/_d$=systolic and diastolic, respectively. SV=stroke volume. $\dot{Q}$=cardiac output. Mean values±SD (HTR $n=21$; CTL $n=10$)

Ventilation

A striking finding is the increased minute ventilation ($\dot{V}_E$) in patients with orthotopic cardiac transplants which is even more pronounced during exercise. Similar observations have previously been reported (Savin et al. 1980; Cerretelli et al. 1988) but others have failed to detect an increased ventilatory response to exercise after cardiac denervation (Shea et al. 1988; Banner et al. 1989). Unlike the combined heart-lung transplant operation, orthotopic cardiac transplantation results in complete denervation of the heart but the pulmonary innervation, lymphatic system and the bronchial circulation remain unaffected and the altered ventilatory response would not be expected to be of pulmonary origin. While the slightly elevated ventilation at rest in our study may have been an effect of instrumentation, the excessive ventilation during exercise present in our study may be a consequence of other factors, such as lack of physical training and/or metabolic (lactacid) acidosis (the latter may, however, have contributed less because [LA] during exercise was only about 2.5 times above resting levels; see Fig. 9, below). As a consequence of the enhanced ventilation $P_{E'O_2}$ is higher and $P_{E'CO_2}$ lower in HTR compared to CTL and similar values were maintained by both groups during exercise.

Metabolic Variables

O_2 uptake ($\dot{V}_{O_2}$) and CO_2 output ($\dot{V}_{CO_2}$) were essentially the same in the two groups studied. For the same work load (50 W) imposed, both groups responded with similar levels of absolute $\dot{V}_{O_2}$ but $\dot{V}_{O_2}$ per unit body mass was slightly higher in HTR (14.0 *vs* 12.7 $ml \cdot min^{-1} \cdot kg^{-1}$). Due to the excessive ventilatory response, the gas exchange ratio had remained elevated but this finding may in part be attributed to non-steady state conditions resulting from delayed $\dot{V}_E$, $\dot{V}_{O_2}$ and $\dot{V}_{CO_2}$ readjustment rates at the onset of exercise (see below).

Cardiovascular System

Heart Rate

The high heart rate (HR) during rest and submaximal work load is characteristic of the chronically denervated heart with absence of autonomic reinnervation (Stinson et al. 1972; Pope et al. 1980; Kavanagh et al. 1988). Following denervation resting heart rate is similar to the rate achieved by combined vagal and β-adrenergic blockade and thus may be attributed to revelation of the "intrinsic" rate of the sinuatrial node (Jose and Collinson 1970) which decreases with age (de Marneffe et al. 1986). No significant correlations were found between resting heart rate and either age of patient, time elapsed between surgery and assessment, or baseline levels of circulating catecholamines.

Upon onset of rectangular 5 min 50 W exercise HR did not change for the first minute and thereafter increased almost linearly with time. The delay for HR to increase 5% above resting levels was of the order of 120 sec. At the offset of exercise HR remained unchanged for 1–2 min and gradually decelerated approaching pre-exercise levels varying from 5–25 min. The average ($\pm$ SD) relative increases of HR for the 1st and 2nd 5 min 50 W work rates were $17.8 \pm 8.9\%$ and $8.9 \pm 6.1\%$ in HTR compared to $32.0 \pm 8.0\%$ and $27.7 \pm 9.5\%$ in CTL. Heart rate was the same at the end of the two submaximal 50 W work loads performed sequentially but separated by 5 min recovery in both HTR and CTL although the absolute values, about 120 min^{-1} in HTR and 100 min^{-1} in CTL, were quite different. In the patients undergoing testing by two different submaximal work rates HR was 120 ± 7 min^{-1} at 50 W and 134 ± 12 min^{-1} at 75 W.

Stroke Volume and Cardiac Output

Cardiac output ($\dot{Q}$) was essentially the same between HTR and CTL at rest but stroke volume (SV) as a result of higher resting heart rate in HTR was less compared to CTL (Table 1). On 50 W exercise $\dot{Q}$, for the same level of $\dot{V}_{O_2}$ in HTR exceeded that of CTL but SV was essentially similar in the two groups. The steady state values of stroke index and cardiac index at the various stages of the experimental protocol (E1 and E2 refer to 1st and 2nd 50 W testing, R1 and R2 pertain to recovery from the two exercise bouts) are shown in Fig. 4. The steady state response of stroke index is practically the same during repetitive exercise testing both in HTR and CTL. However, as a result of higher HR in HTR cardiac index is enhanced above that in normal controls. It would thus seem that heart transplant patients experience "luxury" perfusion at moderate submaximal work loads. Linear regression of the data base relating $\dot{Q}$ to $\dot{V}_{O_2}$ was $\dot{Q} = 9.9\ (\dot{V}_{O_2}) + 5.5\ (r = 0.69)$ in HTR and $\dot{Q} = 8.4\ (\dot{V}_{O_2}) + 5.5\ (r = 0.77)$

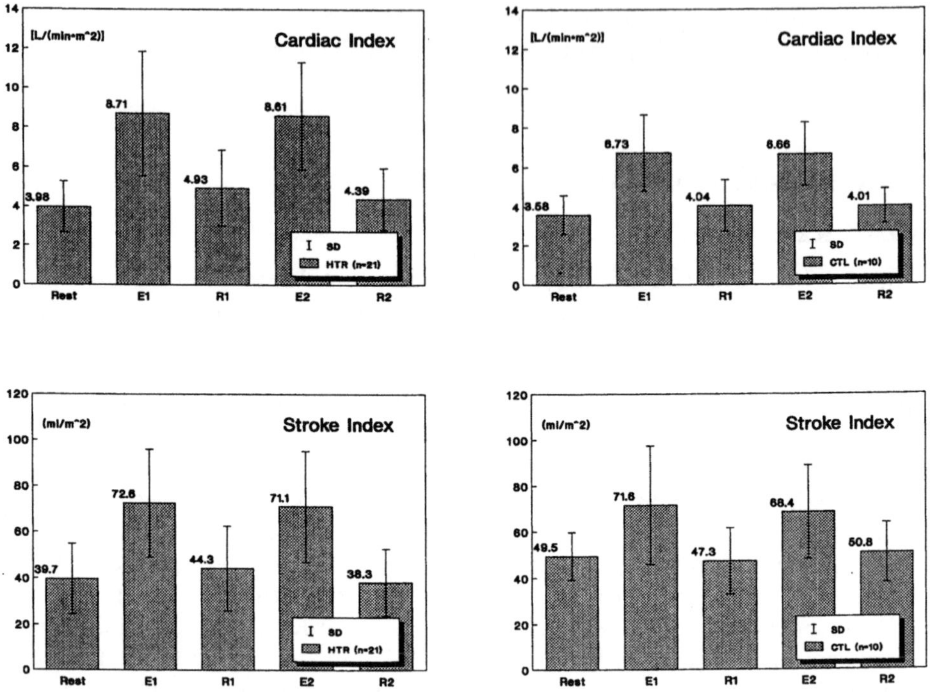

Fig. 4. Cardiac index and stroke index in heart transplant recipients (HTR, *left*) and normal control subjects (CTL, *right*). E1 and E2 refer to 1st and 2nd 50 W exercise runs, R1 and R2 to recovery from the two exercise bouts, respectively (see Experimental Protocol)

in CTL. These figures, both in terms of slope and intercept, are different from those reported recently by Kavanagh et al. (1988): $\dot{Q}=6.1\ (\dot{V}_{O_2}) + 3.29$ (r= 0.88) for HTR and $\dot{Q}=6.0\ (\dot{V}_{O_2}) + 3.87$ (r=0.94) for CTL. In contrast to heart rate which gradually returned to control values, stroke volume and cardiac output approximately approached pre-exercise levels within 5 min of recovery from exercise. Although inconclusive for differences between the present results and those by Kavanagh et al. (1988) it is important to emphasize that different indirect techniques for non-invasive assessment of cardiac output were used: CO_2-rebreathing technique in the study of Kavanagh et al. (1988), beat-by-beat impedance cardiography measurements in the present series.

Systolic Time Intervals

In Fig. 5 pre-ejection period (PEP) and left ventricular ejection time (LVET) are shown as function of heart rate along with the LVET/PEP ratio plotted as function of $\dot{Q}$. Generally, both PEP and LVET are inversely related to HR. The length of PEP is mainly determined by the myocardial contractility and filling volume. The steeper slope of the PEP-HR relationship in HTR reflects the increased venous return and activation of the Frank-Starling mechanism.

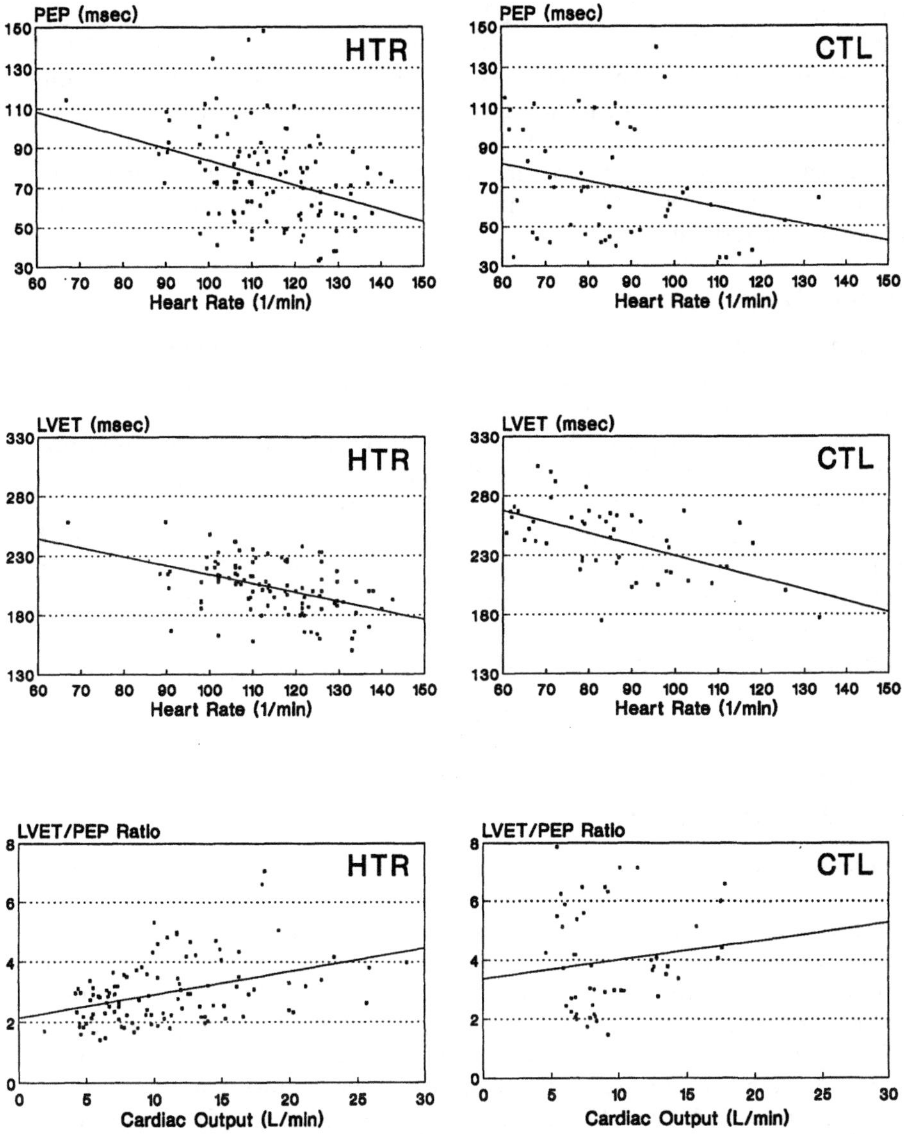

Fig. 5. Pre-ejection period (PEP), left ventricular ejection time (LVET) and LVET/PEP ratio in heart transplant recipients (HTR, *left*) and normal control subjects (CTL, *right*)

The length of LVET in HTR is shortened compared to CTL reflecting the absence of sympathetic stimuli in the denervated heart. During exercise the difference of LVET between HTR and CTL diminishes when HR is increased. The large increase in stroke volume was not associated with a proportionate increase in LVET resulting in considerable enhancement (about 2-fold) of mean systolic ejection rate (SV/LVET). A close correlation is observed between the LVET/PEP ratio and $\dot{Q}$ in HTR which is less obvious in CTL. LVET/PEP is generally considered as a sensitive index of ventricular function. For a given $\dot{Q}$ the LVET/PEP ratio is less in HTR compared with CTL. It is, however, important to recognize that ejection phase indices determined by impedance cardiography measurements are limited for assessment of true ventricular contractility because of complex interactions between contractile state and pre- and afterload conditions.

Systemic Blood Pressure

Elevated systolic and diastolic resting and exercise systemic blood pressures are often seen in HTR (*cf.* Table 1). The resting hypertension may result from long-term preoperative congestive heart failure associated with chronic elevation of plasma norepinephrine levels or may reflect side effects of immunosuppressive medication by cyclosporine and prednisone. Systemic hypertension is a common complication of cyclosporine treatment in cardiac transplant patients (Bantle et al. 1985; Goldman et al. 1985). Given the normal or elevated cardiac output and normal to elevated systemic arterial blood pressure it would seem that peripheral vascular resistance, unlike in normal exercising man, had remained inordinately high or unchanged. Probably both cardiac and peripheral vascular components contribute to changes of resting and exercise blood pressure responses.

Cardiorespiratory Dynamics at Onset and Offset of Exercise

Cardiorespiratory dynamics during exercise and recovery were expressed as half-time (t½, sec) of the $\dot{V}_E$, $\dot{V}_{O_2}$, $\dot{V}_{CO_2}$ and $\dot{Q}$ on- and off-response curves (*cf.* Figs. 1 and 3), i.e., the time required to reach 50% of the asymptotic (steady state or peak) level starting from rest or after 5 min recovery from the 1st 50 W exercise test. The shape of the on-response curves, generally approximating a monoexponential function in normal subjects, appears to be preserved in HTR. Mean values for HTR and CTL are shown for 50 W loads in Table 3. The results demonstrate that in HTR the kinetics of adjustment of $\dot{Q}$ is only moderately impaired, probably resulting from delayed onset of venous return, in contrast to the significantly slower (about 85%) kinetics of respiratory gas exchange. By and large cardiorespiratory readjustment in response to exercise is, unexpectedly, only slightly delayed in HTR. The kinetics for repetitive 50 W exercise testing were essentially similar and were not different at two different (50 and 75 W) work rates (Table 4). The delayed kinetics of adjustment of respiratory gas exchange at the onset of rectangular work loads would be expected of the slightly slower $\dot{Q}$ readjustment rate. The present data demonstrate the sustained capacity of the transplanted human heart and gas exchange at the lungs to adjust appropriately to the metabolic demands of exercise. It would seem reasonable to assume that, during moderate exercise, the

Table 3. Cardiopulmonary dynamics at the onset and offset of rectangular 50 W cycloergometric exercise in heart transplant recipients (HTR) and normal control subjects (CTL)

	HTR ($n=21$)		CTL ($n=10$)	
	$t_{1/2}$ – on	$t_{1/2}$ – off	$t_{1/2}$ – on	$t_{1/2}$ – off
$\dot{V}_E$	77±16***	55±16***	42±10	30± 6
$\dot{V}_{O_2}$	53±10***	46±10***	31±10	25± 6
$\dot{V}_{CO_2}$	79±13***	57±15***	41±11	30± 7
$\dot{Q}$	52±16°	44±15*	40±17	31±14

Cardiopulmonary dynamics are quantified by the half-times ($t_{1/2}$, in sec) required for ventilation ($\dot{V}_E$), O_2 uptake ($\dot{V}_{O_2}$), CO_2 output ($\dot{V}_{CO_2}$) and cardiac output ($\dot{Q}$) to attain 50% of the steady state values following a square-wave increase of power (50 W). Mean values±SD. ° $P>0.05$, * $P<0.05$, *** $P<0.001$

Table 4. Cardiopulmonary dynamics during 50 W and 75 W work load in heart transplant recipients

	50 W		75 W	
	$t_{1/2}$ – on	$t_{1/2}$ – off	$t_{1/2}$ – on	$t_{1/2}$ – off
$\dot{V}_E$	66±15	47±15	71±16	45±16
$\dot{V}_{O_2}$	51±10	44± 7	48± 7	42± 7
$\dot{V}_{CO_2}$	72±15	48±12	68±11	54±15
$\dot{Q}$	42±17	40±17	50±27	62±39

Kinetics of adjustment is determined by the half-times ($t_{1/2}$, sec) required for cardiopulmonary parameters to attain 50% of the steady state values following a square-wave increase of 50 W or 75 W power. Mean values±SD ($n=8$). No statistical differences were detectable for any of the parameters

limiting role of $\dot{Q}$ for the individual's physical performance in HTR does not prevail over that in normal subjects.

The mechanism underlying the pattern of response of cardiac output of the denervated heart is almost the complete opposite of that of the innervated. The innervated heart responds to exercise with an almost instantaneous increase in heart rate with little or no increase in stroke volume. In the normal heart the Frank-Starling mechanism is important only with severe exertion. In the denervated heart the increase in cardiac output early in exercise appears to be almost entirely mediated through an increase in stroke volume as a result of increased venous return, i.e., augmented preload, and the Frank-Starling mechanism (Starling 1918, 1920). The increase of cardiac output later in exercise likely results from a combination of chronotropic and inotropic effects of rising levels of circulating catecholamines. The unique dependence of the transplanted heart on preload as a means of increasing cardiac output in response to work load and effective functioning of the Frank-Starling mechanism is clearly demonstrated by the recording of Fig. 3.

It is of interest to recognize that the transplanted denervated heart by virtue of augmented preload and the Frank-Starling principle achieves a normal cardiac output during dynamic exercise but fails to maintain an adequate increase of cardiac output during isometric exercise when preload and heart rate remain unchanged (Robson et al. 1989). Isometric exercise testing would thus constitute a simple test to demonstrate lack of reinnervation in a heart transplant patient.

Control of Heart Rate After Cardiac Transplantation

Catecholamines

The time course of HR exhibiting a gradual and prolonged acceleration during exercise, in the absence of evidence (in contrast to dogs) for autonomic reinnervation of the human orthotopic transplant (Stinson et al. 1975; Mc Laughlin et al. 1978; Horak 1984), suggests the operation of humoral adrenergic mechanisms. Normal subjects are known to exhibit increased catecholamine levels during exercise. Similarly, a substantial increase of plasma norepinephrine has been observed in HTR during severe exercise (Pope et al. 1980). Moreover, it has been demonstrated recently that the denervated human heart

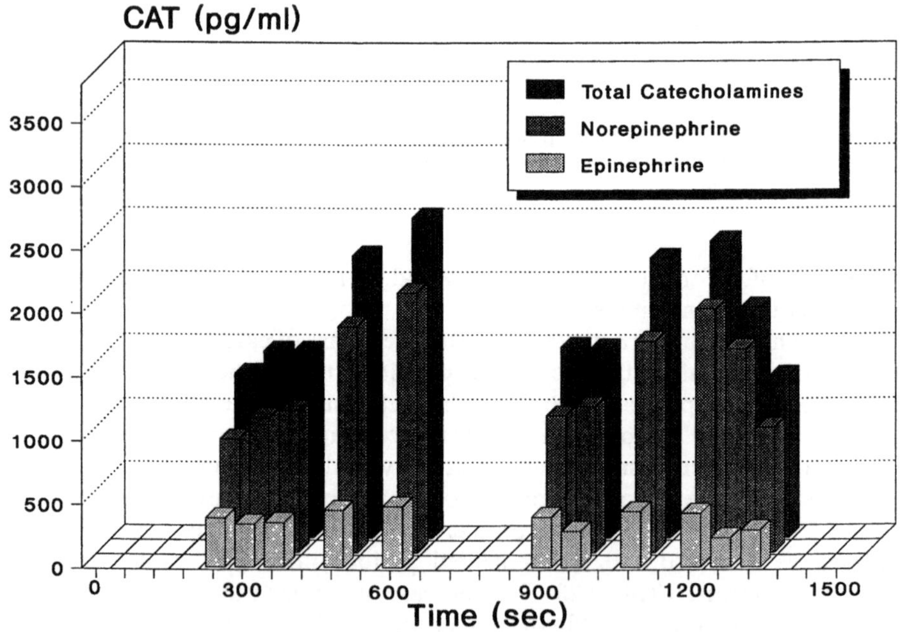

Fig. 6. Time course of circulating catecholamines in heart transplant recipients during submaximal cycloergometric exercise. Mean values from 10 subjects

develops an increased sensitivity to circulating catecholamines (Yusuf et al. 1987).

Circulating plasma catecholamines determined at various stages of the experimental protocol of the present study are shown in Fig. 6. The data relating circulating catecholamine levels to the time of exercise demonstrate rapid changes associated with exercise and recovery periods. The major changes of blood-borne catecholamines are almost exclusively attributable to changes of norepinephrine levels, representing a constant fraction ($77.3 \pm 5.0\%$, means $\pm$ SD) of total catecholamines. Resting plasma norepinephrine levels (means $\pm$ SD) were 853 ± 434 pg/ml, about 4-times higher than previously reported in HTR (Pope et al. 1980; Degre et al. 1987) and in cardiac patients with intact neural control (Thomas and Marks 1978), approaching 2043 ± 1002 pg/ml, respectively 1914 ± 1056 pg/ml, at the end of the two 50 W exercise bouts. Upon recovery from exercise catecholamines rapidly returned to control values.

The role of catecholamines in the control of HR is demonstrated by the close relationship between norepinephrine levels and heart rate (Fig. 7). It is important to emphasize that this relationship applies to the early phase of exercise only; during recovery where HR remains elevated and during repetitive or prolonged exercise other factors (see below) likely contribute to the control of heart rate.

Evidence for catecholamine sensitivity varying among heart transplant subjects is presented in Fig. 8 where the relative change of HR, ΔHR, per unit

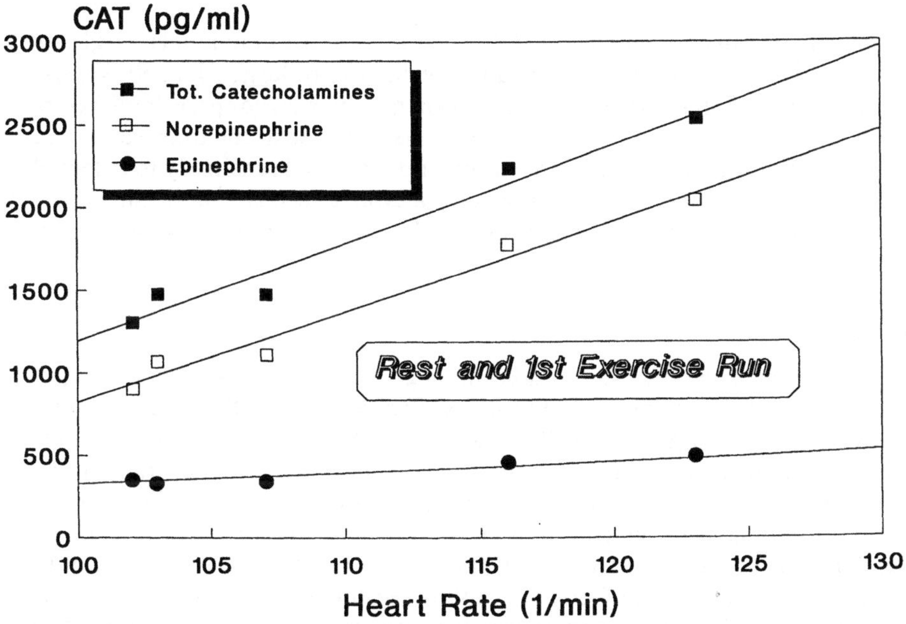

Fig. 7. Relationship between heart rate and circulating catecholamines during rest and early phase of exercise. Mean values from 10 heart transplant patients

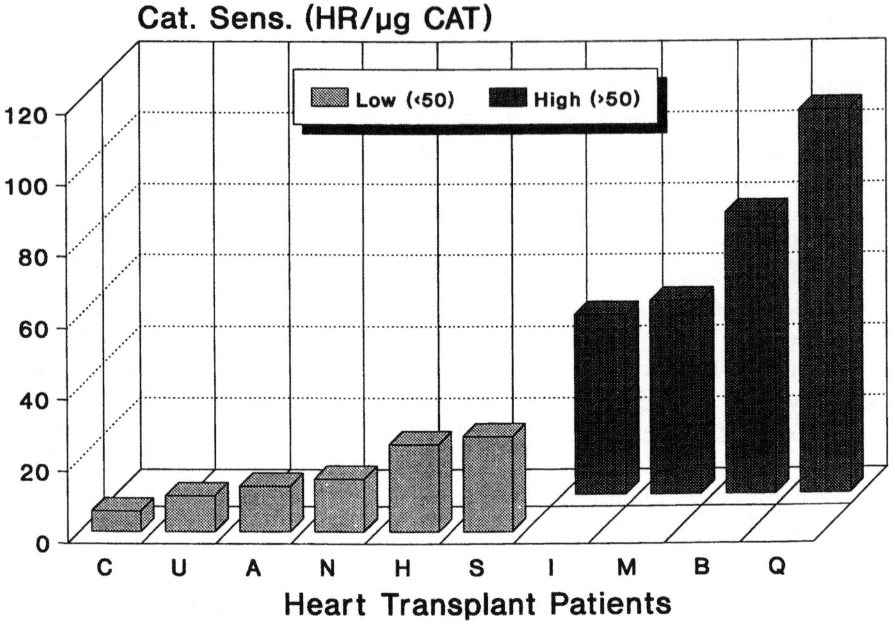

Fig. 8. Catecholamine sensitivity in heart transplant recipients. The sensitivity towards circulating catecholamines is defined as the relative change of heart rate (ΔHR) per unit change of catecholamines (ΔCAT, in µg)

increment of catecholamines, ΔCAT, is shown for 10 individuals. High and low sensitivity is arbitrarily assigned to a value less or larger than 50 beats/µg catecholamine. Interestingly, no correlation among subgroups, established on the basis of their catecholamine sensitivity, is found with the time elapsed between surgery and assessment. Increased and/or varied sensitivity to catecholamines probably represents an important adaptive mechanism of the chronically denervated heart to compensate for the lack of sympathetic nerve stimulation.

Lactate

At the onset of exercise O_2 uptake through the lungs lags behind the performance of mechanical work and is insufficient to meet the energy requirement of the working muscles. Thus an O_2 debt is incurred early in exercise which is repaid later during offset of exercise. The missing energy fraction that is not available from external gas exchange results from phosphocreatinine breakdown, anaerobic glycolysis associated with formation of lactic acid, and depletion of O_2 stores. In the recovery phase of exercise phosphocreatinine levels and O_2 stores of the body are rapidly reestablished to pre-exercise levels while removal of lactate by oxidation or reconversion to glycogen proceeds at much slower rate.

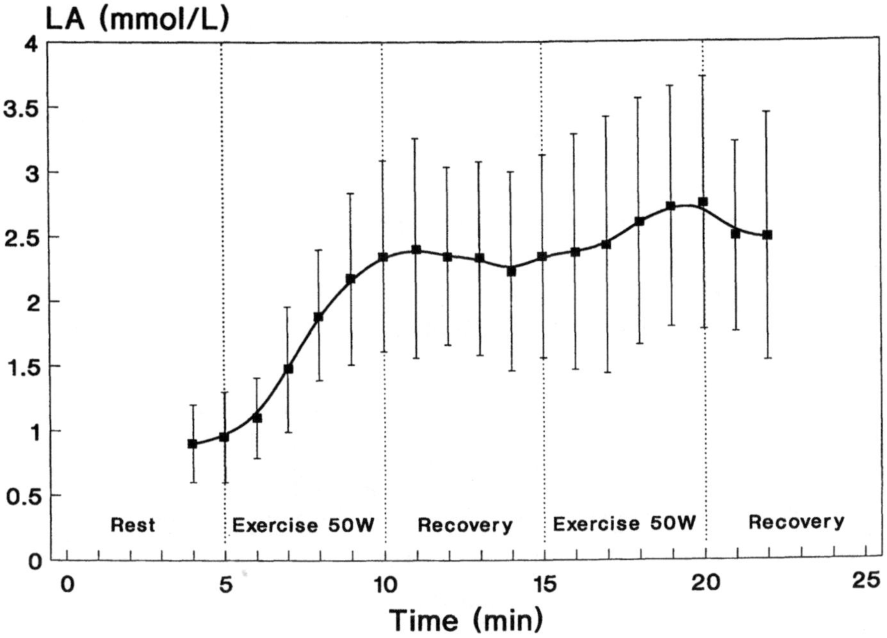

Fig. 9. Time course of lactic acid accumulation in blood in heart transplant recipients during repetitive 50 W cycloergometric exercise

The time course of lactate ([LA]) accumulation in blood is shown in Fig. 9. Resting levels of [LA] were 0.9 ± 0.3 mmol/L (means $\pm$ SD) and peak values of 2.4 ± 0.9 mmol/L and 2.7 ± 0.9 mmol/l were approached with a half-time of about 150 s in the 1st and 2nd 50 W exercise runs, respectively. Moreover, the data demonstrate absence of a massive "early" lactate accumulation within the first 60–90 s after onset of rectangular work that would be expected from early glycolysis if the on-response of cardiac output were seriously delayed.

The metabolic anaerobic threshold is conventionally defined by the maximal work load compatible with a given [LA] level (typically 2–4 mmol/L). Figure 9 suggests that the heart transplant patients of the present study did not experience excessive accumulation of lactate in blood and were exercising at or below their anaerobic threshold. The profile of [LA] in HTR appears to be not materially different from that of sedentary untrained normal subjects. It may be concluded that the cardiorespiratory response to the stress of the level of exercise imposed was fully adequate.

Accumulation of lactate in blood may be important in the control of heart rate later in exercise or during prolonged or repetitive periods of exercise. The time course of heart rate, circulating catecholamines and lactate is shown in Fig. 10. Early in exercise HR is seen to exhibit a pattern similar to that of circulating catecholamines while increase of [LA] lags behind. During recovery catecholamines approximately return to pre-exercise levels but HR remains

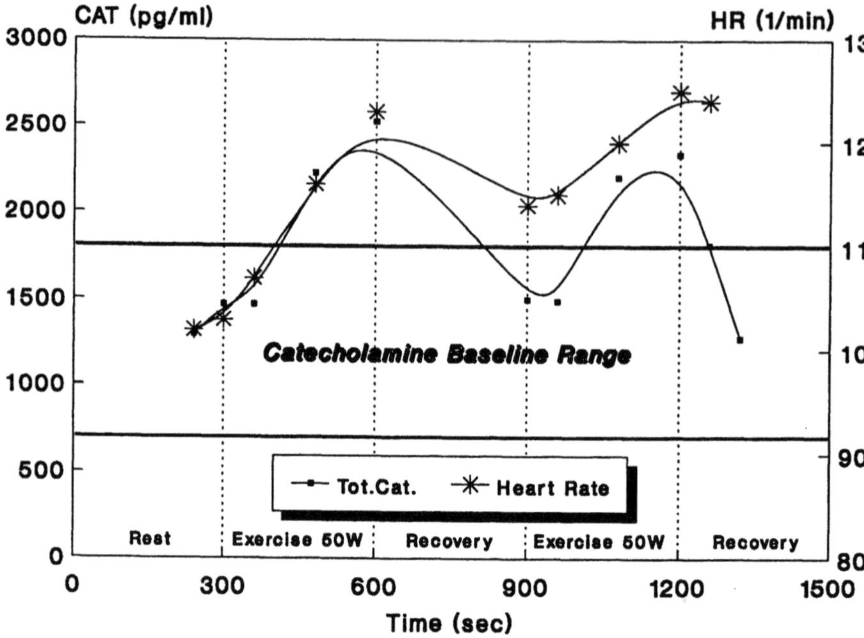

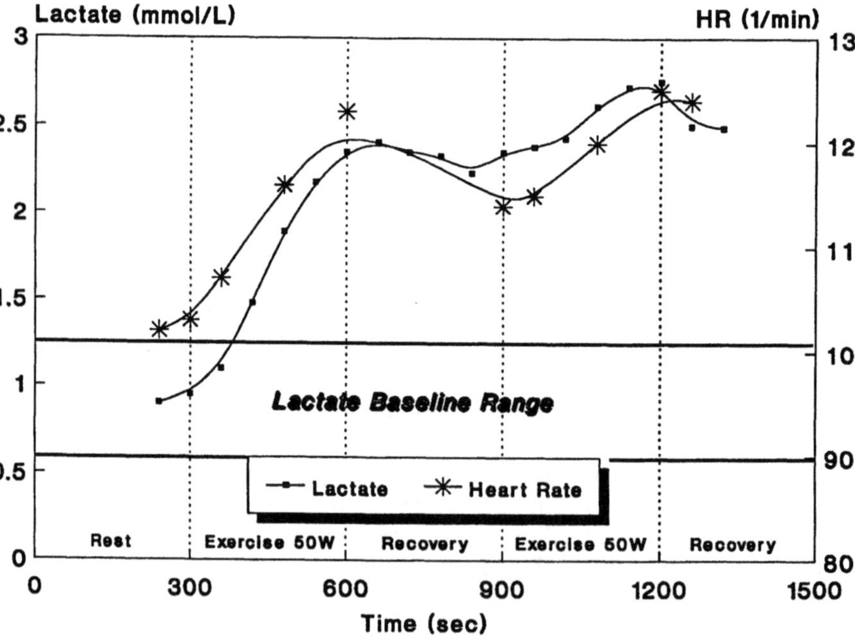

Fig. 10. Time course of circulating catecholamines *(upper panel)*, lactate *(lower panel)* and heart rate *(both panels)* in heart transplant recipients during two-stage submaximal exercise protocol. See text for details

persistently elevated. For the later part of the exercise protocol HR closely approximates the pattern of lactate changes in blood. The data suggest that dissociation of heart rate and catecholamines occurs during recovery from exercise or during sustained periods of exercise while lactate (possibly H^+) and/or other unknown factors take over control of heart rate.

Limiting Factors of Physical Performance in Heart Transplant Recipients

The present study has demonstrated that the cardiorespiratory response in cardiac transplant patients is fully adequate to retain a virtually normal capacity for submaximal exercise. Indeed, the excellent degree of rehabilitation from end-stage cardiac disease in most cardiac transplant patients is truly impressive (*cf.* Kavanagh et al. 1986).

A major conclusion from this study is that the kinetics of adjustment of cardiac output elicited by augmented preload and the Frank-Starling mechanism is not materially impaired. Hence O_2 transport to tissues would not be expected to be limited by the transplanted heart or gas exchange occurring at the lungs. The dependence of the transplanted heart on the Frank-Starling mechanism as a means of increasing cardiac output differs substantially from the normal heart with intact neural control.

It is important to emphasize that our conclusions pertain to conditions of moderate submaximal exercise only and should not be extrapolated to conditions of maximal power output. The present findings do not provide or suggest evidence for the limiting factors of the impaired *maximum* physical performance generally observed in heart transplant patients. Specifically, our findings of relatively rapid cardiorespiratory adjustment in response to submaximal exercise would not exclude the possibility that the major functional limitation for maximal power output is imposed by a reduced maximal cardiac output.

In the present study physiological variables of the cardiorespiratory system of HTR have been assessed during steady state conditions as well as during the transition from rest to exercise and compared with normal individuals. Differences were observed between the two groups for some of the parameters of interest but generally the differences observed were small and were indicative of an altered rather than abnormal response of the transplanted heart.

Assessment of Physical Performance in HTR: Problems and Perspectives

Comparison of cardiac transplant patients with normal controls furthermore involves a number of problems. Generally cardiac patients have experienced a long history of limited activity and physical deconditioning which may have involved morphological and structural changes of skeletal muscles and functional changes of blood flow distribution and vasodilator response. A reduction of muscle mass presents a common observation in HTR and likely plays a major role in limiting maximum exercise performance. It is interesting to note that HTR undergoing cycloergometric exercise testing often complain of leg muscle fatigue and results from a 2-year exercise rehabilitation program have demonstrated that strengthening of peripheral muscles rather than improvement of central hemodynamics played a major role in improving the heart transplant patient's physical ability (Kavanagh et al. 1988). The delayed kinetics of the $\dot{V}_{O_2}$-response seems to be more compatible with a peripheral than a central impairment.

Of the primary determinants of the cardiac output response to exercise, heart rate, preload, afterload and contractility constitute potential limiting factors. The increase of peripheral resistance as a result of systemic hypertension elicited or contributed to by the effects of immunosuppressive drug treatment is of substantial concern (Yacoub et al. 1985). Other factors include chronic anemia resulting from cyclosporine treatment (Myers et al. 1984), coronary artery narrowing due to chronic graft rejection and graft atherosclerosis (Griepp et al. 1977) ultimately leading to left ventricular dysfunction. Exercise capacity in HTR is significantly reduced in HTR by β-blocking agents (Bexton et al. 1983) which should be used with caution when treatment of hypertension or myocardial ischemia is required in heart transplant patients.

A major problem for studies addressing the exercise response of heart transplant recipients resides in the difficulty of obtaining a suitable control group. Typically, heart transplant patients are compared with age-matched normal control subjects or controls matched for donor heart age. Usually the "younger" donor heart is faced with the enhanced aortic outflow impedance of the "older" recipient's cardiovascular system and the donor left ventricle, i.e., the transplanted heart, becomes hypertrophic. Most obviously, the appropriateness of control subjects presents a problem that is difficult to overcome. Comparative assessment of patients chronically undergoing immunosuppressive therapy for other reasons or patients with complete heart block would help to address some of the issues in heart transplant patients that are difficult to appreciate.

Exercise testing in heart transplant patients should generally follow established guidelines but it is important to emphasize that the transplanted heart does not sense anginal pain as a result of myocardial ischemia. Moreover, the sluggish heart rate response of the denervated heart to exercise renders pulse counting less accurate as a measure of exercise intensity.

Summary

Assessment of the cardiorespiratory response to submaximal exercise in heart transplant patients may be summarized as follows. Heart rate during rest and exercise is elevated in HTR. Ventilation is enhanced during rest and exercise associated with lower end-tidal P_{CO_2}. Cardiac output during moderate work load is larger than in normal control subjects for a given level of O_2 uptake. The increase of cardiac output at the onset of exercise is mainly due to an increase of stroke volume (Frank-Starling mechanism). The sluggish increase of heart rate during the early phase of exercise is mediated by circulating catecholamines. Dissociation of heart rate and catecholamine levels occurs during recovery from exercise and during repetitive exercise tests when other factors (lactate ?) take over control of heart rate. Adjustment of pulmonary gas exchange is delayed in HTR. Adjustment of cardiac output is only moderately impaired at onset of and recovery from exercise. The limiting role of cardiac output for the individual's physical performance in heart transplant recipients does not seem to prevail over that in normal subjects.

References

Banner N, Guz A, Heaton R, Innes JA, Murphy K, Yacoub M (1988) Ventilatory and circulatory responses at the onset of exercise in man following heart or heart-lung transplantation. J Physiol (London) 399:437–449

Banner NR, Lloyd MH, Hamilton RD, Innes JA, Guz A, Yacoub MH (1989) Cardiopulmonary response to dynamic exercise after heart and combined heart-lung transplantation. Br Heart J 61:215–223

Bantle JP, Nath KA, Sutherland DER, Najarian JES, Ferris TF (1985) Effects of cyclosporine on the renin–angiotensin–aldosterone system and potassium excretion in transplant recipients. Arch Intern Med 145:505–508

Bexton RS, Milne JR, Cory-Pearce R, English TAH, Camm AJ (1983) Effect of beta blockade on exercise response after cardiac transplantation. Br Heart J 49:584–588

Borow KM, Neumann A, Arensman FW, Yacoub MH (1985) Left ventricular contractility and contractile reserve in humans after cardiac transplantation. Circulation 71:866–872

Buxton M, Acheson R, Caine N, Gibson S, O'Brien B (1985) Cost of the heart transplant programmes at Harefield and Papworth Hospitals. Her Majesty's Stationary Office, London

Campeau L, Pospisil L, Grondin P, Dyrda I, Lepage G (1970) Catheterization findings at rest and after exercise in patients following cardiac transplantation. Am J Cardiol 25:523–528

Carleton RA, Heller SJ, Najafi H, Clark JG (1969) Hemodynamic performance of a transplanted human heart. Circulation 40:447–452

Clark DA, Schroeder JS, Griepp RB, Stinson EB, Dong E, Shumway NE, Harrison DC (1973) Cardiac transplantation in man: review of seven years' experience. Am J Med 54:563–576

Cerretelli P, Grassi B, Colombini A, Carù B, Marconi C (1988) Gas exchange and metabolic transients in heart transplant recipients. Respir Physiol 74:355–371

Degre SG, Niset GL, De Smet JM, Ibrahim T, Stoupel E, Le Clerc JL, Primo G (1987) Cardiorespiratory response to early exercise testing after orthotopic cardiac transplantation. Am J Cardiol 60:926–928

de Marneffe M, Jacobs P, Haardt R, Englert M (1986) Variations of normal sinus node function in relation to age: role of autonomic influence. Eur Heart J 7:662–672

Dempsey PJ, Cooper T (1968) Supersensitivity of the chronically denervated feline heart. Am J Physiol 215:1245–1249

Donald DE (1968) Capacity for exercise after denervation of the heart. Circulation 38:225–226

Evans RW, Manninem DL, Overcast TD, Garrison LP, Yagi J, Marrikin K, Johnsen AR (1984) The National Heart Transplantation Study: final report. Battelle Human Affairs Research Center, Seattle

Goldman MH, Barnhart G, Mohanakumar T, Wetstein L, Szentpetery S, Wolfgang TC, Lower RR (1985) Cyclosporine in cardiac transplantation. Surg Clin N Am 65(3):637–659

Griepp RB, Stinson EB, Dong E, Clark DA, Shumway NE (1971) Hemodynamic performance of the transplanted human heart. Surgery 70:88–96

Griepp RB, Stinson EB, Stieber CP, Reitz BA, Copeland JG, Oyer PE, Shumway NE (1977) Control of graft arteriosclerosis in human heart transplant recipients. Surgery 81:262–269

Horak AR (1984) Physiology and pharmacology of the transplanted heart. In: Cooper DKC, Lanza RP (eds) Heart transplantation. MTP press, Lancaster, pp 147–156

Jose A, Collinson D (1970) The normal sinus node function in relation to age: role of autonomic influence. Cardiovasc Res 4:160–167

Kavanagh T, Yacoub MH, Campbell R, Mertens D (1986) Marathon running after cardiac transplantation: a case history. J Cardiopulmonary Rehab 6:16–20

Kavanagh T, Yacoub MH, Mertens DJ, Kennedy J, Campbell RB, Sawyer P (1988) Cardiorespiratory responses to exercise training after orthotopic cardiac transplantation. Circulation 77:162–171

Kubicek WG, Karnegis JM, Patterson RP, Witsoe DA, Mattson RH (1966) Development and evaluation of an impedance cardiac output system. Aerosp Med 37:1208–1212

Lamberts R, Visser KR, Zijlstra WG (1984) Impedance cardiography. Van Gorcum, Assen

Lurie KG, Bristow MR, Reitz BA (1983) Increased β-adrenergic receptor density in an experimental model of cardiac transplantation. J Cardiovasc Surg 86:195–201

Macoviak JA, Oyer PE, Stinson EB, Jamieson SW, Baldwin JC, Shumway NE (1985) Four-year experience with cyclosporine for heart and heart-lung transplantation. Transplant Proc 17 (suppl 2):97–101

Mc Laughlin PR, Leiman JH, Martin RP, Doherty PW, Reitz B, Stinson EB, Daughters GT, Ingels NB, Alderman EL (1979) The effect of exercise and atrial pacing on left ventricular volume and contractility in patients with innervated and denervated hearts. Circulation 58:476–483

Mertens D, Kavanagh T, Yacoub M (1987) Long term exercise training and cardiac output following cardiac transplantation. J Am Coll Cardiol 9:235 [Abstract]

Mohapatra SN (1981) Non-invasive cardiovascular monitoring by electrical impedance technique. Pitman Medical, London

Myers BD, Ross J, Newton L, Luetscher J, Perlroth M (1984) Cyclosporine related chronic nephropathy. N Engl J Med 311:699–705

Pope SE, Stinson EB, Daughters GT, Schroeder JS, Ingels NB, Alderman EL (1980) Exercise response of the denervated heart in long-term cardiac transplant recipients. Am J Cardiol 46:213–218

Reid CJ, Yacoub M (1988) Determinants of left ventricular function one year after cardiac transplantation. Br Heart J 59:397–402

Robson SC, Furniss SS, Heads A, Boys RJ, Mc Gregor C, Bexton RS (1989) Isometric exercise in the denervated heart: a Doppler echocardiographic study. Br Heart J 61:224–230

Savin WM, Haskell WL, Schroeder JS, Stinson EB (1980) Cardiorespiratory responses of cardiac transplant patients to graded, symptom-limited exercise. Circulation 62:55–60

Schroeder JS (1979) Hemodynamic performance of the human transplanted heart. Transplant Proc 11:304–308

Schroeder JS, Rider AK, Stinson EB, Shumway NE (1976) Cardiac transplantation: review of seven years' experience. Transplant Proc 8:5–8

Shaver JA, Leon DF, Gray S, Leonard JJ, Bahnson HT (1969) Hemodynamic observations after cardiac transplantation. N Engl J Med 281:822–827

Shea SA, Horner RL, Banner NR, Mc Kenzie E, Heaton R, Yacoub MH, Guz A (1988) The effect of human heart-lung transplantation upon breathing at rest and during sleep. Respir Physiol 72:131–150

Starling EH (1918) The Linacre Lecture on the Law of the Heart. Longmans, London
Starling EH (1920) On the circulatory changes associated with exercise. J Roy Army Med Corps 34:258–272
Stinson EB, Caves PK, Griepp RB, Oyer PE, Rider AK, Shumway NE (1975) Hemodynamic observations in the early period after human heart transplantation. J Thorac Cardiovasc Surg 69:264–270
Stinson EB, Griepp RB, Schroeder JS, Dong E, Shumway NE (1972) Hemodynamic observations one and two years after cardiac transplantation in man. Circulation 45:1183–1194
Theodore J, Morris AJ, Burke CM, Glanville AR, Van Kessel A, Baldwin JC, Stinson EB, Shumway NE, Robin ED (1987) Cardiopulmonary function at maximum tolerable constant work rate exercise following human heart-lung transplantation. Chest 92:433–439
Yacoub MH, Alivizatos PA, Khaghani A, Mitchell A (1985) The use of cyclosporine, azathioprine, antithymocyte globulin with or without low-dose steroids for immunosuppression of cardiac transplant patients. Transplant Proc 17:221–222
Yusuf S, Theodoropoulos S, Mathias CJ, Dhalla N, Wittes J, Mitchell A, Yacoub M (1987) Increased sensitivity of the denervated transplanted human heart to isoprenaline both before and after beta-adrenergic blockage. Circulation 75:696–704

Subject Index

GPSR Compliance

The European Union's (EU) General Product Safety Regulation (GPSR) is a set of rules that requires consumer products to be safe and our obligations to ensure this.

If you have any concerns about our products, you can contact us on ProductSafety@springernature.com

In case Publisher is established outside the EU, the EU authorized representative is:

Springer Nature Customer Service Center GmbH
Europaplatz 3
69115 Heidelberg, Germany

Batch number: 10723233

Printed by Printforce, the Netherlands